American Academy of Pediatrics

DEDICATED TO THE HEALTH OF ALL CHILDREN™

Pediatric Education

FOURTH EDITION

FOR PREHOSPITAL PROFESSIONALS

Editors

Susan Fuchs, MD, FAAP, FACEP

Mike McEvoy, PhD, NRP, RN, CCRN

JONES & BARTLETT
LEARNING

World Headquarters
Jones & Bartlett Learning
25 Mall Road
Burlington, MA 01803
978-443-5000
info@jblearning.com
www.jblearning.com
www.psglearning.com

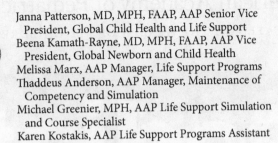

American Academy of Pediatrics
DEDICATED TO THE HEALTH OF ALL CHILDREN™

American Academy of Pediatrics
345 Park Boulevard
Itasca, IL 60143
http://www.PEPPSite.com
http://www.aap.org

Janna Patterson, MD, MPH, FAAP, AAP Senior Vice President, Global Child Health and Life Support
Beena Kamath-Rayne, MD, MPH, FAAP, AAP Vice President, Global Newborn and Child Health
Melissa Marx, AAP Manager, Life Support Programs
Thaddeus Anderson, AAP Manager, Maintenance of Competency and Simulation
Michael Greenier, MPH, AAP Life Support Simulation and Course Specialist
Karen Kostakis, AAP Life Support Programs Assistant

Jones & Bartlett Learning books and products are available through most bookstores and online booksellers. To contact Jones & Bartlett Learning Public Safety Group directly, call 800-832-0034, fax 978-443-8000, or visit our website, www.psglearning.com.

Substantial discounts on bulk quantities of Jones & Bartlett Learning publications are available to corporations, professional associations, and other qualified organizations. For details and specific discount information, contact the special sales department at Jones & Bartlett Learning via the above contact information or send an email to specialsales@jblearning.com.

23826-6

Production Credits
General Manager and Executive Publisher: Kimberly Brophy
VP, Product Development: Christine Emerton
Senior Managing Editor: Donna Gridley
Product Manager: Tiffany Sliter
Product Development Manager: Jennifer Deforge-Kling
Editorial Assistant: Alexander Belloli
VP, Sales, Public Safety Group: Matthew Maniscalco
Project Specialist: Kathryn Leeber
Digital Project Specialist: Angela Dooley
Director of Marketing Operations: Brian Rooney

Production Services Manager: Colleen Lamy
VP, Manufacturing and Inventory Control: Therese Connell
Composition: S4Carlisle Publishing Services
Cover and Text Design: Scott Moden
Media Development Editor: Troy Liston
Rights Specialist: Maria Leon Maimone
Cover Image (Title Page): © Jones & Bartlett Learning. Courtesy of MIEMSS.
Printing and Binding: Strategic Content Imaging (SCI)

Library of Congress Cataloging-in-Publication Data
Names: Fuchs, Susan, editor. | McEvoy, Mike, editor. | Pediatric Education for Prehospital Professionals (Program) | American Academy of Pediatrics, issuing body.
Title: Pediatric Education for Prehospital Professionals (PEPP) / editors, Susan Fuchs, Michael McEvoy ; American Academy of Pediatrics.
Other titles: PEPP
Description: Fourth edition. | Burlington, Massachusetts : Jones & Bartlett Learning, [2021] | Includes bibliographical references and index.
Identifiers: LCCN 2019053393 | ISBN 9781284194579 (paperback) | ISBN 9781284194593 (ebook)
Subjects: MESH: Emergencies | Infant | Child | Emergency Medical Services--methods | Emergency Medical Technicians--education | Pediatrics
Classification: LCC RJ370 | NLM WS 205 | DDC 618.92/0025--dc23
LC record available at https://lccn.loc.gov/2019053393

6048

Printed in the United States of America
26 25 24 23 22   10 9 8 7 6 5 4 3 2

© Jones & Bartlett Learning. Courtesy of MIEMSS.

Brief Contents

Chapter 1   Pediatric Assessment...................................... 1

Chapter 2   Using a Developmental Approach 31

Chapter 3   Respiratory Emergencies 49

Chapter 4   Shock.. 75

Chapter 5   Resuscitation and Dysrhythmias 93

Chapter 6   Medical Emergencies................................. 111

Chapter 7   Trauma 137

Chapter 8   Toxic Emergencies 161

Chapter 9   Behavioral Emergencies 179

Chapter 10   Children with Special Health Care Needs 193

Chapter 11   Child Maltreatment.................................... 213

Chapter 12   Emergency Delivery and Newborn Stabilization 233

Chapter 13   Sudden Unexpected Infant Death and Death of a Child ... 259

Chapter 14   Children in Disasters 271

Chapter 15   Medicolegal and Ethical Considerations 291

Chapter 16   Transportation Considerations......................307

Chapter 17   Making a Difference..............................319

Procedures 335

Medication Formulary   **445**

Glossary   **459**

Index   **473**

© Jones & Bartlett Learning. Courtesy of MIEMSS.

Contents

PEPP Steering Committee . . . . **x**

Acknowledgments . . . . **xii**

Foreword . . . . **xvii**

Chapter 1 Pediatric Assessment 1

Introduction 2

Summary of Assessment Flowchart 2

Scene Size-Up 3

The Pediatric Assessment Triangle 3

Primary Assessment 11

Primary Assessment: The Transport Decision:
  Stay or Go? 19

Summary of Primary Assessment 19

Secondary Assessment: History Taking 20

Physical Examination 21

Additional Monitoring Devices 26

Ongoing Reassessment 26

Summary 27

Chapter 2 Using a Developmental
            Approach 31

Introduction 31

Pediatric Calls and Response From Family
  and Providers 32

Communication With the Child and Family
  or Caregiver 33

Vital Signs Through the Ages 33

Anatomic Changes 35

Summary of Changes in Vital Signs
  and Anatomy Through Childhood 37

Infants 37

Assessment of the Infant 38

Toddlers 39

Assessment of the Toddler 40

Preschoolers 40

Assessment of the Preschooler 41

School-Aged Children 41

Assessment of the School-Aged Child 42

Adolescents 42

Assessment of the Adolescent 43

Children With Special Health
  Care Needs 43

Assessment of a CSHCN 44

Tips for the EMS Provider 45

Summary 45

Chapter 3 Respiratory Emergencies 49

Introduction 49

Respiratory Distress and Failure 50

Prearrival Preparation 51

Scene Size-Up 51

General Assessment: The PAT 51

Primary Assessment: The ABCDEs 52

General Noninvasive Treatment 54

Summary of General and Initial Respiratory
  Assessment and General
  Noninvasive Treatment 56

Specific Treatment for Respiratory Distress 56

Summary of Specific Treatment for
  Respiratory Distress 65

Management of Acute Respiratory
Distress: CPAP 66

Management of Respiratory Failure 66

Summary of Management of
Respiratory Failure 70

Primary Assessment: The Transport Decision—
Stay or Go? 70

Additional Assessment 71

Chapter 4 Shock 75

Introduction 75

Prearrival Preparation 76

Scene Size-Up 76

General Assessment: The Pediatric
Assessment Triangle 76

Primary Assessment: The ABCDEs 77

Additional Assessment 79

Summary of Cardiovascular Assessment 80

Using the Assessment to Identify Shock 80

Hypovolemic Shock 81

Distributive Shock 82

Cardiogenic Shock 83

Obstructive Shock 85

General Noninvasive Treatment of Suspected
Shock of All Types 85

Specific Treatment of Hypovolemia 86

Treatment of Septic Shock 87

Specific Treatment of Hypotensive
(Decompensated) Distributive Shock 88

Treatment of Cardiogenic Shock 88

Primary Assessment: Transport
Decision 89

Summary of Shock States 89

Chapter 5 Resuscitation
and Dysrhythmias 93

Introduction 94

Prearrival Preparation 94

Scene Size-Up 94

General Assessment: The PAT 94

Primary Assessment: The ABCDEs 95

Additional Assessment 96

Summary of Cardiovascular Assessment 96

Dysrhythmias 97

Summary of Dysrhythmias 102

Cardiac Arrest 102

Presenting Cardiac Arrest Rhythm
and Treatment 103

Summary of Cardiac Arrest 107

Congenital Heart Disease 107

Drowning 108

Chapter 6 Medical Emergencies 111

Introduction 111

Medication Dosing 112

Seizures 113

Assessment and Treatment of the
Actively Seizing Child 116

Assessment of the Postictal Child 119

Summary of Seizures 120

Altered Mental Status (AMS) 120

Diabetes Mellitus 123

Hypoglycemia 123

Congenital Adrenal Hyperplasia 124

Cortisol Deficiency 125

Panhypopituitarism 125

Summary of Altered Mental Status
and Endocrine Disorders 126

Fever 126

Summary of Fever 127

Nausea, Vomiting, and Diarrhea
(Gastroenteritis) 128

Sepsis and Meningitis 129

Heat-Related Emergencies 130

Summary of Heat-Related Emergencies 131

Cold-Related Emergencies 132

Summary of Cold-Related Emergencies 133

Bites and Stings 133

Summary of Bites and Stings 134

Chapter 7 Trauma 137

Introduction 137

Fatal Injury Mechanisms 138

Unique Anatomic Features of Children:
Effect on Injury Patterns 138

Mechanism of Injury: Effect on Injury
Patterns 142

Assessment of the Injured Child 143

The General Assessment 144

The Primary Assessment 145

Summary of Primary Assessment 152

Special Airway Considerations
in Pediatric Trauma 152

The Primary Assessment 153

Additional Assessment 153

Summary of Additional Assessment 154

Spinal Motion Restriction
and Splinting for Transport 154

Pediatric Burn Patients 155

Summary of Burns 158

Chapter 8 Toxic Emergencies 161

Introduction 161

Age-Related Differences 161

Summary of Age-Related Differences 163

Prearrival Preparation and Scene Size-Up 164

Role of the Poison Center 165

Assessment of the Child with a Possible
Toxic Exposure 165

Summary of Assessment of the Child
With a Possible Toxic Exposure 170

Toxicologic Management 170

Organophosphates 174

Summary of Toxicologic Management 174

Medicolegal Issues 174

Chapter 9 Behavioral Emergencies 179

Introduction 179

Common Pediatric Psychiatric
and Behavioral Conditions 180

Suicide Attempt/Intentional Ingestions
or Exposures 185

Adverse Reactions of Psychiatric Medications 186

Assessment and Transport of the Child
with a Behavioral Emergency 187

Chapter 10 Children with Special Health Care Needs 193

Introduction 193

Cognitive and Physical Disabilities 194

Assessment of CSHCN 195

Summary of Assessment of CSHCN 198

Transport 198

Summary of Transport 199

Children Assisted by Technology 199

Summary of Children Assisted
by Technology 208

The Medical Home for CSHCN 209

Additional EMS Considerations for CSHCN 209

Chapter 11 Child Maltreatment 213

Introduction 213

Background, Cost, and Definition 213

Definition of Child Maltreatment 214

High-Risk Groups 215

Duties and Communication by the
Prehospital Professional 216

Communicating With the Child
and Caregivers 218

Patient Assessment 218

Summary of Duties, Communication,
and Assessment in Suspected
Maltreatment 223

Legislation, Principles, and Protocols 223

Pediatric Human Trafficking 225

Chapter 12 Emergency Delivery and Newborn Stabilization 233

Introduction 233

Obstetric Delivery in the Prehospital Setting 234

Complications During Pregnancy 234

Triage of a Patient in Labor 236

Summary of Triage of Patient in Labor 239

Preparation for Delivery 240

Performing the Delivery 242

Summary of Vaginal Delivery 245

Immediate Care of the Newborn 246

General Principles of Newborn
Resuscitation 248

Specific Newborn Complications 251

Summary of Resuscitation of the Newborn 254

Transport Considerations 254

Summary 255

Chapter 13 Sudden Unexpected Infant Death and Death of a Child 259

Introduction 259

Definition of SUID 259

SUID Epidemiology.............................. 260

Common Clinical Presentation of SUID... 260

Actions in Suspected SUID..................... 261

Summary of SUID................................ 263

Definition of Brief Resolved
Unexplained Event 264

Common Clinical Presentation of BRUE 264

Actions in Suspected BRUE 264

Summary of BRUE 265

Responses to an Infant Death.................. 265

Critical Incident Stress 267

Chapter 14 Children in Disasters.......... 271

Children in Disasters............................. 271

What Is a Disaster?.............................. 272

Roles of the Prehospital Professional in
a Disaster................................... 273

Pediatric Response Considerations.............. 274

Vulnerable Pediatric Physiologic
and Psychologic Characteristics
in Disasters 280

Effects of Chemical, Biologic, Radiation,
Nuclear, and Explosive Disasters
on Children.................................. 281

Summary.. 287

Chapter 15 Medicolegal and Ethical
Considerations................ 291

Introduction..................................... 291

Consent... 291

Summary of Consent 295

Confidentiality.................................. 295

Respect for Cultural or Religious Differences 295

Patient Rights and Advocacy.................... 296

End-of-Life Issues............................... 296

Pediatric Policies and Procedures 301

Medical Control for Pediatrics.................. 302

Summary of Rationale for Protocols,
Policies, and Procedures 303

Chapter 16 Transportation
Considerations................ 307

Pediatric Transport.............................. 307

How to Begin Transport......................... 308

Taking Caregivers in the Ambulance 309

Child Restraint Systems in Ambulances 310

Transport Mode 315

Transport Destination........................... 315

Multiple Patients................................ 315

Summary of Transport Mode
and Multiple Patients 315

Chapter 17 Making a Difference 319

Introduction..................................... 319

Emergency Medical Services for Children 320

Summary of EMSC............................... 320

Public Health Interface.......................... 322

Prevention and Injury Control................... 322

Summary of Prevention and Injury Control....... 325

The Medical Home 325

Summary of the Medical Home.................. 326

Quality and Safety in EMSC 326

Data and Information Management 328

Summary of Quality, Safety, Data Collection,
and Information Management................. 329

Prevention: The Prehospital
Professional's Role 329

Summary of Roles in Prevention 331

Call to Action: Advocacy for EMSC 331

Procedures.....................................335

1 Field Reporting 336

2 Length-Based Resuscitation Tapes............ 340

3 Oxygen Delivery 342

4 Suctioning.................................. 347

5 Airway Adjuncts 353

6 Foreign Body Obstruction.................... 356

7 Bronchodilator Therapy 360

8 Bag-Mask Ventilation........................ 363

9 Pulse Oximetry 367

10 Orogastric and Nasogastric
Tube Insertion 369

11 Endotracheal Intubation 373

12 Confirmation of Endotracheal Intubation
and End-Tidal Capnography.................. 383

13 Advanced Airway Techniques................. 389

14 Intramuscular Injections 398

15 Intranasal Medication Administration 402

16 Intravenous Access 405

17 Intraosseous Needle Insertion................409

18 Cardiopulmonary Resuscitation..............415

19 AED and Defibrillation......................420

20 Endotracheal Tube Drug Instillation..........425

21 Rectal Administration of Benzodiazepines.....427

22 Spinal Motion Restriction...................430

23 Needle Thoracostomy.......................435

24 Removing and Replacing a
   Tracheostomy Tube.........................437

25 Tourniquet Application......................441

Medication Formulary...........................**445**

Glossary.......................................**459**

Index..**473**

PEPP Steering Committee

Jennifer F. Anders, MD, FAAP
Chair, PEPP Steering Committee
Representative – AAP Section on Emergency
  Medicine
Assistant Professor of Pediatrics
Johns Hopkins University School of Medicine
Associate State Medical Director for Pediatrics
Maryland Institute of EMS Systems
Baltimore, Maryland

S. Heath Ackley, MD, MPH, FAAP
Representative – AAP Section on Emergency
  Medicine
Clinical Associate Professor
Pediatric Emergency Medicine
Seattle Children's Hospital
Seattle, Washington

Thomas Breyer, FF/NRP, MSHS
Representative – International Association
  of Fire Fighters
Director of Fire & EMS Operations
Washington, DC

Kathleen M. Brown, MD, FACEP, FAAP
Representative – American College of Emergency
  Physicians
Professor of Pediatrics and Emergency Medicine
The George Washington University School of
  Medicine
Associate Division Chief, Medical Director
  of Quality
Division of Emergency Medicine
Children's National Medical Center
Washington, DC

Ann Dietrich, MD, FACEP, FAAP
Representative – National Association of Emergency
  Medical Technicians
Associate Professor of Pediatrics and Emergency
  Medicine
Ohio University Heritage College of Medicine
Pediatric Medical Advisor, Medflight of Ohio
Medical Director, The Franklin County Firefighters
  Grant Medical Center EMS Education Program
Columbus, Ohio

J. Joelle Donofrio-Odmann, DO, FAAP, FACEP, FAEMS
Representative – National Association of EMS
  Physicians
EMS Medical Director, Rady Children's Hospital
  of San Diego
Associate Medical Director, San Diego Fire-Rescue
Assistant Professor, Departments of Pediatrics and
  Emergency Medicine
UCSD School of Medicine
San Diego, California

Joyce Foresman-Capuzzi, MSN, APRN, CCNS, CEN, CPEN, CTRN, TCRN, CPN, EMT-P, FAEN
Representative – Emergency Nurses Association
Clinical Nurse Educator
Lankeanu Medical Center
Prospect Park, Pennsylvania

Susan Fuchs, MD, FAAP, FACEP
Co-Editor, *PEPP, Fourth Edition*
Representative – American Heart Association
Professor of Pediatrics, Northwestern University
  Feinberg School of Medicine
Attending Physician, Division of Emergency Medicine
Ann & Robert H. Lurie Children's Hospital of Chicago
Chicago, Illinois

Brandon Kelley, NRP
Representative – National Association of State
    EMS Officials
EMS Supervisor
Wyoming Department of Health, Emergency
    Medical Services
Cheyenne, Wyoming

Corolla Lauck, NRP
Representative – National Association of State
    EMS Officials
Program Director
South Dakota Emergency Medical Services for
    Children Program
Sioux Falls, South Dakota

Rich Martin
Representative – International Association
    of Fire Chiefs
Deputy Chief of Operations
Castle Rock Fire and Rescue Department
Castle Rock, Colorado

Mike McEvoy, PhD, NRP, RN, CCRN
Co-Editor, *PEPP, Fourth Edition*
EMS Coordinator, Saratoga County, New York
Executive Editor, *Journal of Emergency Medical
    Services (JEMS)*
EMS Editor, *Fire Engineering Magazine*
Nurse Clinician, Adult & Pediatric Cardiac Surgical
    ICUs, Albany Medical Center
Chief Medical Officer, West Crescent Fire
    Department
Chair, EMS Section Board – International
    Association of Fire Chiefs
Waterford, New York

Toni M. Petrillo, MD, FAAP
Representative – AAP Section on Critical
    Care/Transport Medicine
Pediatric Critical Care Fellowship Director
Medical Director of Transport
Professor of Pediatrics
Division of Pediatric Critical Care
Emory University and Children's Healthcare
    of Atlanta
Atlanta, Georgia

Michael J. Stoner, MD, FAAP
Representative – AAP Section on Emergency
    Medicine/Transport Medicine
Assistant Professor of Pediatrics
The Ohio State University College of Medicine
Section Chief of Emergency Medicine
Nationwide Children's Hospital
Columbus, Ohio

Michael H. Stroud, MD, FAAP
Representative – AAP Section on Critical
    Care/Transport Medicine
Associate Professor
Pediatric Critical Care
University of Arkansas for Medical Sciences
Associate Medical Director
Angel One Transport
Little Rock, Arkansas

Keith Widmeier, BA, NRP, FP-C
Representative – National Association
    of EMS Educators
Simulation Educator
Children's Hospital of Philadelphia
Center for Simulation, Advanced Education, &
    Innovation
Philadelphia, Pennsylvania

Acknowledgments

Editors

Susan Fuchs, MD, FAAP, FACEP

Mike McEvoy, PhD, NRP, RN, CCRN

Authors

The American Academy of Pediatrics and editors acknowledge with appreciation the contributions of the following individuals in the development of this resource.

Michael R. Aguilar, AA, EMT-P
EMS Adjunct Faculty
Kirkwood Community College
Regional Center for EMS Education
Cedar Rapids, Iowa

Jennifer F. Anders, MD, FAAP
Chair, PEPP Steering Committee
Representative – AAP Section on Emergency
   Medicine
Assistant Professor of Pediatrics
Johns Hopkins University School of Medicine
Associate State Medical Director for Pediatrics
Maryland Institute of EMS Systems
Baltimore, Maryland

S. Heath Ackley, MD, MPH, FAAP
Representative – AAP Section on Emergency
   Medicine
Clinical Associate Professor
Pediatric Emergency Medicine
Seattle Children's Hospital
Seattle, Washington

Victoria Barnes, RN, BSN, EMT
Program Coordinator
Connecticut Emergency Medical Services
   for Children
New Haven, Connecticut

Andrew Bartkus, RN, MSN, JD, CEN, CCRN, CFRN, NREMT-P, FP-C
Emergency Department Director
Sandoval Regional Medical Center
Rio Rancho, New Mexico

Kathleen M. Brown, MD, FACEP, FAAP
Representative – American College of Emergency
   Physicians
Professor of Pediatrics and Emergency Medicine
The George Washington University School of
   Medicine
Associate Division Chief, Medical Director of Quality
Division of Emergency Medicine
Children's National Medical Center
Washington, DC

Tabitha Cheng, MD
UCSD EMS Fellow
Emergency Department Physician
San Diego, California

Sharon Chiumento, BS, BSN, EMT-P
EMS Representative – NYS EMSC Committee
Adjunct Faculty – Monroe Community College
Rochester, New York

Ann Dietrich, MD, FACEP, FAAP
Representative – National Association of Emergency
  Medical Technicians
Associate Professor of Pediatrics and Emergency
  Medicine
Ohio University Heritage College of Medicine
Pediatric Medical Advisor, Medflight of Ohio
Medical Director, The Franklin County Firefighters
  Grant Medical Center EMS Education Program
Columbus, Ohio

J. Joelle Donofrio-Odmann, DO, FAAP, FACEP, FAEMS
Representative – National Association of EMS
  Physicians
EMS Medical Director, Rady Children's Hospital
  of San Diego
Associate Medical Director, San Diego Fire-Rescue
Assistant Professor, Departments of Pediatrics and
  Emergency Medicine
UCSD School of Medicine
San Diego, California

Wm. Travis Engel, DO, MSc
Paramedic, FP-C, CCP-C
Advocate Children's Hospital
Park Ridge, Illinois

John A. Erbayri, MS, NRP, CHSE
Emergency Care Program Manager
Children's Hospital of Philadelphia
Paramedic/Field Training Officer
Marple Township Ambulance Corps
Ridley Park, Pennsylvania

**Joyce Foresman-Capuzzi, MSN, APRN, CCNS, CEN, CPEN,
  CTRN, TCRN, CPN, EMT-P, FAEN**
Representative – Emergency Nurses Association
Clinical Nurse Educator
Lankeanu Medical Center
Prospect Park, Pennsylvania

Susan Fuchs, MD, FAAP, FACEP
Co-Editor, *PEPP, Fourth Edition*
Representative – American Heart Association
Professor of Pediatrics, Northwestern University
  Feinberg School of Medicine
Attending Physician, Division of Emergency
  Medicine
Ann & Robert H. Lurie Children's Hospital
  of Chicago
Chicago, Illinois

**J. Hudson Garrett Jr., PhD, MSN, MPH, MBA, FNP-BC, PLNC,
  IP-BC, AS-BC, NREMT, VA-BC, FACDONA, FAAPM, FNAP**
Adjunct Assistant Professor of Medicine
Division of Infectious Diseases
University of Louisville School of Medicine
Medical Reserve Corp
Pro Care Emergency Medical Services
Atlanta, Georgia

Thomas Herron, Jr. AAS, NRP
EMS Faculty/Clinical Coordinator
Roane State Community College
Knoxville, Tennessee

Will Krost, MD, MBA, NRP
Emergency Medicine & Flight Physician
Bon Secours Mercy Health, St. Vincent
Department of Emergency Medicine
Toledo, Ohio

David LaCovey, BS, EMT-P
EMS Specialist
Benedum Pediatric Trauma Program
UPMC Children's Hospital of Pittsburgh
Pittsburgh, Pennsylvania

Corolla Lauck, NRP
Representative – National Association of State
  EMS Officials
Program Director
South Dakota Emergency Medical Services for
  Children Program
Sioux Falls, South Dakota

Rich Martin
Representative – International Association
  of Fire Chiefs
Deputy Chief of Operations
Castle Rock Fire and Rescue Department
Castle Rock, Colorado

Mike McEvoy, PhD, NRP, RN, CCRN
Co-Editor, *PEPP, Fourth Edition*
EMS Coordinator, Saratoga County, New York
Executive Editor, *Journal of Emergency Medical
  Services (JEMS)*
EMS Editor, *Fire Engineering Magazine*
Nurse Clinician, Adult & Pediatric Cardiac Surgical
  ICUs, Albany Medical Center
Chief Medical Officer, West Crescent Fire
  Department
Chair, EMS Section Board – International
  Association of Fire Chiefs
Waterford, New York

Mary Otting, RN, BSN, CEN
EMS Coordinator
Ann & Robert H. Lurie Children's Hospital
  of Chicago
Chicago, Illinois

Sylvia Owusu-Ansah, MD, MPH, FAAP
Assistant Professor of Pediatrics
EMS/Prehospital Medical Director
UPMC Children's Hospital of Pittsburgh
Pediatric Liaison – Division of EMS
Department of Emergency Medicine, University
  of Pittsburgh
National Registry of EMTs Physician Board Member
Pittsburgh, Pennsylvania

Ali Paplaskas, Pharm. D., BCCCP
Emergency Medicine Pharmacy Specialist
Mercy Health St. Vincent Medical Center
Toledo, Ohio

Toni M. Petrillo, MD, FAAP
Representative – AAP Section on Critical
  Care/Transport Medicine
Pediatric Critical Care Fellowship Director
Medical Director of Transport
Professor of Pediatrics
Division of Pediatric Critical Care
Emory University and Children's Healthcare of
  Atlanta
Atlanta, Georgia

Claudia L. Phillips, MSN-Ed, RN, CEN, CPEN
Emergency Department Registered Nurse
Sandoval Regional Medical Center
Rio Rancho, New Mexico

Michael S. Riley, NRP, EMSI
Senior Emergency Care Educator
Children's Hospital of Philadelphia
Emergency Care Programs
Philadelphia, Pennsylvania

Saranya Srinivasan, MD, FAAP
Medical Director
Los Angeles County Paramedic Training Institute
Santa Fe Springs, California

Jennifer L. Stafford, BSN, CEN, CFRN
Unit Based Educator: Emergency Department
UNM Sandoval Regional Medical Center
Rio Rancho, New Mexico

Michael J. Stoner, MD, FAAP
Representative – AAP Section on Emergency
  Medicine/Transport Medicine
Assistant Professor of Pediatrics
The Ohio State University College of Medicine
Section Chief of Emergency Medicine
Nationwide Children's Hospital
Columbus, Ohio

Matthew R. Streger, Esq, MPA, NRP
Partner
Keavney & Streger, LLC
Princeton, New Jersey

Michael H. Stroud, MD, FAAP
Representative – AAP Section on Critical
  Care/Transport Medicine
Associate Professor
Pediatric Critical Care
University of Arkansas for Medical Sciences
Associate Medical Director
Angel One Transport
Little Rock, Arkansas

Sam Vance, MHA, LP
Lead Project Manager
Prehospital Domain Lead
State Partnership Co-Domain Lead
National EMS for Children Innovation
  and Improvement Center
Houston, Texas

Keith Widmeier, BA, NRP, FP-C
Representative – National Association of EMS
  Educators
Simulation Educator
Children's Hospital of Philadelphia
Center for Simulation, Advanced Education, &
  Innovation
Philadelphia, Pennsylvania

Board Reviewer

The editors would like to acknowledge the work of the American Academy of Pediatrics Board-appointed reviewer.

Wendy S. Davis, MD, FAAP
American Academy of Pediatrics
District I Chairperson
Larner College of Medicine at the University
  of Vermont
Burlington, Vermont

EMS Reviewers

David Anderson
North Gilliam County Health District
Arlington, Oregon

Ryan K. Batenhorst, MEd, NRP, EMSI
Southeast Community College
Lincoln, Nebraska

James Blivin
Training 911
Chambersburg, Pennsylvania

Rob Bozicevich, NRP
MetroAtlanta EMS Academy
Marietta, Georgia

Jason Brooks
University of South Alabama Department
    of EMS Education
Mobile, Alabama

Joshua Chan, BA, FP-C, CCP-C
Glacial Ridge Health System
Glenwood, Minnesota

Ted Chialtas, BA, EMT-P
San Diego Fire-Rescue Department EMS
    Training Facility
San Diego, California

Kent Courtney, NRP
EMS/Fire/Rescue Educator
Essential Safety Training and Consulting
Rimrock, Arizona

Lyndal M. Curry, MS, NRP
Southern Union State Community College
Auburn, Alabama

Kevin Curry, AS, NRP, CCEMT-P
Augusta Fire Rescue
Augusta, Maine

William Faust, MPA, NRP
Western Carolina University
Cullowhee, North Carolina

Lori Gallian, BS, EMT-P
Summit Sciences
Citrus Heights, California

Fidel O. Garcia, EMT-P
Professional EMS Education
Grand Junction, Colorado

Rodney Geilenfeldt II, BS, EMT-P
EMSTA College
Santee, California

Jeffery D. Gilliard, FPM/CCEMTP/NRP
EMETSEEI Institute, Inc.
Rockledge, Florida

Keith B. Hermiz, NREMT-A, I/C
Grafton Rescue Squad, Inc.
Grafton, Vermont

Michele M. Hoffman, MSEd, RN, NREMT
James City County Fire Department
Williamsburg, Virginia

Michael Hudson, NR-P, NJ MICP
Sea Bright Ocean Rescue
Edison, New Jersey

Sandra Hultz, NRP
Holmes Community College
Ridgeland, Mississippi

Joseph Hurlburt, BS, NRP
North Flight EMS Wexford County
Manton, Michigan

Timothy M. Kimble, BA, AAS, CEM, NRP
Craig Co Emergency Services
New Castle, Virginia

Mark King
MEEMS Paramedic
Kennebec Valley Community
Winthrop, Maine

Christopher Maeder, BA, EMT-P
Chief
Fairview Fire District
Poughkeepsie, New York

Gregory S. Neiman, MS, NRP, NCEE
Center for Trauma and Critical Care Education
Virginia Commonwealth University
Richmond, Virginia

Sean Newton
Mesa Community College
Mesa, Arizona

Laurie Oelslager, EdD, NRP, CP
South Central College
North Mankato, Minnesota

Keito Oritz, Paramedic, NAEMSE II
Jamaica Hospital Medical Center
Jamaica, New York

Scott A. Smith, MSN, APRN-CNP, ACNP-BC, NRP, I/C
Atlantic Partners EMS, Inc.
Lisbon, Maine

Mark A. Spangenberg, CCP, ECG-BC, I/C
Milwaukee Area Technical College
Milwaukee, Wisconsin

Michael E. Tanner, FP-C, NRP, MCCP
WV Public Service Training, Waverly Vol. Fire Co.,
     Air Evac Lifeteam
Waverly, West Virginia

Jennifer TeWinkel Shea, BA, AEMT
Regions Hospital Emergency Medical Services
Oakdale, Minnesota

Antoinette Tharrett, MSN, RN-BC, CCEMT-P, NRP
Lake Cumberland Regional Hospital
Russell Springs, Kentucky

A. Elizabeth Trujillo, NRP, B.S.
Fielding Fire Department
Fielding, Utah

Scott Vanderkooi, MEd, NRP
Blue Ridge Community College
Weyers Cave, Virginia

Tom Watson, AS, AAS, Paramedic
Chesapeake, Virginia

Rekeisha A. Watson-Love, AAS, NRP
Henderson, Nevada

Raymond C. Whatley, Jr., MBA, NRP, TP-C
George Washington University
Washington, DC

Keri Wydner Krause
Lakeshore Technical College
Cleveland, Wisconsin

Andy Yeoh, NRP, EFOP, BS
Pima Community College
Vail, Arizona

Video Shoot Acknowledgments

We would like to thank the following institutions for their collaboration on the video and photo shoot for this project. Their assistance is greatly appreciated.

Lifespan Medical Simulation Center
Providence, Rhode Island

East Kingston Fire Department
East Kingston, Rhode Island

East Providence Fire Department
Providence, Rhode Island

Warwick Fire Department
Warwick, Rhode Island

Foreword

PEPP, Fourth Edition . . .Written by EMS for EMS

In celebration of the 20th Anniversary of the PEPP program, we are thrilled to bring you the *PEPP, Fourth Edition*, providing prehospital professionals with education that has become known as the gold standard in pediatric emergency care. As has always been our primary focus, content within this manual has been authored by a team of EMS professionals and physicians with expertise in prehospital care.

The Provider Manual serves as the core of the PEPP course and has been completely updated and revised to include many exciting new additions and enhancements.

All NEW Content

- **New chapter on behavioral emergencies**
- **New procedures on tourniquet application and intranasal medication administration**
- Enhanced section on supraglottic airways, to include i-gel
- Enhanced section on intraosseous infusion, to include EZ-IO

- Information on active threat/hostile threat and human trafficking
- Updated images

Enhanced Course Features

- An **Enhanced Hybrid course format**, featuring all new small-group, case-based discussions
- **Nine new procedural skills video clips** including Narcan, epinephrine, and albuterol administration; tourniquet application; intranasal medication administration; intraosseous needle insertion; supraglottic airways; spinal motion restriction; and length-based resuscitation tape
- **New case-based scenario lectures**
- **Interactive course activities**
- Optional materials you can use to customize and supplement your courses

We hope you find all the enhancements and improvements to the *Fourth Edition* to be dynamic, innovative, and flexible to better meet your continuing education needs.

Susan Fuchs, MD, FAAP, FACEP
Mike McEvoy, PhD, NRP, RN, CCRN

© Eddie M. Sperling.

CHAPTER 1

Pediatric Assessment

Ann Dietrich, MD, FACEP, FAAP

Keith Widmeier, BA, NRP, FP-C

LEARNING OBJECTIVES

1. Describe *Pediatric Education for Prehospital Professionals (PEPP)* as a program that meets national education priorities in the emergency care of children.
2. Discuss the special challenges for the prehospital professional in pediatric assessment.
3. Recognize the key features of prearrival preparation and the scene size-up.
4. Differentiate the three elements of the Pediatric Assessment Triangle (PAT).
5. Describe the important pediatric considerations for each step in the hands-on ABC sequence of the primary assessment.
6. Recognize clinical situations requiring pain assessment and management.
7. Discuss guidelines for when to stay on scene and treat, and when to immediately transport an ill or injured child, including appropriate mode of transport.
8. Outline the unique considerations in the additional assessment of a child, including history taking, secondary assessment, monitoring devices, and ongoing reassessment.

CASE STUDY 1

A 9-year-old unhelmeted boy rode his bicycle out of his driveway into the path of an oncoming car. According to witnesses, the car was moving about 25 mph (40 kph), the victim was struck and thrown approximately 15 ft (4.5 m), and he was unconscious for 1 minute. On your arrival, he is crying and anxious but responds appropriately to questions. He is complaining that his stomach hurts. He has no abnormal airway sounds, grunting, flaring, or retracting. His skin is pale. The respiratory rate is 30 breaths/min, there are equal breath sounds with good air exchange, and the pulse oximetry reading is 98% on room air. His heart rate is 140 beats/min, and his blood pressure is 80/40 mm Hg. Capillary refill time is 4 seconds.

1. How badly injured is this child, and which physiologic process requires your emergent attention?
2. Should this child's pain be treated?

Introduction

Caring for a critically ill or injured infant or child is one of the most stressful duties of the prehospital professional. Key history may be unreliable or unknown because the patient may be too young to have descriptive language, or the child may be afraid and unable to accurately recount the key events. The caregiver may be sobbing, frightened, and anxious for reassurance. Examination may be limited because of the child's small size and resistance to hands-on evaluation. **Vital signs** may be deceptive because of normal age-based variations and the difficulty in obtaining them accurately. It is the job of the prehospital professional to bring comfort to the child, caregiver, or family and to bring order to the chaos on scene. The prehospital professional must conduct an accurate assessment and deliver effective emergency treatment to the child.

The *Pediatric Education for Prehospital Professionals (PEPP)* course, developed by the American Academy of Pediatrics (AAP), provides the core cognitive knowledge and skills to prepare prehospital professionals for comprehensive assessment and management of any ill or injured infant and child. PEPP materials are designed to meet the national emergency medical services (EMS) education standards for all levels of emergency medical provider, as established by the United States Department of Transportation's National Highway Traffic Safety Administration (NHTSA). Therefore, some of the terminology previously used in PEPP (general, initial, and additional assessment) has been modified to reflect the national EMS core content and the Definitions and Assessment Approaches for Emergency Medical Services for Children document.

Effective emergency care of children involves many professionals inside and outside of the hospital setting. Two of the most important concepts for comprehensive and high-quality prehospital pediatric emergency care are teamwork and prevention. Teamwork involves professionals working together to develop and implement comprehensive clinical services, professional education, and appropriate administrative oversight specifically for children. A Pediatric Emergency Care Coordinator (PECC) can act as a liaison between EMS agencies and the hospital setting. Agency PECCs can help with protocol development, pediatric case reviews, agency pediatric quality assurance/quality improvement (QA/QI), ensure the presence of adequate pediatric supplies, assist in injury prevention activities, help promote family-centered care, identify local pediatric trends, and coordinate with emergency departments (EDs).

Prevention involves professionals recognizing the limitations of an emergency care system oriented toward treatment after an illness or injury occurs and working to change potentially dangerous conditions before an event of this type occurs. Of all community activities that can improve children's overall health and well-being, prevention of acute injury and illness is by far the most cost-effective. "Making a difference," as described in detail in Chapter 17, involves new roles for prehospital professionals in injury and illness prevention, in their professional day-to-day duties, and as part of their activities as community leaders and health advocates

Accurate assessment of a child with an illness or injury requires special knowledge and skills. For patients of all ages, the prehospital professional's evaluation includes four steps: (1) scene size-up; (2) use of the **Pediatric Assessment Triangle (PAT)**; (3) primary assessment using the ABCDE assessment, vital signs, and pulse oximetry; and (4) **secondary assessment**, including a focused history, focused examination, monitoring devices, ongoing reassessment of physiologic status, and response to treatment. The primary and secondary assessments have well-defined components that follow the same sequence used for adult patients. However, all four steps in the primary assessment have important pediatric modifications. The tertiary assessment includes laboratory and radiologic tests that can include point-of-care labs in the prehospital setting, but are usually performed in the ED.

Summary of Assessment Flowchart

This chapter introduces a flowchart that reflects the sequence of pediatric assessment taught by the PEPP course. The flowchart reinforces the interconnecting relationships of the different assessment components. Sometimes the assessment sequence must be stopped after the primary assessment to allow the prehospital professional to treat potentially life-threatening problems and initiate transport. For example, when a child has a critical injury, the secondary assessment must be deferred until after the child has been resuscitated and stabilized. Reassessment, however, is required in every case to monitor response to treatment, guide further interventions, and assist with transport and triage decisions. Monitoring devices such as a pulse oximeter or end-tidal CO_2 monitor and bedside glucose checks may provide valuable adjunctive data to confirm and guide treatment in the prehospital setting.

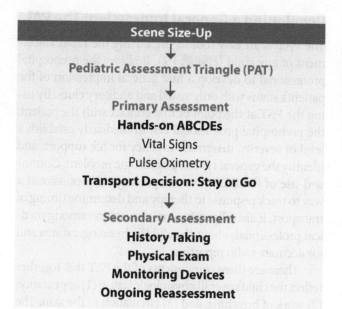

Scene Size-Up

↓

Pediatric Assessment Triangle (PAT)

↓

Primary Assessment

Hands-on ABCDEs

Vital Signs

Pulse Oximetry

Transport Decision: Stay or Go

↓

Secondary Assessment

History Taking

Physical Exam

Monitoring Devices

Ongoing Reassessment

FIGURE 1-1 Environmental assessment.

Courtesy of Rhonda J. Hunt.

Scene Size-Up

On the way to the scene, prepare mentally to approach and treat an infant or child, and to interact with a distressed family. This means planning for a pediatric scene size-up, pediatric equipment and medication requirements, and age-appropriate assessment. All pediatric equipment and medications should be routinely checked, as they are less often used by most prehospital professionals and it is easy to forget their application. The information from dispatch on age and gender of the child, location of the scene, and chief complaint or mechanism of injury (or both) is the basis for prearrival preparation.

At the scene, begin the size-up by looking for possible safety threats to the prehospital professionals, child, caregiver, and/or bystanders. Examples of safety threats include spilled toxins, open containers of alcohol, drug paraphernalia, weapons, or fire. The child actually may be a safety threat if he or she has an infectious disease, such as varicella or meningococcemia.

> **TIP**
>
> On the way to the scene, mentally rehearse your approach to the assessment and treatment of an infant or child and the expected interaction with a caregiver or family. Dispatch information, when available, about the child's age can be helpful to mentally prepare for age-appropriate developmental considerations and for anticipating equipment and medication requirements for assessment and treatment.

Evaluating the setting includes an inspection of the physical environment and watching family–child or caregiver–child interactions (**FIGURE 1-1**). For example, documenting observations of dangerous scene conditions and inappropriate statements from caregivers greatly assists child protective services if the child is later determined to be a victim of inflicted injury or negligence. On the scene, be like a sponge; soak up as much useful information as possible. Also, ensure scene safety for both your team and the child.

The Pediatric Assessment Triangle

After the scene size-up, begin an assessment of the child, which must have a developmentally appropriate approach. This assessment includes a visual and auditory general impression of the child and uses the PAT as a standardized method to gather this information.

Rapid assessment is essential to determine the level of acuity and urgency for treatment and transport. Ask yourself, "Is the patient sick or not sick?" In the case of a child who is a victim of trauma with a known mechanism of injury, or of a child with a clear-cut complaint of pain in a specific anatomic location, the assessment may be straightforward. Still, careful evaluation is needed to identify less obvious, but potentially serious, injuries or physiologic instability. For a child with an illness, the assessment may be much trickier. The prehospital professional must elicit information on the onset, duration, severity, and progression of symptoms, often from a child who cannot accurately provide such history. Moreover, illness complaints may be vague and less specific to an anatomic region. Whether the child has an injury or an illness, the PAT helps to identify physiologic instability, direct resuscitation priorities, and determine the timing of transport.

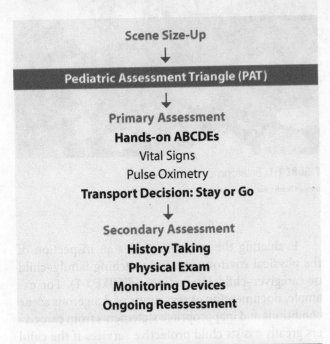

Scene Size-Up
↓
Pediatric Assessment Triangle (PAT)
↓
Primary Assessment
Hands-on ABCDEs
Vital Signs
Pulse Oximetry
Transport Decision: Stay or Go
↓
Secondary Assessment
History Taking
Physical Exam
Monitoring Devices
Ongoing Reassessment

TIP

Use the PAT at the point of initial contact with every child, regardless of age or presenting complaint.

Developing a General Impression: The PAT

The PAT is an easy tool to use during the rapid assessment of any child (**FIGURE 1-2**). It allows the prehospital professional to develop a first general impression of the patient's status with only visual and auditory clues. By using the PAT at the point of first contact with the patient, the prehospital professional can immediately establish a level of severity, determine urgency for life support, and identify the general type of physiologic problem. Continued use of the PAT gives the prehospital professional a way to track response to therapy and determine timing of transport. It also allows for communication among medical professionals about the child's physiologic status and for accurate radio reporting.

There are three components of the PAT that together reflect the child's overall physiologic status: (1) appearance, (2) work of breathing, and (3) circulation to the skin. The PAT is based on listening and seeing and does not require a stethoscope, blood pressure cuff, cardiac monitor, or pulse oximeter. The PAT should be completed in less than 30 seconds and is designed to organize a time-honored process of "across the room assessment," an intuitive process that experienced pediatric providers do instinctively.

TIP

The elements of the PAT incorporate auditory and visual clues that should be obtained from "across the room," without appearing threatening to an already anxious child.

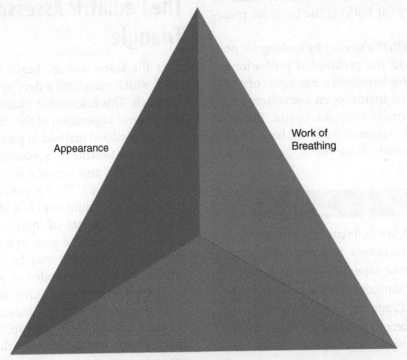

Appearance

Work of Breathing

Circulation to Skin

FIGURE 1-2 Pediatric Assessment Triangle (PAT).

The PAT

Together, the physical characteristics of the PAT provide an accurate initial picture of the child's underlying cardiopulmonary status and level of consciousness. Although the PAT does not necessarily lead to a diagnosis, it identifies the general category of the physiologic problem and establishes urgency for treatment or transport. The PAT does not replace traditional vital signs and the ABCs, which are part of the primary assessment in the next phase of the physical evaluation.

The patient characteristics emphasized by the three arms of the PAT did not originate with PEPP. Experienced pediatric health care providers developed these characteristics to share the intuitive assessment skills to obtain a rapid first general impression of ill or injured children. What is unique about the PAT is its systematic approach to making, integrating, and communicating these observations. The PAT is the cornerstone of the PEPP course. Use the PAT in every encounter with every child. Over time, it will become an indispensable and spontaneous method for making a rapid initial "sick or not sick" assessment of ill or injured children of all ages.

Appearance

Characteristics of Appearance. The child's general appearance is the most important factor in determining the severity of the illness or injury, the need for treatment, and the response to therapy. Appearance reflects the adequacy of ventilation, oxygenation, brain **perfusion**, body **homeostasis**, and **central nervous system (CNS)** function. There are many characteristics of appearance; the most important are summarized in the "tickles" (TICLS) mnemonic: tone, interactiveness, consolability, look/gaze, and speech/cry (**TABLE 1-1**).

Identifying abnormal appearance is a better way to detect subtle abnormalities in behavior than the conventional **"alert, verbal, painful, unresponsive" (AVPU) scale** or the Pediatric Glasgow Coma Scale (GCS) for neurologic evaluation. Most children with mild to moderate illness or injury are "alert" on the

> ### CAUTION
>
> In assessing patients with mild to moderate illness or injury, numerical "scoring" methodologies and severity scales for levels of consciousness are rarely useful. These classical neurologic evaluation systems work best in patients with severe injury or illness as a tool to monitor for changes in children with serious brain dysfunction.

AVPU or "15" on the Pediatric GCS. Children with an abnormal appearance must be assumed to have a potentially serious underlying problem. Therefore, assessing a child's appearance is the most useful first thing to do in evaluating every pediatric patient.

> ### TIP
>
> Never ignore the pale infant, the "nobody home stare," or the infant who does not respond appropriately to stimulation.

Techniques to Assess Appearance. Assess the child's appearance from the doorway. This is Step 1 in the PAT. Techniques for assessment of a conscious child's appearance

---

TABLE 1-1 Characteristics of Appearance: The "Tickles" (TICLS) Mnemonic

	Characteristic Features
▪ Tone	Is she moving or vigorously resisting examination? Does she have good muscle tone? Or is she limp, listless, or flaccid?
▪ Interactiveness	How alert is she? How readily does a person, object, or sound distract her or draw her attention? Will she reach for, grasp, and play with a toy or examination instrument, such as a penlight? Or is she uninterested in playing or interacting with the caregiver?
▪ Consolability	Can she be consoled or comforted by the caregiver? Or is her crying or agitation unrelieved by gentle reassurance?
▪ Look/Gaze	Does she fix her gaze on a face? Or is there a "nobody home," glassy-eyed stare?
▪ Speech/Cry	Is her speech or cry strong and spontaneous? Or is it weak, muffled, or hoarse?

Adapted from Dieckmann RA, Brownstein D, Gausche-Hill M. The Pediatric Assessment Triangle: a novel approach to pediatric assessment. *Pediatr Emerg Care.* 2010:26;312–315.

include observing from a distance; allowing the child to remain in the caregiver's lap or arms; using distraction tools, such as bright lights or toys, to measure the child's ability to interact; and kneeling down to be at eye level with the child. An immediate "hands-on" approach may cause agitation and crying and may complicate the assessment. Unless a child is unconscious or obviously critically ill, get as much information as possible by observing the child before touching the child or taking vital signs.

One example of a child with a normal appearance is an infant who holds himself or herself upright in the mother's arms, makes good eye contact, and has good color (**FIGURE 1-3**). An example of an infant with a worrisome appearance is an infant who makes poor eye contact with the caregiver or prehospital professional and is pale and listless (**FIGURE 1-4**).

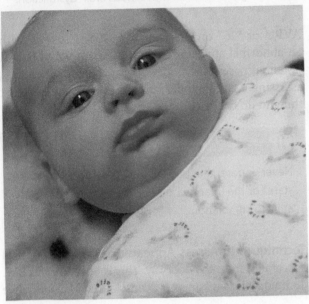

FIGURE 1-3 A child making good eye contact is normal and a sign of a good appearance.
© Photos.com.

FIGURE 1-4 A limp, pale child unable to make eye contact or a child with retractions may be critically ill or injured.
© CGN089/Shutterstock.

> **TIP**
>
> The child's general appearance is the single most important feature when assessing severity of illness or injury, need for treatment, and response to therapy.

An abnormal appearance may have many causes: inadequate oxygenation, ventilation, or **brain perfusion**; systemic abnormalities, such as poisoning, infection, or **hypoglycemia**; or acute or chronic brain injury. Regardless of the cause, a child with a grossly abnormal appearance is seriously ill or injured and needs immediate life support efforts to increase oxygenation, ventilation, and perfusion.

> **CAUTION**
>
> Although an alert, interactive child is usually not critically ill, there are some exceptions to the reliability of general appearance as an indicator of stable cardiopulmonary and neurologic function. The most common exceptions are ingestions with delayed physiologic effects and blunt injury with slow internal bleeding.

Although an alert, interactive child is usually not critically ill, there are some cases where a child may have life-threatening problems despite an initially normal appearance. Toxicologic or traumatic emergencies are good examples:

1. A child with **acetaminophen**, iron, or a **cyclic antidepressant** overdose may not show symptoms immediately after ingestion. Despite the child's normal appearance, he or she may develop deadly complications in the coming minutes or hours.
2. A child with blunt trauma and solid organ injury may be able to maintain adequate **core perfusion**, despite internal bleeding, by increasing cardiac output and systemic vascular resistance; therefore, he or she may appear normal during the primary assessment. However, when these **compensatory mechanisms** fail, the child may acutely "crash," with rapid progression to **decompensated shock**. Pallor may be the only finding on the PAT that suggests impending disaster.

A benign appearance should never justify a denial of transport. However, a normal appearance usually means that a transport with lights and siren is not necessary.

Age differences are associated with important developmental differences in psychomotor and social skills. "Normal" appearance and behavior vary by age group, as discussed in Chapter 2. Children of all ages engage their environment: newborns do this through energetic sucking and crying; older infants, by smiling or tracking a light; toddlers through physical exploration; and adolescents through speech. Knowledge of normal child development through the age groups should guide the assessment of appearance and result in more accurate treatment and transport decisions. Although appearance reflects the severity of illness or injury, it does not identify the cause. Appearance is the "screening" portion of the PAT. The other elements of the PAT (work of breathing and circulation to the skin) provide more specific information about the type of physiologic derangement, while giving additional clues about severity.

Work of Breathing

Characteristics of Work of Breathing. In children, work of breathing is a more accurate indicator of oxygenation and ventilation than respiratory rate or breath sounds on auscultation, the standard measures of breathing effectiveness in adults. Work of breathing reflects the child's attempt to compensate for abnormalities in oxygenation and ventilation, and it is a proxy for the effectiveness of gas exchange. This component of the PAT requires listening carefully for abnormal airway sounds and looking for signs of increased breathing effort. It is another "hands-off" evaluation method that does not require a stethoscope or pulse oximeter. TABLE 1-2 summarizes the key characteristics of work of breathing.

Abnormal Airway Sounds. Examples of abnormal airway sounds that can be heard without a stethoscope are snoring, muffled or hoarse speech, stridor, grunting, and wheezing. Abnormal airway sounds provide information about the physiology and anatomic location of the breathing problem.

Snoring, muffled or hoarse speech, and stridor suggest an upper airway obstruction. Snoring or gurgling occurs when the oropharynx is partially obstructed by the tongue and soft tissues. Muffled or hoarse speech reflects inflammation of the glottis or supraglottic structures. Stridor is a high-pitched sound heard on inspiration, or during inspiration and expiration, reflecting an obstruction at the level of the glottis or subglottic trachea. All of these sounds reflect abnormal airflow through partially obstructed upper airway structures. Obstruction of the upper airway passages can occur in a variety of illnesses and injuries, including croup, foreign body aspiration, and bacterial upper airway infections, or as a result of bleeding or edema.

Abnormal lower airway sounds that may be heard during the PAT include grunting and wheezing. Grunting is a sound produced by partial closure of the glottis on the end of expiration. Grunting is a form of auto positive end-expiratory pressure, a way to distend lower respiratory tract air sacs (alveoli) to promote maximum gas exchange. Grunting involves exhaling against a partially closed glottis. This short, low-pitched sound is best heard at the end of the exhalation and is easily mistaken for whimpering.

Grunting is often present in children with moderate to severe hypoxia, and it reflects poor gas exchange because of obstruction in the lower airways and alveoli. Conditions that cause hypoxia and grunting are pneumonia, pulmonary contusion (bruising of the lungs), and pulmonary edema (fluid in air sacs).

Wheezing is the result of movement of air across partially blocked small airways. At first, wheezing usually occurs during exhalation and can be heard only by auscultation of the chest with a stethoscope. As the airway obstruction increases and breathing requires more work, wheezing is often present during inhalation and exhalation. With more obstruction, wheezing may be audible without a stethoscope. Finally, if respiratory failure develops, work of breathing may

TABLE 1-2 Characteristics of Work of Breathing	
Characteristic	**Features to Look For**
Abnormal airway sounds	Snoring, muffled or hoarse speech, stridor, grunting, wheezing
Abnormal positioning	Sniffing position, tripoding, refusing to lie down
Retractions	Supraclavicular, intercostal, or substernal retractions of the chest wall; head bobbing in infants
Flaring	Flaring of the nares on inspiration

TIP

Grunting is the only airway sound noted that is not where the problem is occurring (i.e., upper airway sound with lower lung tissue disorder).

TIP

Abnormal airway sounds can provide excellent information about breathing effort, type of breathing problem, location of the breathing problem, and potential degree of hypoxia.

FIGURE 1-5 The sniffing position opens up the airways to improve patency.

diminish and the wheezing may not be heard at all. The most common cause of wheezing in childhood is **asthma**, although wheezing may also be associated with **bronchiolitis** (a viral respiratory infection in infants) and lower airway foreign body aspiration.

Visual Signs of Increased Work of Breathing.
There are several useful visual signs of increased work of breathing. These signs reflect an increased breathing effort by the child to improve oxygenation and ventilation. The presence of certain physical features, such as abnormal positioning, retractions, and nasal flaring, reflects overall illness or injury severity. Abnormal positioning is usually evident from the doorway. There are several types of abnormal postures that can indicate the child is struggling to improve airflow. A child who is in the **sniffing position** is trying to align the axes of the airways to improve patency and increase airflow (**FIGURE 1-5**). This position is usually the result of severe upper airway obstruction. The child who refuses to lie down, or who leans forward on outstretched arms (**tripoding**), is creating optimal mechanical positioning to use accessory muscles of respiration (**FIGURE 1-6**). The sniffing position and tripoding are abnormal and indicate airway obstruction, increased work of breathing, and severe respiratory distress.

Retractions are physical signs of increased work of breathing. Retractions represent the recruitment of accessory muscles of respiration to provide more "muscle power" to move air into the lungs in the face of airway or lung disease or injury. To optimally observe

FIGURE 1-6 The abnormal tripod position indicates the patient's attempts to maximize accessory muscle use.

retractions, expose the child's chest. Retractions are a more useful measure of work of breathing in children than in adults, because a child's chest wall is less muscular and the inward excursion of skin and soft tissue between the ribs is more apparent. Retractions may be in the **supraclavicular** area (above the clavicle), the **intercostal** area (between the ribs), or the **substernal** area (under the sternum), as illustrated in **FIGURE 1-7**. Another form of accessory muscle use seen only in infants is "**head bobbing**," which is the use of neck muscles to assist breathing during times of severe hypoxia. The infant extends the neck as he or she inhales and then allows the head to fall forward as he or she exhales.

Nasal flaring is another sign of increased work of breathing (**FIGURE 1-8**). **Nasal flaring** is the exaggerated opening of the nostrils during labored inspiration and indicates moderate to severe hypoxia. It reflects the child's extra effort to breathe during **hypoxic stress**,

TIP

Head bobbing is a form of accessory muscle use specific to infants and is indicative of increased work of breathing.

FIGURE 1-7 Retractions indicate increased work of breathing and may occur in the supraclavicular, intercostal, and substernal areas.

© AePatt Journey/Shutterstock.

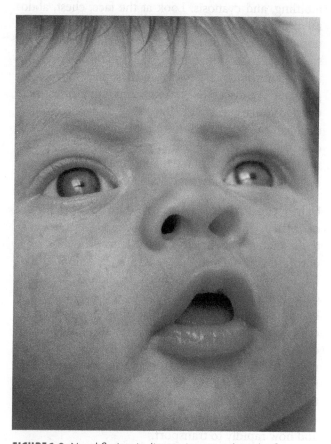

FIGURE 1-8 Nasal flaring indicates increased work of breathing and moderate to severe hypoxia.

© Hemera/Thinkstock.

usually caused by such conditions as croup, pneumonia, asthma, bronchiolitis, or pulmonary contusion.

Techniques to Assess Work of Breathing. Step 2 in the PAT is assessing work of breathing. Begin by listening carefully from a distance for abnormal airway sounds. Next, look for key physical signs. Note if the child has an abnormal posture, most notably the

sniffing position or tripoding. Next, have the caregiver uncover the chest of the child for direct inspection, or have the child undress on the caregiver's lap. Look for intercostal, supraclavicular, and substernal retractions, and note if there is head bobbing in infants. After examining for retractions, inspect for nasal flaring. This stepwise process is critical for gathering accurate information. After an infant or child begins to cry, assessment of work of breathing becomes more difficult.

Children may have increased work of breathing because of abnormalities anywhere in their upper or lower airways, alveoli (air sacs), **pleura** (membrane surrounding the lungs and lining the walls of the pleural cavity), or chest wall. The type of abnormal airway sounds gives an important clue to the anatomic location of the illness or injury process, whereas the number and type of physical signs of increased work of breathing help in determining the degree of physiologic stress.

Combining assessment of appearance and work of breathing can also help establish the severity of the child's illness or injury. A child with a normal appearance and increased work of breathing is in respiratory distress. An abnormal appearance and increased work of breathing suggest respiratory failure. An abnormal appearance and abnormally decreased work of breathing imply impending respiratory arrest.

Circulation to Skin

Characteristics of Circulation to Skin. The goal of rapid circulatory assessment is to determine the adequacy of cardiac output and core perfusion or perfusion of the vital organs. The child's appearance is one indicator of brain perfusion, but abnormal appearance may be caused by other conditions unrelated to circulation, such as hypoxia, hypoglycemia, brain injury, or intoxication. For this reason, other signs of adequacy of perfusion must be added to the evaluation of appearance to assess the child's true circulatory status.

An important sign of core perfusion is circulation to the skin. When cardiac output is inadequate, the body shuts down circulation to nonessential anatomic areas, such as the skin and mucous membranes, to preserve blood supply to the most vital organs (brain, heart, and kidneys). Therefore, circulation to the skin reflects the overall status of core circulation. **Pallor**, **mottling**, and **cyanosis** are key visual indicators of reduced circulation to the skin and mucous membranes. **TABLE 1-3** summarizes these characteristics.

Pallor may be the first sign of poor skin or mucous membrane perfusion; it may be the only visual sign apparent in a child with compensated shock and indicates reflex peripheral vasoconstriction to shunt blood away from the skin to the core. Pallor may also

TABLE 1-3 Characteristics of Circulation to Skin

Characteristic	Features to Look For
Pallor	White or pale mucous membrane coloration from inadequate blood flow
Mottling	Patchy skin discoloration caused by vasoconstriction or vasodilation
Cyanosis	Bluish discoloration of skin and mucous membranes

be a sign of anemia or hypoxia. Mottling is another sign of inadequate skin perfusion, reflecting vasomotor instability (abnormal blood vessel tone) in the capillary beds of the skin. Mottled skin has patchy areas of **vasoconstriction** (pallor) mixed with areas of **vasodilation** (cyanosis or erythema). Mottling may also be a normal physiologic response in a child exposed to cold environmental temperatures.

Cyanosis is blue discoloration of the skin and mucous membranes. It is the most extreme visual indicator of poor perfusion or poor oxygenation. Do not confuse **acrocyanosis** (blue hands and feet in a newborn or infant less than 2 months of age) with true cyanosis. Acrocyanosis is a normal finding when a young infant is cold, and it reflects **vasomotor** instability rather than hypoxia or shock. True cyanosis is a late finding of respiratory failure or **shock**. A hypoxic child is likely to show other physical abnormalities long before turning blue. These abnormalities may include abnormal appearance with agitation or lethargy and increased work of breathing. A child in shock may also have pallor or mottling. Never wait for cyanosis to begin treatment with supplemental oxygen. However, the presence of cyanosis is always a critical sign that requires immediate intervention with breathing support.

Abnormal circulation to the skin, in combination with an abnormal appearance, suggests shock. However, the abnormalities in appearance in early phases of compensated shock may be subtle, and some children may remain alert. As perfusion worsens and compensatory mechanisms fail, appearance becomes abnormal, reflecting inadequate delivery of oxygen and glucose to the brain. Another clue to the presence of shock is **effortless tachypnea**, or **tachypnea** without signs of increased work of breathing. Effortless tachypnea is a reflex mechanism that allows the body to blow off carbon dioxide to compensate for the metabolic **acidosis** caused by poor peripheral perfusion (**lactic acidosis**). **Hypocarbia** (low blood CO_2

levels) generates a respiratory alkalosis and helps to restore normal pH (blood acid–base balance). Effortless tachypnea is different from the rapid and labored respirations that are present with illnesses and injuries associated with airway or lung pathology.

Techniques to Assess Circulation to Skin. Step 3 in the PAT is evaluating circulation to the skin. Be sure the child is exposed long enough for visual inspection but not long enough to become cold. A cold child may have normal core perfusion but abnormal circulation to the skin. Cold circulating air temperature is the most common reason for misinterpretation of skin signs, and an exposed young infant may become hypothermic quickly, even at normal ambient temperatures.

Inspect the skin and mucous membranes for pallor, mottling, and cyanosis. Look at the face, chest, abdomen, and extremities, and then inspect the lips for cyanosis. In dark-skinned children, circulation to the skin is sometimes more difficult to assess, and the lips, mucous membranes, and nail beds are the best places to look for pallor or cyanosis (**FIGURE 1-9**). Combining assessment of appearance and circulation to the skin can also help establish the severity of the child's illness or injury. A child with a normal appearance and poor circulation to the skin is possibly cold. An abnormal appearance and circulation to the skin suggests the child is in shock.

Using the PAT to Evaluate Severity and Illness or Injury. The PAT provides a general impression of the pediatric patient. The intent is to provide a standardized approach to the "general impression" and an immediate picture of the child's physiologic status. By combining the three components of the PAT, the prehospital professional should be able to answer three critical questions: (1) How severe is the child's illness or injury? (2) What is the most likely physiologic abnormality? (3) What is the urgency for treatment? This information helps the prehospital professional select the most important actions: how fast to intervene, what type of general and specific treatments to give, and how rapidly to transport.

The three elements of the PAT work together and allow a rapid assessment of the child's overall physiologic stability. For example, if a child is interactive and pink, but has mild intercostal retractions, the prehospital professional can take time to approach the child in a developmentally appropriate manner to complete the primary assessment. However, if the child is limp, with unlabored rapid breathing and pale or mottled skin, shock is likely. In this case, the prehospital professional must move rapidly through the primary assessment and begin resuscitation. A child who has an abnormal appearance, but normal work of

FIGURE 1-9 In dark-skinned children, circulation to the skin is sometimes more difficult to assess, and the lips, mucous membranes, and nail beds may be the best places to look for pallor or cyanosis.

breathing and normal circulation to skin, probably has a primary brain dysfunction or a major metabolic or systemic problem, such as **postictal state**, **subdural hemorrhage**, **concussion**, intoxication, hypoglycemia, or **sepsis**.

The PAT has two important advantages. First, it allows the examiner to quickly obtain critical information about the child's physiologic status before touching or agitating the child. Second, the PAT helps set priorities for the rest of the hands-on primary assessment. The PAT takes only seconds, it helps to identify the need for lifesaving interventions, and it assists in the transition into the next phase of hands-on physical assessment.

The three components of the PAT (appearance, work of breathing, and circulation to the skin) can be assessed in any sequence, unlike the ordered ABCDEs of resuscitation discussed next.

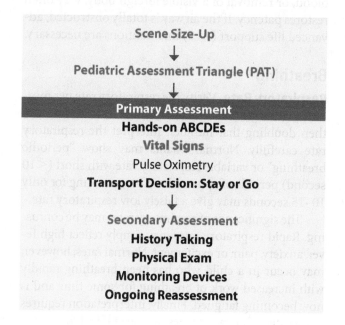

TIP

By combining the three components of the PAT, the prehospital professional can answer three critical questions: (1) How sick or injured is the child? (2) What is the most likely physiologic abnormality? (3) What is the urgency for treatment?

Primary Assessment

Hands-on ABCDEs

The primary assessment continues the process of identifying life-threatening conditions using an ordered hands-on physical evaluation of the ABCDEs.

It provides a prioritized sequence of life-support interventions to reverse critical physiologic abnormalities. As in adults, there is a specific order for treating life-threatening problems as they are identified, before moving to the next step. The steps are the same, but there are important pediatric differences in anatomy, physiology, and signs of distress. ABCDE assessment involves the following components:

1. Airway
2. Breathing
3. Circulation
4. Disability
5. Exposure

Airway

The PAT may identify the presence of an airway obstruction based on the presence of abnormal airway sounds. However, the loudness of the stridor or wheezing is not necessarily related to the amount of airway obstruction. For example, children with asthma in severe distress may have little or no wheezing. Similarly, children with an upper airway foreign body below the **vocal cords** may have minimal stridor. Abnormal positioning and retractions provide further information about the degree of obstruction, as does the quality of air entry on auscultation during the hands-on assessment.

If the airway is open, ensure that the chest rises with each breath. If a child has assumed a position that maximizes his or her ability to maintain a spontaneously open airway, allow the child to remain in that position of comfort. If gurgling is present, there may be mucus, blood, or a foreign body in the mouth or upper airway. Oropharyngeal suctioning of mucus or blood, or removal of a visible foreign body, very often restores patency. If the airway is totally obstructed, advanced life support (ALS) interventions are necessary.

Breathing

Respiratory Rate. Verify the respiratory rate per minute by counting the number of chest rises in 30 seconds, then doubling that number. Interpret the respiratory rate carefully. Normal infants may show "periodic breathing" or variable respiratory rate with short (<10 second) periods of apnea. Therefore, counting for only 10–15 seconds may give a falsely low respiratory rate.

The significance of respiratory rates may be confusing. Rapid respiratory rates may simply reflect high fever, anxiety, pain, or excitement. Normal rates, however, may occur in a child who has been breathing rapidly with increased work of breathing for some time and is now becoming fatigued. Finally, interpretation requires knowledge of normal values for age (**TABLE 1-4**).

> ### TIP
>
> "Red flag" respiratory rates are less than 20 breaths/min for children younger than 6 years of age and less than 12 breaths/min for children between 6 and 18 years of age.

Serial assessment of respiratory rates may be especially useful, and the trend is sometimes more accurate than any single value. A sustained increase or decrease in respiratory rate is usually significant.

Pay close attention to extremes of respiratory rate. A very rapid respiratory rate (>60 breaths/min for any

TABLE 1-4 Normal Respiratory Rate for Age	
Age	**Respiratory Rate (breaths/min)**
Infant	30–60
Toddler	24–40
Preschooler	22–34
School-aged child	18–30
Adolescent	12–16

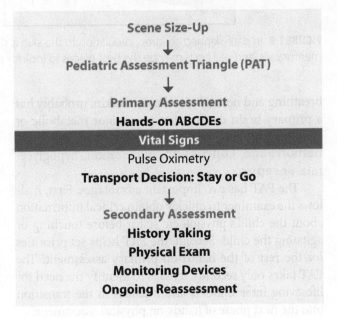

Scene Size-Up
↓
Pediatric Assessment Triangle (PAT)
↓
Primary Assessment
Hands-on ABCDEs

Vital Signs

Pulse Oximetry

Transport Decision: Stay or Go
↓
Secondary Assessment
History Taking
Physical Exam
Monitoring Devices
Ongoing Reassessment

age), especially with abnormal appearance or marked retractions, indicates respiratory distress and possibly respiratory failure. An abnormally slow respiratory rate is always worrisome because it might mean respiratory failure. Red flags are respiratory rates less than 20 breaths/min for children younger than 6 years of age and less than 12 breaths/min for children between 6 and 18 years of age. A normal respiratory rate alone never guarantees adequate oxygenation and ventilation. The respiratory rate must be interpreted along with appearance, work of breathing, and air movement.

Pulse Oximetry

Oxygen Saturation. Pulse oximetry is an excellent tool to assess how well a child is oxygenating. **FIGURE 1-10** illustrates the technique of placing a pulse oximetry probe on a young child. In infants and younger children, the patient may tolerate the probe more readily if a wrap around probe is used and it is placed around the toe or

A

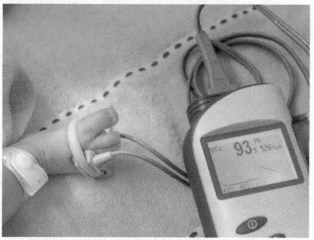

B

FIGURE 1-10 A. Various pulse oximeter probes wrap around or clip onto digits or earlobes. **B.** Pulse oximetry is an excellent tool for assessing the effectiveness of oxygenation.

B: tnkorn yangaun/Shutterstock.

the foot. Covering the extremity with a blanket, sock, or towel may also help improve tolerance of the probe. A pulse oximetry reading above 94% saturation on room air indicates good oxygenation. Be careful not to underestimate respiratory distress in a child with a reading above 94%. Sometimes the child can compensate for hypoxia by significantly increasing work of breathing and respiratory rate, and pulse oximetry may not reflect the true severity or urgency of the respiratory problem. As with any other measurement, interpret pulse oximetry in the context of the "big picture," including work of breathing, appearance, and circulation.

Although pulse oximetry is quite helpful in identifying a child with moderate respiratory distress, it can also help identify the child in respiratory failure. When the pulse oximetry reading is below 90% saturation in a child on 100% oxygen by a nonrebreathing mask, this usually represents respiratory failure requiring **assisted ventilation**. However, sometimes a child in severe respiratory distress or early respiratory failure may maintain measured oxygen saturation by increasing work of breathing and respiratory rate. This child may not appear to be critically ill by

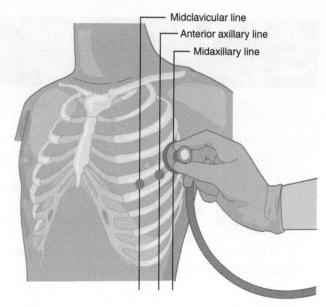

FIGURE 1-11 Listen for air movement over the midaxillary line.

pulse oximetry alone. Again, interpret pulse oximetry together with the rest of the assessment to accurately evaluate the degree of respiratory distress or failure.

Auscultation. Listen with a stethoscope over the midclavicular and **midaxillary lines** during inhalation and exhalation to hear abnormal lung sounds, such as **crackles** and wheezing (**FIGURE 1-11**). **Inspiratory** crackles indicate disease in the alveoli (air sacs) themselves. Often, crackles are not heard on auscultation, even when the child has a pathologic condition, such as pneumonia. The younger the child, the more difficult it is to appreciate abnormal sounds during auscultation. Expiratory wheezing indicates lower airway obstruction. Auscultation also helps evaluate the volume of air movement and effectiveness of work of breathing. A child with increased work of breathing and poor air movement may be in impending respiratory failure.

TABLE 1-5 lists abnormal breath sounds, their causes, and common examples of associated disease processes.

Circulation

The PAT provides important visual clues about circulation to the skin. Information obtained from the hands-on evaluation of heart rate, pulse quality, skin temperature, capillary refill time, and blood pressure provides further information on the adequacy of perfusion.

Heart Rate. Methods used to assess adult circulatory status (heart rate and blood pressure) have important limitations in children. First, normal heart rate varies with age, as noted in **TABLE 1-6**. Second, tachycardia may be an early sign of hypoxia or poor perfusion,

TABLE 1-5 Interpretation of Abnormal Breath Sounds

Sound	Cause	Examples
Stridor	Upper airway obstruction	Croup, foreign body aspiration, retropharyngeal abscess
Wheezing	Lower airway obstruction	Asthma, foreign body, bronchiolitis
Expiratory grunting	Inadequate oxygenation	Pulmonary contusion, pneumonia, drowning
Inspiratory crackles	Fluid, mucus, or blood in airway	Pneumonia, pulmonary contusion
Absent breath sounds despite increased work of breathing	Severe airway obstruction (upper or lower airway)	Physical barrier to transmission of breath sounds, foreign body, severe asthma, hemothorax, pneumothorax, pleural fluid, pneumonia

TABLE 1-6 Normal Heart Rate for Age

Age	Heart Rate (beats/min)
Infant	100–160
Toddler	95–150
Preschooler	80–140
School-age child	70–120
Adolescent	60–100

but it may also reflect fever, anxiety, pain, and excitement. Like respiratory rate, interpret heart rate within the context of the overall history, PAT, and primary assessment. A trend of increasing or decreasing heart rate may be quite useful: It may suggest worsening hypoxia or shock or improvement after treatment. When hypoxia or shock becomes critical, the heart rate falls,

TIP

A rapid initial respiratory rate may simply reflect high fever, anxiety, pain, excitement, and not any real physiologic or anatomic problem. Noting a trend of an abnormal respiratory rate is more useful for indicating true **pathology**.

leading to frank bradycardia. **Bradycardia** indicates critical hypoxia or ischemia. With tachycardia greater than 180 beats/min, an electronic monitor is necessary to accurately determine heart rate.

Pulse Quality. Feel the pulse to ascertain pulse quality. Normally, the brachial pulse is palpable in the medial aspect of the **antecubital fossa** (**FIGURE 1-12**). Note the quality as either weak or strong. If the brachial pulse is strong, the child is probably not hypotensive. If a peripheral pulse cannot be felt, attempt to find a central pulse. Check the femoral pulse in infants and young children or the carotid pulse

CASE STUDY 2

A 3-year-old boy was found face down in the family swimming pool. He was under water for no more than 1 minute but required cardiopulmonary resuscitation by the mother to get him breathing again. On arrival of EMS, the child is alert, pink, and clinging to his mother. Respirations appear regular and nonlabored. When you examine him further, he screams and fights you. His respiratory rate is 26 breaths/minute, but you are unable to obtain a blood pressure or heart rate or assess lung sounds. The mother is sobbing and frightened.

1. How useful is the PAT in evaluating severity of illness and urgency for care?
2. How is the PAT different from the ABCDEs in the primary assessment?

FIGURE 1-12 The anatomic position of the brachial pulse is in the medial aspect of the antecubital fossa.

in an older child or adolescent. If there is no pulse, or the pulse is low (<60 beats/min) and the child is symptomatic with poor circulation, start cardiopulmonary resuscitation (CPR) (see Chapter 5 for more information).

Skin Temperature and Capillary Refill Time. Next, do a hands-on evaluation of circulation to the skin. Although children with normal circulation may have cool hands and feet, the skin should be warm above the wrists and ankles. With decreasing perfusion, the extremities become cooler proximally. Check capillary refill time in a fingertip, toe, or heel or on the pads of the fingertips. Normal capillary refill time is less than 2 to 3 seconds. The value of measuring capillary refill time is controversial for several reasons: the peripheral perfusion baseline may vary from child to child; environmental factors, such as cold room temperature, may complicate interpretation; and it may be difficult for the prehospital professional to accurately count seconds under critical circumstances. The capillary refill time is just one element in the assessment of circulation. It must be evaluated in the context of the PAT and other perfusion characteristics, such as heart rate, pulse quality, and blood pressure.

Signs of circulation to the skin (skin temperature, capillary refill time, and pulse quality) are helpful tools to assess a child's circulatory status, especially when performed consecutively on a child who is not cold.

Blood Pressure. Blood pressure determination and interpretation may be difficult in children because of the lack of patient cooperation, confusion about proper cuff size, and problems remembering normal values for age. **FIGURE 1-13A** illustrates the different sizes of blood pressure cuffs, and **FIGURE 1-13B** demonstrates the technique for getting a correct blood pressure in the arm or thigh. Always use a cuff with a width of two-thirds the length of the upper arm or thigh. For patients 3 years of age or younger, technical difficulties reduce the value of a blood pressure in the field. When shock is suspected in this age group based on other assessments (e.g., history, mechanism, PAT), consider attempting blood pressure once on scene, but do not delay treatment or transport. In a child who is clearly unstable (requiring assisted ventilation, absent radial or femoral pulses), begin immediate resuscitation and delay blood pressure until child is in a more stable condition. For stable patients older than 3 years of age, try one blood pressure measurement in the field, then move on to the rest of the assessment.

For children older than 1 year of age, an easy formula for determining the lower limit of acceptable blood pressure by age is as follows: minimal systolic blood pressure should be greater than 70 + (2 × age in years). For example, a 2-year-old toddler with a

A

B

FIGURE 1-13 A. There are several different blood pressure (BP) cuff sizes: neonatal, infant, child, and adult. **B.** To obtain an accurate BP reading, use a cuff that is two-thirds the length of the child's upper arm.

B. © Jones & Bartlett Learning. Courtesy of Glen Ellman.

systolic blood pressure of 65 mm Hg is hypotensive. **TABLE 1-7** shows approximate normal minimal systolic blood pressure values for different ages. High blood pressure is usually not a clinical problem for children in the field. Assume that a blood pressure is within normal limits if an infant or young child is agitated, is crying, has pink skin, and has easily palpable peripheral pulses. In a patient with this clinical profile,

TABLE 1-7 Minimum Systolic Blood Pressure by Age

Age	Minimal Systolic Blood Pressure (mm Hg)
Infant (birth to 12 mo)	>60
Toddler (1–3 yr)	>70
Preschooler	>75
School-age child	>80
Adolescent	>90

do not delay transport to obtain a blood pressure. Remember, a normal blood pressure measurement may be misleading. Although a low blood pressure definitely indicates hypotensive shock, a "normal" blood pressure frequently exists in children with compensated shock.

Note that a widening pulse pressure (systolic pressure minus diastolic pressure) may occur secondary to increased intracranial pressure and early septic shock; a narrowing pulse pressure may be seen early in hypovolemic shock.

TIP

For patients younger than 3 years of age, the value of obtaining a blood pressure in the field may be outweighed by the technical difficulties of getting an accurate measurement. Focus on immediate resuscitation in a child with an unstable airway, tachycardia and poor perfusion or absent radial or femoral pulses, and delay blood pressure until child's condition stabilizes.

CAUTION

Do not depend on blood pressure readings to diagnose shock. A "normal" blood pressure frequently exists in compensated shock.

Disability

Assessment of disability, or neurologic status, involves quick evaluation of the two main parts of the CNS: the cerebral cortex and the brainstem. First assess neurologic status, which is controlled by the cerebral cortex, by looking at appearance as part of the PAT; then assess the level of consciousness using the AVPU scale (**TABLE 1-8**). Evaluate the brainstem by checking the responses of each pupil to a direct beam of light. A normal pupil constricts after a light stimulus. Pupillary response may be abnormal in the presence of drugs, ongoing seizures, hypoxia, or impending brainstem herniation. Next, evaluate motor activity. Look for symmetric movement of the extremities, seizures, posturing, or flaccidity.

CAUTION

Neither the AVPU scale nor the Pediatric GCS allows assessment of restless or agitated behavioral states.

TABLE 1-8 AVPU Scale

Category	Stimulus	Response Type	Reaction
Alert	Normal environment	Appropriate	Normal interactiveness for age
Verbal	Simple command or sound stimulus	Appropriate or inappropriate	Responds to name; nonspecific or confused
Painful	Pain	Appropriate, inappropriate, or pathologic	Withdraws from pain or sound or motion without purpose or localization of pain; posturing
Unresponsive			No perceptible response to any stimulus

AVPU Scale. The AVPU scale is a standardized method of assessing the level of consciousness in all patients. It helps categorize motor response based on simple responses to stimuli. The patient is either alert, responsive to verbal stimuli, responsive only to painful stimuli, or unresponsive.

Abnormal Appearance and the AVPU Scale. Assessment of appearance using the PAT provides different information than assessment using the AVPU scale. A child with an altered mental status (AMS) on the AVPU scale always has an abnormal appearance in the PAT, because such a child almost always has a serious or critical condition. However, a child with a mild to moderate illness or injury may be alert on the AVPU scale, but have an abnormal appearance in the PAT. Assessing appearance using the PAT may provide an earlier indication of the presence of serious illness and injury.

The accuracy of the AVPU scale is controversial, and it has a few important limitations. Its ability to predict the extent of neurologic compromise has not been well tested in children. Its scope is limited in the evaluation of children with restless or agitated states. The scale only addresses decreased levels of responsiveness, a problem common to all of the current prehospital methods for disability assessment. However, it is easy to remember (there are no numbers to recall) and to use. The more complicated Pediatric GCS involves memorization and numerical scoring, tasks that may be hard to remember and apply in critical situations (**TABLE 1-9**). Recent data suggest that the motor component of the GCS alone is the best predictor of neurologic outcome. The much simpler-to-administer motor component of the GCS may be adequate for mental status evaluation in the field. The motor categories of the GCS from lowest point value to highest are (1) no response, (2) **extensor posturing**, (3) flexor posturing, (4) withdrawing, (5) **localizing**, and (6) obeying instructions (as age-appropriate). Like the AVPU scale, the GCS does not address degrees of neurologic disability in children who are restless, agitated, or combative.

Exposure

Proper exposure of the child is necessary for completion of the primary physical assessment. The PAT requires that the caregiver remove part of the child's clothing to allow careful observation of the face, chest wall, and skin. Completing the ABCDE components of the primary assessment may require further exposure to fully evaluate physiologic function, anatomic abnormalities, and unsuspected injuries. Pay attention to the need for privacy, even for prepubescent children, when possible.

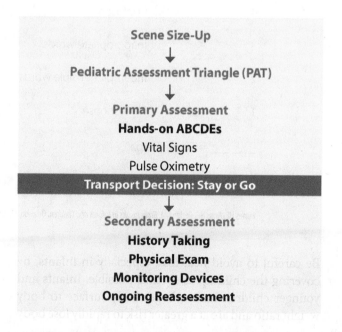

Scene Size-Up
↓
Pediatric Assessment Triangle (PAT)
↓
Primary Assessment
Hands-on ABCDEs
Vital Signs
Pulse Oximetry
Transport Decision: Stay or Go
↓
Secondary Assessment
History Taking
Physical Exam
Monitoring Devices
Ongoing Reassessment

TABLE 1-9 Pediatric Glasgow Coma Scale

Score	Child	Infant
Eyes		
4	Opens eyes spontaneously	Opens eyes spontaneously
3	Opens eyes to speech	Opens eyes to speech
2	Opens eyes to pain	Opens eyes to pain
1	No response	No response
_____ = Score (Eyes)		
Motor		
6	Obeys commands	Spontaneous movements
5	Localizes	Withdraws to touch
4	Withdraws	Withdraws to pain
3	Flexion	Flexion (decorticate)
2	Extension	Extension (decerebrate)
1	No response	No response
_____ = Score (Motor)		
Verbal		
5	Oriented	Coos and babbles
4	Confused	Irritable cry
3	Inappropriate words	Cries to pain
2	Incomprehensible words	Moans to pain
1	No response	No response
_____ = Score (Verbal)		
_____ = **Total Score (Eyes, Motor, Verbal). Scores will range from 3 to 15.**		

James HE, Anas NG, Perkin RM. *Brain Insults in Infants and Children.* Orlando, FL: Grune & Stratton; 1985. Reprinted with permission.

Be careful to avoid heat loss, especially in infants, by covering the child up as soon as possible. Infants and younger children have a larger body surface to body weight ratio and are at a greater risk to rapidly lose body heat when left exposed. Cold stress in critically ill or injured patients can increase metabolic demands, worsen the effects of hypoxia and hypoglycemia, and adversely affect the response to resuscitative efforts.

Primary Assessment: The Transport Decision: Stay or Go?

After completing the PAT and the hands-on ABCDEs and beginning resuscitation as necessary, the prehospital professional must make a crucial decision: should he or she immediately transport the child to the ED, or should he or she continue with the additional assessment and treatment on scene? Should he or she transport the child, or is there a more appropriate mode of transport available (e.g., aeromedical services, pediatric specialty transport teams)? Should the child be transported to a local community hospital, for either treatment or stabilization, or does the child need to go directly to a trauma center or pediatric specialty hospital? This decision process is different for each child and for each EMS system. While vital signs and pulse oximetry are listed in the primary assessment, the transport decision can be made if the prehospital provider determines the need for expedited transport after using the PAT and evaluating the ABCDEs.

> **TIP**
>
> Deciding when to go and when to stay is different for each child and for each EMS system.

> **TIP**
>
> If the child is physiologically unstable, defer or omit history taking and physical examination on scene and perform en route.

Expected Benefits of Treatment

The time it takes to reach definitive care in the hospital has a major effect on the outcomes of children with serious injuries. The time it takes to reach hospital care may also significantly affect the outcomes of children with certain medical illnesses. For example, a child in cardiogenic shock benefits most from rapid transport to definitive care, because the hospital is the best place for lifesaving treatments of this rare and complex condition.

However, some critically ill children benefit from basic life support (BLS) and ALS treatment on scene. For example, for a child who is seizing, early treatment with a benzodiazepine is the best hope to get the seizure under immediate control and avoid additional anticonvulsant administration and advanced airway management. A child with an anaphylactic reaction requires an intramuscular (IM) epinephrine injection from an autoinjector or drawn up by a BLS or ALS provider. Similarly, the risk of brain injury is decreased if glucose is administered to the unconscious diabetic child at the time that the prehospital professional recognizes hypoglycemia with a bedside test.

EMS System Regulations

The decision to stay or go often is defined by EMS system regulations about treatment and transport. For example, some systems allow prehospital professionals to treat a child in cardiopulmonary arrest with ALS interventions until either the resuscitation is successful or death is declared. Other systems require transport after initial resuscitation is under way, with the decision to discontinue efforts left to the ED staff.

Comfort Level

Whenever a prehospital professional believes that the illness or injury requires a higher level of care, it is best to initiate transport quickly. Moreover, whenever the prehospital professional feels uncomfortable with a critical intervention, it is best to transport and attempt the intervention on the way to the ED, rather than on scene. For example, a child with hypotensive (decompensated) shock usually deserves one attempt at vascular access on scene, then fluid administration on the way to the ED. The time spent on multiple intravenous attempts on scene might be better spent in transporting the child to definitive care, where the underlying cause of shock can be more appropriately addressed.

Transport Time

The time to the nearest ED is another key factor. A shorter transport time ordinarily supports a shorter scene time. For example, if a child has ingested a potentially lethal poison, immediate transport is prudent if the ED is close by, because of the complications related to delay of definitive care. However, if transport time is long, consider initiating treatment on scene. Prehospital providers should also consider the pediatric capabilities of the area EDs compared to the criticality of the pediatric patient. While pediatric patients are best served at pediatric hospital EDs, the criticality of the patient may cause the prehospital provider to transport a critical pediatric patient to the closest ED so he or she can be stabilized before being transported to a pediatric hospital.

Summary of Primary Assessment

The components of the pediatric primary assessment include the PAT, the ABCDEs, immediate resuscitation needs, and transport decision. The PAT is the basis for the general impression. It includes evaluation of the characteristics of appearance, work of breathing, and circulation to the skin and uses clues obtained by looking and listening from across the room. The primary assessment includes a hands-on evaluation of pediatric-specific indicators of cardiopulmonary or neurologic abnormalities. Although vital signs can be useful in the primary assessment, they can also be misleading. They must be interpreted in the context of age and the overall general and primary assessments. Interventions may be necessary at any point in the ABCDE sequence. After the ABCDEs, another crucial decision is whether to stay on scene and begin treatment or transport immediately. The type of clinical problem, the expected benefits of earlier transport, the local EMS policies, the prehospital professional's comfort level, and the transport time are all important elements in the transport decision.

TIP

Always perform reassessment to track problems and monitor response to treatment.

Scene Size-Up
↓
Pediatric Assessment Triangle (PAT)
↓
Primary Assessment
Hands-on ABCDEs
Vital Signs
Pulse Oximetry
Transport Decision: Stay or Go
↓
Secondary Assessment
History Taking
Physical Exam
Monitoring Devices
Ongoing Reassessment

Secondary Assessment: History Taking

History taking has two objectives and should be performed on both medical and trauma patients:

1. To obtain a complete description of the main complaint
2. To determine the mechanism of injury or circumstances of illness

If the child seems to be physiologically unstable based on the primary assessment, the prehospital professional may decide to transport immediately and defer the history and secondary assessment. If the child is stable and the scene is safe, the prehospital professional should obtain a thorough history and complete the secondary assessment on the scene and before transport. As opposed to the primary assessment, which focuses on physiologic problems that may be immediately life-threatening, this secondary assessment focuses on anatomic abnormalities, which are rarely life-threatening.

A history should be obtained from the caregiver of the pediatric patient or from the caregiver and the older child or adolescent. In some cases, it may be helpful to interview the adolescent separate from the caregiver; many adolescents are hesitant to disclose information about drug use or sexual activity (as it relates to the current illness or injury) in front of their caregiver. The history provides important information that assists the prehospital professional in analyzing assessment findings. The SAMPLE mnemonic may be used to elicit information: Signs and Symptoms, Allergies, Medications, Past medical problems, Last food or liquid, and Events leading up to this illness or injury (**TABLE 1-10**).

TABLE 1-10 Pediatric SAMPLE Components

Component	Explanation
Signs and symptoms	Onset and nature of symptoms of pain or fever Age-appropriate signs of distress
Allergies	Known drug reactions or other allergies
Medications	Exact names and doses of ongoing drugs Timing and amount of last dose Timing and dose of analgesics or antipyretics
Past medical problems	History of pregnancy, labor, delivery Previous illness or injuries Immunizations
Last food or liquid	Timing of the child's last food or drink, including bottle or breastfeeding
Events leading to the injury or illness	Key events leading to the current incident Fever history

Children with special health care needs often require additional history collection, but the type of history necessary is dependent on the underlying illness or condition. The use of an **Emergency Information Form (EIF)** can be extremely helpful in obtaining critical information about these patients. More information about children with special health care needs can be found in Chapter 10.

If a child has an apparently minor condition (e.g., low-grade fever, feeding difficulties, fussiness, minor trauma), be careful not to overlook clues to possible serious underlying conditions. Ingestions, metabolic problems, and systemic infections may present with nonspecific findings in infants and toddlers. Consider child maltreatment when the physical findings are not logically related to the complaint leading to the call or if the history is implausible or changes.

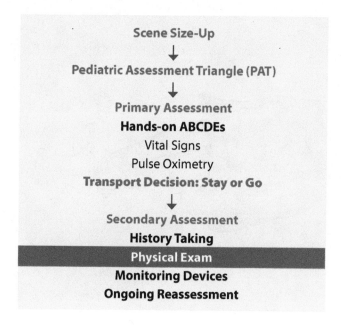

Physical Examination

Often, this portion of the assessment is not possible because of transport and treatment priorities. Sometimes it is unnecessary because the problem has been fully evaluated in earlier phases of the assessment or the complaint and history are minor or well localized (e.g., minor laceration or twisted ankle).

If the child with traumatic injuries is stable on scene and does not need resuscitation after the primary assessment, or if he or she is on the way to the hospital but does not require ongoing treatment, perform a detailed secondary assessment. This physical evaluation must include all anatomic areas affected and builds on the findings of the primary assessment and history taking.

Use the toe-to-head sequence for the detailed secondary assessment of infants, toddlers, and preschoolers. This approach allows the prehospital professional to gain the child's trust and cooperation and increases the accuracy of the physical findings. Ask for the assistance of the caregiver in the assessment. Note the following special anatomic characteristics of children when performing the secondary assessment.

General Observations

Observe the clothing for any unusual odors or for stains that might suggest a poison. If poisoning is suspected, remove soiled or dirty clothing and save it, and wash the child's skin with soap and water.

Skin

Observe the skin carefully for rashes and bruising patterns that may suggest maltreatment, as discussed in Chapter 11. Look for bite marks; straight line marks from cords or straps; pinch marks; or hand, belt, or buckle pattern bruises. Patterned injuries, or those with a geometric shape, are often indicative of abuse. Inspect for nonblanching **petechial** or **purpuric** lesions (which may indicate severe infections), and look for any new lesions that develop during transport.

Head

The younger the infant or child, the larger the head is in proportion to the rest of the body (**FIGURE 1-14**). This disproportionate size increases the risk for head injury with deceleration, such as in motor vehicle crashes. Look for bruising, swelling, and **hematomas**. Significant blood can be lost between the skull and scalp of a small infant. Assessment of the anterior **fontanelle** in infants younger than 9–18 months old can provide helpful information (**FIGURE 1-15**). If possible, the fontanelle should be assessed with the infant in a sitting position, and when not crying. A bulging and **nonpulsatile fontanelle** suggests elevated intracranial pressure caused by **meningitis**, **encephalitis**, or **intracranial** bleeding. A sunken fontanelle suggests dehydration.

Eyes

A thorough evaluation of pupil size, reaction to light, and symmetry of **extraocular** muscle movements may be difficult to perform in infants. Gently rocking infants in the upright position often gets them to open their eyes. A colorful distracting object can then be used to help assess eye movements.

FIGURE 1-14 The relationship of the head to the body changes with advancing age.

Modified from McKinney ES et al: *Maternal child nursing*, ed 3, St. Louis, 2009, Saunders.

2 Months (fetal) | 5 Months (fetal) | Newborn | 2 years | 6 years | 12 years | 25 years

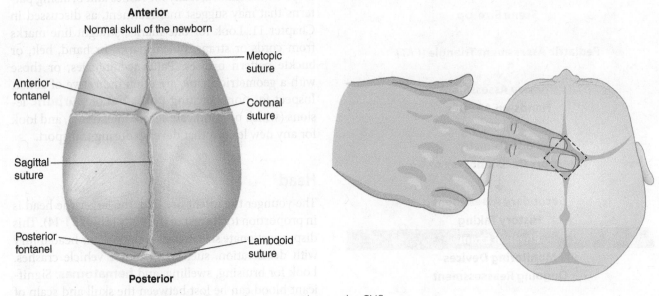

Anterior
Normal skull of the newborn

Metopic suture
Anterior fontanel
Coronal suture
Sagittal suture
Posterior fontanel
Lambdoid suture
Posterior

FIGURE 1-15 The anterior fontanelle of the infant is a window to the CNS.

Nose

Young infants preferentially breathe through their noses, so nasal congestion with mucus can cause marked respiratory distress. Gentle bulb or catheter suction of the nostrils may bring relief (**FIGURE 1-16**). In a trauma patient, leaking blood (**rhinorrhea**) or cerebrospinal fluid (CSF) suggests a **basilar skull fracture**.

Ears

Look for any drainage from the ear canals (**otorrhea**). Bruises to the ear pinna, especially in a nonambulatory child, may suggest inflicted trauma. Leaking blood or

FIGURE 1-16 Gentle bulb suction may bring relief to the infant.

CSF suggests a basilar skull fracture. Check for bruises behind the ear or **Battle sign**, another indicator of basilar skull fracture. The presence of **pus** may indicate an ear infection or perforation of the eardrum (tympanic membrane).

Mouth

In the trauma patient, look for active bleeding and loose teeth. In nonambulatory children, mouth trauma may be a sign of inflicted trauma. Note the smell of the breath. Some ingestions are associated with identifiable odors, such as **hydrocarbons**. Acidosis, as in **diabetic ketoacidosis**, may impart a sweet or "fruity" smell to the breath.

Neck

Examine the **trachea** for **edema** or bruising. Listen with a stethoscope over the trachea at the midline (**FIGURE 1-17**). This is a quick and easy way to differentiate between very proximal airway obstruction (usually mucus in the nose) and true wheezing or stridor. The neck should also be assessed for a tracheal shift or jugular vein distention (JVD). These are classic signs of tension pneumothorax, but occur late in the physiologic process. JVD may not be present if there are other injuries present that have led to hypovolemia. Assess for neck tenderness.

FIGURE 1-17 Listen at the trachea to distinguish the origin of abnormal airway sounds.

The National Association of State EMS Officials currently recommend spinal motion restriction for children with neck pain, an inability to move the neck, focal neurologic deficit, altered mental status, high-risk mechanism (i.e., high-speed motor vehicle collision, diving), torso trauma, or a predisposing condition.

Chest

Reexamine the chest for penetrating injuries, lacerations, bruises, or rashes. If the child is injured, feel the **clavicles** and every rib for tenderness or deformity.

Back

Inspect the back for lacerations, penetrating injuries, bruises, or rashes.

Abdomen

Inspect the abdomen for any bruising, swelling, deformities, or rashes. Multiple bruises or bruises in different stages of healing on the chest or abdomen may be associated with inflicted injury. In the trauma patient, redness or bruising under the site of protective straps, or "seat belt sign," may be apparent. A "handlebar" mark may also be present if a child had contact with the handlebar of a bicycle during an accident. Both seat belt marks and handlebar injuries are associated with significant internal injuries. Also, inspect the abdomen for **distention**. Gently palpate the abdomen, and watch closely for guarding or tensing of the abdominal muscles, which may suggest infection, obstruction, or **intra-abdominal** injury. Note any tenderness or masses. If an infant or toddler has been crying for a prolonged period of time, or if a child's respiratory effort has been supported with a bag-mask device, this may also lead to abdominal distention because of air that has been pushed into the stomach.

Extremities

Assess for **symmetry**. Compare both sides for color, warmth, size of joints, and tenderness. Put each joint through a full range of motion while watching the eyes of the child for signs of pain; understandably, if there is obvious deformity of the extremity suggesting a fracture, this technique should not be used, and the extremity should be splinted. If there is a suspected fracture present, assess for a pulse, capillary refill, motor function, and sensation distal to the injury.

Fractures in nonambulatory children are suspicious for inflicted trauma.

Additional Vital Signs

Although pulse and respirations have been assessed in the primary assessment, they may or may not have been formally counted and recorded because of circumstances of resuscitation or brevity of transportation. It is important to obtain and record these vital signs to assess and monitor the child's changing condition. When resuscitation is necessary, pulse and respirations should be monitored frequently, but additional vital signs may be deferred until the child has stabilized or the transportation is completed.

Assessment of Pain

It is easy for the prehospital professional to ignore, underestimate, or misinterpret the signs and symptoms of pain in infants and young children. Children are much less likely to receive effective pain medications than adults. Studies have demonstrated reluctance by all levels of emergency care personnel to administer medications to children for control of pain and anxiety. The younger the child, the less likely the child will receive effective **analgesia** and **anxiolysis**. However, adult and pediatric experience has validated the effectiveness of analgesia in the prehospital setting to decrease pain, without causing respiratory depression or interference with the accuracy of physical assessment.

Pain is present with most types of injuries and with many illnesses. Inadequate treatment of pain has many adverse effects on the child and family. Pain itself causes significant morbidity and misery for the child and family or caregivers and interferes with the prehospital professional's accurate assessment of physiologic abnormalities. Children who do not receive appropriate analgesia are more likely to have exaggerated pain responses to subsequent painful procedures. Even neonates have demonstrable chronic changes in pain perception when they are subjected to painful

procedures without the benefit of analgesia. Posttraumatic stress is also more common among children who experience pain during acute illness and injury and do not receive pharmacologic relief. Hence, just as with adults, it is essential to carefully assess pain in all children and to consider effective methods to provide relief from suffering when appropriate.

Local EMS protocols now require that prehospital professionals assess and manage pain as a part of the secondary assessment. Indeed, evaluation of pain has become a new vital sign in all ages, including children. Appropriate pain management relieves distress of the child and family or caregivers and facilitates communication, physical assessment, and ease of transport.

Assessment of pain must take into consideration the developmental age of the patient. The ability to recognize pain improves as the age of the child increases. For example, in a preverbal infant, crying and agitation unrelieved by being held by the caregiver may be caused by hunger, hypoxia, or pain. In infants, further assessment is essential to identify sources of pain before administration of analgesia. In contrast, verbal children older than 3 years of age are usually quite vocal about pain. Therefore, in older children, pain scales using pictures of facial expressions (Wong-Baker FACES Scale) or **visual analogue scores (VAS)** may be helpful in assessing the need for pharmacologic relief of pain. **FIGURE 1-18** illustrates the Wong-Baker FACES Scale. Although such "self-report" scales have not yet been extensively used in the prehospital environment, they have been validated in other settings to provide an immediate evaluation of intensity of pain and to monitor response to treatment.

There is much overlap between the management of fear and anxiety and the management of pain in infants and young children. Many nonpharmacologic and pharmacologic methods relieve anxiety and reduce the perception of pain, as summarized in **TABLE 1-11**. Remaining calm and providing quiet, professional reassurance to caregivers and child are the first important steps. A calm caregiver helps to make the child calm and more at ease. Distraction techniques may be

0	2	4	6	8	10
NO HURT	HURTS LITTLE BIT	HURTS LITTLE MORE	HURTS EVEN MORE	HURTS WHOLE LOT	HURTS WORST

FIGURE 1-18 Wong-Baker FACES Pain Rating Scale for self-assessment of pain.

Wong-Baker FACES Foundation (2019). Wong-Baker FACES® Pain Rating Scale. Retrieved with permission from http://www.WongBakerFACES.org.

TABLE 1-11 Methods of Prehospital Analgesia and Anxiolysis
Nonpharmacologic
Calm manner
Caregiver assistance through presence or holding
Distraction techniques with "toolbox" of toys
Ice
Visual imagery
Pacifier
Music
Splinting of fractures
Pharmacologic
Morphine
Fentanyl
Midazolam
Ketamine
Nitrous oxide
Benzodiazepines
12%–25% sucrose for neonates
Acetaminophen
Ibuprofen (no ibuprofen for infants <6 months)

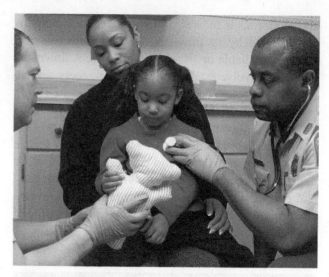

FIGURE 1-19 Use distraction techniques to help reduce the child's pain.

TIP

Pain is often considered an additional vital sign. Pain management can help relieve distress of the child and family, greatly facilitate communication and physical assessment, assist in timely provision of necessary interventions, and ease the transport process.

CONTROVERSY

Although "self-report" pain scales have not yet been extensively used for pediatric patients in the prehospital environment, they have been validated in other clinical settings. They can help provide an immediate evaluation of pain intensity, and they can aid in monitoring response to treatment.

extremely helpful in reducing pain. Many prehospital providers learn to use toys, "magic tricks," or engaging stories to provide distraction. Some EMS systems have developed a "toolbox" with distraction equipment to facilitate pain relief (**FIGURE 1-19**). Keeping the caregiver with the child and sometimes holding the child are also useful strategies.

In older children, visual imagery techniques can often be helpful. Ask the child where he or she would most prefer to be at the present time, then assist the child in closing his or her eyes and visualizing a more tranquil or enjoyable environment. Music is also a very effective distraction.

Pharmacologic methods for reducing pain are also a standard of prehospital care. **Opiates**, benzodiazepines, **ketamine**, and **nitrous oxide** are available to prehospital professionals in many EMS systems. **Intramuscular medications** are less effective because children fear needles, and the injection site pain may last for days. Analgesic and anxiolytic drugs may be easily delivered through inhalation techniques, by the **transmucosal** (e.g., sublingual, intranasal, and rectal) route, or by the **transdermal** route, although experience is still limited. Several techniques, such as inhaled nitrous oxide, intranasal fentanyl, inhaled midazolam, and rectal **diazepam**, have had excellent success in prehospital pediatric care. However, the fastest method for administration of analgesia and anxiolysis is by way of the intravenous route. Intravenous delivery provides the most effective and most controllable or **titratable** method. A downside is it does involve establishing vascular access, which, like the IM route, is usually painful. Also, the child's response to pain and anxiolytic medication is sometimes unpredictable and must be carefully weighed against unwanted side effects. Medications to reduce pain also cause sedation and can result in respiratory depression, bradycardia, **hypoxemia**, **hypotension**, and even loss of protective airway reflexes. Occasionally, anxiolytic drugs cause a paradoxical worsening of agitation.

TIP

Analgesic and anxiolytic drugs may be easily delivered through inhalation, transmucosal (e.g., intranasal, sublingual, rectal), or transdermal routes. Several techniques, such as inhaled nitrous oxide, intranasal fentanyl, intranasal midazolam, inhaled naloxone, and rectal diazepam, have had excellent success in prehospital pediatric care.

Assessment of pain has become a "vital sign," and management of pediatric pain and anxiety must be a routine part of field care in all EMS systems. This entails a thorough understanding of available non-pharmacologic techniques, medications, potential medication contraindications and complications, and management of those complications.

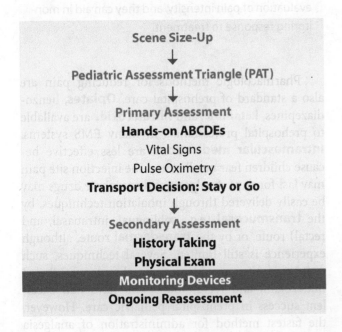

Additional Monitoring Devices

The prehospital professional can perform some types of specific testing in the field, such as rapid glucose determinations, point-of-care lactate, 12-lead electrocardiogram monitoring, waveform capnography, and other specialty testing available based on local protocols.

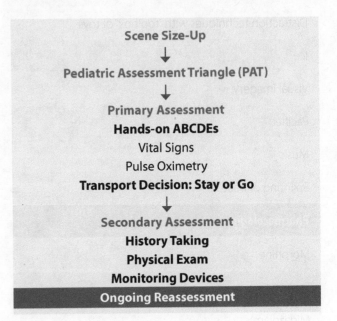

Ongoing Reassessment

Perform reassessment of all patients to gauge the response to treatment and to track the progression of identified physiologic and anatomic problems. New problems may also be identified on reassessment. Data from the reassessment will guide ongoing treatment. The elements in the reassessment are as follows:

1. The PAT
2. The ABCDEs with repeat vital signs
3. Assessment of positive anatomic findings
4. Review of the effectiveness and safety of treatment

The elements in the reassessment are also the basis for determination of an appropriate transport destination and for accurate, pediatric-specific radio or telephone communications with medical oversight or the ED.

Radio Reporting

Proper radio reporting promotes a seamless transfer of care from the prehospital to the ED setting, maximizing the ability of all clinicians to provide efficient and effective care. A good radio report transmits

CASE STUDY 3

You are called to the home of a 1-month-old boy who stopped breathing and turned blue, according to his babysitter. He reportedly had a fever all day. The infant is lying supine; his skin is pale and mottled. When touched, the infant becomes extremely irritable and exhibits a high-pitched, screeching cry. When left alone, he appears lethargic and poorly responsive. There is no abnormal positioning and no abnormal airway sounds, stridor, nasal flaring, or grunting. His color is pale. The respiratory rate is 60 breaths/min and unlabored. The heart rate is 200 beats/min. His peripheral pulses are weak and his extremities are cool to the touch. Capillary refill time is approximately 5 seconds.

1. Does this infant's appearance suggest a serious problem?
2. Is this infant in shock?

vital data completely and concisely, highlighting pediatric-specific information to allow the ED team to best prepare for the patient's arrival. If available, provide the ED a patient weight, as reported by the caregiver or as obtained by a length-based resuscitation tape. For a step-by-step explanation, see **Field Reporting, Procedure 1**.

Summary

After the primary assessment, and before beginning any necessary resuscitative efforts, the prehospital professional must determine the severity of the illness or injury and make a decision regarding mode and timing of transport. If additional evaluation is appropriate, perform a detailed history and secondary assessment either on scene or on the way to the ED. These additional phases of assessment are not indicated if there is an acute life-threatening or limb-threatening problem that requires the prehospital professional's ongoing attention. The secondary assessment is more for the detection of anatomic problems than for evaluation of physiologic abnormalities. Always perform reassessments to observe the patient's response to interventions and to guide changes in treatment, transport, and triage. Diagnostic testing refers to laboratory and radiographic evaluation to determine causation and mainly occurs after arrival in the ED and during hospitalization for admitted patients.

CASE STUDY ANSWERS

CASE STUDY 1

Beware of the pale child! Consider any child who has experienced significant trauma and is pale at the scene to have significant blood loss until proven otherwise. Children are able to compensate for blood loss and hypovolemia through catecholamine surges, which cause tachycardia and peripheral vasoconstriction. These reflexes inhibit the circulation to the skin and result in a pale patient. Although this child could have had a significant head injury based on mechanism of injury, his level of consciousness is normal; therefore, the initial issue needing emergent attention is hemorrhagic shock. Abdominal injuries with blunt trauma to the liver or spleen can result in significant internal bleeding without external signs of injury. Many children with internal bleeding do not always have abdominal tenderness. Indicators of suspected hemorrhagic shock are tachycardia, weak pulses, and delayed capillary refill, and a late sign is a decrease in the blood pressure (80 mm Hg/palp). This child requires timely transport to a trauma center with pediatric capabilities. Delay vascular access until the child is en route to the hospital.

This child is also clearly in pain. However, weigh the benefits of pharmacologic therapy to relieve pain against the potential for circulatory collapse, delay in transport, and the need to effectively assess appearance. Use opiate analgesics, such as morphine, in patients with suspected compensated hemorrhagic shock cautiously because of morphine's vasodilatory effect.

CASE STUDY 2

The PAT is an accurate tool to evaluate severity of illness or injury and to determine the urgency for providing lifesaving care. Upon arrival at the scene of this patient, it is quite reassuring to find the toddler alert, pink, and with nonlabored respirations. His vigorous responses make it difficult to perform the conventional ABCDE assessment. Because this child clearly has no serious immediate cardiorespiratory problems, is alert and awake, and fights your examination, history taking and secondary assessment can occur. However, the prehospital professional should transport every infant or child who has had a submersion injury to a hospital for observation of progression of symptoms. Still, the findings on the PAT allow the prehospital professional to slow the pace and get more information while on the scene. There is no need for immediate resuscitative interventions, and the prehospital professional can avoid the risk of "lights and siren" transport.

Any time there is an unwitnessed submersion event, consider that a traumatic injury may be present. The usual mechanism of a toddler pool drowning involves falling less than 3 ft (1 m) into a body of water. In this scenario, it is unlikely that he has sustained a significant head or spinal injury. Furthermore, if he is moving his neck without apparent discomfort while in his mother's arms, but then vigorously screams and fights when you attempt to examine him, it is unlikely that spinal motion restriction will be helpful (and may prove more harmful and distressing than not). Local protocols govern this decision. Although treatment and transport of this patient are not emergent, ongoing assessment during transport is necessary. Pulmonary complications of submersion, primarily hypoxia, may have a delayed presentation.

CASE STUDY 3

Any infant who has a brief resolved unexplained event, who reportedly stopped breathing or turned blue, deserves EMS transport, regardless of his or her appearance on your arrival. In this case, the need for urgent treatment and transport is obvious. One of the PAT indicators of shock in this infant is altered appearance. Although that finding could be due to causes other than poor brain perfusion (e.g., infection, trauma, toxins, hypoxia), the presence of effortless tachypnea and pale, mottled skin supports the diagnosis of shock. Alternating lethargy and irritability may progress to unresponsiveness as perfusion worsens.

The hands-on examination confirms the suspicion of shock. This patient's heart rate is rapid at 200 beats/min, with weak peripheral pulses, cool extremities, and delayed capillary refill. Even without a blood pressure, the abnormal appearance and skin findings suggest that he should be treated for hypotensive shock. Although the cause of shock is unknown, treatment of any type of hypotensive shock includes vascular access and 20-mL/kg boluses of crystalloid fluid. Make one attempt at vascular access on scene and then rapidly transport this patient to definitive care. Reassess his response to therapy frequently en route.

SUGGESTED REFERENCES

Textbooks

Aehlert B. *Mosby's Comprehensive Pediatric Emergency Care*. Sudbury, MA: Elsevier; 2006.

American Academy of Orthopaedic Surgeons. *Emergency Care and Transportation of the Sick and Injured*. 11th ed. Burlington, MA: Jones & Bartlett Learning; 2016.

American Academy of Pediatrics and the American College of Emergency Physicians. *APLS: The Pediatric Emergency Medicine Resource*. 5th ed. Burlington, MA: Jones & Bartlett Learning; 2012.

Anne M, Agur A, Dalley A. *Grant's Atlas of Anatomy*. 11th ed. Philadelphia, PA: Lippincott Williams & Wilkins; 2004.

Bledsoe B, Porter R, Cherry R. *Paramedic Care: Principles & Practice*. 5th ed. London, UK: Pearson, 2017.

Chameides L, Samson RA, Schexnayder SM, Hazinski MF. *PALS Provider Manual*. American Heart Association; 2011.

Zitelli and Davis' Atlas of Pediatric Physical Diagnosis, 7th ed. Zitelli B, McIntire S, Nowalk AJ, ed. Philadelphia: Elsevier Saunders 2017.

Articles

American Academy of Pediatrics. Emergency information forms and emergency preparedness for children with special health care needs (policy statement). *Pediatrics*. 2010;125:829–837.

Fernandez A, Ares MI, Gasrcia S, Martinez-Indart L. The validity of the pediatric assessment triangle as the first step in the triage process in a pediatric emergency department. *Pediatr Emerg Care*. 2017;33(4):234–238.

Fernandez A, Benito J, Minegi S. Is this child sick? Usefulness of the Pediatric Assessment Triangle in emergency settings. *J Pediatr*. 2017;93(Suppl 1): 60–67.

Fleming S, Gill PJ, Van den Bruel A, Thompson M. Capillary refill time in sick children: a clinical guide for general practice. *Br J Gen Pract*. 2016;66(652):587.

Fuchs S, Terry M, Adelgais K, et al. Definitions and assessment approaches for emergency medical services for children. *Pediatrics*. 2016:138(6);e20161073.

Gausche M. Out-of-hospital care of pediatric patients. *Pediatr Clin North Am*. 1999;46(6):1305–1327.

Hoffmann F, Schmalhofer M, Jehner M, Zimatschek S, Grote V, Reiter K. Comparison of the AVPU scale and the Pediatric GCS in prehospital setting. *Prehosp Emerg Care*. 2016;20(4):493–498.

Proehl JA. Initial assessment and resuscitation. In: Hoyt KS, Selfridge-Thomas J, eds. *Emergency Nursing Core Curriculum*. 6th ed. St. Louis, MO: Saunders Elsevier; 2007:125.

Thompson DO, Hurtado TR, Liao MM, Byyny RL, Gravitz C, Haukoos JS. Validation of the Simplified Motor Score in the out-of-hospital setting for the prediction of outcomes after traumatic brain injury. *Ann Emerg Med*. 2011;58:417–425.

Warren J. Guidelines for the inter- and intrahospital transport of critically ill patients. *Crit Care Med*. 2004;32(1):256–262.

Other Resources

United States Department of Transportation, National Highway Traffic Safety Administration. National EMS Education Standards (2009). https://www.ems.gov/pdf/811077a.pdf. Accessed October 13, 2019.

© Ralph125/E+/Getty Images.

CHAPTER 2

Using a Developmental Approach

David LaCovey, BS, EMT-P

Sylvia Owusu-Ansah, MD, MPH, FAAP

LEARNING OBJECTIVES

1. Discuss the communication challenges in handling the emotional responses of a family with a child who is ill or injured.

2. List the expected changes in vital signs with advancing age.

3. Describe key growth and development characteristics for the following groups: infants, toddlers, preschoolers, school-aged children, adolescents, and children with special health care needs.

4. Explain unique anatomic and physiologic characteristics that influence assessment of children in each group.

Introduction

Infants and children constitute a small percentage of all patients seen in an emergency medical services (EMS) system. An even smaller percentage require advanced life support (ALS). EMS providers must become comfortable with pediatric-specific information to promote success while interacting with this special patient population. Because of the unique anatomic, physiologic, and developmental differences in children, EMS

CASE STUDY 1

You receive a 9-1-1 call about a fussy infant. On your arrival, a crying mother meets you at the door with her 2-week-old daughter in her arms. The infant is crying inconsolably. She has no retractions, but her skin is mottled on both the trunk and the extremities. Her arms and legs are cool. The mother tells you that the baby has been fussy all day and vomiting all her feedings, and the mother thinks her stomach looks big.

1. What are the steps to assess and treat this child, and how will you address the mother's concerns?

2. What are the worrisome findings in this infant?

providers must be well versed in normal developmental changes in infants and children. To successfully complete a pediatric patient assessment, the provider must be able to incorporate an understanding of how a child's physical growth and psychosocial development relate to his or her condition.

In addition to knowing the growth and developmental characteristics of the different age groups, the prehospital professional must be aware of special considerations when assessing a child with special health care needs (CSHCN). Sometimes the chronologic age of the CSHCN does not correspond with his or her developmental stage, and physical growth may not reflect emotional maturity.

Caring for a child also includes caring for the family. Caregivers, friends, and siblings may be present, in addition to parents. Each person may have a different response to the child who is ill or injured, and the prehospital professional must be prepared to care for the entire "extended" family of friends and relatives. Communication skills are often as important as assessment and treatment skills in establishing an atmosphere of trust and comfort. Creating such an atmosphere requires that the prehospital provider have a confident and professional attitude toward children's care and use age-appropriate pediatric skills. Communication skills become especially important in the event of a mass-casualty incident or natural disaster (see Chapter 14).

This chapter addresses age-specific growth characteristics and assessment techniques for physiologically stable children from infancy to adolescence, and for CSHCN. Chapter 1 addresses general assessment techniques for the acutely ill or injured child, and Chapter 10 expands the discussion on CSHCN.

Pediatric Calls and Response From Family and Providers

Every family responds differently when a child is ill (**FIGURE 2-1**). Having an ill child places immense pressure on the family unit. Common responses are reviewed in **TABLE 2-1**. Although some caregivers'

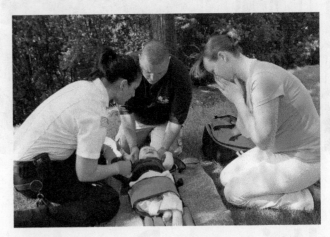

FIGURE 2-1 Every family responds differently to a child's illness or injury.
© Jones & Bartlett Learning. Courtesy of Glen Ellman.

TABLE 2-1 Common Responses of Caregivers to Acute Illness or Injury in a Child	
Response	**Description**
Disbelief	Caregivers may be struggling with a child's illness or injury. They may seem too calm or unconcerned.
Guilt	Caregivers may be horrified that they were unable to recognize the serious nature of their child's condition or that they were unable to prevent an injury. They may focus their attention on what should have been done, rather than on the child's immediate situation.
Anger	Caregivers may show their concern as anger, and they may direct their anger at the prehospital professional. Caregivers may become hostile when the prehospital professional makes efforts to stabilize their child. They may attempt to refuse transport.
Physical symptoms	Caregivers may have tachycardia, nausea, headache, chest pain, sweaty palms, dry mouth, or hyperventilation.

TIP

A family's response to a child's illness or injury is influenced by the child's developmental level, previous experience with the medical system, coping strategies, culture, availability of support systems, and nature of the emergency.

responses may seem too emotional or illogical, listen to their concerns. Acting as an advocate for proper care allows the EMS provider to best approach the pediatric patient. Caregivers usually know the patient best and can provide vital information that allows the EMS interaction to be successful. Children, even infants, can quickly sense emotions in adults.

EMS providers, similar to family members, may respond emotionally to a pediatric patient. EMS providers may also experience any of the emotional responses as outlined in Table 2-1. Acting in a calm, professional manner gains trust from the family or caregivers and also helps the EMS crew to establish control of a potentially emotional situation. This approach also allows the providers to gain as much valuable information as possible from the family or caregivers, which ultimately helps triage the patient to the correct emergency department or include the most accurate differential diagnosis as part of the patient assessment.

The best way to reduce provider stress related to patient interactions is to remain current with pediatric patient assessment and treatment standards. Being familiar with the currently stocked pediatric equipment and medications, as well as their locations, can also decrease stress while interacting with an ill child. Because of the limited number of pediatric calls, being well versed with the pediatric devices on an EMS unit becomes increasingly important.

Often, providers feel guilt after interacting with a sick infant or child. It is common for providers to think about the pediatric situation after the call. Depending on the situation, a single patient interaction can cause reflection for days, weeks, or months.

> **TIP**
>
> Any provider can experience difficult emotions after a stressful pediatric call. EMS providers should seek professional help from a licensed mental health professional when unresolved stress results from these interactions.

Communication With the Child and Family or Caregiver

To effectively approach infants and children, EMS providers should account for developmental information as it relates to the patient assessment at hand. Similar to interaction with adults, each pediatric patient is unique with a distinct personality that can impact the EMS provider's ability to obtain pertinent assessment information. Calling 9-1-1 is often a stressful situation for the patient and family. Approaching the patient gently and at his or her eye level is important to initiating communication with the child. The best policy is to be honest with a child because distrust can interfere with effectively finding important information about the situation at hand. Observing the patient's behavior can provide clues to age-specific actions. It may also be possible to notice nonverbal clues that providers can pick up from across the room as they approach the patient.

In addition to communication with the pediatric patient, communication with the caregiver or family is also important. Children seek clues from their parents regarding safety. Infants and children are never a single-patient EMS call. The family and caregivers must be treated as therapeutic allies in the situation because their involvement can provide necessary information to properly handle the situation. Whenever possible, the pediatric patient and family or caregiver should be kept together. A successful pediatric patient interaction includes information gathering from family and primary caregivers. Effective communication is the cornerstone of effective prehospital care.

> **TIP**
>
> Communication skills are often as important as assessment and treatment skills.

Vital Signs Through the Ages

A common challenge in evaluating infants and children is determining when vital signs are normal based on the age of the patient. Respiratory rate, heart rate, blood pressure, and temperature all change with age. The presence or absence of fever, anxiety, or pain and the child's activity level also affect vital signs. In ill or injured children, the prehospital professional must distinguish the impact of these outside influences on vital signs from changes caused by pathologic processes. Chapter 1 presents key physical characteristics and assessment techniques that assist the prehospital professional in separating a "sick" child from a "not sick" child.

Respiratory Rate

Although normal values for vital signs vary with age, there are a variety of physiologic or anatomic bases for these changes. The normal range of respiratory rate slows with age because of an increase in the number of **alveoli** and increasing lung volume and lung compliance with physical growth. **TABLE 2-2** lists the normal respiratory rate for age.

At times, there is a problem with accurate counting of the rate, especially if the count is done in a 15-second interval. In infants, observe and count **abdominal excursions** (belly breathing) for 30 seconds to obtain an accurate respiratory rate. As a child grows, breathing becomes less dependent on abdominal muscles and the diaphragm and more dependent on the chest muscles. Observing **thoracic excursions** (movement of the chest wall) for 15–30 seconds provides an accurate respiratory rate in an older child. Use

TABLE 2-2 Normal Respiratory Rate for Age

Age	Respiratory Rate (breaths/min)
Infant (birth–12 mo)	30–60
Toddler (1–3 yr)	24–40
Preschooler (3–5 yr)	22–34
School-aged child (6–12 yr)	18–30
Adolescent (13–18 yr)	12–16

TABLE 2-3 Normal Heart Rates for Age

Age	Heart Rate (beats/min)
Infant (birth–12 mo)	100–160
Toddler (1–3 yr)	90–150
Preschooler (3–5 yr)	80–140
School-aged child (6–12 yr)	70–120
Adolescent (13–18 yr)	60–100

FIGURE 2-2 Electrocardiogram (ECG) of a sinus arrhythmia.

Arrhythmia Recognition: The Art of Interpretation, courtesy of Tomas B. Garcia, MD.

> **TIP**
>
> In infants, observe abdominal excursions and count rate for 30–60 seconds to obtain an accurate respiratory rate.

of accessory muscles to breathe, such as intercostal and subcostal muscles, is never normal when examining a child for normal respirations.

Heart Rate

The baseline heart rate of infants and children slows with age, reflecting increasing control of the heart rate by the **vagus nerve**. The vagus nerve transmits **cholinergic impulses**, which slow the beating of the heart. **TABLE 2-3** lists normal heart rates for age. In addition, by 2 years of age, a **circadian rhythm** in heart rate is present, seen in a fall of 10–20 beats/min, while the child is asleep. One confusing factor in

assessing a child's heart rate during different phases of the sleep-wake cycle, or during different phases of respiration, is that the child's rhythm is more irregular than an adult's. This **sinus arrhythmia** is more prominent in toddlers to school-aged children and is caused by immature vagus nerve control (**FIGURE 2-2**).

Blood Pressure

A child's **blood pressure** increases with age (**TABLE 2-4** lists minimum systolic blood pressure values for age). A quick formula for the minimum systolic blood pressure is 70 + (2 × age in years). The measured blood pressure is affected by equipment size. A cuff that is too small gives falsely elevated readings, whereas one that is too large gives readings that are too low. If **diastolic pressure** cannot be **auscultated**, obtain a systolic pressure by palpating the pulse. This value is approximately 10 mm Hg lower than an auscultated pressure because of the relative insensitivity of **palpation** in appreciating initial pulsations as the cuff is deflated.

TABLE 2-4 Minimal Systolic Blood Pressure Values for Age

Age	Minimal Systolic Blood Pressure (mm Hg)
Newborn (birth–1 mo)	>60
Infant (1–12 mo)	>65
Toddler (1–3 yr)	>70
Preschooler (3–5 yr)	>75
School-aged child (6–12 yr)	>80
Adolescent (13–18 yr)	>90

Temperature

Body temperature also varies with age and site of measurement. Newborn temperatures are often higher than those of older children, averaging 37.5°C (99.5°F) during the first 6 months of life. After 3 years of age, the temperature falls to below 37.2°C (99°F), and finally to 36.7°C (98°F) by 11 years of age. There is also a circadian rhythm to body temperature that develops by 5 years of age. This results in a lower temperature at night and a higher temperature during the day. In infants, when a recorded temperature is important to the assessment and the child is stable, ask the caregiver to obtain a rectal temperature. A rectal temperature is the accepted standard. A **tympanic temperature** may be acceptable in older children (>1 year), but may not be accurate based on the technique of the caregiver. Temperature may also be obtained with temporal artery thermometers. These devices use infrared technology to measure temperature in the superficial temporal artery. If obtained with good technique, these are quite accurate. An **axillary temperature** is approximately 1°C (2°F) lower than the rectal temperature. Normal body temperature decreases with increasing distance from the central circulation.

Growth Rates

Physical growth of infants and children includes body (somatic) growth and organ system growth. Skeletal and muscular growth has two spurts, the first from birth to 4 years of age and the second in adolescence (ages 9–14 for girls, ages 10–16 for boys). Brain, spinal cord, and nerve growth occurs maximally in the first few years of life and reaches adult proportions by 10 years of age.

The presence or absence of key secondary sex characteristics, especially pubic hair, marks a physiologic turning point for children. Genital growth begins about 8 years of age in girls and 9 years of age in boys, but there is significant variation. When children have visible pubic hair, they have usually attained adult physiology.

Anatomic Changes

Neck and Airway

The neck is short in infancy and elongates during childhood because of vertebral growth. As this occurs, anatomic landmarks also change in shape, size, and location. The **epiglottis** changes from a U-shape to the longer and thinner adult structure (**FIGURE 2-3**). It also moves in location from the level of the C1 vertebra to the C3 vertebra as the child's height increases. At birth, the **larynx** is only one-third the adult size. It becomes wider and longer until 3 years of age and undergoes another growth spurt during puberty. At birth, the **trachea** is one-third the adult length and increases 300% in circumference by puberty.

Chest and Lungs

At birth, the chest wall is round (anteroposterior, or AP, diameter equals lateral diameter). As the infant grows, it flattens out (lateral growth exceeds AP growth). Because an infant's chest wall is thin, heart and lung sounds are transmitted throughout the chest. Breath sounds are often audible on inspiration and expiration (**bronchovesicular**). In addition, secretions present anywhere in the respiratory tract are often heard throughout the chest. In an infant, respirations are mainly abdominal because of the greater role of the **diaphragm** in breathing mechanics. By 6 years of age, breathing becomes more thoracic in origin because of the development of chest wall musculature.

The lung tissue itself also changes with age. At birth, an infant has only 8% of the adult number of alveoli. The number of alveoli increases until 8 years of age, after which they increase in size but not number.

Heart

At birth, the right **ventricle** is the same size as the left ventricle, a function of the demands of fetal circulation. This accounts for right axis deviation seen on **electrocardiograms (ECGs)** in infants. However, the

U-shaped
and more
floppy epiglottis

More anterior
and higher
airway

Smaller diameter
more flexible

Tongue

Narrowest

Vocal cords

Cricoid ring

Trachea

Longer
epiglottis

Narrowest

Tongue

FIGURE 2-3 Differences between the child and adult airways.

left ventricle quickly grows in size and muscle mass and greatly outsizes the right ventricle with age. The left ventricle reaches adult proportions of 2:1 by 1 year of age.

Abdomen

A newborn infant has a protuberant abdomen for numerous reasons: The liver is relatively large, the stomach is more horizontal, and the lungs expand downward with a movement of the diaphragm. There is also less coverage of the abdominal solid organs (liver and spleen) by mature abdominal muscles. The stomach capacity increases from 30–90 mL at birth, to 210–360 mL by 1 year of age, and 500 mL by 2 years of age. It assumes a more vertical position and reaches an adult volume of 750–900 mL during childhood. The abdomen also seems protuberant in toddlers because of a normal lumbar **lordosis** (curvature) of the spine. The abdomen becomes more **scaphoid** (flat) in school-aged children.

Musculoskeletal System

In infants and young children, new longitudinal bone growth occurs in secondary centers of **ossification** at the end of the long bones, in **vertebral bodies**, and

the **cranium (physeal plates)**. These **cartilaginous growth plates** are relatively weak and are vulnerable to fractures exclusive to childhood. Bone growth ends with the ossification of the growth cartilage and union of the **epiphysis** and **diaphysis**. Growth in children is asymmetric, with the lower extremities, especially the **distal extremities** (e.g., feet), growing before puberty and the trunk during puberty.

Muscle growth includes an increase in the size of muscle cells. There is a growth spurt in the number of muscle cells at 2 years of age, with a maximal increase during puberty. The proportion of muscle mass to body weight changes during childhood, going from 1:5 at birth to 1:3 in adolescence.

Nervous System

The growth of the nervous system occurs rapidly during infancy. It is 25% the adult size at birth, 50% by 1 year of age, 80% by 3 years of age, and 90% by 7 years of age. This includes the growth of **glial cells**, **dendrites**, and **synaptic connections**. This growth is associated with a rapid increase in fine motor, gross motor, and language skills of infants and toddlers. These changing competencies impact the type of assessment techniques appropriate for evaluating children of different ages.

Summary of Changes in Vital Signs and Anatomy Through Childhood

Vital signs are useful for assessment but are sometimes difficult to obtain and difficult to interpret. Not only do normal vital signs change significantly with age, but respiratory and heart rates are especially sensitive to **adrenaline** release because of fear, pain, anxiety, cold, or high activity level. Other anatomic changes in the airway, chest, heart, abdomen, musculoskeletal system, and nervous system occur throughout childhood and require adaptations in assessment techniques.

Infants

Developmental Characteristics

Neonates range in age from birth to 28 days. They do not elicit interactive behavior, and therefore communicate predominantly by crying, though they are able to recognize their mother's voice. Neonates are physiologically immunodeficient. Infants are ages 1 month to 12 months, and their development varies dramatically by age in months. Infants are vulnerable and have a limited number of behaviors (**FIGURE 2-4**). Infants younger than 2 months spend most of their time sleeping or eating. They are not yet able to tell the difference between parents and other caregivers or strangers. They need to be kept warm, dry, and fed. They experience the world through their bodies. Being held, cuddled, or rocked soothes the infant. Hearing is also well developed at birth, and calm and reassuring talk is often helpful.

FIGURE 2-4 Infants are vulnerable, with a limited number of behaviors.
© Ascent/PKS Media Inc./Stockbyte/Getty Images.

Infants between 2 and 6 months of age are more active, which makes them easier to evaluate. They spend more time awake, they begin to make eye contact, and they recognize caregivers. Healthy infants in this age group have a strong suck, active extremity movement, and a vigorous cry. They may follow a bright light or toy with their eyes or turn their heads toward a loud sound or the caregiver's voice.

Between the ages of 6 and 12 months, most infants learn to talk or babble, sit unsupported, reach for toys, move objects from one hand to another, and put things in their mouths. At approximately 1 year of age, most infants start to scoot or crawl, pull themselves to a standing position, "cruise" furniture, and possibly start to walk.

At 7–8 months, infants show a clear preference for their parents or caregivers, and by the age of 9–10 months demonstrate stranger anxiety, making separation of the child and caregiver for the purposes of assessment or transport especially problematic. They are most easily comforted by their parent or by a familiar adult. **TABLE 2-5** summarizes anatomic and physiologic differences that are important in the assessment and care of the infant.

TABLE 2-5 Anatomic and Physiologic Features of Infants

- Infants are nose breathers for the first several months of life. Obstruction of the nose from secretions, blood, or edema may cause respiratory distress.

- The muscles of the infant's chest wall are not yet developed, and the abdominal muscles are the main muscles used for breathing. "Belly breathing" is normal in infants and may become exaggerated as breathing becomes more rapid.

- Retractions are easily seen in the infant with respiratory distress.

- A faster metabolic rate increases the need for oxygen and nutrients.

- Because of immature temperature regulation and high body surface-to-mass ratio, infants are at risk for heat loss and hypothermia if left undressed.

- The head is large in proportion to the body (**FIGURE 2-5**) and may be a potential source of significant heat loss.

The infant's capacity to interact with the environment is limited, and signs and symptoms of illness are not always easy to appreciate. Because of these factors, always take the caregiver's perception that "something is wrong" seriously. *A neonate or infant in the first 3 months of life who is reported to be fussier than usual, feeding poorly, or sleeping excessively, or who has a temperature greater than 38°C (100.4°F), must be seen by a physician.* It is important to find out if there has been a recent history of trauma, how the infant was acting before the event, and if the infant has been healthy since birth. Find out if the infant was born at term and if there were any problems during pregnancy, labor, delivery, or immediately after the birth.

In the first few months of life, excessive irritability or sleeping, fever, and poor feeding may be symptoms of a very serious illness, such as **sepsis** or **congenital heart disease**. **Apnea** is a common chief complaint in the infant. Periods of apnea may be a sign of infection; heart disease; seizure activity; head injury; or a metabolic problem, such as **hypoglycemia**. As the infant grows older and the behavioral repertoire expands, making the "sick" versus "not sick" decision potentially easier.

Common Conditions in Infants

- Viral syndromes (vomiting and diarrhea)
- Respiratory problems
- Fever
- Ear infections
- Sudden unexpected infant death syndrome (SUIDS)
- Child maltreatment

Assessment of the Infant

Conduct the assessment of the infant using the following principles:

- Obtain the name of the patient, and use it while interacting with him or her.
- Obtain the normal disposition of the patient, and compare it to the current behavior being displayed. Any acute change in disposition should

FIGURE 2-5 The infant's head is disproportionately large compared to older children and adults. The head may be a source of significant heat loss.

be noted and relayed during the transfer-of-care report. Communicate with the infant using a confident but smiling face directed at him or her.

- Have the caregiver hold the infant while the EMS provider completes the assessment. Unless the infant requires a lifesaving intervention, the infant is better assessed in the arms of someone with whom he or she is familiar.
- Observe, auscultate, and palpate, in that order, to get the most information with the least amount of stress to the infant (**FIGURE 2-6**).
- Approach the infant slowly and calmly, because loud voices and quick movements may frighten him or her.
- Squat down or sit at "baby level."
- Observe the interaction of the infant with the caregiver. At 7–8 months, infants may begin to show stranger anxiety.
- A comfortable environment is important. An infant who is happily snuggled in a caregiver's arms

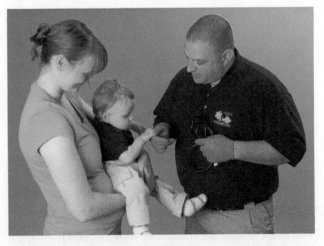

FIGURE 2-6 Approaching an infant: Observe the infant in the caregiver's arms before palpating or auscultating.

may become fussy and cry when unwrapped and placed on cold sheets.

- If the infant begins to cry, a pacifier, blanket, or favorite toy may help to calm him or her. Avoid feeding the infant who is seriously ill or injured.
- Perform the assessment based on the infant's activity level. For example, if the infant is calm, get the respiratory rate and auscultate lung sounds at the beginning of the assessment.
- Make nonthreatening physical contact first, such as touching an extremity to assess warmth and capillary refill. Perform the most upsetting parts of the examination last.
- Use a warmed stethoscope and warm hands and handle the infant gently. Avoid doing anything potentially painful or distressing until near completion of the assessment. It is difficult to assess heart and lung sounds or to palpate the abdomen when the infant is crying.
- Consider offering the infant a toy as a distraction.
- In the older infant who may have stranger anxiety, have the caregiver remove the baby's clothing. Remove one item of clothing at a time, and then replace it, if possible, to avoid heat loss and hypothermia.

CAUTION

The older infant is fearful of separation and develops stranger anxiety. Approach slowly and assess the infant while he or she is being held by the caregiver.

Toddlers

Developmental Characteristics

Toddlers (ages 1–3 years) experience rapid changes in growth and development. Developmentally, it is a critical time in brain development and learned behaviors. By approximately 18 months of age, the toddlers are able to run, feed themselves, play with toys, and communicate with others. They begin making their own decisions and asserting their independence. The "terrible two" stage actually begins at about 1 year of age and often lasts into the third year. Toddlers are mobile and opinionated and may be terrified of strangers. They are illogical by nature and are intensely curious, but lack a sense of danger. Problem-solving is concrete because toddlers cannot reason abstractly. Learning is done by trial and error, with little anticipation of consequences. Toddlers are playful, magical thinkers and are tremendously self-centered. They understand ownership and label things (e.g., toys) as "mine."

Language capabilities vary widely. Some toddlers utter only single words, whereas others may speak in paragraphs. They often understand what is being said, even if they cannot respond with words. Older toddlers may remember earlier experiences with doctors or nurses, such as vaccinations or stitches, and be fearful about being examined.

The toddler's anatomy and physiology are much like the infant's, notably a large head and use of abdominal muscles to breathe. **Thermoregulation** is better, and limb muscles are more developed.

Common Ailments in Toddlers

- Viral syndromes (vomiting and diarrhea)
- Respiratory problems
- Febrile seizures
- Ear infections
- Child maltreatment
- Unintentional ingestions
- Open wounds

CAUTION

Do not separate the older infant or toddler from the caregiver.

CASE STUDY 2

You respond to a call for a 2-year-old who is having respiratory difficulty. On your arrival, you hear a barking cough from the child's room. When you enter, the child is sitting up in bed; he starts to cry and hides behind his mother. With crying, his breathing becomes noisier, and he becomes more anxious. Even though he has pajamas on, you can see **suprasternal retractions**. His skin is pink. His mother states he was fine today, but suddenly woke up during the night "gasping for air."

1. Is this appropriate behavior for this child?
2. How can you assess this child without making him more upset?

Assessment of the Toddler

Conduct the assessment of the toddler using the following principles:

- Obtain the name of the patient, and use it while interacting with him or her.
- Obtain the normal disposition of the patient, and compare it to the current behavior being displayed. Any acute change in disposition should be noted and relayed during the transfer-of-care report.
- Approach the toddler slowly, and keep physical contact to a minimum until he or she is familiar with you. Watch the toddler's activity level and behavior as you approach.
- Communicate with the toddler using a confident but friendly tone of voice.
- Sit or squat, and use a quiet, soothing voice. Allow the toddler to remain on the caregiver's lap.
- Use play and distraction tools, such as a penlight or teddy bear, to help with the assessment (**FIGURE 2-7**). Introduce equipment slowly, and encourage the toddler to hold it.
- Talk to the toddler, preferably about himself or herself. Admire his or her clothes; ask about pets or recent events. A toddler is the center of his or her universe.
- Give the toddler limited choices, such as "Do you want me to listen to your belly or your heart first?" This provides the toddler with a sense of control.
- Avoid questions that the toddler can answer with "no."
- Use simple, concrete terms. Provide a lot of reassurance and praise.
- Perform the most critical parts of the assessment first, working from toe to head, with the head and neck last.

- Ask for caregiver assistance with the assessment. The toddler is often less upset if the caregiver removes the toddler's clothes or administers oxygen.
- If necessary, ask the caregiver to gently palpate the toddler's extremity to test for pain.
- Do not expect toddlers to sit still and cooperate. Be flexible, but thorough.
- In certain situations, the toddler may be extremely difficult to examine. If he or she is alert but resists the examination, determine the need for transport based on history. Use of lights and sirens during transport may increase the toddler's level of fear.

Preschoolers

Developmental Characteristics

Preschoolers (ages 3–5 years) are creative, illogical, and literal thinkers (**FIGURE 2-8**). They are not always able to distinguish between fantasy and reality, and they have many misconceptions about illness, injury, and bodily functions. For example, a preschooler might think of a cut as "my insides leaking out." If you tell a preschooler you are going to take his or her pulse, they may ask, "Where are you going to take it and will I get it back?" Common fears for this age group include body mutilation, loss of control, death, darkness, and being left alone. Attention span is short. It is always best to maintain honesty about painful procedures. Information should be told as close to the procedure as possible to avoid miscommunication and increased anxiety. Preschool patients can be easily distracted by caregivers or friendly EMS providers. Positively rewarding these patients can help them maintain a good memory about interacting with EMS.

FIGURE 2-7 Approaching a toddler: Offer a toy or distraction tool to help with the assessment.

FIGURE 2-8 Preschoolers are creative and illogical thinkers.

Common Ailments in Preschoolers

- Unintentional ingestions
- Respiratory problems
- Febrile seizures
- Viral syndromes (vomiting and diarrhea)
- Open wounds
- Child maltreatment

> **TIP**
>
> Preschoolers are creative thinkers who fear the loss of control. Explain procedures in simple terms, allow them to handle equipment, and assess from toe to head.

Assessment of the Preschooler

Conduct the assessment of the preschooler using the following principles:

- Obtain the name of the patient, and use it while interacting with him or her.
- Obtain the normal disposition of the patient, and compare it to the current behavior being displayed. Any acute change in disposition should be noted and relayed during the transfer-of-care report.
- Use simple terms to explain procedures.
- Choose words carefully, using language that is age-appropriate and that does not induce fear.
- Clarify any apparent misconceptions.
- Use dolls or puppets, if available, to explain what you are doing.
- When appropriate, allow the child to handle equipment (**FIGURE 2-9**). Allow the patient to help.
- Set limits on behavior—for example, "You can cry or scream, but don't bite or kick."

- Praise good behavior.
- Use games or distraction tools.
- Use dressings or bandages freely.
- Focus on and carry out one thing at a time.

School-Aged Children

Development Characteristics

School-aged children are talkative, analytical, and able to understand the concept of cause and effect (**FIGURE 2-10**). They feel a sense of accomplishment as they acquire new skills. Their knowledge of how bodies work may be sketchy, and they have limited ability to gauge the seriousness of a particular illness or injury. With a careful choice of words, they can understand simple explanations about their bodies, and they like to be involved in their own care.

Common fears include separation from parents and friends, loss of control, pain, and physical disability. They are often afraid to talk about their feelings and may be unable to put their feelings into words. As they become more mobile and more independent, they begin to take more risks. They live in the present. Belonging and peer group support are important.

The anatomy and physiology of a child are similar to an adult's by about 8 years of age.

Common Conditions in School-Aged Children

- Poisonings/ingestion
- Respiratory problems
- Fractures (e.g., sports injuries)
- Open wounds
- Viral syndromes (vomiting and diarrhea)

FIGURE 2-9 When approaching a preschooler, allow the child to handle the equipment.

FIGURE 2-10 School-aged children are talkative, analytical, and able to understand the concept of cause and effect.
© Hero Images/Getty Images.

Assessment of the School-Aged Child

Conduct the assessment of the school-aged child using the following principles:

- Obtain the name of the patient, and use it while interacting with him or her.
- Obtain the normal disposition of the patient, and compare it to the current behavior being displayed. Any acute change in disposition should be noted and relayed during the transfer-of-care report.
- Speak directly to the child, and then include the caregiver. Be careful not to offer too much information.
- Anticipate the child's questions and fears, and discuss them immediately.
- Explain in simple terms what is wrong and how it will affect them. For example, when speaking to a 5-year-old, you may explain, "Your arm bone is broken, but the doctor will be able to fix it good as new. We'll give you some medicine in your arm to help stop it from hurting so much."
- Explain procedures immediately before doing them. Never lie to a child, telling the child that something will not hurt or that you are almost finished if this is not true. Remember that the child may not ask questions, even if he or she has real concerns.
- Ask the older school-aged child if he or she would like to have the caregiver present.
- Provide privacy. Children in this age group are modest. Expose the child for physical assessment as necessary, and cover him or her up when done.
- If physical restraint is necessary to complete a procedure or to guarantee the safety of the child or crew, tell the child what is going to happen and then do it.
- Do not negotiate unless the child really has a choice. For example, it is okay to ask the child if he or she would like the intravenous (IV) line in the right or left hand, but not to ask if it is okay to start an IV when it must be done.
- Let the child be involved in his or her own care. Children in this age group are afraid of being out of control (**FIGURE 2-11**).
- Reassure the child that being ill or injured is not a punishment.
- Praise the child for cooperating. Be careful not to be irritable if the child does not cooperate.
- The physical assessment can usually be done in the head-to-toe format.

FIGURE 2-11 Approaching a school-aged child: Let the child be involved in his or her own care.

FIGURE 2-12 Adolescence is a time of experimentation and risk-taking behaviors.
© yanik88/Shutterstock.

Adolescents

Growth and Development Characteristics

Adolescents sometimes seem to share some characteristics of toddlers: They are very mobile but may lack common sense. However, adolescents are rational, understand cause and effect, and are able to express themselves with words. Adolescence is a time of experimentation and risk-taking behaviors (**FIGURE 2-12**). Adolescents often believe they are immune to danger, that they are "indestructible." They gradually shift from relying on family to relying on friends for psychological support and social development.

- Adolescents struggle with independence, loss of control, body image, sexuality, and peer pressure. Anything that makes them different from their peers causes anxiety. Psychosomatic complaints are common in this age group. They may have mood swings or depression and when ill or injured may act younger than their age, leaving a scared child in an adult body.

- Respect is an important part of the relationship and interaction with the adolescent patient, as it may enable an opportunity to gain information needed to provide the appropriate care for this patient population in a short period of time. An example may be a situation with the need to determine use of drugs and which drug may have been used. Most toxicology drug screens detect only a small number of common drugs used, but not drugs such as synthetic marijuana. An adolescent may be able to guide you in the right direction if there is a trusting relationship developed in a short period of time.

> **TIP**
>
> Adolescents struggle with independence, loss of control, body image, sexuality, and peer pressure. Provide concrete information, respect their privacy, and speak to them directly.

Common Conditions in Adolescents

- Poisonings/drug ingestion
- Respiratory problems
- Fractures (e.g., sports injuries)
- Open wounds

Assessment of the Adolescent

Conduct the assessment of the adolescent using the following principles:

- Obtain the name of the patient, and use it while interacting with him or her.
- Obtain the normal disposition of the patient, and compare it to the current behavior being displayed. Any acute change in disposition should be noted and relayed during the transfer-of-care report.
- Provide accurate information about the illness or injury, normal body functions, and interventions. Explain what you are doing and why.
- Encourage the patient to ask questions and to be involved in his or her own care.
- Show respect. Speak directly to the adolescent. Do not turn to the caregiver for initial information (**FIGURE 2-13**).

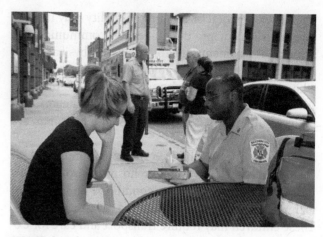

FIGURE 2-13 Approaching an adolescent: Speak to him or her directly.

- Respect the adolescent's modesty, privacy, and confidentiality unless it places him or her at risk.
- Be honest and nonjudgmental.
- Do not be misled by the adolescent's size or make assumptions about his or her comprehension of events. Adolescents may misinterpret the seriousness of the situation. They may also have many fears about permanent injury, disfigurement, or "being different" as a result of the illness or injury. Give adolescents accurate information, and anticipate their questions or fears.
- Avoid becoming frustrated or angry if the adolescent does not talk or is uncooperative.
- Enlist the adolescent's friends to help persuade the adolescent to cooperate with the assessment or treatment, if he or she resists.
- Be mindful of their modesty.

Children With Special Health Care Needs

Growth and Development Characteristics

When working with **children with special health care needs (CSHCN)**, it is important to consider developmental age, rather than chronologic age. Information about the patient should be obtained from caregivers. If an EMS provider does not fully understand the child's medical or developmental history, *it is better to be honest than to feign understanding and potentially place the patient at risk.* CSHCN may have any type of chronic condition that affects health, normal growth, or development. This may include physical disability, developmental or learning disability, technologic dependency, or chronic illness.

The developmental or learning disability may include mental impairment, difficulties in communication, sensory impairment, or limitations in physical activity. The child who is technology dependent may have a home **ventilator**, **tracheostomy**, **gastric feeding tube**, or long-term IV device. Specific categories of patients and methods of assessment and treatment are discussed in Chapter 10.

The number of children in the community with special needs is growing. Prehospital professionals must be familiar with the conditions and types of technology used in assessing and treating CSHCN. These children may require transport and care for exacerbation of their illness or for an unrelated illness or injury.

Unique aspects related to children with special needs include the following:

- Baseline vital signs may be outside the age-appropriate values.
- Weight may be significantly higher or lower than expected.
- Standard prehospital quick reference guides may be inaccurate.
- The child may have a limited ability to endure respiratory distress or shock.
- Be alert for a latex allergy.

CAUTION

Do not assume that a child with a physical disability is cognitively impaired. Always ask the caregiver to clarify the child's normal level of functioning and interaction.

TIP

Even if a disabled child cannot talk or interact, show your respect by introducing yourself, explaining what you are doing, and providing verbal reassurance.

Assessment of a CSHCN

Conduct the assessment of CSHCN using the following principles:

- Obtain the name of the patient, and use it while interacting with him or her.
- Obtain the normal disposition of the patient, and compare it to the current behavior being displayed.

Any acute change in disposition should be noted and relayed during the transfer-of-care report. Include the impressions of the caregiver in chart documentation. Ask the caregiver what he or she thinks of the child's condition, activity, and behaviors. Find out if the caregiver believes that the child is "not acting right."

- Get a careful history from the caregiver. The caregiver can provide detailed information about the child's medical history, medications, and current complaints. He or she is also aware of how best to approach the child and of typical responses and behaviors.
- Approach the child with a developmental delay gently, and use techniques appropriate to his or her developmental level not chronologic age. Use language and techniques tailored to the child's cognitive level to communicate.
- Do not assume that the child with a physical disability is mentally impaired (**FIGURE 2-14**). Ask the caregiver about the child's level of function and interaction with others. To get at baseline functional level you might query, "What would Johnny be doing right now if he was feeling well?"
- Use polite, professional behavior; acknowledge the caregivers' expertise; and take their concerns seriously. Families of chronically ill children usually have had extensive experience with the medical system. If most of their experiences have been good, they will very likely perceive the prehospital professional as an ally. However, if they have had bad experiences, they may feel a need to be very vigilant in protecting their child and be perceived as difficult or controlling.

FIGURE 2-14 Approaching CSHCN: Obtain a thorough history, and identify developmentally appropriate approaches that work best with the child.

© Judith Haeusler/Cultura/Getty Images.

■ Keep in mind the amount of stress that the caregiver of a CSHCN may be experiencing and be sympathetic. It is often helpful to acknowledge their stress about the care being provided.

Tips for the EMS Provider

Infant (0–12 months):
- Be diligent about keeping infants warm and dry to limit hypothermia.
- This is a particularly stressful time for parents adjusting to the eating, sleeping, and crying cycle; sometimes this is complicated by postpartum depression, which can be a risk factor for abuse.
- Persistent crying, irritability, or feeding difficulties can be a symptom of serious illness.
- Although infants sleep a lot, they should rouse easily; inability to rouse an infant should be considered an emergency.
- Head control is limited until closer to 6 months, so when handling an infant, make sure to support the head and neck well.
- By 6 months, infants should make eye contact; lack of eye contact in a sick infant could be a sign of significant illness, depressed mental status, or delayed development.
- By 6–12 months, infants are at risk for foreign body aspiration and poisoning because of the exploration of the environment (by crawling, using their hands, etc.) and placing objects into their mouths.
- Reduce separation anxiety by keeping the child and parent together during an evaluation and involving the parent in the treatment if appropriate.
- Crawling and walking can increase exposure to physical dangers and injuries.

Toddlers (12–36 months):
- Persistent crying or irritability can be a symptom of serious illness.
- Due to a lack of molars, there is an increased risk of choking because children may not be able to grind up food before swallowing.
- Increased mobility increases exposure to physical dangers and injury.
- Distracting a child with a flashlight or toy may aid in physical examination.
- Allow a child to hold objects of importance to him or her (e.g., blanket).
- Try to make the interaction as positive as possible; painful procedures make for lasting impressions.

Preschool children (3–5 years):
- The rapid increase in language means they understand much of what is said if simple terms are used.
- Respect the patient's modesty, and cover him or her up after the physical examination.
- Foreign body airway obstruction risk continues to be high.
- Offer choices to the patient if appropriate (e.g., "Should I listen to your front first or the back?").
- Do not waste time trying to use logic to convince preschoolers; they are concrete thinkers. Avoid frightening or misleading comments.
- Appealing to their magical thinking may allow you to do more (e.g., "This magic mist [nebulizer] will help you breathe better.").
- Communicate about procedures as close to doing them as possible.
- Respect modesty.

School-aged children (6–12 years):
- Provide simple explanations for illness and treatments.
- Be honest about painful procedures.
- If possible, provide sense of control by giving choices.
- Respect modesty.
- Ask about school/sports/activities or interests to allow patients to warm up to you faster.

Adolescents (13–18 years):
- Explain things as clearly and honestly as you would to an adult.
- Give choices when appropriate.
- Respect modesty.
- Be honest about procedures that will cause discomfort.
- Address concerns and fears about the lasting effects of their injuries.
- Adolescence includes hormonal surges, emotions, and peer pressure; there is an increased risk for substance abuse, self-endangerment, pregnancy, and dangerous sexual practices.

Summary

Understanding the developmental characteristics of each age group is essential for accurate assessment and treatment of the child in the prehospital environment. Good field care requires good communication with the child and family. The family may include a large number of people, all of whom become "patients." CSHCN pose additional challenges in assessment, but

CASE STUDY 3

You respond to a park where a 15-year-old was doing skateboard tricks and fell. He was not wearing a helmet and had a brief loss of consciousness. He now complains that his wrist hurts but wants to stay with his friends. A friend had called 9-1-1. He does not want to be examined, definitely does not want to go to the hospital, and starts to leave the scene as you approach him.

1. Is this teenager's reaction normal?
2. What techniques can help you adequately assess his injuries?

their caregivers can be a great asset in guiding field evaluation and management.

Every call experience offers the ability for an EMS provider to learn something. With pediatric patients, the opportunities are larger than with adults. Postcall self-evaluation and call critique can offer providers an opportunity to identify ways to improve for the next pediatric patient interaction.

CASE STUDY ANSWERS

CASE STUDY 1

Even though the mother is crying, it is important to get additional history: Was the infant full-term? Did she have any problems with delivery or after birth? Has she had feeding problems or vomiting in the past? Any fever or diarrhea?

Infants in the first few months of life have a limited range of behaviors, so anything out of the ordinary in the child's feeding, sleeping, or basic activity level is concerning for serious underlying illness or injury.

Reassuring the mother is important, but this infant may be critically ill and requires rapid assessment and transport. Although an infant's extremities may be mottled because of cold, mottling of the trunk is an extremely worrisome sign, reflecting poor perfusion. The possibility of **hypovolemic shock** is supported by the infant's cool extremities and history of vomiting. Furthermore, although infants can develop abdominal distention because of crying and swallowing air, abdominal distention in association with vomiting and signs of shock (abnormal appearance and abnormal circulation to the skin) suggest serious pathology, such as intestinal obstruction.

Move the infant quickly into the ambulance, explaining what you are doing and why to the mother. If local protocol permits, allow the mother to ride with you to the hospital. The infant should be transported and secured on the stretcher. It is never okay to allow a parent or caregiver to hold an infant on his or her lap while on the stretcher. Treatment of this infant includes administration of oxygen by a face mask and rapid transport to an emergency department. Prevention of heat loss by swaddling and applying a hat is important because **hypothermia** is a risk for a small infant. Consider vascular access en route, with a bolus of 20 mL/kg of crystalloid fluid.

CASE STUDY 2

Toddlers are often fearful of strangers, so enlisting the help of parents or caregivers makes patient assessment much easier. Allow the child to remain with the parent. Sit on the bed or crouch down to the child's eye level, and use a calm soothing voice. You can use distractions, such as a penlight, or ask about a stuffed animal on the bed to gain the child's attention and to evaluate interactivity. Ask the parent to remove the child's pajamas, and observe the work of breathing, including suprasternal, subcostal, or intercostal retractions, and respiratory rate. Although your main concern is the child's respiratory status, you may have to perform other portions of the hands-on examination, such as touching or tickling the child's toes before you get to the chest. When listening to breath sounds, warm the stethoscope beforehand and explain what you are doing. If the child resists, you may be able to listen to a stuffed animal first, and allow the child to do the same, before resuming your examination.

Your assessment reveals the child's respiratory rate is 32 breaths/min and heart rate is 128 beats/min. You decide to give the child oxygen, but he refuses to keep the oxygen mask in place even with his mother's help, a response you recognize is typical of a toddler who is not seriously ill. For transport to the hospital, you secure the child on the stretcher, allowing his mother to accompany you in the ambulance, and direct blow-by oxygen in his direction.

CASE STUDY 3

This teenager is asserting his independence but is not legally able to give consent or refuse care, unless he is emancipated. He may not realize the risks of occult injury. Show respect, be honest and nonjudgmental, and speak directly to him. Explain why it is important to check him for potentially serious injuries, and offer him the privacy of the ambulance to conduct the examination. If he still refuses care, attempt to contact his parents or caregivers or enlist the assistance of the police.

SUGGESTED REFERENCES

Textbooks

American Academy of Pediatrics, American College of Emergency Physicians. *APLS: The Pediatric Emergency Medicine Resource*. 5th ed. Burlington, MA: Jones & Bartlett Learning; 2012.

Kliegman R, St Geme J. *Nelson Textbook of Pediatrics*. 21st ed. Philadelphia, PA: Elsevier; 2020.

Chameides L, Samson RA, Schexnayder SM, Hazinski MF. *PALS Provider Manual*. Dallas, TX: American Heart Association; 2011.

Marx JA, Hockberger RS, Walls RM. *Rosen's Emergency Medicine Concepts and Clinical Practice*. 7th ed. Philadelphia, PA: Mosby; 2009.

Tittinalli J. *Emergency Medicine: A Comprehensive Study Guide*. 7th ed. Columbus, OH: McGraw Hill; 2011.

Zitelli B, Davis H, McIntire S, Nowalk AJ. *Zitelli and Davis' Atlas of Pediatric Physical Diagnosis*. 6th ed. Philadelphia, PA: Elsevier; 2012.

Other Resources

Code Green Campaign (first responder mental health advocacy and education): www.codegreencampaign.org

Fire/EMS Helpline: 1-888-731-FIRE (3473)

CHAPTER 3

Respiratory Emergencies

Ann Dietrich, MD, FACEP, FAAP

Joyce Foresman-Capuzzi, MSN, APRN, CCNS, CEN, CPEN, CTRN, TCRN, CPN, EMT-P, FAEN

LEARNING OBJECTIVES

1. Describe how to assess airway and breathing, including interpreting information from the Pediatric Assessment Triangle and the ABCDEs.

2. Differentiate among respiratory distress, respiratory failure, and respiratory arrest based on history, physical examination, and physiologic monitoring.

3. Define the physiologic information provided by pulse oximetry and capnometry, recognize situations in which each should be used, and recognize appropriate management responses to abnormal measurements.

4. Outline a general treatment strategy, going from the least to the most invasive, for children with respiratory compromise.

5. Contrast the key signs, symptoms, and management of upper airway obstruction versus lower airway obstruction.

6. Discuss possible complications of assisted ventilation, and outline strategies to identify and correct these complications.

Introduction

The most common chief complaints for prehospital providers are traumatic injury (28%), general illness (10%), and respiratory distress (9%). Of all conditions causing respiratory disease in children, asthma is the most common noninfectious cause. However, respiratory distress may also be associated with a myriad of other conditions, including viral illnesses, pneumonia, foreign bodies, and trauma. Good assessment and early intervention for pediatric respiratory problems can avert serious illness and preventable death and may shorten treatment time in the emergency department (ED).

Focusing on certain key physical signs and symptoms allows the prehospital professional to rapidly assess the effectiveness of gas exchange in the airways and lung alveoli. Using the Pediatric Assessment Triangle (PAT) is an important first step in determining the severity of disease, localizing the physiologic problem, and beginning treatment. Of the three aspects of the PAT, appearance and work of breathing are essential to the initial impression for a child in respiratory distress. Appearance reflects the overall state of ventilation and oxygenation. Increased work of breathing indicates either airway obstruction at some level or a problem in gas exchange at the alveolar level; it is often an early sign of hypoxia or hypercapnia. Fading respiratory effort is a sign of severe hypoxia or hypercapnia. Cyanosis of the skin or mucous membranes also indicates severe hypoxia and is part of the third aspect of the PAT, circulation to the skin.

After utilizing the PAT to establish an initial impression, the primary assessment provides a more detailed assessment and includes assessing the work of breathing (this can be done in a nonthreatening manner by asking the parent or caregiver to lift the child's shirt or clothing), counting the respirations, performing hands-on chest auscultation, evaluating the heart rate, and obtaining pulse oximetry. This assessment not only provides a picture of respiratory function but also helps prioritize general and specific treatments, interventions, and timing of transport.

Respiratory Distress and Failure

Respiratory distress, failure, and arrest are three points on a continuum of physiologic response to different types of hypoxic stress. Using PAT, respiratory distress is characterized by increased work of breathing and normal appearance. An abnormal appearance with increased work of breathing is consistent with respiratory failure/arrest. In addition, cyanosis may also occur. Causes of hypoxic stress are variable and include asthma, bronchiolitis, croup, pneumonia, and chest wall injury. Although these three points in the continuum (respiratory distress, failure, and arrest) have different clinical characteristics in theory, in reality they are part of a spectrum that is not black or white.

Respiratory distress is an abnormal physiologic condition identified by increased work of breathing. Increased respiratory rate; supraclavicular, suprasternal, intercostal, or subcostal retractions; use of accessory muscles; and nasal flaring are signs that, alone or in combination, indicate increased work of breathing. These physical signs represent the patient's attempt to make up for decreased gas exchange in the lungs and airways and to maintain oxygenation and ventilation.

The child's appearance is relatively normal because oxygen delivery is still adequate.

Respiratory failure occurs when the infant or child exhausts his or her energy reserves and can no longer maintain oxygenation and ventilation. Respiratory failure may occur when chest wall muscles get tired after a long period of increased work of breathing (e.g., a child with severe asthma who is very tight and has been working hard to breathe for several hours), when the insult is severe and progressive (e.g., **fulminant pneumonia**), or when there is a failure of central respiratory drive (e.g., a child with a severe closed-head injury). An abnormal appearance (fussy, poor feeding) or cyanosis in a child with an increased work of breathing indicates respiratory failure. An abnormally low respiratory rate and decreased respiratory effort, usually with a decreasing heart rate, also indicate respiratory failure. Respiratory failure must be treated immediately to restore good oxygenation and ventilation and to prevent respiratory arrest.

Signs of failure are decreased level of consciousness, slow to agonal respirations, grunting, decreasing pulse oximetry, and bradycardia or inappropriate slowing of the heart rate.

Respiratory arrest means absence of effective breathing. If ventilation and oxygenation are not immediately supported, respiratory arrest rapidly progresses to full cardiopulmonary arrest. Most episodes of cardiac arrest in pediatric patients begin as respiratory arrest. Intervening at this point may prevent cardiac arrest.

Early intervention for children with respiratory distress may prevent progression to respiratory failure and arrest. If the child presents in respiratory failure, aggressive intervention will provide a far better chance of producing neurologically intact survivors than treatment of cardiac arrest, which has an extremely low probability of survival.

CASE STUDY 1

You are dispatched to the home of a 32-month-old boy who is having difficulty breathing. His mother says that for 2 days he has had a slight fever and has been "wheezing." He suddenly awoke tonight acutely short of breath and now is making a very loud noise each time he breathes in. The child has no prior history of wheezing or respiratory illness.

The child is sitting on his mother's lap looking anxious but makes eye contact and cries when you approach. He makes loud, harsh noises with each inspiration. His color is pink, but he has marked supraclavicular and suprasternal retractions and nasal flaring. Respiratory rate is 38 breaths/min, and the heart rate is 160 beats/min. The blood pressure is not obtained. His skin is warm, and he has strong pulses and normal capillary refill time. He has good air movement with loud, harsh breath sounds heard on each inspiration.

1. How sick is this child?
2. Are this child's findings more likely to be caused by upper airway or lower airway obstruction, and how will you manage him in the field?

Prearrival Preparation

Based on dispatch information and while en route to the scene, prepare mentally for management of respiratory distress and failure by reviewing the appropriate assessment techniques and treatment options for the child's age. This includes recalling an age-based approach to assessment, as outlined in Chapter 1; equipment needs; and the likely treatment and transport options. Also, anticipate the determinants of whether to stay on scene and treat or to manage the airway and transport immediately to the ED.

Scene Size-Up

Be sure the scene is safe and that there are no obvious illness or injury threats. Assess the environment for foreign body risks, medications, noxious gases, fumes, chemicals, or smoke. Document scene conditions if environmental factors may be contributing to anticipated respiratory problems. If indicated, make sure to wear personal protective equipment (PPE); question how many patients are in the home or facility; determine if additional resources are needed; and attempt to determine mechanism of injury (MOI), nature of illness (NOI), and the need for cervical spine precautions or immobilization.

General Assessment: The PAT

Evaluating the Presenting Complaint

Find out the nature of the presenting complaint by asking several directed questions, as suggested in **TABLE 3-1**. After the primary assessment, in patients with mild distress, there is time to get a more complete SAMPLE history on scene as part of the focused history. If the child is in respiratory failure, do this later, while en route to the ED.

Assessment of Respiratory Status

Using the PAT

Begin the assessment with the PAT, as discussed in the chapter on patient assessment. Carefully evaluate appearance, work of breathing, and circulation to the skin. The PAT helps establish how sick the child is, an overall impression of the child, and the need for emergent intervention. Table 1-2 in Chapter 1 lists physical features in the child to help make these clinical distinctions by simple observation and listening.

TABLE 3-1 Key Questions About the Presenting Complaint

Key Question	Possible Medical Problem
Has your child ever had this kind of problem before?	Asthma, chronic lung disease
Is this the first time that your child has had trouble breathing?	Asthma, foreign body aspiration, bronchiolitis
Is your child taking any medications?	Asthma, chronic lung disease, congenital heart disease
Has your child had a fever?	Pneumonia, bronchiolitis, viral infections such as croup
Did your child suddenly start coughing/choking/gagging?	Foreign body aspiration or ingestion
Has your child had an injury to his or her chest?	Pulmonary contusion, pneumothorax

Appearance

Appearance reflects the adequacy of oxygenation and ventilation in a child with difficulty breathing. If the child is compensating effectively for the respiratory insult, the appearance is fairly normal, and the TICLS mnemonic (see Table 1-1 in Chapter 1) shows an interactive child with good tone and color, with normal vocalizations, who looks or gazes at someone. If the child is not compensating, the appearance is abnormal, and the child has abnormal findings in the TICLS mnemonic because his or her brain is impaired from hypoxia or hypercapnia. Abnormal appearance is a spectrum of clinical states, so that the severity of respiratory failure determines how abnormal the child appears. Also, assessing appearance guides urgency of basic life support (BLS) versus advanced life support (ALS) treatment. Even if ALS procedures are required, start with BLS procedures while preparing to implement ALS procedures based on local protocol.

Example 1: A 3-year-old child who has stridor and retractions, but is running around the room and has a normal appearance, requires general noninvasive treatment and transport. The child is compensating effectively and is only in respiratory distress.

Example 2: An 8-year-old child who is anxious and quiet, with wheezing and increased work of breathing, has an abnormal appearance and is probably hypoxic. The child is beginning to decompensate and is in early respiratory failure. In addition to general noninvasive treatment, this child requires immediate specific ALS treatment on scene with a bronchodilator, then rapid transport to an ED.

Example 3: A 3-year-old child who has been working hard to breathe for hours and is now sleepy or poorly responsive has an abnormal appearance. The altered mental status is the result of severe hypoxia or hypercapnia, reflecting respiratory failure and impending respiratory arrest. These patients require immediate assisted ventilations with airway adjuncts, such as oropharyngeal airway or nasopharyngeal airway, using a bag-mask device on scene and possibly advanced airway procedures. This may include endotracheal intubation, supraglottic airways, or laryngeal tube (e.g., dual lumen airway).

Work of Breathing

To assess for adequate breathing, sometimes the patient needs to be appropriately exposed. Attempt to visualize the thorax in a nonthreatening manner while keeping the child warm. Look for signs of increased work of breathing:

1. Abnormal positioning (tripoding, "sniffing" position)
2. Abnormal airway sounds (e.g., snoring, stridor, wheezing, or grunting)
3. Retractions (suprasternal, supraclavicular, intercostal, subcostal)
4. Head bobbing in infants
5. Nasal flaring

The significance of each of these findings is discussed in Chapter 1. These indicators of breathing effort help to identify the anatomic location of the problem (upper airway, lower airway, or lung alveoli), the severity of the physiologic dysfunction (respiratory distress, failure, or arrest), and the urgency for treatment (immediate resuscitation, general treatment only on scene with specific treatment en route, general and specific treatment on scene). In addition to abnormal airway sounds (stridor, wheezing, and grunting), retractions and the use of accessory muscles may help localize the site of airway problems. Use of the accessory muscles of the neck and suprasternal and supraclavicular retractions occur more often with upper airway obstruction. Predominant subcostal and intercostal retractions and the use of abdominal muscles tend to localize an obstructive process to the lower airways. It is hard to recognize some of these signs when the child has on clothing; if needed, appropriately remove clothing to ascertain these other clinical signs.

Circulation to Skin

Finally, evaluate skin color. Cyanosis is an ominous sign, signaling profound hypoxia and the need for assisted ventilation. However, a child may have severe hypoxia without an obvious change in skin color. Pulse oximetry is very helpful; use it whenever available in a child with respiratory distress or respiratory failure.

Primary Assessment: The ABCDEs

After the PAT, perform the second portion of the primary assessment, the hands-on ABCDEs. There are three parts to the "B" or breathing evaluation:

1. Respiratory rate
2. Auscultation for air movement and abnormal breath sounds
3. Pulse oximetry

Respiratory Rate

In the noncritical patient, determine respiratory rate by sitting the child in the caregiver's lap and exposing the patient's chest. Count the rise and fall of the abdomen over 30 seconds, and then double that number. Normal respiratory rates vary in children of different ages (see Table 1-4 in Chapter 1). Always think about respiratory rates in the context of the PAT and the overall clinical assessment. Respiratory rate may be affected by level of activity, fever, anxiety, and metabolic state.

A respiratory rate of greater than 60 breaths/min is abnormal in a child of any age and should be a signal for careful evaluation for other signs of respiratory or circulatory problems. Even more dangerous is a rate that is too slow for age. A respiratory rate of less than 20 breaths/min in a sick child younger than 6 years of age, or a rate of less than 12 breaths/min in a sick child between 6 and 15 years of age, may be a sign of respiratory failure, and immediate intervention may be required.

Auscultation for Air Movement and Abnormal Breath Sounds

Assess air movement by placing the stethoscope and listening for the amount of air movement with each breath (**FIGURE 3-1**). Poor air movement may exist in children with respiratory problems for many reasons, as outlined in **TABLE 3-2**.

Assessing air movement, or the volume of air exchanged with each breath, allows clinical estimation of **tidal volume**. Tidal volume is one of two factors that determine minute ventilation (the volume of air exchanged per minute). **Minute ventilation** is the basis for gas exchange in the lungs.

$$\text{Minute Ventilation} = \text{Tidal Volume} \times \\ \text{Respiratory Rate}$$

This equation shows the connection between tidal volume and respiratory rate. A child may not have enough gas exchange if tidal volume is low, even with a normal or fast respiratory rate. Also, a normal or increased tidal volume does not mean there is enough gas exchange if the respiratory rate is too slow.

While listening for air movement, also listen for abnormal breath sounds. Table 1-5 in Chapter 1 summarizes the types and causes of abnormal breath sounds. Stridor, which is usually inspiratory in nature (at least initially), is indicative of upper airway obstruction, whereas crackles and wheezes are associated with lower airway processes.

FIGURE 3-1 Assess air movement by placing the stethoscope and listening for the amount of movement with each breath (remember to use a small diaphragm and compare breath sounds side to side). In infants, if the chest is noisy, consider suctioning the nose and listening again.

© Jones & Bartlett Learning. Courtesy of Glen Ellman.

Pulse Oximetry

Pulse oximetry is a useful tool for detecting and measuring hypoxia. **FIGURE 3-2** illustrates possible sites for placement of the oximetry probe. **Pulse Oximetry, Procedure 9**, explains how to use a pulse oximeter. The pulse oximeter emits red light of two different wavelengths. These are absorbed differently by saturated and desaturated hemoglobin. The sensor on the pulse oximeter measures the transmission of the two wavelengths of red light, and a computer in the machine then determines the percentage of hemoglobin saturated with oxygen. When properly applied, *and if there is a good arterial tracing*, a reading of 95% or higher means normal blood oxygen saturation. *A value of 94% or less on room air is abnormal and is a signal to give supplemental oxygen.* A reading of less than 90% in a patient on 100% oxygen usually indicates respiratory failure, unless the child has a chronic respiratory problem.

Patients with uncorrected cyanotic heart disease and some patients with chronic respiratory problems (e.g., cystic fibrosis) have a low oxygen saturation at baseline. In this type of patient, obtain the baseline value from the caregiver and attempt to provide enough oxygen to get the child to his or her baseline pulse oximetry level. Providing more oxygen than is needed to achieve the baseline pulse oximetry level may actually suppress ventilation by reducing the child's hypoxic drive to breathe. In normal children, hypercapnia or increased carbon dioxide pressure stimulates the drive to breathe, but in some children with chronic respiratory disease, hypercapnia is a constant state. In such cases, hypoxia becomes the stimulus to breathe. The preferred saturation rate is between 94% and 99%.

TABLE 3-2 Causes of Poor Air Movement in Children	
Functional Problem	**Possible Causes**
Obstruction of airway	Asthma, bronchiolitis, croup, foreign body
Restriction of chest wall movement	Chest wall injury, severe **scoliosis** or kyphosis
Chest wall muscle fatigue	Prolonged increased work of breathing, muscular dystrophy
Decreased central respiratory drive	Head injury, intoxication
Chest injury	Rib fractures, pulmonary contusion, pneumothorax

FIGURE 3-2 Possible sites for placement of the oximetry probe.

One must be careful not to overinterpret low oxygen saturation. Pulse oximetry is merely an adjunct to physical assessment. Falsely low readings are common with pulse oximetry. Movement by the child, cold extremities or a cold ambient temperature, and interference by light in the child's surroundings all may cause inaccurate pulse oximetry readings. Check probe placement, the quality of the tracing, and the child's clinical state before treating. Inaccurate readings or the inability to obtain a reading may also occur in children in shock with poor perfusion. However, give these children oxygen even if they do not have respiratory distress and regardless of pulse oximeter readings. It is also important not to underinterpret a normal pulse oximetry reading. *Sometimes, an apparently normal oxygen saturation (above 94%) may be present in a child with significant respiratory distress who is compensating by increased work of breathing.* Always use pulse oximetry in combination with physical assessment to ensure accurate interpretation of adequacy of breathing.

TIP

Remember, the pulse oximeter does not tell about adequacy of ventilation. A patient who is receiving supplemental oxygen may have a normal pulse oximeter reading but not have adequate ventilation. Capnometry, which quantitatively measures exhaled carbon dioxide, monitors carbon dioxide levels and adequacy of ventilation and provides a minute-by-minute picture of ventilatory status.

CAUTION

Be careful not to overinterpret low or normal oxygen saturation. Match with the physical findings.

General Noninvasive Treatment

For every child in respiratory distress, begin general noninvasive treatment. *The general noninvasive treatment of every noncritical patient is the same—allow the patient to assume a position of comfort and supply oxygen, if tolerated* (**FIGURE 3-3**). This is the only treatment for patients in respiratory distress without upper or lower airway obstruction. If the child is in respiratory failure or arrest, perform assisted ventilation immediately with airway adjuncts and consider advanced airways based on local protocols.

Positioning

A child in respiratory distress naturally moves into the position that provides the best air exchange, called the position of comfort. For example, a child with severe upper airway obstruction may get into the sniffing position to straighten the airway and open the air passages (**FIGURE 3-4**). A child with severe lower airway obstruction may voluntarily take the tripod posture (sitting up and leaning forward on outstretched arms) to help accessory muscles (**FIGURE 3-5**). Infants and toddlers may be most comfortable in their caregiver's arms or lap. Do not move a child from his or her position of comfort, as this might worsen the respiratory distress. In the ambulance, keep the dyspneic child safely restrained in an upright position, unless the child requires assisted ventilations or has other physiologic problems that require treatment in a supine position.

Oxygen

Treatment with high-flow oxygen is usually safe. If the child has chronic respiratory illness, be careful not to administer too much oxygen. The prehospital professional must weigh the possible benefits of

FIGURE 3-3 Always keep a child with respiratory distress in his or her position of comfort.

© Jones & Bartlett Learning. Courtesy of Glen Ellman.

FIGURE 3-5 Tripod position.

FIGURE 3-4 Sniffing position.

FIGURE 3-6 If the child resists application of a mask or nasal cannula, administer oxygen through a nonthreatening object, such as a cup.

© Jones & Bartlett Learning. Courtesy of Glen Ellman.

CAUTION

Do not move a child from his or her position of comfort.

giving oxygen against the risks of agitating the child and worsening the respiratory distress. This is a special concern in a child with an unstable airway. Infants with respiratory distress, cyanosis, or other signs of respiratory disease require high-flow, 100% oxygen.

Because of concerns about oxygen toxicity in newborns, those without signs of hypoxia no longer require 100% oxygen, as explained in Chapter 12. For premature newborns in respiratory distress, start at 21% oxygen and titrate as needed to achieve an oxygen saturation of 94% or greater.

Most children accept oxygen therapy, especially if the prehospital professional is creative in the approach. This often means getting the help of the caregiver. If a child resists the use of a mask or **nasal cannula**, have the caregiver give blow-by oxygen from the end of the oxygen tubing or from tubing inserted into a cup (**FIGURE 3-6**).

Oxygen Delivery

Give oxygen to any child with clinical signs of cardiopulmonary distress or failure or with a history suggesting possible abnormalities in gas exchange. The delivery method should provide the concentration of oxygen most appropriate for the child's condition, degree of cooperation, respiratory effort, and age. For a step-by-step explanation of this procedure, see **Oxygen Delivery, Procedure 3**.

Summary of General and Initial Respiratory Assessment and General Noninvasive Treatment

The PAT is a good tool for determining the effectiveness of gas exchange, based on observation of appearance and work of breathing. If the PAT suggests respiratory distress, begin general noninvasive treatment with oxygen and keep the child in his or her position of comfort. The PAT also identifies the critical child in respiratory failure who requires immediate assisted ventilation. Obtaining the respiratory rate, listening for air movement, and determining oxygen saturation by pulse oximetry work in concert with the PAT. The primary assessment should allow an evaluation of severity and urgency for treatment and should establish if specific treatment for upper or lower airway obstruction is indicated.

Specific Treatment for Respiratory Distress

After completing the primary assessment, consider specific treatment. The PAT and ABCDE assessment help determine whether the child has an upper or lower airway obstruction, lung disease, or disordered control of breathing (from such conditions as brain or nerve injury, poisoning, or sepsis). Snoring or stridor indicates upper airway obstruction; wheezing indicates lower airway obstruction. It can be difficult to separate true stridor from upper airway noise because of nasal congestion. Breath sounds may also make it difficult to tell the difference between upper airway noise and true wheezing. Listen for breath sounds in the second or third intercostal space at the midaxillary line bilaterally (**FIGURE 3-7**). Consider the auscultation of breath sounds posteriorly between the scapula and spine bilaterally and lower lobes directly above the kidneys. At this location, it is easier to distinguish upper airway congestion from lower airway obstruction. When abnormal airway sounds are loudest with the stethoscope held near the child's nose rather than over the lungs, nasal congestion/obstruction is the likely cause.

The presence of abnormal breath sounds in a child with hypoxia and increased work of breathing suggests lung disease, such as pneumonia. Lastly, a child with

Midclavicular line
Anterior axillary line
Midaxillary line

FIGURE 3-7 Listen for breath sounds.

hypoxia and *decreased* work of breathing may have either respiratory failure from airway obstruction or lung disease or disordered control of breathing from another insult to the brain or metabolic system.

> **TIP**
>
> When abnormal airway sounds are loudest with the stethoscope held near the child's nose rather than over the lungs, nasal congestion/obstruction is the likely cause.

Upper Airway Obstruction

Proximal Airway Obstruction

In a patient with neurologic impairment, loss of oropharyngeal muscle tone may cause upper airway obstruction and stridor because of the tongue and **mandible** falling back and partially blocking the **pharynx**. This is a common problem in children during and after seizures. The head-tilt/chin-lift maneuver (**FIGURE 3-8**) or jaw-thrust maneuver (**FIGURE 3-9**) may relieve this **proximal** airway obstruction. At times, it may be helpful or even necessary to have two rescuers assist with the jaw-thrust maneuver. The use of airway adjuncts based on level of consciousness may help with keeping the airway open, especially in larger children, children who are actively seizing, or children receiving positive-pressure ventilation (**FIGURE 3-10**).

Sometimes secretions, blood, or foreign bodies block the proximal upper airway. This is an important concern in the child with closed-head injury or seizures. Suctioning alone often relieves the upper airway

FIGURE 3-8 Use the head-tilt/chin-lift maneuver to place the airway in a neutral position.

FIGURE 3-9 Use the jaw-thrust maneuver in a child with possible spinal injury.

FIGURE 3-10 Two-rescuer technique for the jaw-thrust maneuver and positive-pressure ventilation.

obstruction caused by fluids or occluding objects in the mouth, pharynx, or nose.

Maintenance of an adequate airway may require placement of an oropharyngeal airway, a nasopharyngeal airway, an endotracheal tube, or other approved advanced airways. The role of endotracheal intubation of children in the prehospital setting has been brought into question by data demonstrating significant failure rates, induced hypoxia, airway injury, and endotracheal tube dislodgement. *Bag-mask ventilation is the key lifesaving technique that should be mastered by all prehospital providers and provides adequate airway management for most pediatric patients.*

Alternative advanced airways, including supraglottic airways and laryngeal tubes, can be considered in the early treatment of the child in respiratory failure or arrest. The particular type and brand are based on local emergency medical services (EMS) protocols.

Airway Obstruction Above the Thoracic Inlet

Upper airway obstruction beyond the proximal upper airway may result from a variety of causes. It is not necessary to make an exact diagnosis to provide appropriate management to children with upper airway obstruction. In most of these cases, simply allow the child to maintain his or her position of comfort and provide supplemental oxygen by the least-invasive and least-threatening means possible. Causing the child to become more agitated or struggle may worsen the airway obstruction and precipitate the onset of a severe airway obstruction, leading to respiratory failure or respiratory arrest.

In an awake, alert child, upper airway obstruction and stridor are usually caused by croup, a viral disease with inflammation, edema, and narrowing of the larynx or trachea. Croup usually affects infants and toddlers. Most children with croup have had several days of cold symptoms. The cold symptoms are followed by the development of a barking or "seal-like" cough, stridor, and various levels of respiratory distress. There is usually a low-grade fever, and symptoms are often worse at night. The severity of symptoms varies widely among patients, but they usually progress over days, rather than hours.

Treatment. In the prehospital setting, the use of cool mist, either in the form of humidified oxygen or nebulized saline, may provide some comfort for the child. Having the caregiver assist by holding the nebulizer may be of benefit. If the child does not tolerate the treatment, transport in a position of comfort (**FIGURE 3-11**).

FIGURE 3-11 Use the caregiver to assist in the administration of oxygen or nebulized saline.

ALS

Pharmacologic Treatment of Croup. Nebulized epinephrine is a specific treatment for the upper airway inflammation associated with croup. Epinephrine is a potent α- and β-agonist and works through vasoconstriction to decrease the upper airway edema causing partial obstruction. If local EMS protocols permit, consider nebulized epinephrine therapy for children with stridor, increased work of breathing, poor air movement, blood oxygen saturation less than 94%, or altered appearance. Nebulized epinephrine has two formulations, and either is acceptable: racemic epinephrine and L-epinephrine.

Side effects of nebulized epinephrine include tachycardia, tremor, and vomiting. Children who receive nebulized epinephrine need a period of observation in the ED because of possible return of stridor after the medicine wears off. Very few children with croup require assisted ventilation in the prehospital setting. In the rare case of a child with croup and respiratory failure, begin assisted ventilation and reassess. Two-person bag-mask ventilation technique may be necessary.

Invasive Airway Management for Croup. Perform endotracheal intubation only in the unusual case of the child with respiratory failure who does not respond to bag-mask ventilation. Preparation for intubation includes choosing an endotracheal tube that is one or two sizes smaller than normal for age or length. Inflammation of the trachea at the subglottic level makes it difficult or impossible to use an endotracheal tube of normal size. Refer to local protocols when making the decision for drug-assisted intubation (DAI; formerly called rapid sequence intubation). Other advanced airways should also be considered based on local protocols and availability.

CAUTION

Stridor is often mistaken for wheezing. Stridor is an inspiratory sign of upper airway obstruction and may improve with an agent with vasoconstrictive properties, such as nebulized epinephrine.

TIP

Position of comfort, humidified oxygen, and avoiding agitation are the best treatments for suspected croup.

Bacterial Upper Airway Infections

Bacterial infections may also cause upper airway obstruction in children. Unlike viral croup, these infections tend to progress rapidly, with severe respiratory compromise developing over hours. The child with a bacterial upper airway infection usually is older than 12 months, appears ill or toxic, has pain on swallowing, and may drool. Stridor may be present, but the child does not have the barking cough that is common with croup.

There are several possible causes of bacterial upper airway infections. Epiglottitis, inflammation of the epiglottis, is now extremely rare because of widespread vaccination of infants against the bacteria *Haemophilus influenzae* type B. A retropharyngeal abscess involves swelling of the retropharyngeal nodes that are located between the cervical vertebrae and esophagus. It usually occurs in children younger than 4 years and can mimic the presentation of epiglottitis. The child may have torticollis, and there may be swollen cervical lymph nodes. A peritonsillar abscess is a collection of pus adjacent to the tonsil. It tends to occur more often in adolescents and is often caused by group A streptococcus (so the child may be on antibiotics for a strep throat). The child complains of trouble speaking, is unable to open his or her mouth fully, and often drools. Tracheitis can occur in two forms. In the child without a tracheostomy, it can mimic the presentation of epiglottitis; in a child with a tracheostomy, it results in increased thick airway secretions.

Treatment. When a bacterial upper airway infection is suspected, give only general noninvasive treatment with high-flow oxygen in a position of comfort. Avoid agitating the child by trying to place an intravenous line or attempting another maneuver, and quickly transport. If the child is in respiratory failure, initiate bag-mask ventilation and consider endotracheal intubation.

Foreign Body Aspiration

Foreign body aspiration may cause mechanical obstruction anywhere in the airway, from the pharynx to the bronchus. A retained esophageal foreign body can also cause respiratory distress in an infant or young child. This happens because the trachea is pliable and can be compressed by the adjacent distended esophagus. A typical history of foreign body aspiration includes the sudden onset of coughing, choking, gagging, and shortness of breath in a previously well child without a fever or other symptoms of upper respiratory tract infection. Older infants and toddlers, who explore their world by placing things in their mouths, are at highest risk.

Treatment. If the child can still cough, cry, or speak, the airway is only partially obstructed. Stridor may be present. Immediately transport these children, who are considered to have mild upper airway obstruction. Use only general noninvasive treatment, avoid agitating the child, and keep the child in a position of comfort.

If the child has severe respiratory distress and is at risk for getting worse during transport, be prepared to perform foreign body airway obstruction (FBAO) maneuvers for severe airway obstruction, as illustrated in **FIGURES 3-12** and **3-13**. **TABLE 3-3** summarizes these maneuvers. Consider these FBAO maneuvers if the child cannot cough, cry, or speak. *Never perform FBAO procedures if the child has mild airway obstruction (i.e., can cough, cry, or speak).*

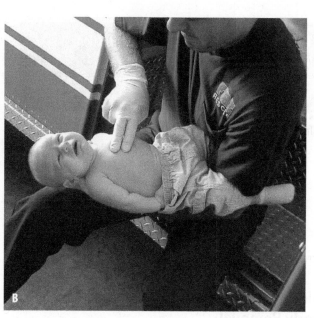

FIGURE 3-12 Foreign body airway maneuvers for a conscious infant. **A.** Use five back blows (slaps), followed by **B.** five chest compressions in infants with severe airway obstruction.

CASE STUDY 2

Your unit is dispatched to a child care center for a child in respiratory distress. On arrival you and your partner find an 18-month-old girl who is very cyanotic and grasping her throat. The child care worker states that she believes the child choked on a grape. The child is making no audible noises and seems desperate for help.

1. What is the most important thing for you to do at this time?
2. What would you do if your initial steps failed? What would you do next?

FIGURE 3-13 Foreign body airway maneuvers for a conscious child. Use abdominal thrusts to treat severe airway obstruction in the conscious child in the standing position.

TABLE 3-3	Foreign Body Airway Obstruction Maneuvers
Age	**Technique**
Infant (<12 months)	Five back blows (slaps), followed by five chest compressions until unresponsive, then start CPR
Child (>1 year)	Abdominal thrusts until unresponsive, then start CPR

CPR, cardiopulmonary resuscitation.

Airway Obstruction and Foreign Body Removal

In the setting of severe airway obstruction, prehospital professionals can make the difference between life and death. Immediate removal of an airway foreign body can often be achieved using BLS procedures while the child is still conscious. Sometimes basic maneuvers are unsuccessful. In such cases, pediatric Magill forceps along with direct laryngoscopy may be the only option for removal. For a step-by-step explanation of this procedure, see **Foreign Body Obstruction, Procedure 6**.

Foreign Body Airway Obstruction Maneuvers.
If the child has severe airway obstruction and BLS

maneuvers fail to dislodge the foreign body to the mouth, where it can be easily removed, and the patient loses consciousness, begin cardiopulmonary resuscitation (CPR) with chest compressions, then open the airway. If the foreign body can be seen at or above the level of the larynx, remove it using pediatric Magill forceps if at the level of a paramedic. If not at the paramedic level, continue CPR and look for airway obstruction before delivering ventilations. Finger sweep FBAO only if the object is seen. If the child has severe airway obstruction and neither FBAO maneuvers nor direct laryngoscopy relieves the obstruction, attempt bag-mask ventilation, using the two-person technique whenever possible (**FIGURE 3-14**). If bag-mask ventilation fails to achieve chest rise, consider endotracheal intubation, if in your scope of practice. Suction should be readily available when performing unconscious airway maneuvers.

Based on local protocols, cricothyrotomy might be considered for obstructions that cannot be removed.

Specific Treatment of Upper Airway Obstruction

When transporting any child with suspected mild upper airway obstruction, have airway equipment immediately available. Consider transporting the caregiver with any conscious child with airway obstruction, because this may keep the child calm. Also, the caregiver can help administer oxygen.

CAUTION

Never perform airway obstruction procedures if the child has only mild airway obstruction and can still cough, cry, or speak.

FIGURE 3-14 Two-person bag-mask ventilation technique.

© Jones & Bartlett Learning. Courtesy of Glen Ellman.

Lower Airway Obstruction

Bronchiolitis and asthma are the most common conditions causing lower airway obstruction in children. Foreign body aspiration is much less common and usually occurs in toddlers who have been otherwise well, and then suddenly start choking, coughing, or wheezing. *Wheezing is the clinical hallmark of lower airway obstruction of any cause.* Pneumonia can also cause lower airway disease, but usually without obstruction. A specific diagnosis of lower airway obstruction in the field is not necessary, and many times it is impossible to tell which of the three main conditions the child is experiencing: (1) bronchiolitis, (2) asthma, or (3) foreign body aspiration.

> **TIP**
>
> Attempt BLS maneuvers first in a child with suspected foreign body aspiration and critical airway obstruction.

Asthma

Asthma is the most common chronic disease of childhood, affecting almost 5 million children in the United States. The ED admission rate for children with asthma younger than 5 years of age is more than twice the national average for all ages, and the mortality rate for children is rising. One-half of all pediatric asthma deaths occur in the out-of-hospital setting. The length of the final attack is less than 1 hour in many children, and less than 2 hours in one-half of children with asthma who die. Common reasons for an asthma attack include upper respiratory infection and exercise. Exposure to cold air, emotional stress, and passive exposure to smoke also may trigger attacks.

Asthma is a disease of small airway inflammation. The inflammatory reaction leads to bronchoconstriction, mucosal edema, and profuse secretions. These three factors in combination cause airflow obstruction and **ventilation-perfusion mismatch**. Clinically, children having an asthma attack show different degrees of tachypnea, tachycardia, increased work of breathing, and wheezing on exhalation; however, inspiratory wheezes can also be present. Pulse oximetry may be normal or low.

Carefully assess air movement by auscultation both anteriorly and posteriorly; this helps to distinguish not only sounds, but also tidal volume. The person with asthma complaining of shortness of breath, but without wheezing on auscultation, may have too much airway obstruction to wheeze. Aggressive bronchodilator treatment may improve airflow and increase audible wheezing. Beware of the following features of the primary assessment, which suggest severe bronchospasm and respiratory failure:

- Altered appearance
- Exhaustion
- Inability to recline
- Interrupted speech
- Severe retractions
- Decreased air movement

In the focused history, several things suggest that a severe or potentially fatal attack may occur. These include the following:

- Prior intensive care unit admissions or intubation
- More than three ED visits in a year
- More than two hospital admissions in past year
- Use of more than one metered-dose inhaler canister in the last month
- Use of bronchodilators more frequently than every 4 hours
- Progressive symptoms despite aggressive home therapy

Home therapy of asthma has several goals: preventing and controlling asthma symptoms, reducing the number and severity of attacks, and reversing existing airflow obstruction. Some children with a history of severe or frequent asthma attacks are on daily medications, but most children receive treatment only during serious attacks. **TABLE 3-4** lists the medications frequently used in home asthma therapy for quick relief. Some patients may think they will obtain quick relief from medications that do not have a quick onset of action and delay calling for help.

Treatment of Lower Airway Obstruction

For all children with lower airway obstruction, give general noninvasive treatment as the first field action.

ALS

Asthma Treatment

Specific field treatment of wheezing includes either inhaled bronchodilators or intramuscular (IM) epinephrine. In patients with asthma, treatment with corticosteroids in the ED has been shown to result in decreased need for admission and more rapid time to resolution of symptoms. Based on this evidence, some prehospital protocols now include corticosteroid treatment as an option in patients with asthma. However, the effect of prehospital corticosteroid treatment on patient outcome is not known. **FIGURES 3-15, 3-16,** and **3-17** illustrate administration of inhaled bronchodilators.

TABLE 3-4 Asthma: Common Home Therapy Quick-Relief Medications for Acute Asthma Attacks

Class of Medication	Medication	Mechanism of Action
β_2 agonists	Inhaled bronchodilators (**albuterol** [salbutamol]), levalbuterol	Relax bronchiole smooth muscle; prevent bronchospasm; rapid onset of action
Anticholinergics	Inhaled anticholinergics (**ipratropium**)	Relax bronchiole smooth muscle; decrease secretions; rapid onset of action
Anti-inflammatory medications	Oral corticosteroids (prednisone)	Block allergic response; reduce airway hyperresponsiveness; improve response to bronchodilators; delayed onset of action (2–12 hours)

FIGURE 3-15 A nebulized bronchodilator can also be given without a mask using a blow-by technique.

FIGURE 3-17 One method for delivering a bronchodilator is with an oxygen-powered nebulizer.

FIGURE 3-16 A. A metered-dose inhaler and spacer can be used with or without a mask. **B.** A metered-dose inhaler with spacer and mask can be used in children as young as 6 months.

Bronchodilators. Early bronchodilator therapy, on the scene and on the way to the ED, helps immediately open airways, relieve respiratory distress, and improve oxygen delivery in asthma. In unstable or critical patients, continuous inhaled treatment with a β-agonist is the preferred approach, although IM epinephrine is acceptable in some patients who cannot cooperate with inhalation therapy, have severe respiratory distress, or have signs or symptoms consistent with anaphylaxis. For a step-by-step explanation of this procedure, see **Bronchodilator Therapy, Procedure 7** and **Intramuscular Injections, Procedure 14.** An in-line bronchodilator used with continuous positive airway pressure (CPAP) can be used on older children based on local protocols.

Pharmacologic Treatment of Wheezing. Albuterol (salbutamol) is the most commonly used inhaled bronchodilator. Because of its selective action on the bronchiole smooth muscles and its minimal effect on cardiac rate, the drug has a high margin of safety. In a critical child with wheezing, treat with the highest dose and give continuous treatment. Unit dose vials of albuterol (salbutamol) premixed with saline are used by most prehospital systems. These vials provide 2.5 mg of albuterol (salbutamol) in a total volume of 3 mL. One vial is an acceptable initial dose for almost all children and adolescents. For critical patients, the nebulizer may be refilled continuously, or two vials may be placed in the nebulizer initially and given immediately. Levalbuterol is an isomer of albuterol that has not been studied in the prehospital setting and has not been shown to offer any benefit over albuterol in the hospital setting.

Depending on local protocols, give ipratropium with albuterol (salbutamol). Ipratropium is an anticholinergic that may provide additional bronchodilatation in addition to β-agonists. Precautions include sensitivity to the effects of ipratropium or atropine. Adverse reactions include dry mouth, headache, cough, hoarseness, blurred vision, tachycardia, and occasionally flushing. Add it to a unit dose vial of albuterol (salbutamol), and administer together by nebulizer. Multiple doses of ipratropium provide added benefit in asthma exacerbations.

If a child cannot tolerate nebulized drug therapy or is moving air so poorly that the drug is not being inhaled, or in cases of possible anaphylaxis, give IM epinephrine. Transport with cardiac monitoring if frequent nebulized treatments or IM epinephrine is necessary. **TABLE 3-5** summarizes the drugs and doses for field bronchodilator therapy.

In most cases of known asthma, begin a bronchodilator on scene before transport and then give additional doses en route, as indicated.

TABLE 3-5 Management of Wheezing: Bronchodilator Treatment

Bronchodilator	Dose
Albuterol (salbutamol)	Nebulized solution (1.25 mg/3 mL, 2.5 mg/3 mL, 5 mg/mL) Minimum dose: 2.5–5 mg every 20 minutes for three doses. Repeat dose every 1–4 hours as needed. If not already prediluted, dilute in minimum of 2–3 mL saline for adequate nebulization. May use continuously for critical patients.
Ipratropium bromide inhalation solution	Nebulized solution (0.5 mg/2.5 mL). Children <12 years: 0.25 mg nebulized every 20 minutes for three doses. Children >12 years: 0.5 mg nebulized every 20 minutes for three doses.
Albuterol (salbutamol) metered-dose inhaler	90 mcg per puff. 4–8 puffs every 15–20 minutes for three doses.

Unit dose vials of 2.5 mg of albuterol (salbutamol) premixed with saline to a total volume of 3 mL may be used as an initial dose for children and adolescents of all ages. In critical patients, doses may be repeated continuously en route to the ED.

TIP

When a child fails to respond to assisted ventilation with improvement in clinical status, quickly assess your equipment—from the oxygen tank to the patient—for mechanical failure.

IM Injections. IM administration allows the medication to absorb slowly but steadily. The IM route may result in pain at the site (**FIGURE 3-18**). For a step-by-step explanation of this procedure, see **Intramuscular Injections, Procedure 14.**

Assisted Ventilation. Because of the severe air trapping associated with bronchospasm, assisted ventilation may be associated with many complications and death. Positive-pressure ventilation requires very high inspiratory pressures and may result in pneumothorax

Vastus lateralis

Deltoid

FIGURE 3-18 Common sites for IM injections.

or **pneumomediastinum**. Consider bag-mask ventilation and endotracheal intubation of a wheezing child only if the child is in respiratory failure and has failed to respond to high-flow oxygen and maximal bronchodilator therapy. While assisting ventilation in any patient with lower airway obstruction, slow rates (12–15 breaths/min in older children and adolescents, and a maximum rate of 20–30 breaths/min in infants) with long expiratory times are useful in minimizing barotrauma and complications.

Bronchiolitis

Bronchiolitis is a viral lower respiratory infection, which usually affects infants and children younger than 2 years of age. Often caused by **respiratory syncytial virus (RSV)**, this infection is widespread in the winter months. The infection leads to destruction of the lining of the bronchioles, profuse secretions, and bronchoconstriction. Infants are particularly likely to develop the infection because of their small airway size, high resistance to airflow, and poor airway clearance. Airway edema and debris from sloughed cells and mucus are much more important in the pathophysiology of this infection than bronchospasm and smooth muscle contraction.

Presenting complaints of bronchiolitis include upper respiratory infection symptoms, fever, cough, vomiting, poor feeding, poor sleep, and trouble breathing. Assessment shows variable degrees of increased work of breathing, tachypnea, diffuse wheezing, inspiratory crackles, and tachycardia.

Historic risk factors for respiratory failure in infants with suspected bronchiolitis include age younger than 2 months, history of prematurity, underlying lung disease, congenital heart disease, and immune deficiency. **TABLE 3-6** lists important clinical predictors of respiratory failure in children with suspected bronchiolitis. BLS treatment can include nasopharyngeal suctioning with a bulb syringe (see **Suctioning, Procedure 4**).

In the past, treatment of bronchiolitis included the use of bronchodilators, but studies have shown no benefit from their use in bronchiolitis. The most important treatment is bulb suctioning of the infant's nose. If the oxygen saturation is less than 94%, supply oxygen via nasal cannula or face mask.

Foreign Body Aspiration

Children with lower airway obstruction caused by foreign body aspiration usually are only mildly ill. Unlike foreign bodies in the upper airway, it is rare to develop respiratory failure or severe airway obstruction from a small foreign body in the lower airway. Foreign body aspiration is most common in older infants and toddlers (**FIGURE 3-19**). Often, there is an abrupt onset of coughing or choking that may be followed by a period of relatively few symptoms. Tachypnea, increased work of breathing, and wheezing or decreased breath sounds, which are usually unilateral unless the foreign body is in the trachea, may develop rapidly or over a period of hours to days. The absence of a history of asthma or the symptoms of an upper respiratory infection in a child of the right age should suggest the possibility of foreign body aspiration. General noninvasive treatment, including allowing the child to assume a position of comfort and providing oxygen if tolerated, should be given to all patients. A trial of inhaled bronchodilators is reasonable if the diagnosis is unclear, but do not delay transport. Additional diagnostic tests may be done after arrival at the ED.

TABLE 3-6 Predictors of Respiratory Failure in Suspected Bronchiolitis
Respiratory rate >60 breaths/min with increased work of breathing
Heart rate >200 beats/min or <100 beats/min
Poor appearance (using PAT)
Blood oxygen saturation <90% on supplemental oxygen

FIGURE 3-19 Examples of foreign bodies that can obstruct the airway.

© Jones & Bartlett Learning. Photographed by Kimberly Potvin.

Lung Disease

In children, most lung disease is caused by pneumonia. Pneumonia may cause symptoms of lower airway disease and respiratory distress or failure in children. Almost all children with pneumonia have fever or a history of fever at some point in their illness. Most pneumonias in children are caused by viruses such as influenza. These children generally have symptoms that are less severe and of a more gradual onset than children with bacterial pneumonia.

Bacterial pneumonia in children occurs after aspiration or hematogenous seeding of bacteria into the lung. This is followed by an acute inflammatory reaction leading to the accumulation of fluid within the airspaces of the lung. At times, this may be accompanied by the development of a pleural effusion, or collection of fluid in the pleural space outside the lung parenchyma. Children with bacterial pneumonia usually have symptoms including fever; shaking; chills; tachypnea; and frequently nonspecific complaints such as lethargy or irritability, poor appetite, and occasionally chest pain. Cough may not develop until after a period of other, more nonspecific symptoms.

Physical findings may include fever, tachypnea, increased work of breathing, decreased breath sounds, and rales. Grunting respirations are relatively common in young children with any form of lung disease. Wheezes may be heard, especially with viral infections, but are not as common as rales or decreased breath sounds. In the absence of underlying illness, disability, or very young age, it is unusual for a child to abruptly develop respiratory failure caused by pneumonia. Respiratory distress is more likely.

Approach children with suspected pneumonia like any patient with symptoms of lower airway disease. Making the diagnosis is not as important as providing good supportive care. Give general, noninvasive treatment to all patients. If the patient has wheezing, try bronchodilators. Patients with signs of respiratory failure may need assisted ventilation. Respiratory failure from lung disease is more commonly seen in young infants, children with underlying neurologic or pulmonary disease, and children who have been ill for several days. There is no specific prehospital therapy for children with pneumonia.

Disordered Control of Breathing

Sometimes hypoxia or respiratory insufficiency is caused by problems in control of breathing. This category of respiratory disease includes that resulting from brain injury, spinal injury, poisoning, metabolic problems (e.g., botulism, Guillain-Barré syndrome), postictal state, or sepsis. The hallmark of patients with disordered control of breathing is inadequate minute volume, from poor tidal volume or slow breathing rate. This can lead to hypoventilation, hypercarbia, and hypoxemia. Treatment includes opening the airway, ventilatory support with oxygen, bag-mask ventilation, and occasionally endotracheal intubation or other advanced airways.

Summary of Specific Treatment for Respiratory Distress

After identifying respiratory distress or failure and beginning general supportive measures, assess whether the anatomic level of the respiratory problem is in the upper or lower airway, using the PAT and the hands-on ABCDEs. Stridor is the hallmark of upper airway obstruction, wheezing is the hallmark of lower airway obstruction, grunting is the hallmark of lung disease, and inadequate minute volume and decreased work of breathing are the clinical markers for disordered control of breathing.

The most common cause of upper airway obstruction is croup. Specific treatment of croup includes nebulized epinephrine. Rarely, foreign bodies lodged at or above the vocal cords may be the cause of stridor in infants and toddlers. Frequent causes of lower airway obstruction are asthma and bronchiolitis—a disease of infants. Asthma is the most likely cause of wheezing in all children from infancy to adulthood. A nebulized bronchodilator, delivered continuously if necessary, is the specific treatment for asthma. Albuterol (salbutamol) and epinephrine have similar effectiveness as bronchodilators, and the anticholinergic ipratropium provides added benefit in patients with asthma. Start treatment on scene in those with asthma.

CASE STUDY 3

A caregiver calls 9-1-1 because a 4-month-old girl has had 3 days of cough, runny nose, and low-grade fever. The caregiver is concerned because the child seems to be working harder to breathe and is having a hard time taking feedings. On arrival, the child is found lying on the caregiver's lap. She appears sleepy and does not make eye contact or respond to examination. You note her neck and belly muscles are pulling in. She has audible wheezing and deep subcostal and intercostal retractions. There is nasal flaring. Her skin is mottled. On a more detailed assessment, her respiratory rate is 70 breaths/min and heart rate is 170 beats/min. She has only fair air movement, and you hear high-pitched, inspiratory and expiratory wheezes throughout. Pulse oximetry in room air is 78% with a pulse that corresponds to the patient's pulse on examination.

1. Is this child in respiratory distress or respiratory failure, and what is the level of airway obstruction?
2. What are the first steps in the management of this child?

Foreign body aspiration and pneumonia may present as lower airway problems, but there is no specific treatment for these conditions in the prehospital setting other than the general noninvasive measures for respiratory distress. Disordered control of breathing has many causes and often requires general ventilatory support.

Management of Acute Respiratory Distress: CPAP

In children, severe respiratory distress may be challenging to manage. Escalating therapy may mitigate or delay the need for invasive interventions such as endotracheal intubation. CPAP and noninvasive ventilation may provide a way to support and manage a child in acute respiratory distress and provide airway support. CPAP attempts to open the peripheral airways in the lungs (**FIGURE 3-20**). Increased airway pressure may also support peripheral small airways during expiration.

Although the literature is not robust, there is evidence to suggest that CPAP may improve breathing in children with a variety of respiratory diseases, particularly bronchiolitis and asthma. The utilization of CPAP may allow for airway support and potentially improvement in the child's status.

Management of Respiratory Failure

Regardless of the cause, initially treat every cooperative child in respiratory failure with general noninvasive measures. If upper or lower airway obstruction is present, attempt specific treatment. However, if the

FIGURE 3-20 A disposable, single-use CPAP device.
Mercury Medical.

child has altered appearance or altered mental status and has signs of increased or decreased work of breathing (e.g., flaring, grunting, gasping, apnea, or cyanosis), or if the child has a documented blood oxygen saturation of less than 90% on 100% oxygen via nonrebreathing mask, the child is in respiratory failure or respiratory arrest. For this child, bypass general noninvasive treatment and consider immediately beginning assisted ventilation.

First, position the patient to maintain an open airway, then use suction. Suctioning is a basic technique to maintain an open airway. Children have tiny airways that are easily obstructed by secretions, vomitus, pus, blood, or foreign bodies. For a step-by-step explanation, see **Suctioning, Procedure 4**.

If the patient is unresponsive, use an airway adjunct. Adjuncts may immediately improve the child's spontaneous ventilation. In addition, they may allow more effective bag-mask ventilation and reduce gastric inflation. For a step-by-step explanation of this procedure, see **Airway Adjuncts, Procedure 5**.

Next, deliver assisted ventilation or **positive-pressure ventilation** using a bag-mask device. Bag-mask ventilation is usually the best method for providing oxygenation and ventilation during stabilization and transport. Use an age-appropriate rate of 30 breaths/min in infants and 20 breaths/min in older children. Saying the words, "squeeze, release, release" helps time the ventilations to avoid a rate that is too rapid. Ensure that there is good chest rise. Good bag-mask technique decreases the risk of gastric distention, a common complication leading to elevation of the **diaphragm**, decreased lung compliance, and increased risk of vomiting and aspiration of gastric contents. With severe, lower airway obstruction, slower rates and longer expiratory times are indicated. Consider placing a nasogastric (NG) tube.

TIP

For an older child in respiratory failure who has increased work of breathing, ventilating at a rate of 20 breaths/min may assist the patient's respiratory effort.

Bag-Mask Ventilation

Bag-mask ventilation is one of the prehospital professional's most useful skills in pediatric prehospital care. Although the technique does not provide the definitive airway control that endotracheal intubation does, in most cases bag-mask ventilation is the best technique for providing oxygenation and ventilation during resuscitation and transport. For a step-by-step explanation of this procedure, see **Bag-Mask Ventilation, Procedure 8**.

CAUTION

Minimize gastric distention during bag-mask ventilation with good bagging technique.

TIP

If the child does not respond to bag-mask ventilation, or if there is a long transport time with a critically ill or injured child who has an unstable airway, consider endotracheal intubation.

ALS

Management With Endotracheal Intubation

The indications for endotracheal intubation of a child in the prehospital setting are limited and based on a careful and thorough assessment of risk versus benefit. Potential advantages of intubation include definitive airway control, decreased risk of aspiration, and ease of assisted ventilation. Potential complications include transient hypoxia and hypercapnia caused by prolonged intubation attempts; unrecognized misplacement of the tube; elevation of intracranial pressure; aspiration of stomach contents; and injury to the teeth, mouth, tongue, palate, larynx, and soft tissues of the pharynx and neck.

Dislodgment of the tube from the trachea during patient movement or transport is common and may be catastrophic. If an intubated patient fails to respond with improved color, oxygen saturation, heart rate, and appearance, the DOPE mnemonic may help to identify potential technical problems (**TABLE 3-7**). Most EMS systems require constant monitoring of proper placement of endotracheal tubes. Alternative advanced airways are also considerations for the treatment of ventilatory support; refer to local protocols and procedures.

CONTROVERSY

Avoid inserting a nasogastric or orogastric tube unless ventilation is impaired by a distended stomach and there is no facial trauma.

Nasogastric and Orogastric Insertion

During positive-pressure ventilation, it is common to inflate the stomach and the lungs with air. Gastric inflation with air slows downward movement of the diaphragm and decreases tidal volume, making ventilation more difficult and necessitating higher inspiratory pressures. In addition, inflation of the stomach with air increases the risk that the patient will vomit and aspirate. Gastric intubation with an NG or orogastric tube takes air from the stomach and helps positive-pressure ventilation. However, only use this technique if there is difficulty ventilating the patient. Insertion may be painful and frightening to the child and family. For a step-by-step explanation of this procedure, see **Orogastric and Nasogastric Tube Insertion, Procedure 10**.

TABLE 3-7 Troubleshooting the Endotracheal Tube: DOPE

	Problem	Assessment	Intervention
Dislodgments	Esophageal intubation	End-tidal carbon dioxide monitor or detector reads no or low carbon dioxide or has poor waveform, or no color change Oxygen saturation <90% Bradycardia Lack of chest rise with ventilation Auscultation of bubbling over the stomach	Extubate Bag-mask ventilation Reintubate
	Mainstem bronchus intubation	Asymmetric chest rise Asymmetric breath sounds	Pull tube back until breath sounds and chest rise are symmetric
	Accidental extubation	End-tidal carbon dioxide monitor/detector reads no or low carbon dioxide level, or has poor waveform, or no color change Oxygen saturation <90% Bradycardia Lack of chest rise with ventilation Poor or absent air movement on auscultation	Bag-mask ventilation Reintubate
Obstruction	Tube blocked with blood, secretions, or kink	Decreased chest rise Decreased breath sounds bilaterally Oxygen saturation <90% End-tidal carbon dioxide monitor/detector has abnormal waveform Increased resistance to bagging	Suction; if no improvement, extubate Bag-mask ventilation Reintubate
Pneumothorax	Tension pneumothorax, spontaneous or induced, compromises air exchange and may lead to decreased cardiac output	Asymmetric chest rise Asymmetric breath sounds Shock Oxygen saturation <90% *Jugular venous distention *Tracheal deviation	Needle thoracostomy
Equipment	Big air leak around tube Activated pop-off valve on resuscitator Oxygen tubing disconnected Oxygen tank empty	Oxygen saturation <90%	Check equipment, "patient-to-tank"

* Not easily assessed in young children.

Endotracheal Intubation

Successful endotracheal intubation allows optimal oxygenation and ventilation, provides a tube for medication delivery, and decreases the risk of aspiration and loss of airway control. A properly placed and secured endotracheal tube is a good tool for managing critical patients, but the procedure can take a long time, and there can be frequent and serious complications. Every placement of an advanced airway must be confirmed for proper placement of the device. Exhaled carbon dioxide colorimetric devices or in-line capnometry or capnography should be used during the confirmation process. For a step-by-step explanation of this procedure, see **Endotracheal Intubation, Procedure 11.**

Alternative Breathing and Intubation Techniques

Rarely, standard bag-mask ventilation fails and endotracheal intubation is difficult or impossible. Examples of such patients are children with massive head trauma and airway edema or hematoma of the mouth or upper airway, or infants with significant congenital or acquired airway abnormalities who cannot be ventilated. In such dire circumstances, some EMS systems allow prehospital professionals to perform advanced breathing techniques. These include use of a supraglottic airway, laryngeal tube, or dual lumen airway. Additional adjuncts to assist in endotracheal intubation include the gum elastic bougie and **drug-assisted intubation (DAI)**. Needle cricothyrotomy is another option, if necessary. None of these techniques has been well evaluated in children in the prehospital setting.

TABLE 3-8 summarizes the advantages and disadvantages of these alternative techniques. For a step-by-step explanation of supraglottic airways (LMA, i-gel), laryngeal tubes (King Airway), and gum elastic bougie, see **Advanced Airway Techniques, Procedure 13. Needle Thoracostomy, Procedure 23,** explains needle cricothyrotomy.

Confirmation of Endotracheal Tube Placement

Several products are currently available for confirming proper placement of the endotracheal tube. These include quantitative end-tidal carbon dioxide monitors or capnometers, which reflect the blood carbon dioxide tension (**FIGURE 3-21**), and colorimetric

TABLE 3-8 Advantages and Disadvantages of Rescue Breathing Techniques

Technique	Advantages	Disadvantages
Supraglottic airway devices (LMA, SALT, King LAD, i-gel)	Simple insertion Good airway seal Adapts to bag-mask equipment	Does not prevent aspiration
Gum elastic bougie	May facilitate endotracheal tube insertion	No equipment or data in infants and young children Prolonged attempts may worsen hypoxia
Dual lumen airway (e.g., Combitube), pharyngeotracheal lumen airway	Effective isolation of the airway Reduced risk of aspiration More reliable ventilation relative to bag-mask ventilation Does not require visualization of the glottis	Fatal complications may occur if the position of esophageal-tracheal tube is identified incorrectly Potential for esophageal trauma
Laryngeal tube/supralaryngeal airway (e.g., King LT-D)	Effective isolation of the airway Reduced risk of aspiration More reliable ventilation relative to bag-mask ventilation Does not require visualization of the glottis Less complicated to insert than esophageal-tracheal tube	Limited data published on the use of the laryngeal tube in children Potential for esophageal trauma
Drug-Assisted Intubation (DAI)	Paralyzes child and eliminates muscle resistance Improves visualization Allows mild hyperventilation	Drugs remove spontaneous breathing Drugs may decrease blood pressure or respiratory rate **Succinylcholine** may cause high potassium
Cricothyrotomy	Provides tiny airway for lifesaving oxygenation or ventilation Bypasses obstruction	Technically difficult Bleeding Injury to other neck structures

FIGURE 3-21 Normal end-tidal carbon dioxide waveform.

end-tidal carbon dioxide detectors that give a qualitative reading.

The optimal method for tube confirmation in children in the prehospital setting is continuous wave form capnometry. Because the child's airway is so short, even slight movement of the endotracheal tube can lead to extubation or mainstem intubation. If capnometry shows no carbon dioxide, or if the colorimetric detector fails to change color with ventilation, these are indications that the endotracheal tube may not be in the trachea. In such cases, remove the endotracheal tube, perform bag-mask ventilation, and reintubate after 1–2 minutes of oxygenation and ventilation.

The only exception to this approach is the patient in full cardiopulmonary arrest, where pulmonary circulation may be too low to generate detectable expired carbon dioxide. In this case, if the capnometer shows a low or absent end-tidal carbon dioxide reading, or if the colorimetric device shows a tan color (low carbon dioxide), observe for chest rise, auscultate bilaterally for air movement, and attempt to visualize the tube passing through the vocal cords by direct laryngoscopy. If the endotracheal tube seems to be in proper position, leave the tube in place.

TIP

The optimal method for tube confirmation in children in the prehospital setting is continuous waveform capnometry.

For a step-by-step explanation of these confirmation procedures, see **Confirmation of Endotracheal Tube Placement and End-Tidal Capnography, Procedure 12.**

Summary of Management of Respiratory Failure

Respiratory failure or arrest can result from many different insults to the airway, mechanics of breathing, or gas exchange. Infection, trauma, and bronchospasm are important causes in children. Think respiratory failure when primary assessment reveals a child with altered appearance in the setting of significantly increased or decreased work of breathing. Bradycardia, poor air movement, and low oxygen saturation are key findings. In a child with respiratory failure or respiratory arrest, immediately begin assisted ventilation with a bag-mask device at an age-appropriate rate. Avoid gastric insufflation. Add specific treatment for airway obstruction, such as an inhaled bronchodilator, if indicated. Perform endotracheal intubation cautiously and be alert for the frequent DOPE complications in the intubated child who suddenly worsens or fails to respond. Always confirm proper placement of the endotracheal tube with capnometry, colorimetric carbon dioxide detection, or an esophageal bulb or syringe. In some EMS systems, advanced or alternative breathing techniques are options in the child who cannot be ventilated by bag-mask ventilation or endotracheal intubation.

Primary Assessment: The Transport Decision—Stay or Go?

When a child has respiratory distress, begin general noninvasive treatment (position of comfort and oxygen) and consider specific treatment on scene. Never transport a child who is in respiratory failure without assisted ventilations. Also, never transport a child with a severely obstructed airway until after performing FBAO maneuvers. Immediate on-scene care to support breathing improves the outcomes of children with many respiratory emergencies. After opening the airway and providing assisted ventilation when necessary, or after simply giving general treatment, the prehospital professional must decide whether to stay on scene to assess further and treat specifically, or to go.

If the PAT and ABCDEs are normal and the child has no history of serious breathing problems, the child does not usually require urgent treatment or immediate transport. Take the time to get a focused history and physical examination and perform a detailed physical examination (trauma patient) on the scene if possible.

If the child has respiratory distress and signs of upper airway obstruction, transport is usually indicated after general noninvasive treatment. Consider specific treatment of suspected croup with a dose of nebulized epinephrine on the way to the ED, if available. *If the child has asthma and has lower airway obstruction with wheezing, begin specific treatment with bronchodilators on scene, and continue treatment during transport to the closest medical facility.* Call in advance and let the ED know what kind of patient is being transported to their facility.

For critical children, consider endotracheal intubation or other advanced or alternative airways if the child is in respiratory failure and ventilation by bag-mask device is ineffective, or if an airway is difficult to maintain. However, endotracheal intubation increases scene time and delays the time to definitive care at the ED. There has been a high rate of complications documented in prehospital studies of endotracheal intubation in children. Intubation skills tend to extinguish rapidly because they are used infrequently. In most cases, bag-mask ventilation is probably a better option.

Additional Assessment

If the child has minimal respiratory distress and there are no immediate safety concerns for the child or prehospital professional, consider obtaining the focused history and physical examination and performing a detailed physical examination (trauma patient) on scene. Use the SAMPLE mnemonic to find important features of the complete respiratory history. **TABLE 3-9** gives examples of a focused history in a child with a breathing problem.

> **TIP**
>
> When a child fails to respond to assisted ventilation with improvement in clinical status, quickly assess your equipment from the oxygen tank to the patient for mechanical failure.

Perform vigilant ongoing assessment of all children with respiratory distress or failure while on the way to the ED. Use the PAT to recall observational indicators of effective gas exchange, and watch respiratory rate, heart rate, and pulse oximetry. Be prepared to increase the level of respiratory support or to correct complications of therapy if the child worsens or fails to respond.

TABLE 3-9 SAMPLE Components in a Child With Respiratory Distress

Component	Explanation
Signs and symptoms	Onset and nature of shortness of breath Presence of hoarseness, stridor, or wheezing Presence and quality of cough; chest pain
Allergies	Known allergies: food, medications, environmental Cigarette smoke exposure
Medications	Exact names and doses of ongoing drugs, including metered-dose inhalers and over-the-counter medications Recent use of steroids Timing and amount of last dose Timing and dose of analgesics and antipyretics
Past medical problems	History of asthma, chronic lung disease, or heart problems or prematurity Prior hospitalizations for breathing problems Prior intubations for breathing problems Immunizations
Last food or liquid	Timing of the child's last food or drink, including bottle or breastfeeding
Events leading to the injury or illness	Evidence of increased work of breathing Fever history

CASE STUDY ANSWERS

CASE STUDY 1

The child's general appearance is normal: he looks anxious, but makes eye contact and cries when you approach. The child's work of breathing is increased with marked supraclavicular and suprasternal retractions and nasal flaring. His color is pink. He has a normal circulatory status (pink with good perfusion).

This child is in respiratory distress, but does not seem to have progressed to respiratory failure. He is exhibiting many of the signs and symptoms of upper airway obstruction. His loud, harsh inspiratory breath sounds are consistent with stridor. This sound, along with the supraclavicular and suprasternal retractions, help localize the obstruction to the upper airway. He has increased work of breathing, but does not show any signs of hypoxia or hypercapnia (carbon dioxide retention). Upper airway obstruction and stridor in a young child after a few days of an upper respiratory infection are most consistent with croup, a swelling in the trachea below the area of the vocal cords caused by a viral infection. Other problems that may cause upper airway obstruction include foreign bodies, bacterial infections (e.g., epiglottitis or retropharyngeal abscess), and airway edema caused by allergic reactions.

Regardless of the cause, the management of children with upper airway obstruction is similar and is based on the severity of the symptoms. Keep this patient in a position of comfort, give oxygen for a pulse oximetry of <94%, and transport to an ED for further care.

Nebulized medications (e.g., epinephrine or racemic epinephrine) act as vasoconstrictors and decrease airway edema. These may be helpful en route to the ED. The child should be closely monitored because his upper airway obstruction may progress and respiratory failure may develop.

CASE STUDY 2

This is a choking child who needs BLS maneuvers first and, if unsuccessful, progression to ALS maneuvers by removing the FBAO using pediatric Magill forceps. This cannot be accomplished until the patient becomes unconscious. If the level of training prohibits the use of ALS skills, rapid transport to the ED while continuing chest compressions and ventilation or calling for an ALS intercept should be considered.

CASE STUDY 3

Using the PAT, this child has an increased work of breathing, abnormal appearance, and poor circulation to the skin. She is in respiratory failure. Her wheezes and subcostal and intercostal retractions localize her airway obstruction to her lower airways. In the setting of preceding upper respiratory symptoms, fever, and progressive lower airway obstruction, the child probably has bronchiolitis. Open the child's airway, suction her nose, give high-flow oxygen, and begin bag-mask ventilation. Do not delay transport because the child is not likely to have an easily reversible condition. This is unlike the child with asthma, who will likely benefit from a dose of a bronchodilator begun on scene, before transport.

SUGGESTED REFERENCES

Textbooks

American Heart Association. *Textbook of Pediatric Advanced Life Support*. Dallas, TX: American Heart Association; 2011.

Gausche M. *Pediatric Airway Management for the Prehospital Professional*. Burlington, MA: Jones and Bartlett Learning; 2004.

Articles

Anders J, Brown K, Simpson J, Gausche-Hill M. Evidence and controversies in pediatric prehospital airway management. *Clin Pediatr Emerg Med.* 2014;15(1):28–37.

Bhende MS, Thompson AE, Orr RA. Evaluation of an end-tidal CO$_2$ detector during pediatric cardiopulmonary resuscitation. *Pediatrics.* 1995; 96(5 Pt 1):983.

Brownstein D, Shugerman R, Cummings P. Prehospital endotracheal intubation of children by paramedics. *Ann Emerg Med.* 1996;28:34–39.

Gausche M, Lewis R, Stratton S, et al. Effect of out-of-emergency department pediatric tracheal intubation on survival and neurologic outcome: controlled clinical trial. *JAMA*. 2000;283:783–790.

Jat KR, Mathew JL. Continuous positive airway pressure (CPAP) for acute bronchiolitis in children. *Cochrane Database Syst Rev*. 2019;1:CD010473. doi: 10.1002/14651858.CD010473.pub3.

Kellner JD, Ohlsson A, Gadomski AM, et al. Efficacy of bronchodilator therapy in bronchiolitis—a meta-analysis. *Arch Pediatr Adolesc Med*. 1999;153(4):430.

Lerner EB, Dayan PS, Brown K, et al. Characteristics of the pediatric patients treated by the Pediatric Emergency Care Applied Research Network's affiliated EMS agencies. *Prehosp Emerg Care*. 2014; 18(1):52–59. doi: 10.3109/10903127.2013.836262.

Menon K, Sutcliffe T, Klassen T. A randomized trial comparing the efficacy of epinephrine with salbutamol in the treatment of acute bronchiolitis. *J Pediatr*. 1995;126:1004–1007.

Qureshi F, Pestian J, Davis P, et al. Effect of nebulized ipratropium on hospitalization rates of children with asthma. *N Engl J Med*. 1998;339:1030–1035.

Sharieff GQ, Rodarte A, Wilton N, et al. The self-inflating bulb as an airway adjunct: is it reliable in children weighing less than 20 kilograms? *Acad Emerg Med*. 2003;10:303–308.

Vitaliti G, Vitaliti MC, Finocchiaro MC, et al. Randomized comparison of helmet CPAP versus high-flow nasal cannula oxygen in pediatric respiratory distress. *Respir Care*. 2017;62(8):1036–1042. doi: 10.4187/respcare.05384.

Zar HJ, Ferkol TW. The global burden of respiratory disease-impact in children. *Pediatr Pulmonol*. 2014; 49(5):430–434. DOI: 10.1002/ppul.23030.

© Kali9/E+/Getty Images.

CHAPTER 4

Shock

Kathleen M. Brown, MD, FACEP, FAAP

Michael S. Riley, NRP, EMS-I

LEARNING OBJECTIVES

1. Describe how to assess circulation using the PAT, ABCDEs, and additional assessment.
2. Explain the relationship between shock and blood pressure.
3. Differentiate between compensated and hypotensive (decompensated) hypovolemic shock, and discuss appropriate management.
4. Distinguish the types of shock (hypovolemic, distributive, cardiogenic, and obstructive), and outline treatment.
5. Review septic shock, and discuss need for rapid recognition and therapy.

Introduction

Emergencies involving shock, or inadequate perfusion, may be the result of hypovolemia, increased vascular permeability, cardiac failure, output obstruction, or a combination of any or all of these causes. **Hypovolemia** is the most common cause of inadequate perfusion in children, often precipitated by acute gastrointestinal losses from viral illnesses. Traumatic hemorrhage is a less frequent **etiology** for severe hypovolemia in children. Regardless of the type of emergency involving hypoperfusion, early recognition and timely management can reduce the likelihood of serious morbidity or mortality.

Most perfusion problems in children arise from loss of intravascular fluid. The child's young, healthy cardiovascular system compensates for fluid loss by increasing heart rate and reducing blood flow to

CASE STUDY 1

A father calls 9-1-1 about a 6-month-old boy with a fever of 6 hours duration. On your arrival, the child is listless. He will not interact and cries inconsolably when held. There are no abnormal airway sounds. Breathing is rapid without retractions or flaring. There is a purplish rash of the face, trunk, and legs. The brachial pulse is faint, the skin is warm to touch, and **capillary refill time (CRT)** is approximately 4 seconds. Respiratory rate (RR) is 60 breaths/min, and blood pressure is 50 mm Hg by palpation. The cardiac monitor shows a heart rate (HR) of 190 beats/min.

1. What type of shock is present?
2. What differs in the management of this case versus treatment of pure hypovolemic or cardiogenic shock?

nonessential anatomic areas through the mechanism of **peripheral vasoconstriction**, or "clamping down." Vasoconstriction limits blood flow to less essential peripheral sites, such as the skin, and preserves blood flow to the "core" organs, such as the brain, heart, lungs, and kidneys. The physiologic process of restricting circulation to such areas as the skin and mucous membranes results in important physical signs of **hypoperfusion**. Children have a great ability to compensate for hypovolemia using these mechanisms and may maintain a normal blood pressure for age despite significant hypovolemia. However, if not treated, they can quickly decompensate; at that point, hypovolemic resuscitation efforts may be less successful. **Early recognition of hypoperfusion is critical.**

Distributive shock is less common in children and is usually caused by **sepsis**. This type of shock primarily involves loss of vascular tone. Additionally, distributive shock can result from anaphylaxis, spinal cord injury, and toxin exposures.

Cardiogenic shock is unusual in pediatrics, except in children with **congenital heart disease**, **dysrhythmias**, or acquired **viral myocarditis**. Cardiogenic shock results from heart rates that are either too fast or too slow to support perfusion or from primary congestive heart failure. Regardless of the underlying cause, cardiac output is insufficient to meet perfusion requirements.

Obstructive shock is the rarest of all shock types in children. It is caused by **pericardial tamponade** or **tension pneumothorax**, secondary to injury to the chest. A third cause, pulmonary emboli, is extremely rare in children.

Identifying the type of shock can be difficult, especially when the **pathophysiology** is mixed. For example, bacterial toxins or ingested poisons may have adverse effects on **vascular tone** and **myocardial function**; sepsis may involve a volume deficit from third spacing (loss of plasma from the vascular space because of leaky blood vessels) and loss of vascular tone and **myocardial depression**. However, a careful history and physical assessment usually identify the cause of shock and drive appropriate management. Shock from any cause, if unrecognized or inadequately treated, may advance to cardiac arrest. After arrest has occurred, successful resuscitation is unlikely.

Prearrival Preparation

Based on the dispatch information, prepare mentally for the assessment and management of a child with circulatory problems en route to the scene. Recall appropriate techniques for assessment; the role of vital signs; and the possible equipment, drug, and fluid requirements of the child. Consider when to stay and treat on scene and when to transport immediately.

Scene Size-Up

Be sure that the scene is safe. Evaluate the environment, and document potentially important features, especially concerns for child maltreatment.

General Assessment: The Pediatric Assessment Triangle

Evaluating the Presenting Complaint

On arrival, determine the child's presenting complaint. Key questions include the onset of illness, presence of fever, risk factors for sepsis, frequency and amount of fluid losses (vomiting and diarrhea), when the child last ate or drank, and prior history of possible congenital or cardiovascular problems. Ask if the child has been injured. In children with mild circulatory compromise who are not in shock, obtain a more complete SAMPLE history during the additional assessment.

Assessment of Circulation

Using the Pediatric Assessment Triangle

The Pediatric Assessment Triangle (PAT) is the first step in assessment of perfusion, as outlined in Chapter 1. The PAT evaluates three characteristics: (1) appearance, (2) work of breathing, and (3) circulation to skin. Knowing these characteristics helps to determine whether the child is sick or not sick, the type of physiologic abnormality, and the urgency for treatment. Circulatory problems affect each of these characteristics in identifiable patterns.

Appearance

First, assess the child's appearance. A child with decreased core circulation from any shock type may have signs of poor brain perfusion. The abnormality in the child's appearance will be variable, depending on the type of perfusion problem; the degree of circulatory insufficiency; and the presence of associated problems, such as fever, head trauma, or intoxication. Abnormalities in the appearance of a child with decreased core circulation include the following:

- Lethargy or listlessness
- Decreased motor activity

- Diminished interactiveness with caregivers, the prehospital professional, and the environment (**FIGURE 4-1**)
- Inconsolability
- Poor eye contact
- Weak cry

Sometimes the child in shock is restless and inconsolable. Appearance alone, however, is not a very accurate sign of inadequate perfusion. An abnormal appearance may be caused by many different things, such as poor oxygenation and ventilation, head trauma, hypothermia, drugs, or fever. Assessing appearance is a good way to tell if the child is ill, but not a good way to identify the physiologic cause. Assessment tools other than the PAT, such as the hands-on ABCDE assessment, help distinguish the type of physiologic problem and the presence or absence of abnormal perfusion.

Work of Breathing

Next, assess the work of breathing. If circulation to vital organs is decreased, the child's respiratory rate increases. "Effortless tachypnea," sometimes known as "silent tachypnea," is a fast respiratory rate without increased work of breathing. Effortless tachypnea is a common but nonspecific sign of shock. It reflects the child's attempt to blow off carbon dioxide and reduce the **metabolic acidosis** created by decreased perfusion to cells. Signs of increased work of breathing, such as abnormal positioning, retractions, flaring, or abnormal airway sounds (e.g., grunting, stridor, or wheezing) are not usually present in a child without a corresponding respiratory problem. These signs reflect poor gas

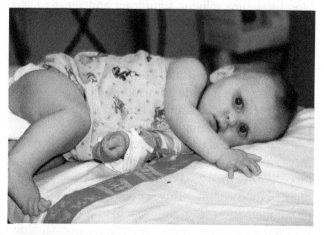

FIGURE 4-1 A child with decreased core circulation and too little blood and oxygen to the brain has an abnormal appearance. This dehydrated child has listlessness, poor motor activity, and decreased interactiveness.

Courtesy of Ronald A. Dieckmann.

exchange and **hypoxia**, typically from a primary lung problem. Although increased work of breathing is most commonly a function of respiratory disease, these signs may also occur with hypoxia and **pulmonary edema**, when cardiogenic shock results from **congestive heart failure**, or in anaphylaxis when the respiratory system is a target organ.

Circulation to Skin

After assessing appearance and work of breathing, assess circulation by looking at skin color. This is difficult to interpret if the environmental temperature is low, because **vasoconstriction**, as a reflexive effort to preserve heat, falsely alters skin findings, especially in infants. If possible, disrobe the child and look for mottling, pallor, and cyanosis, which reflect peripheral vasoconstriction or clamping down of nonessential skin perfusion to maintain essential core circulation. If a child has abnormal appearance and abnormal skin signs in a warm ambient environment, the child may be in shock.

Primary Assessment: The ABCDEs

After the PAT, perform the hands-on ABCDE assessment. After evaluating airway and breathing, as described in the previous chapters, assess circulation. There are four parts to the assessment of circulation: (1) HR, (2) pulse quality, (3) skin temperature and CRT, and (4) blood pressure.

Heart Rate

First, measure HR by feeling a pulse for 30 seconds, and then double the number. A normal HR is between 60 and 160 beats/min, depending on the child's age (see Chapter 2, Table 2-3, for a list of vital sign ranges in children). The radial or brachial areas are preferred sites to measure the pulse rate in infants and children. The carotid pulse is acceptable in older children and adolescents, but it is hard to locate in infants. If a pulse is difficult to feel, determine HR by listening to the heart sounds directly with a stethoscope placed on the medial side of the child's left nipple. However, be aware that the presence of a "normal" HR by auscultation does not necessarily reflect adequate cardiac output and perfusion.

Interpreting HR may be difficult, as explained in Chapter 1. Ranges of normal HR change inversely with advancing age. Also, many conditions can increase HR, ranging from serious physiologic problems to noxious stimuli that are rarely life threatening. Stimuli that can cause **tachycardia** include pain, fever, fear, cold, and anger. Interpret HR in the context of overall signs of perfusion, age, presence or absence of noxious stimuli, and observed trends. Although a single measurement of HR is usually of limited value in determining the degree of physiologic derangement, a trend of mounting tachycardia, or a HR that is falling below the lower limits of normal, suggests a serious physiologic problem. In addition, sustained tachycardia is a worrisome sign. Finally, be extremely vigilant when the child has **bradycardia**. This may indicate hypoxia or an advanced state of hypoperfusion.

Pulse Quality

Presence of a strong central pulse (carotid, femoral, or brachial in infants) with a strong peripheral pulse (**brachial**, **radial**, or **pedal** in children) suggests an adequate blood pressure. A strong central pulse with a weak peripheral pulse indicates a shock-like state. If a brachial pulse is not palpable, the child is probably hypotensive and in hypotensive (decompensated) shock.

> **TIP**
>
> Tachycardia is often the first sign of shock in a pediatric patient.

Skin Temperature and Capillary Refill Time (CRT)

The next part of the hands-on cardiovascular assessment involves evaluating skin signs. Check skin temperature for warmth at the hands, feet, thighs, or forearms. Cool hands and feet may be normal, but cool proximal extremities reflect poor perfusion and shunting of blood to the core. Determine CRT by pressing firmly on the skin. CRT should be less than 2–3 seconds in a child who is not cold (**FIGURE 4-2**). Again, inadequate core perfusion results in peripheral vasoconstriction, which manifests as cool skin and delayed CRT. Although CRT is a good test of circulation in children, it must be interpreted in the context of overall signs of perfusion. The prehospital professional can become comfortable with the technique and interpretation of the key skin findings by practicing on every child.

Blood Pressure

Last, consider taking a blood pressure. A high blood pressure value is not clinically significant in the field, unless the child has a history of hypertension, known

A

B

FIGURE 4-2 To determine CRT, first depress the skin **(A)**, and then count the seconds before color returns **(B)**. Capillary refill time should be less than 2–3 seconds in a child who is not cold.

renal disease, or acute head injury. However, a low blood pressure value is significant and means hypotensive (decompensated) shock. A normal blood pressure does not rule out a shock-like state. **Children in significant shock may have normal blood pressures until they decompensate.** The challenges in the prehospital setting include knowing when to get a blood pressure reading, obtaining the blood pressure correctly, and interpreting it accurately.

Systolic blood pressure does not accurately reflect **intravascular volume** status until the acute volume loss is greater than 25%–35% of normal circulating pediatric blood volume. This is because of the efficiency of compensation in a child, including vasoconstriction and an increase in HR. Therefore, a normal blood pressure does not mean the child has a normal blood volume or normal perfusion. A normal minimal systolic blood pressure in a child older than 1 year of age is 70 + (2 × years of age). Proper equipment, technique, and patience are required to obtain an accurate blood pressure in an infant or toddler. Because this can be a time-consuming process and may not contribute greatly to the clinical assessment of perfusion, especially in very young children, more time should be spent on assessing other signs of perfusion than on attempting to obtain a blood pressure measurement. Inadequate perfusion is better reflected in the other signs of perfusion described previously (skin color, HR, pulse quality, CRT, and skin temperature). In a child older than 3 years of age, make at least one blood pressure attempt in every patient. Use a cuff with a width two-thirds the length of the upper arm. Applying too large a cuff falsely decreases the blood pressure measurement.

CAUTION

A normal blood pressure does not rule out shock.

TIP

In children, one can use the combination of tachycardia, poor pulse quality, delayed CRT, and decreased mental status to diagnose shock, even with a normal blood pressure.

Additional Assessment

If the child is stable after the primary assessment and does not require immediate treatment, and if there are no immediate safety concerns for the child or prehospital professional, conduct history taking and physical examination and the detailed physical examination (trauma patient) on scene. Use the SAMPLE mnemonic (**TABLE 4-1**) to recall important features of the history in a child with inadequate perfusion. Use age-appropriate approaches to gain the child's trust and speak directly to him or her. Ask the caregiver to add to the child's history. Obtain the history from the caregiver if the child is too young to speak or is unable to cooperate.

After the history, perform a focused examination of the heart, peripheral circulation, and the abdomen. Then, do an anatomic examination of the entire body, as outlined in Chapter 1. If the child has a traumatic injury, also do a detailed physical examination, searching for other injuries.

Perform an ongoing assessment of all children with perfusion problems while on the way to the emergency department (ED). The child's status may

TABLE 4-1 SAMPLE Components in a Child With Hypoperfusion Problems

Component	Features
Signs/ Symptoms	Presence of vomiting or diarrhea Number of episodes of vomiting or diarrhea Vomiting blood or bile External hemorrhage Presence or absence of fever Rash Respiratory distress or shortness of breath (e.g., in cardiogenic shock with congestive heart failure)
Allergies	Known allergies History of anaphylaxis
Medications	Exact names and dosages of ongoing medications Use of laxatives or antidiarrheal medications Chronic diuretic therapy Potential exposure to other medications or drugs Timing and doses of analgesic/antipyretics
Past medical problems	History of heart problems History of prematurity Prior hospitalizations for cardiovascular problems History of cancer, transplant, adrenal problems, or immunosuppressive medication
Last food or liquid	Timing of the child's last food or drink, including bottle or breast feedings
Events leading to the injury or illness	Travel Trauma Fever history Symptoms in family members Potential toxic exposure

change during transport, so observe and document any physiologic trends. Use the PAT to monitor effective perfusion, and watch respiratory rate, HR, blood pressure, and pulse oximetry. Keep a child who is in shock on a cardiac monitor. Be prepared to increase the level of respiratory and cardiovascular support if the child worsens or fails to respond to treatment.

Summary of Cardiovascular Assessment

The PAT provides a good first-line evaluation of perfusion: abnormal appearance, normal work of breathing, and poor circulation to skin suggest a perfusion problem. Pallor, mottling, and cyanosis all indicate poor peripheral perfusion. The circulatory portion of the hands-on ABCDEs consists of evaluating HR, pulse quality, skin temperature, CRT, and blood pressure. These physical features complement the PAT and help identify the type and severity of circulatory compromise. Vital signs can sometimes be misleading and must be correctly obtained and interpreted for age. Trends in vital signs or persistence in abnormal vital signs, such as tachycardia, are more accurate indicators of real physiologic problems than mild vital sign abnormalities on primary assessment.

Using the Assessment to Identify Shock

Shock is inadequate perfusion at the tissue level, with insufficient oxygen delivery to maintain normal cellular function. Oxygenation and ventilation, HR, intravascular volume, myocardial function, and vascular stability are all determinants of effective systemic cardiovascular function. If any one of these factors is impaired by illness or injury, the body attempts to compensate and normalize perfusion through modification of other physiologic components.

In a child, the same physiologic components are at work as in an adult. However, there are some differences. The physiologic compensatory mechanisms, such as vasoconstriction and tachycardia, are very efficient in a child. Vasoconstriction is so efficient that a line of demarcation can sometimes be seen on extremities and mottling may be evident when circulation to the capillary beds has become stagnant. Sweating as

a response to compensation, although common in an adult, does not always occur in a young child. Therefore, most children in shock have cool, dry skin versus pale, cool, diaphoretic skin. By adolescence, sweating as a response to compensation for shock is consistent. The last difference involves the child's energy reserves. A child does not have the amount of energy reserves that are had by an adult. The younger the child, the less is the capacity for energy reserves. Infants in particular have high glucose needs with low energy stores. As a result, compensatory mechanisms, although efficient, cannot last as long as those of an adult. **Checking a blood glucose level is important in any child who is suspected of being in shock.**

Because of these differences, clinical signs of decreased perfusion include altered mental status, persistent tachycardia as a compensatory mechanism, and changes in skin color and temperature as a result of vasoconstriction. Do not expect sweating unless the child has increased work of breathing and is building up body heat. As long as vasoconstriction, increased HR, and increased myocardial contraction are supported by the child's reserves, systolic pressure is maintained and the child compensates. When the body's reserves begin to fail or are exhausted, perfusion to the vital organs, such as the brain, is compromised. Blood pressure falls, mental status is impaired, and organ systems fail.

There are four general classes of shock (hypovolemic, distributive, cardiogenic, and obstructive) (**TABLE 4-2**), reflecting impairment of the three major functional components of circulation: (1) the blood volume (hypovolemic), (2) the vascular system (distributive), and (3) the heart (cardiogenic and obstructive). Studies of hypovolemia (the most common type of pediatric shock) have allowed researchers to describe the clinical signs that characterize the progression of shock from a compensated state (adequate systolic blood pressure) to an uncompensated state (hypotension). However, the clinical signs characterizing the progression of distributive, cardiogenic, or

CASE STUDY 2

9-1-1 receives a call about a lethargic 6-year-old girl. On your arrival, she is lying in bed and barely notices your entrance. There is no increased work of breathing, but you do notice that she is breathing fast. Her color is pale. Vital signs are as follows: HR, 160 beats/min; RR, 40 breaths/min; BP, 70/40 mm Hg; SpO$_2$, 99% in room air. Her capillary refill is 4 seconds. Her mother states that she has been having vomiting and diarrhea for 3 days and cannot keep anything down.

1. Is this patient in shock?
2. If so, what type of shock is this?
3. What is the prehospital treatment?

TABLE 4-2 Summary of Different Types of Shock

Shock Type	Physiologic Insult	Common Causes	Treatment
Hypovolemic	Volume loss	Hemorrhage Gastroenteritis (vomiting, diarrhea) Burns Prolonged poor fluid intake	Rapid transport Oxygen administration Intravenous fluid boluses
Distributive	Decreased vascular tone	Sepsis Anaphylaxis Drug overdose Spinal cord injury (neurogenic shock)	Rapid transport Oxygen administration Fluid administration Epinephrine for anaphylaxis Epinephrine or norepinephrine for septic shock
Cardiogenic	Heart failure	Congenital heart disease Cardiomyopathy Dysrhythmia Drug overdose	Rapid transport Oxygen administration Cautious crystalloid fluid administration, 10 mL/kg Consider a vasopressor, such as dopamine, dobutamine, epinephrine, or norepinephrine For drug overdose, consider antidote therapy
Obstructive	Obstructed blood flow	Pericardial tamponade Pneumothorax	Rapid transport Oxygen administration Needle thoracostomy Fluid administration

obstructive shock are not as well defined. This reflects the complex physiology of these other forms of shock.

Hypovolemic Shock

Hypovolemia (loss of fluid) is the most common cause of shock in children in the prehospital setting. Vomiting and diarrhea from gastroenteritis is the most common cause of hypovolemic shock. Bleeding from blunt injuries, such as falls or vehicle collisions with the child as a pedestrian, bicyclist, or passenger, is the most common cause of hemorrhagic hypovolemic shock.

The signs and symptoms of hypovolemic shock vary with the amount, duration, and timing of fluid loss. As intravascular volume is further compromised by ongoing fluid losses (such as profuse diarrhea or continued bleeding), the child may progress from compensated to decompensated shock.

Compensated Hypovolemic Shock

Children who lose bodily fluids through minor blood loss or dehydration from gastroenteritis usually show no clinically significant effects on circulation. However, if fluid losses are more than about 5% of body weight, the body compensates for decreased blood flow by predictable adjustments in cardiovascular physiology. Sympathetic stimulation results in vasoconstriction and an increase in HR or tachycardia. As long as these processes maintain cardiac output to core organ systems, perfusion is maintained. This is compensated shock.

Vasoconstriction causes the following signs of abnormal circulation to the skin: delayed CRT, decreased pulse strength, poor skin color (pallor or mottling), and dry and cool or cold skin temperature. A cold environment or hypothermia may also cause vasoconstriction as a reflex to maintain body heat, which mimics poor perfusion. **Systolic blood pressure is normal in compensated shock.**

In the compensated stage of hypovolemic shock, appearance may be normal, or the child may appear slightly restless or less interactive. In a child with gastroenteritis, the appearance may be abnormal because of fever, which can alter appearance regardless of the circulatory status.

Hypotensive (Decompensated) Hypovolemic Shock

In hypotensive shock, perfusion is profoundly affected because compensatory mechanisms (increased HR and peripheral vasoconstriction) have failed to maintain sufficient circulation to core organs. The clinical signs are those of organ failure. Although a child in hypotensive shock may still be alert on AVPU, assessment of appearance is abnormal because of inadequate brain perfusion. The child may be restless and agitated, or poorly responsive. Hypotension, or low blood pressure for age, develops when there is about a 25% loss of intravascular volume (blood volume). Other late signs are effortless or silent tachypnea, extreme tachycardia, extreme pallor or presence of mottling, and cold skin temperature. If not reversed, hypotensive shock leads to cardiac failure, with bradycardia and respiratory failure, and then to cardiac arrest.

Although the course is less predictable, decreasing perfusion in children with distributive, cardiogenic, or obstructive shock results in progressive changes in appearance, skin signs, and work of breathing. For example, a child with cardiogenic shock may present only with tachycardia and diminished peripheral perfusion, and then progress to respiratory distress and lethargy as cardiac output worsens and congestive heart failure develops. In all shock types, hypotension is an ominous sign. More than one type of shock can occur concurrently in the same patient, as previously described.

Distributive Shock

In distributive shock, the child has decreased vascular muscle tone (peripheral vasodilation), impaired vascular integrity, or both in the presence of a normal circulating blood volume. This creates a relative hypovolemia, and can be thought of as operating with a "less than full" tank. This change in the capacity of the vascular system and relative hypovolemia leads to hypoperfusion to vital organs because of loss of vascular integrity. Patients with distributive shock may also have a component of hypovolemia. This is the case in a patient with sepsis, who in addition to loss of vascular tone has "capillary leak" caused by the effect of bacterial toxins—or, in the case of anaphylaxis, where capillary leak may occur in the lungs or in the target tissues. In these situations, hypovolemia is the result of "third spacing" of fluid from the vascular space into the surrounding tissues.

The most common cause of distributive shock is sepsis. Identification of patients in early septic shock is challenging, especially in children where hypotension is usually a late finding. However prehospital providers should maintain a high index of suspicion in patients with fever, tachycardia, and signs of poor perfusion. Patients with known risk factors such as cancer and chronic immunodeficiency, including sickle cell disease, are at higher risk, but sepsis can develop in healthy children as well. Recognition is key, as early therapy can improve patients' outcomes.

Other causes of distributive shock include anaphylaxis, chemical intoxication with drugs that decrease vascular tone (e.g., β-blockers, barbiturates), and spinal cord injury (above T6) with interruption of spinal sympathetic nerves to the muscle walls of peripheral arteries.

Special Features in Assessment of Distributive Shock

Signs of distributive shock reflect low peripheral vascular resistance (warm skin, bounding pulses, wide pulse pressure, changes in HR, hypotension) and decreased organ perfusion (abnormal appearance and behavior). These signs may vary with the specific cause, as noted in the descriptions of the three major types of shock. Although the progression of physical signs in distributive shock is not as predictable as that in hypovolemic shock, the late findings are indistinguishable from those of hypotensive shock from any cause: abnormal appearance from poor brain perfusion and hypotension.

Major Types of Distributive Shock
Sepsis

Sepsis occurs when any type of infection, usually bacterial or viral, overwhelms the body's defense system and sets in motion a systemic reaction called systemic inflammatory response syndrome (SIRS). This leads to a generalized breakdown in core organ function, or multiple organ failure. Both can lead to death or serious long-term morbidity.

Distinctive signs of early septic shock are warm skin, tachycardia, and bounding pulses. A septic child's appearance is abnormal and may include listlessness, lethargy, decreased interactiveness, restlessness, and poor consolability. Rash, fever, poor feeding, vomiting, diarrhea, and fussiness may also be present. This early phase may be brief, and patients with sepsis shock often present with signs of poor perfusion, similar to those with hypovolemic shock.

Ill children usually like to be held and cuddled. If a child with a fever does not want to be held but is more comfortable when left alone, the child may have paradoxical irritability. This may be a sign of meningitis, where movement irritates the inflamed meninges (membranes covering the spinal cord and brain).

Sometimes, a septic child has a petechial rash or purpura (nonblanching dark red or purple dots or splotches) (FIGURE 4-3). These skin lesions are the result of toxins that cause inflammation of the blood

FIGURE 4-3 Purpura.
© Jonathan ORourke/Alamy Stock Photo.

vessels and leakage of blood into the skin. Consider a child with shock in association with a rash and fever to be septic. He or she may require aggressive volume resuscitation in the field, and prehospital professionals should use strict infection-control practices, including masks, to decrease their risk of infection.

Anaphylaxis

Anaphylaxis is a major allergic reaction that involves a generalized, multisystem response to an **antigen** (foreign protein). The airways and cardiovascular system are important sites of this often life-threatening reaction. Common causes include insect stings by bees, wasps, or fire ants; peanuts; latex; or medication. A child in anaphylactic shock has hypoperfusion and possibly additional signs, such as stridor or wheezing, with increased work of breathing. The child also has altered appearance with restlessness and agitation and sometimes a sense of impending doom. **Hives** (an intensely itchy skin rash) (**FIGURE 4-4**) and angioedema

FIGURE 4-4 Hives suggest an allergic reaction and are usually present with anaphylaxis, the most extreme form of an allergic reaction.
© nidchita/Shutterstock.

TABLE 4-3 Drug Intoxications That May Cause Shock
Antihypertensives
β-blockers
Calcium antagonists
Clonidine
Cyclic antidepressants
Iron
Opioids
Phenothiazines

(flushed, swollen skin) are also common. Signs and symptoms of anaphylactic shock are dependent on the target organ. This is why some victims of anaphylaxis present with vomiting, diarrhea, and hives, whereas others have angioedema, wheezing, and stridor.

Shock From Drug Intoxication

There are numerous cardiovascular drugs that can cause loss of vascular tone and hypoperfusion when ingested. **TABLE 4-3** lists common agents. The mechanism usually involves direct depressant effect on the cardiovascular system (slowing of the HR, decreased strength of contraction, and vasodilation).

Neurogenic Shock

Neurogenic shock is rare in children. It results from a mechanism of injury that involves the back, neck, or both and that interrupts nervous system pathways. There is a loss of the autonomic nervous system's sympathetic control of circulation. This is observed when the injury occurs at T6 or above. The result is vasodilation and impaired sympathetic stimulation of the heart. The child has motor paralysis and is hypotensive and bradycardic, with loss of the normal tachycardic response to actual or relative hypovolemia. With loss of the normal vascular reflex to maintain body heat, the body also loses heat to the environment.

TIP
If a trauma patient has a normal or slow HR and low blood pressure, think spinal cord injury and neurogenic shock.

Cardiogenic Shock

Cardiogenic shock is uncommon in children and is rarely diagnosed in the prehospital arena unless the child has a known cardiac history. In fact, the child's condition may be misdiagnosed as septic or hypovolemic shock, resulting in the administration of fluid boluses and **adrenergic agents**. The most likely cause is congenital heart disease, dysrhythmia, or cardiomyopathy from **myocarditis**. Myocarditis is a disease of the heart muscle, usually caused by a virus. A **dysrhythmia**, such as **supraventricular tachycardia (SVT)** or bradycardia (HR <60/min), may also cause cardiogenic shock. Overdose with a **cardiac medication**, such as a **calcium channel blocker** or β-blocker, is another possible etiology.

Special Features in Assessment of Cardiogenic Shock

A history from the caregiver usually reveals that the child has had nonspecific symptoms, such as loss of appetite, poor feeding, lethargy, irritability, and inappropriate sweating over a period of days. The sweating is caused by the increased workload (work of breathing or work of the heart) and is an attempt to cool off the body. This is true of children with myocarditis and congenital heart disease. There is often a history of congenital heart disease or the presence of a midline chest scar from heart surgery (**FIGURE 4-5**). **TABLE 4-4** summarizes the common symptoms and signs of cardiogenic shock.

> **TIP**
>
> Cardiogenic shock can occur from HRs that are too fast or too slow.

FIGURE 4-5 A midline sternal scar is an indicator of a cardiac history.
© Perboge/iStock/Getty Images.

TABLE 4-4 Symptoms and Signs of Cardiogenic Shock

Possible Historical Findings in Cardiogenic Shock

1. Preceding history of chest pain

2. Previous history of flulike symptoms associated with weakness and fatigue

3. Difficulty feeding because of fatigue and sweating during feeding in the breast- or bottle-fed infant

4. No history of fever

5. No history of volume loss (e.g., diarrhea, vomiting, or blood loss)

6. Positive history of congenital heart disease

7. No history of asthma despite wheezing on examination

8. Persistent wheezing despite the administration of β-agonist (e.g., **albuterol** [salbutamol])

9. History of cyanosis

10. Recent history of exercise intolerance

Possible Physical Findings

1. Tachypnea or grunting with clear lungs on examination

2. Unexplained dysrhythmias in the presence of a flulike illness

3. Tachycardia disproportionate to the degree of fever

4. Persistent or worsening tachycardia despite fluid administration

5. Heart murmur, friction rub, or gallop on examination

6. Presence of cyanosis that does not improve with the administration of oxygen

7. Crackles on lung examination

8. Peripheral edema or pitting edema

9. Hepatomegaly

Cardiogenic shock may develop from left heart failure, as impaired left heart function causes decreased core organ perfusion. On physical assessment, the child may appear abnormal—sluggish, irritable, or agitated—and the skin color mottled or cyanotic. Heart rate is rapid; blood pressure may be high (early), normal, or low (late). The skin is cool and the child may be **diaphoretic** (not dry as with hypovolemic shock) related to the increased work load. Pulmonary edema causes increased work of breathing and inspiratory crackles or wheezing. The increased work load may deplete energy stores, resulting in hypoglycemia. Checking blood glucose levels is recommended.

Increased right-sided cardiac pressures are also present in cardiogenic shock and result in liver enlargement (**hepatomegaly**). Hepatomegaly is an especially useful finding in infants and toddlers. Peripheral edema and **jugular venous distention** are rare in children. Cardiogenic shock can also occur from HRs that are too fast or too slow. Because the origin of a rate-related problem is often congenital, assessment and treatment are discussed under congenital cardiac problems.

Obstructive Shock

Several pathologic conditions may obstruct blood flow from the heart and cause shock. Pericardial tamponade and tension pneumothorax are two acute conditions that cause dramatic development of shock after blunt or penetrating injuries to the chest wall. **Hemopericardium** develops quickly after a gunshot or sharp object penetrates into a blood-filled heart chamber, usually the right ventricle. Blunt trauma to the chest at just the right time during the cardiac cycle can produce pressures great enough to rupture the tendons stabilizing the cardiac valves or rupture the tissue between the chambers of the heart. The hole in the wall of the heart provides a route for blood to escape into the space between the two pericardial membranes. Because the membranes do not stretch quickly, blood collects and collapses the right ventricle (tamponade). This interrupts venous return to the right heart and produces a profound drop in cardiac output.

Rarely, pericardial tamponade may develop after an infectious or inflammatory process in the chest. Cancer, chronic renal failure, or rheumatologic disease may cause pericardial fluid accumulation. This type of fluid accumulation is slow, and the membranes around the heart stretch. Therefore, obstructive shock caused by infectious or inflammatory processes rarely occurs.

Tension pneumothorax develops after a penetration into the pleural space. Sometimes blunt injury to the chest wall can also rupture alveoli, causing a pneumothorax, which may rapidly progress to a tension pneumothorax when vigorous ventilation with a bag-mask device occurs. Air and sometimes blood (hemothorax) collect in between the two membranes of the pleura. When the pressure increases enough to cause a shift of the **mediastinum**, venous return to the right heart is impaired. This causes a drop in cardiac output and hypoperfusion.

In children or adolescents with cystic fibrosis, the lung may have blebs that rupture spontaneously, resulting in a pneumothorax, which can progress to a tension pneumothorax.

Special Features in Assessment of Obstructive Shock

Penetrating injuries to the chest wall are often deceptive. The appearance of the wound may be benign and seem superficial. Consider all gunshot wounds or stab wounds to the chest as major penetrations into the heart or pleura. Other types of penetrations from sticks or sharp objects may also cause severe internal injury. Be especially vigilant when the penetration has an entry site in the area between the two nipples and the clavicles, because this is a high-risk location for cardiac injury. Blunt chest injury may also cause a pneumothorax that may progress to a tension pneumothorax. Suspect this condition in a child with a significant blunt mechanism of injury and signs of obstructive shock.

The cardinal features of obstructive shock are signs of decreased circulation in an injured child with increased jugular venous distention. The increased jugular pressures reflect the obstruction to venous return to the right ventricle. Sometimes, however, blood loss into the chest (hemothorax) or other related injuries may be associated with hemorrhage, so that jugular venous distention is not apparent. In the case of a tension pneumothorax, in addition to signs of obstructive shock, lung sounds are unequal or absent on the affected side, and ventilation is increasingly difficult.

General Noninvasive Treatment of Suspected Shock of All Types

Begin general noninvasive treatment of every child with suspected hypoperfusion after completing the PAT and initiating the hands-on ABCDEs. The general treatment is always the same: Allow the child to assume a position of comfort if the cause is medical (in the case of blunt trauma, spinal motion restriction should be considered [see Chapter 7]) and supply oxygen, as tolerated.

Positioning

Infants and toddlers may be most "comfortable" in their caregiver's arms or lap during assessment. If the primary assessment indicates that the child is physiologically unstable, place the child in a position of comfort that decreases his or her anxiety and activity. This is usually the supine position (**FIGURE 4-6**). Elevating the legs when the child is in the supine position is not effective. Putting the child in a head-down position is not known to improve outcomes. In a head-down position, the internal organs of the abdomen put pressure on the diaphragm, interfering with breathing; the resulting agitation increases oxygen demand and complicates treatment. In the supine position, alignment of the airway is aided by placing a towel under the shoulders and trunk of the child. This helps with ease of breathing. Keep the child warm because children have a high surface-to-volume ratio and can lose body heat rapidly.

Oxygen

Treat all children in shock with high-flow oxygen. The prehospital professional must weigh the potential benefits of oxygen administration against the risk of agitating the child. "Blow-by" may be the only mechanism for delivering supplemental oxygen without upsetting the child and increasing his or her oxygen consumption.

> **TIP**
>
> Provide high-flow oxygen to all children in shock.

FIGURE 4-6 A. Treat suspected hypovolemic shock with high-flow oxygen and supine positioning. **B.** Keep the patient warm.

Specific Treatment of Hypovolemia

After the primary assessment and general supportive measures, provide additional specific treatment of shock. If the child has hypovolemic shock, consider how to stop the child's fluid losses and whether to attempt to replace them. In trauma patients, always look carefully for bleeding sites and assume there may be internal bleeding. Apply direct pressure to stop external bleeding. Consider spinal motion restriction when appropriate and splinting of injured extremities, as described in Chapter 7.

ALS

If the child has severe fluid losses from vomiting or diarrhea, consider obtaining vascular access to give fluids. If the child has hypotensive shock from illness, attempt an intravenous (IV) placement once in the field. Any further attempts should be made during transport to avoid a prolonged scene time. If the child is in extremis or unconscious, consider an intraosseous (IO) needle insertion.

Intravenous Access

IV access makes it easier to give medications and provides a way to give fluid therapy in severe blood or fluid loss. IV delivery is the gold standard for giving medication, because it permits rapid drug and fluid treatment and allows titration of important drugs. See **Intravenous Access, Procedure 16**.

IV Fluid Treatment of Compensated Hypovolemic Shock

If the child has mild to moderate volume losses as determined by HR, pulse quality, CRT, and skin temperature, and has a normal blood pressure, he or she is in compensated shock. Make one attempt on scene to perform IV insertion and fluid administration. If unsuccessful, on the way to the hospital, obtain vascular access and give IV crystalloid fluid at 20 mL/kg boluses to stabilize the patient. Reassessment should be completed after each bolus, and the patient may require additional fluid boluses to correct the perfusion abnormalities.

IV Fluid Treatment of Hypotensive (Decompensated) Shock

If the child has hypotensive shock from illness, make one attempt on scene to establish vascular access. If the child is injured, delay all vascular access attempts until en route to the ED. This is in contrast to ongoing traumatic hemorrhage, where the value of establishing access and initiating volume resuscitation at the scene may be outweighed by continued blood loss. Once access is established during transport, give 20 mL/kg boluses of IV crystalloid fluid as fast as possible. Consider IO needle insertion if vascular access cannot be obtained quickly and the child is unconscious. Repeat boluses (20 mL/kg up to 60 mL/kg) as needed to stabilize perfusion, based on ongoing reassessment of the PAT and vital signs.

IO Needle Insertion

Using an IO needle to give drugs or fluids is an excellent alternative to cannulating peripheral veins. The IO space is highly vascularized and functions as a noncollapsible vein. Needle insertion into this space is quick, simple, effective, and usually safe. Complications are infrequent and usually minor. See **Intraosseous Needle Insertion, Procedure 17**.

Treatment of Septic Shock

The mainstays of treatment are rapid administration of IV fluids and antibiotics. Timely antibiotic treatment has been shown to decrease mortality. An alert by EMS to the receiving ED has been shown to improve time to antibiotics and fluid resuscitation in adult patients; for a child in whom you suspect sepsis, rapid transport to the ED and alerting the ED that the patient may have sepsis can improve outcomes.

CAUTION

In a child with hypovolemic shock, crystalloid fluid boluses need to be given as fast as possible. Do not let the fluid just drip in.

CASE STUDY 3

A 6-year-old boy at a birthday party is having trouble breathing, so 9-1-1 is called. On your arrival, the boy has swollen eyes but answers your questions about his name and age. He has increased work of breathing with audible wheezing. There are hives on his face and arms. The adult is not sure if he has a peanut allergy, and he may have eaten a birthday cake with nuts. Vital signs are as follows: HR, 150 beats/min; RR, 50 breaths/min; BP, 90/50 mm Hg; SpO_2, 90% in room air.

1. Is this child in shock?
2. What is the appropriate prehospital therapy?

Specific Treatment of Hypotensive (Decompensated) Distributive Shock

The primary difference between treatment of distributive and hypovolemic shock is the potential need for a vasopressor agent to improve vascular tone and heart muscle function when the child has distributive shock. Treat all shock conditions first with general noninvasive measures. Administer 100% high-flow oxygen, and put the poorly responsive child with shock in a supine position.

FIGURE 4-7 An allergic reaction, with edema of face, lips, and tongue.
Courtesy of Susan Fuchs, MD, FAAP.

ALS

Treatment of Distributive Shock

Attempt a vascular access on scene at least once. Deliver fluid boluses, of 20 mL/kg boluses, up to 60 mL/kg of a crystalloid fluid solution on the way to the ED. If the child has lost protective airway reflexes or has refractory shock, support ventilation with a bag-mask device or endotracheal intubation.

If cardiovascular instability (hypotension, markedly increased HR, and poor responsiveness) persists after volume therapy with up to 60 mL/kg of crystalloid fluid, try a vasopressor agent (epinephrine, or norepinephrine). Do not administer a vasopressor agent if you suspect untreated hypovolemia.

Treatment of Anaphylaxis

A child with anaphylaxis requires fluid and special treatment with **epinephrine**, a β-agonist if bronchospasm is present, and methylprednisolone. If hives and angioedema are present, diphenhydramine may also be necessary. Unlike a simple allergic reaction, anaphylaxis has dangerous cardiovascular effects (**FIGURE 4-7**).

Epinephrine is an excellent drug for treatment of anaphylaxis. It stimulates α- and β-adrenergic receptors, leading to two important effects: (1) constriction of the blood vessels to help counter the vasodilation and increased permeability of anaphylaxis (alpha effect), and (2) opening up the airways to help reverse the bronchospasm of anaphylaxis (beta effect). For all children with allergic reactions associated with wheezing, administer epinephrine, 0.01 mg/kg (0.01 mL/kg) of 1 mg/mL concentration (maximum, 0.3 mg or 0.3 mL) intramuscularly (IM). For BLS providers, if the patient or parent has an epinephrine autoinjector, administer the medication IM.

Epinephrine is a short-acting drug. Therefore, it is necessary to follow up with a long-acting steroid, such as **methylprednisolone**. Methylprednisolone (1–2 mg/kg IV/IO; maximum, 60 mg) acts to stabilize mast cell membranes to prevent perpetuation of the reaction by chemicals triggered by the allergic reaction. Research suggests that the earlier the administration of methylprednisolone after treatment of the acute problem, the better the outcome.

If hives or angioedema are present, **diphenhydramine** (1 mg/kg orally, IV, or IO; maximum, 50 mg) may also be necessary. Diphenhydramine works as a histamine blocker, specific for the histamine receptors that reside in the walls of the blood vessels and in the skin. Administration of this medication eases itching.

Treatment of Cardiogenic Shock

If cardiogenic shock is suspected by history or physical assessment, transport after general noninvasive treatment. On the way to the ED, consider vascular access. If the diagnosis of cardiogenic shock is uncertain, give a cautious fluid bolus of only 10 mL/kg of crystalloid fluid, and then reassess appearance, work of breathing, CRT, HR, and blood pressure. If there is no rhythm disturbance on the cardiac monitor (rate-related problems are discussed in Chapter 5) and the child remains poorly perfused after the initial fluid bolus, consider a vasopressor agent (dobutamine, **dopamine**, epinephrine, or norepinephrine) after speaking to medical control, if the transport time is long. Start vasopressors at low doses, based on micrograms per kilogram, and then titrate to achieve acceptable perfusion (improved appearance and skin circulation and decreased HR and respiratory rate). If the child is known to be in congestive heart failure with cardiogenic shock, avoid fluid boluses and consider vasopressor therapy as front-line treatment if perfusion is severely compromised.

The major difference in treatment of hypovolemic, distributive, and cardiogenic shock is the amount of fluid administration and consideration of a vasopressor.

> **CAUTION**
>
> Do not withhold fluid from a child in cardiogenic shock; just give it in boluses of 10 mL/kg and reassess.

`ALS`

Treatment of Obstructive Shock

The additional option for treatment of obstructive shock from a tension **pneumothorax** is needle **thoracostomy** to decrease air pressure, as explained in **Needle Thoracostomy, Procedure 23**.

This technique does not remove blood but relieves pressure in the pleural space. Rapid transport is an essential feature of field management of chest injury.

Primary Assessment: Transport Decision

After completing the primary assessment and beginning general treatment when appropriate, the prehospital professional must decide whether to go or stay on scene. If the PAT and ABCDEs are normal and the child has no history of serious illness or injury mechanism, no anatomic abnormalities, and no pain, the child does not usually require urgent treatment or immediate transport. Take the time to get a history and physical examination, and perform a detailed physical examination (trauma) on scene if possible.

If the child has a serious mechanism of injury, a physiologic or anatomic abnormality, severe pain, or if the scene is not safe, transport immediately. With such patients, do the additional assessment and attempt specific treatment on the way to the hospital, if possible.

The transport decision is sometimes difficult in a child with a suspected cardiovascular problem who needs vascular access. If the child is in compensated shock and has a palpable brachial pulse or normal blood pressure, protect the spine (if the child is injured), manage the airway and breathing, control hemorrhage, and transport immediately. Attempt vascular access for specific treatment on the way to the ED.

If the child is in hypotensive shock, the prehospital professional has several options, depending on the clinical condition of the child, local EMS system regulations, comfort level, and the time to the nearest ED. If the child is injured, always transport immediately. If the child is ill with abnormal appearance and hypotension, consider attempting a vascular access on scene, and then transporting without delay.

Summary of Shock States

There are four major classes of shock seen both in children and adults: (1) hypovolemic, (2) cardiogenic, (3) distributive, and (4) obstructive. Hypovolemic shock is commonly the result of trauma and hemorrhage after injury. Vomiting and diarrhea leading to dehydration is the most common medical cause of hypovolemia. Distributive shock may result from sepsis, anaphylaxis, drug intoxication, or spinal injury. Always suspect sepsis in the infant or toddler who has fever and abnormal appearance. A petechial or purpuric skin rash is a red flag for sepsis. Cardiogenic shock caused by inadequate left ventricular contraction is rare in children and difficult to identify in the field, unless the child has a known congenital cardiac problem. Obstructive shock sometimes occurs in conjunction with significant chest wall injury. Clinical findings may reflect more than one type of shock pathophysiology. Treatment of all shock types includes general noninvasive interventions and then specific treatment based on clinical findings. Consider rapid fluid boluses in children who are hypotensive with an abnormal appearance.

CASE STUDY ANSWERS

CASE STUDY 1

This child has septic or distributive shock. He has hypotensive shock. The rash is an ominous sign, and aggressive treatment is necessary to save the child's life. The appropriate first interventions are oxygen and bag-mask ventilation.

Attempt IV or IO access on scene once, and give a 20 mL/kg crystalloid fluid bolus as fast as possible. Then, transport and deliver 20 mL/kg fluid boluses of crystalloid, to a maximum of 60 mL/kg, while en route as needed to correct perfusion. Reassess after each bolus. Consider giving a vasopressor agent (epinephrine, or norepinephrine) if perfusion remains poor after fluid administration and the transport time is long. Bag mask ventilation or even endotracheal intubation may be necessary.

This case also requires universal precautions to protect the prehospital professional, because the child has a serious communicable disease. Direct specific questions about exposures and prophylactic treatment to your infection control personnel.

CASE STUDY 2

This child is in hypotensive (decompensated) shock, because her blood pressure is low. The etiology is likely hypovolemia, because of the history of vomiting and diarrhea. Her lethargy can be caused by shock, but could also be caused by hypoglycemia. Prehospital treatment is attempt IV or IO access on scene and give a 20 mL/kg normal crystalloid fluid bolus as fast as possible. Begin transport, and reassess. Give additional 20 mL/kg fluid boluses as needed to correct perfusion, to a maximum of 60 mL/kg, while en route to the ED. A bedside glucose can also be obtained, and if it is low, 10% dextrose given in addition to the IV fluids. In this case, her glucose is 50 mg/dL, and her weight is 20 kg, so 100 mL of 10% dextrose can be administered.

CASE STUDY 3

This is a case of anaphylaxis, and although this child is not in shock at this time, it could still develop. Anaphylaxis requires urgent treatment of 0.01 mg/kg of epinephrine of the 1 mg/mL concentration IM. This child weighs 20 kg, so the dose is 0.2 mg (0.2 mL). This medication can be given by the patient's autoinjector, if available, at its prescribed dose. Administration of albuterol via a nebulizer may help his wheezing. Insertion of an IV now can be useful to give IV diphenhydramine and methylprednisolone (if carried). If his blood pressure begins to drop (anaphylactic shock), a rapid infusion of 20 mL/kg normal crystalloid fluid bolus is indicated.

SUGGESTED REFERENCES

Textbooks

American Academy of Pediatrics and the American College of Emergency Physicians. *APLS: The Pediatric Emergency Medicine Resource*. 5th ed. Burlington, MA: Jones and Bartlett Learning; 2012.

American Heart Association. *2010 Handbook of Emergency Cardiovascular Care for Healthcare Providers*. Hazinski MF, Samson R, Schexnayder S, eds. Dallas, TX: American Heart Association; 2010.

Hazinski MF, Mondozzi MA, Baker RA. Shock, multiple organ dysfunction syndrome, and burns in children. In: McCance KL, Heuther SE, Brashers VL, Rote NS, eds. *Pathophysiology: The Biologic Basis for Disease in Adults and Children*. 6th ed. St. Louis, IL: Mosby Elsevier; 2010:1727–1752.

Articles

Brierly J, Carcillo JA, Choong K, et al. Clinical practice parameters for hemodynamic support of pediatric and neonatal septic shock: 2007 update from the American College of Critical Care Medicine. *Crit Care Med.* 2009;37(2):666–688.

DeCaen AR, Maconochie IK, Aickin R, et al. Part 6: Pediatric Basic Life Support and Pediatric Advanced Life Support. 2015 International Consensus on Cardiopulmonary Resuscitation and Emergency Cardiovascular Care Science with Treatment Recommendations. *Circulation.* 2015;132 [suppl 1]: S177–S203.

Fuchs S, Terry M, Adelgais K, et al. Definitions and assessment approaches for emergency medical services for children. Supplemental information. *Pediatrics.* 2016:138(6);e20161073.

Han Y, Carcillo J, Dragotta, et al. Early reversal of pediatric-neonatal septic shock by community physicians is associated with improved outcome. *Pediatrics.* 2003;112(4):793–799.

Kawasaki T. Update on pediatric sepsis: a review. *J Intens Care.* 2017:5:47. https://doi.org/10.1186 /s40560-017-0240-1.

Kleinman, ME, Chameides L, Schexnayder SM, et al. Part 14: Pediatric advanced life support: 2010 American Heart Association Guidelines for Cardiopulmonary Resuscitation and Emergency Cardiovascular Care. *Circulation.* 2010;122(suppl 3):S876–S908.

Morris MC. Pediatric cardiopulmonary-cerebral resuscitation: an overview and future directions. *Crit Care Clin.* 2003;19(3):337–364.

© Kali9/E+/Getty Images.

CHAPTER 5

Resuscitation and Dysrhythmias

John A. Erbayri, MS, NRP, CHSE

Michael H. Stroud, MD, FAAP

LEARNING OBJECTIVES

1. Describe how to assess circulation using the Pediatric Assessment Triangle (PAT), ABCDEs, and additional assessment.
2. Explain when to treat tachycardia and bradycardia, and discuss management.
3. List the links in the pediatric "Chain of Survival."
4. Order the steps in managing pediatric cardiac arrest caused by asystole, pulseless electrical activity (PEA), ventricular fibrillation (VF), and pulseless ventricular tachycardia (VT).
5. Define indications for the use of the automated external defibrillator (AED) in pediatric patients.
6. Describe the causes of primary cardiac arrest in the pediatric patient.
7. Discuss medical issues in children with congenital heart disease who may present to the prehospital professional.

CASE STUDY 1

You have been dispatched for a 9-year-old child who is unconscious and not breathing. You arrive at a baseball field and find the child lying supine on the pitcher's mound. Teammates say he was hit in the chest by a baseball. The child is unresponsive, not breathing, cyanotic, and has no pulse. You begin cardiopulmonary resuscitation (CPR) while your partner attaches the AED.

1. How does management of VF or VT differ from treatment for **pulseless electrical activity (PEA)** or asystole?
2. Why should CPR be started as rapidly as possible and continued without interruptions?

Introduction

Cardiac arrest in pediatrics is uncommon in the prehospital setting. Survival to discharge from out-of-hospital cardiac arrest is 6% (3% for infants and 9% for children and adolescents). The primary cause of arrest in children is usually an asphyxial arrest situation that deteriorates into cardiac arrest.

Although hypoxia leading to pulseless electrical activity (PEA) or asystole is the most common cause of pediatric arrest, a small percentage may demonstrate **ventricular fibrillation (VF)** or **ventricular tachycardia (VT)**. Regardless of the type of cardiovascular emergency, early recognition and timely management can reduce the likelihood for serious morbidity or mortality.

Prearrival Preparation

Based on dispatch information, the provider needs to be prepared to assess, manage, and make transport decisions for a child exhibiting a symptomatic cardiac dysrhythmia, cardiac event, or cardiac arrest. Recall appropriate techniques for assessment; the role of vital signs; and the possible equipment, medications, fluid requirements, automated external defibrillator (AED), and electrical therapy a child may require. Consider when to stay and treat on scene and when to transport immediately.

Scene Size-Up

All providers need to ensure that the scene is safe and note any significant findings that may be contributing factors to the situation. The provider must also assess the scene, as appropriate, for signs of child maltreatment.

General Assessment: The PAT

Evaluating the Presenting Complaint

On arrival, determine the child's presenting complaint. Gathering a complete patient history is a vital component in determining the cardiac event the patient may be experiencing. Attempt to gather a complete SAMPLE history during the primary assessment.

Assessment of Circulation

Using the PAT

The Pediatric Assessment Triangle (PAT) is the first step in assessment of circulation, as outlined in Chapter 1. The PAT evaluates three characteristics: (1) appearance, (2) work of breathing, and (3) circulation to skin. Knowing these characteristics helps to determine whether the child is sick or not sick, the type of physiologic abnormality, and the urgency for treatment. Circulatory problems affect each of these characteristics in identifiable patterns.

Appearance

First, assess the child's appearance. A child with decreased core circulation from any cardiac compromise may have signs of poor brain perfusion. The abnormality in the child's appearance will be variable, depending on the type of perfusion problem and the degree of circulatory insufficiency. Abnormal features in the appearance of a child with decreased core circulation include the following:

- Lethargy or listlessness
- Decreased motor activity for infants, poor muscle tone
- Diminished interactiveness with caregivers, the prehospital professional, and the environment
- Inconsolability
- Poor eye contact
- Weak cry

Sometimes the child with hemodynamic instability will be restless and inconsolable. *Appearance alone, however, is not a very accurate sign of circulatory problems.* Assessing appearance is a good way to tell if the child is ill, but not a good way to identify the physiologic problem. Assessment tools other than the PAT, such as the hands-on ABCDE assessment, will help distinguish the type of physiologic problem and the presence or absence of abnormal perfusion.

Work of Breathing

Next, assess the work of breathing. If circulation to vital organs is decreased, the child's respiratory rate will increase. "**Effortless tachypnea**," or a fast respiratory rate without increased work of breathing, is a common but nonspecific sign of hemodynamic instability. It reflects the child's attempt to blow off carbon dioxide and reduce the **metabolic acidosis** created by decreased perfusion to cells. Signs of increased work of breathing, such as abnormal positioning; retractions; flaring; or abnormal airway sounds, such as grunting, stridor, or wheezing, may or may not be present in a child with a circulatory problem.

Circulation to Skin

After assessing appearance and work of breathing, assess circulation by looking at skin color. This will be difficult to interpret if the environmental temperature is low, because **vasoconstriction**, as a reflexive effort to preserve heat, will falsely alter skin findings, especially in infants. Disrobe the child, and look for mottling, pallor, and cyanosis, which reflect peripheral vasoconstriction or clamping down of nonessential skin perfusion to maintain essential core circulation. If a child has abnormal appearance and abnormal skin signs in a warm ambient environment, the child may be hemodynamically unstable.

Primary Assessment: The ABCDEs

After the PAT, perform the hands-on ABCDE assessment. After evaluating airway and breathing, as described in previous chapters, assess the circulation. There are four parts to the assessment of circulation:

1. Heart rate
2. Pulse quality
3. Skin temperature and capillary refill time
4. Blood pressure

Heart Rate

First, measure heart rate by feeling the pulse for 30 seconds, and then double the number. A normal heart rate is between 60 and 160 beats/min, depending on the child's age, as noted in **TABLE 5-1**. The radial or brachial areas are preferred sites to measure pulse rate in infants and children. The carotid pulse is acceptable in older children and adolescents, but it is hard to locate in infants. Femoral pulses are often easily palpable in neonates and infants. If a pulse is difficult to feel, determine heart rate by listening to the heart sounds directly with a stethoscope placed on the medial side of the child's left nipple. However, be aware that the presence of a "normal" heart rate by auscultation does not necessarily reflect adequate cardiac output and perfusion.

Interpreting heart rate may be difficult, as explained in Chapter 1. Ranges of normal heart rates change inversely with advancing age. Also, many conditions can increase heart rate, ranging from serious physiologic problems to noxious stimuli that are rarely life threatening. Certain common medications may also alter heart rate (high and low). Stimuli that can cause **tachycardia** include pain, fever, fear, and agitation. Interpret heart rate in the context of overall signs of perfusion, age, presence or absence of noxious stimuli, medications, and observed trends. Although a single measurement of heart rate is usually of limited value in determining the degree of physiologic derangement, *a trend of mounting tachycardia, or a heart rate that is falling below the lower limits of normal, suggests a serious physiologic problem*. In addition, sustained tachycardia is a worrisome sign. Finally, be extremely vigilant when the child has **bradycardia**, because this often indicates hypoxia or may be a sign of profound ischemia.

> **TIP**
>
> Bradycardia is always a critical sign in a young child and reflects hypoxia or advanced shock.

Pulse Quality

Presence of a strong central pulse (carotid, femoral, **brachial** in infants) with a strong peripheral pulse (brachial, **radial**, or **pedal** in children) suggests a good blood pressure. A strong central pulse with a weak peripheral pulse indicates compensated shock. If a brachial pulse is not palpable, the child is probably hypotensive and is hemodynamically unstable.

> **CAUTION**
>
> The carotid pulse is an acceptable site for measurement of pulse rate in older children and adolescents, but it is hard to locate in infants.

Skin Temperature and Capillary Refill Time

The next part of the hands-on cardiovascular assessment involves evaluating skin signs. Check skin temperature for warmth at the hands, feet, kneecaps, or forearms. Cool hands and feet may be normal, but cool proximal extremities reflect poor perfusion and shunting of blood

TABLE 5-1 Normal Heart Rate for Age	
Age	**Heart Rate (beats/min)**
Infant (birth–12 months)	100–160
Toddler (1–3 years)	95–150
Preschooler (3–5 years)	80–140
School-aged child (6–12 years)	70–120
Adolescent (13–18 years)	60–100

to the core. **Capillary refill time (CRT)** *should be less than 2 seconds in a child who is not cold.* Inadequate core perfusion results in peripheral vasoconstriction, which will manifest as cool skin and delayed CRT. Although CRT is a good test of circulation in children, it must be interpreted in the context of overall signs of perfusion. The prehospital professional can become comfortable with the technique and interpretation of the key skin findings by practicing on every child.

> **TIP**
>
> Practice CRT and pulse quality on every child. This will help you to become comfortable with the technique and interpret key findings accurately.

> **CAUTION**
>
> CRT is a good test for circulation in children, but do not place heavy emphasis on this sign alone.

Blood Pressure

Last, consider taking a blood pressure. A high blood pressure value in a child is not clinically significant in the field, unless he or she has a history of hypertension, known renal disease, or acute head injury. However, a true low blood pressure value is significant of hemodynamic instability. The challenges in blood pressure measurement in children in the prehospital setting include knowing when to get a blood pressure reading, obtaining the blood pressure correctly, and interpreting it accurately.

A normal minimal systolic blood pressure in a child older than 1 year of age is determined with the following equation: 70 + (2 × years of age). Proper equipment, technique, and patience are required to obtain an accurate blood pressure in an infant or toddler. Because this can be a time-consuming process and may not contribute greatly to the clinical assessment of perfusion, in a child 3 years or younger, attempt a blood pressure measurement only once or skip altogether. Inadequate perfusion will be better reflected in the other signs of perfusion described previously (heart rate, pulse quality, CRT, and skin temperature).

In a child older than 3 years of age, make at least one blood pressure attempt in every patient to provide a baseline for future assessments. Repeated vital signs provide trends that can yield useful information to determine patient severity. Use a cuff with a width that is two-thirds the length of the upper arm. Applying too large a cuff will falsely decrease the blood pressure measurement, and too small a cuff will falsely increase the measurement.

> **TIP**
>
> A normal minimal systolic blood pressure in a child older than 1 year of age is 70 + (2 × years of age). An infant younger than 1 year should have a systolic blood pressure >60.

Additional Assessment

If the child is stable after the primary assessment and does not require immediate treatment, and there are no immediate safety concerns for the child or prehospital professional, conduct the focused history and physical examination and the detailed physical examination on scene. Use the SAMPLE (**TABLE 5-2**) and OPQRST mnemonics (**TABLE 5-3**) to recall important features of the focused cardiovascular history. Use age-appropriate approaches to gain the child's trust and speak directly to him or her. Ask the caregiver to add to the child's history. Obtain the history from the caregiver if the child is too young to speak or is unable to cooperate.

After the focused history, perform a focused examination of the heart, peripheral circulation, and abdomen. Then, do an anatomic examination of the entire body, as outlined in Chapter 1. If the child has a traumatic injury, also do a detailed physical examination, searching for other injuries.

Perform an ongoing assessment of all children with cardiovascular problems while on the way to the emergency department, observing for changes on the cardiorespiratory monitor. The child's status may change during transport, so observe and document any physiologic trends. Use the PAT to monitor effective perfusion and watch respiratory rate, heart rate, blood pressure, and pulse oximetry. Be prepared to increase the level of respiratory and cardiovascular support if the child worsens or fails to respond to treatment.

Summary of Cardiovascular Assessment

The PAT provides a good first-line cardiovascular evaluation: abnormal appearance, normal work of breathing, and poor circulation to skin suggest a perfusion problem. Pallor, mottling, and cyanosis all

TABLE 5-2 SAMPLE Components in a Child With Cardiovascular Problems

Component	Features
Signs/symptoms	Presence of vomiting More cyanotic than usual Lower pulse oximeter reading Number of episodes of vomiting Presence or absence of fever Rash Respiratory distress or shortness of breath (e.g., in cardiogenic shock with congestive heart failure)
Allergies	Known allergies and what reaction occurs History of anaphylaxis
Medications	Exact names and dosages of ongoing medications Chronic diuretic therapy Potential exposure to other medications or drugs Timing and doses of analgesics or antipyretics
Past medical problems	History of heart problems or heart surgery History of prematurity Prior hospitalizations for cardiovascular problems
Last food or liquid	Timing of the child's last food or drink, including bottle or breast feedings
Events leading to the injury or illness	Travel Trauma Fever history Symptoms in family members Potential toxic exposure

TABLE 5-3 The OPQRST of Pain

O—Onset
Key Question: What were you doing when the pain/discomfort started?

P—Provocation/Palliation
Key Questions: What makes the pain/discomfort better or worse? What have you tried to reduce the symptoms? Did it work?
Support Questions: Has this ever happened before? If so, when?

Q—Quality
Key Question: What does the pain feel like?

R—Region/Radiation
Key Question: Can you point with one finger to the main area of pain/discomfort?
Support Questions: Do you feel pain anywhere else? If so, can you show me or tell me where it is?

S—Severity
Key Question: How bad is the pain or chief complaint on a scale of 1 to 10, with 1 being no pain and 10 being extreme pain?
Support Questions: What is the worst pain you have ever experienced? How does this compare?

T—Time Frames
Key Question: When did you first notice the symptoms?
Support Questions: Have the symptoms been continuous? If not, has the feeling come and gone?

indicate poor peripheral perfusion. The circulatory portion of the hands-on ABCDEs consists of evaluating heart rate, pulse quality, skin temperature, CRT, and blood pressure. These physical features complement the PAT and will help identify the type and severity of circulatory compromise. Vital signs can sometimes be misleading and must be correctly obtained and interpreted for age. Trends in vital signs, or persistence in abnormal vital signs, such as tachycardia, are more accurate indicators of real physiologic problems than mild vital sign abnormalities on primary assessment.

Dysrhythmias

Bradycardia

In children, bradycardia usually reflects hypoxia, rather than a primary cardiac problem. It is a prearrest rhythm, and the prognosis is ominous if left untreated. Immediate delivery of high-flow oxygen and **assisted ventilation** are essential. Untreated bradycardia can quickly cause hemodynamic instability and ultimately death. In children with asthma or respiratory distress, bradycardia may indicate profound hypoxia. Pulse oximetry, when available, will help determine the degree of hypoxia in the field.

Congenital heart block is an extremely rare cause of bradycardia in infancy and early childhood. Drug overdose (e.g., β-blockers, calcium channel blockers, digoxin, clonidine) is another possible cause of bradycardia. Bradycardia may also result from vagal stimulation during medical procedures or gastric tube placement. However, although bradycardia that develops during laryngoscopy or suctioning may be the result of vagal stimulation, hypoxia may be the true cause. If bradycardia does occur in this setting, stop the procedure, administer supplemental oxygen, and reassess the patient.

Bradycardia may also be a normal finding, especially in asymptomatic athletic adolescents. If bradycardia is an isolated finding, without signs of hemodynamic instability, in a well-perfused school-aged child or teenager, no treatment is necessary in the field.

Assessment of the Child With Bradycardia

If the child has a heart rate below the normal range for age (see Table 5-1), evaluate carefully for signs of respiratory failure or shock. The PAT and ABCDEs, along with a brief history, will establish the likely cause, the severity of the problem, and the need for urgent treatment.

Treatment of Bradycardia

If the child is asymptomatic, consider no treatment, especially if the child is an adolescent, because slow heart rates are common in athletic teenagers. If the child has bradycardia and a primary assessment demonstrates oxygenation, ventilation, or perfusion abnormalities, provide 100% oxygen with bag-mask ventilation and transport. Check effectiveness of ventilation by observing for chest rise and an improvement in the PAT, heart rate, perfusion, and blood pressure.

In rare situations, chest compressions for bradycardia are necessary. If the heart rate is below 60 beats/min and the child shows signs of poor systemic perfusion after oxygenation and assisted ventilation, begin chest compressions.

ALS

Drug Therapy for Symptomatic Bradycardia.
Oxygenation and ventilation are the primary treatments for bradycardia. If the heart rate does not rise in response to assisted ventilation, in most cases administer epinephrine as the first-line drug at 0.1 mg/mL concentration, 0.01 mg/kg or 0.1 mL/kg intravenous (IV) or intraosseous (IO), every 3–5 minutes. If there is increased vagal tone (or poisoning by cholinergic drugs or agents, such as organophosphates) or an atrioventricular heart block, administer atropine, 0.02 mg/kg IV or IO (maximum dose of 0.5 mg). When the child has a known reason for cholinergic-mediated bradycardia, such as congenital heart block, give atropine and monitor the response; you may repeat once if indicated.

Before administering vasopressor drugs, always assess for mechanical problems with oxygen delivery and ventilation. Check for disconnected oxygen tubing, poor mask seal, airway obstruction, inadequate chest rise, endotracheal tube blockage, or malposition. Other causes of bradycardia from hypoxia or ischemia are pneumothorax, hypovolemia, cardiomyopathy, poisoning, or increased intracranial pressure.

When oxygenation, ventilation, and drug therapy for bradycardia fail, consider external electrical cardiac pacing of the heart.

Endotracheal Administration of Drugs. If neither IV nor IO access is available for giving drugs during resuscitation, the endotracheal route is an alternative for at least four pediatric drugs: (LEAN) lidocaine, epinephrine, atropine, and naloxone. Although endotracheal drugs are probably not as effective as medications delivered by the IV or IO routes, endotracheal delivery is appropriate in the critical patient until IV or IO access is established. Use the technique for endotracheal drug delivery described in **Endotracheal Tube Drug Instillation, Procedure 20**.

When administering epinephrine through an endotracheal tube to a child who has no vascular or IO access, give epinephrine at the higher concentration of 1 mg/mL, and use the higher dose of 0.1 mg/kg (0.1 mL/kg). Note that this is the same total volume of epinephrine as the IV/IO dose, because the 10-fold dose has 10 times the concentration of 0.1 mg/mL. When administering atropine through an endotracheal tube, the dose is two to three times the IV/IO dose (0.04–0.06 mg/kg).

CAUTION

Be extremely careful with IV/IO/endotracheal tube epinephrine, and check doses and concentration.

Tachycardia

Tachycardia may be a nonspecific sign of fear, anxiety, pain, or fever and may not represent serious injury or illness. Tachycardia may also be a sign of a life-threatening problem, such as hypoxia, cardiac abnormality, or hypovolemia. Sinus tachycardia is the most common dysrhythmia in children, and treatment is generally limited to fluid administration, supplemental oxygen, pain medication, and transport.

Assessment of the Child With Tachycardia

Tachycardia must be assessed in conjunction with the PAT and ABCDEs. Always ask about a history of congenital heart disease and check for midline chest scars from cardiac surgery.

There are two characteristics in the child's rhythm strip to measure and use as a basis for treatment, along with the perfusion assessment: (1) the heart rate per minute and (2) the width of the QRS complex. First, establish an accurate heart rate electronically from the rhythm strip. As in the assessment of bradycardia, interpret the heart rate based on knowledge of the normal range for age (see Table 5-1). Second, establish the width of the QRS from the rhythm strip. If the QRS complex is ≤0.09 seconds (<2¼ standard boxes on the rhythm strip), consider the child to have a narrow complex tachycardia. If the width is >0.09 seconds (>2¼ standard boxes on the rhythm strip), consider the child to have a wide complex tachycardia.

TABLE 5-4 distinguishes the features of a narrow complex sinus tachycardia from narrow complex supraventricular tachycardia (SVT) and wide complex VT.

Specific Treatment of Tachycardia

If the child presents with tachycardia, determine the appropriate treatment by establishing perfusion status and by assessing the rhythm strip for heart rate and QRS duration.

Narrow Complex Tachycardia. If the child has a narrow QRS tachycardia (≤0.09 seconds), P waves are present, and the heart rate is variable and less than 220 beats/min in an infant or less than 180 beats/min in a child, the cause is usually sinus tachycardia (**FIGURE 5-1**) from noncardiac conditions (e.g., hypoxia, hypovolemia, hypothermia, hypoglycemia, metabolic abnormalities, toxins, fear, pain, or serious trauma to the chest). No specific cardiac medical management of the sinus tachycardia is needed. Instead, treat with fluids, oxygen, splinting, analgesia, or sedation as indicated by the associated condition. If there is no change in heart rate after treatment, consider other etiologies, such as SVT.

Specific Treatment of SVT. If the QRS is less than or equal to 0.09 seconds, P waves are absent or abnormal, and the rate is not variable, and is ≥220 beats/min in

TABLE 5-4 Features of Sinus Tachycardia, SVT, and VT

	History	Heart Rate	Variability	QRS Interval	Assessment	Possible Treatments
Sinus tachycardia	Fever Volume loss Hypoxia Pain Increased activity or exercise	<220 beats/min (infant) <180 beats/min (child)	Yes	Narrow ≤0.09 seconds	Hypovolemia Hypoxia Painful injury	Fluids Oxygen Splinting Analgesia/ sedation
Supraventricular tachycardia	Congenital heart disease Known SVT Nonspecific symptoms (e.g., poor feeding, fussiness)	≥220 beats/min (often 240–300 beats/min) (infant) ≥180 beats/min (child)	No	Narrow ≤0.09 seconds	CHF may be present	Vagal maneuvers (ice to face) Adenosine (stable) Synchronized cardioversion (unstable)
Ventricular tachycardia	Serious systemic illness	>150 beats/min	Yes	Wide >0.09 seconds	CHF may be present	Synchronized cardioversion Defibrillation (VT without a pulse) Lidocaine Amiodarone

CHF, congestive heart failure; SVT, supraventricular tachycardia; VT, ventricular tachycardia.

FIGURE 5-1 Electrocardiogram of sinus tachycardia.

From *12-Lead ECG: The Art of Interpretation*, courtesy of Tomas B. Garcia, MD.

an infant or ≥180 beats/min in a child, consider SVT as the likely etiology. If the child has no previous history of SVT and is stable, provide oxygen and transport to the emergency department. Delaying specific treatment for SVT until hospital arrival will permit the hospital staff to confirm SVT, and to run a continuous electrocardiogram while actively managing the dysrhythmia. A patient with a confirmed diagnosis of SVT may need long-term treatment with cardiac medications.

ALS

If the patient has a prior history of SVT and is stable, consider a vagal maneuver first. Ice to the face (if available) evokes the "**diving reflex**" and is an effective management tool for SVT in infants and toddlers. Place crushed ice in a plastic bag, glove, or washcloth, and apply firmly over the mid-face (cheeks and bridge of nose) for approximately 15 seconds, until the rhythm changes or the patient's condition dictates immediate cessation of the procedure (**FIGURE 5-2**). Do not occlude the nose (to allow breathing), and provide constant reassurance to the parent and child. Avoid ocular pressure (pressure on the eyeballs) as a method of vagal stimulation in a child. Only attempt a vagal maneuver once.

FIGURE 5-2 Placing a bag of ice on a child's face elicits the "diving reflex" and may convert SVT to sinus rhythm.

ALS

If the patient with narrow complex tachycardia is stable, and the heart rate does not convert to sinus rhythm after one attempt at vagal stimulation, give **adenosine** at 0.1 mg/kg up to a maximum first dose of 6 mg rapid IV or IO push, and follow immediately with a 2- to 5-mL bolus of normal saline. Use an IV/IO nearest to the heart and rapidly push adenosine followed by saline; a three-way stopcock, if available, is a good tool to use when rapidly giving adenosine immediately followed by saline. Double the dose to 0.2 mg/kg if the rhythm does not convert after the first dose of adenosine (maximum second dose = 12 mg). Be prepared to treat the untoward effects of adenosine; it is a very potent cardiac drug. If given properly, it is usually effective in the treatment of SVT. Brief runs of bradycardia or even several seconds of asystole commonly occur with adenosine administration, but sustained or fatal dysrhythmias (e.g., asystole, VT, and VF) are rare. Caution should be used when administering adenosine in children who are already taking carbamazepine (Tegretol) because it can result in prolonged heart block. Monitor the child closely, place defibrillator pads on the child, and have a **defibrillator** and resuscitative drugs within reach.

If a child with suspected SVT has signs of poor perfusion and hemodynamic compromise (abnormal PAT, poor pulse quality, abnormal CRT and skin temperature, hypotension), is in shock, or is unconscious, immediately administer synchronized electrical cardioversion at 0.5–1 joule/kilogram (J/kg) as a starting electrical dose. If the initial shock is ineffective, double to 2 J/kg. If the child is in shock but still conscious and has vascular access, administer sedation, if possible, before delivering the electrical countershock. Do not delay electrical therapy for sedation. If electrical therapy fails to convert the child to sinus rhythm, consider using other antidysrhythmic drugs, such as **amiodarone** (5 mg/kg over 20–60 minutes) or procainamide (15 mg/kg over 20–60 minutes) as per local emergency medical services (EMS) system guidelines. Do not give amiodarone and procainamide together.

TIP

Prehospital personnel must be prepared to treat the adverse drug effects of all cardiac medications, even if the indication, dose, and route of delivery are correct.

Wide Complex Tachycardia. If the patient is conscious and has adequate perfusion, a heart rate of greater than 150 beats/min, and a QRS interval of greater than 0.09 seconds, he or she is probably in stable VT. Sinus tachycardia with a conduction abnormality (bundle branch block) may look like VT, but usually occurs in a child with a history of heart disease or cardiac surgery. Likewise, SVT with aberrant conduction can result in a wide complex rhythm. In such stable cases with wide complex tachycardias, provide oxygen and transport the patient to an appropriate emergency department, with close cardiac monitoring and equipment for defibrillation/cardioversion immediately available.

ALS

If the child has VT, is stable, and the rhythm is monomorphic and regular, try a dose of adenosine first to determine if the rhythm is SVT with aberrant conduction. If the rhythm is VT, an antiarrhythmic can be used per EMS guidelines. If the child has VT and shows signs of poor perfusion, treat with synchronized electrical cardioversion (0.5 to 1 J/kg). If a second shock (2 J/kg) is unsuccessful, or if the tachycardia recurs quickly, consider antidysrhythmic drugs, such as amiodarone (5 mg/kg over 20–60 minutes) or procainamide (15 mg/kg over 30–60 minutes) per local EMS system guidelines. Do not give amiodarone and procainamide together.

If the child has VT and shock, without a pulse, treat as pulseless VT/VF.

Automated External Defibrillator

Cardiac arrest in children is usually the result of profound hypoxia or shock, which leads to **asystole**, or **pulseless electrical activity (PEA)**, the most frequent rhythms of pediatric cardiac arrest. VF, however, does occur in pediatrics. The typical VF case is a child out of the infant age group who has had a witnessed collapse. Etiologies for VF arrest in children include **myocarditis**, an infection of the heart muscle; long QT syndrome, a congenital cardiac conduction problem; and **hypertrophic cardiomyopathy (HCM)**, a hypertrophy of the ventricular septum and ventricles. One other special circumstance for VF arrest is **commotio cordis**, which develops usually in a young athlete who is struck in the chest by a ball, stick, or other blunt object.

Perform rapid assessment for VF on all unresponsive children, begin CPR, and administer defibrillation if VF is present on the cardiac monitor. Be especially vigilant for VF when the child is older and has suffered a witnessed collapse. There is no demonstrated benefit to defibrillation of asystole, and this procedure will only delay the key interventions of chest compressions, ventilation, and oxygenation.

The AED (**FIGURE 5-3**) allows early recognition of VF and rapid defibrillation. The American Heart Association (AHA) guidelines recommend the use of an AED for treatment of VF in children of all ages, including infants. AEDs have been shown to accurately identify VF and VT in young children and are also accurate in identifying pediatric rhythms that do not require defibrillation. When used with a designated pediatric pad-cable system, these AEDs deliver an energy dose that is smaller than that delivered with adult pads. Use a pediatric AED or pediatric AED pads if available;

FIGURE 5-3 An AED.

FIGURE 5-4 Using the AED with CPR in unresponsive children.

© Jones & Bartlett Learning. Courtesy of MIEMSS.

however, an adult AED can be used on a child or an infant (one may consider putting pads anterior–posterior for an infant). For a pediatric arrest, use the AED as soon as possible. Studies show that even school-aged children with no prior experience or education in defibrillation can successfully operate an AED. **FIGURE 5-4** illustrates the use of an AED on a child.

> **TIP**
>
> AEDs can be used on anyone. Preferably use an AED with pediatric attenuator/cables for infants and children, but an adult AED can be used. For an unwitnessed arrest, begin CPR and use an AED as soon as it is available.

Summary of Dysrhythmias

Unlike adults, primary cardiac rhythm disturbances are rare in children. Bradycardia, a prearrest rhythm, almost always reflects profound hypoxia and bag-mask ventilation should be initiated rapidly. Tachycardia is most commonly a sinus rhythm, but may represent SVT or VT. Although children can develop sinus tachycardia greater than 200 beats/min, do a careful evaluation for hypovolemia and hypoxia and other treatable causes, and then treat the

identified causes. Assume all rates over 220 beats/min in infants or over 180 beats/min in children and all wide complex (QRS >0.09 seconds) tachycardias are primary cardiac dysrhythmias. The stable patient may need only general supportive care, regardless of cardiac rhythm. **Symptomatic ventricular dysrhythmias** may require drug therapy, with amiodarone or procainamide, and cardioversion or defibrillation. The AED is an important adjunct for prehospital professionals in unresponsive children with VF.

Cardiac Arrest

The emphasis for patients in cardiac arrest is based on early and excellent compressions. The new "Chain of Survival" has added a fifth component to enhance the postresuscitation care for the patient who has suffered a cardiac arrest.

The Pediatric Chain of Survival is as follows:

- Prevention
- Early CPR
- Early access
- Early advanced life support (ALS)
- Postresuscitation care

Survival from cardiac arrest depends on several factors, including time to CPR and presenting rhythm. The shorter the "downtime" before basic life support (BLS), the better the outcome. As in adults, pediatric patients who present to EMS personnel in VF are more likely to survive than children who present in asystole, as long as there is early CPR and access to early defibrillation.

> **TIP**
>
> The only intervention associated with survival in pediatric asystolic cardiac arrest is time to onset of CPR.

You are volunteering as a health care professional at a local high school track meet when a 14-year-old boy collapses while running the 100-meter dash. You rush to his aid and find him apneic and pulseless. You immediately start CPR.

1. What should be the next step in your assessment/management of this child?
2. At what age is it appropriate to apply an AED to assess for VF in a child?

Causes

In contrast to adults, pediatric cardiac arrest is almost always a secondary event, the result of profound hypoxia or shock. Cardiac arrest in children usually follows a primary respiratory arrest, often from respiratory failure originating from common conditions, such as pneumonia, bronchiolitis, or asthma. **Myocardial infarction** or a **cardiac dysrhythmia**, frequent causes of cardiac arrest in adults, is extremely unusual in young children.

Children can present in arrest from conditions such as HCM, which has a high incidence of sudden death and is the leading cause of cardiac death in both preadolescent and adolescent children. HCM is a condition in which a child has profound hypertrophy of the ventricles and intraventricular septum, which causes an outflow obstruction. It also has effects on the coronary arteries, leading to a thickening of the lining of the artery, a narrowing in the vessel, and a decrease of flow to the myocardium.

Long QT syndrome is a congenital problem with the electrophysiology of the heart that results in an increased risk of dysrhythmias, including bradycardia and VF. **Commotio cordis** is another cause of cardiac arrest that occurs when a child is struck by a nonpenetrating object such as a baseball, hockey puck, or karate blow. The blow is most likely to be critical if it is over the center of the left ventricle. Because this results in VF and collapse, the presence of an AED is critical.

The primary age group for pediatric cardiac arrest is infancy, when **sudden unexpected infant death (SUID)**, infection, or child maltreatment precipitates respiratory failure. In toddlers and school-aged children, however, the causes of cardiac arrest change. In this older age group, the most likely causes are hemorrhagic shock and blunt trauma from either vehicle-related injuries or falls.

Assessment in Cardiac Arrest

A child in cardiac arrest is unresponsive, apneic, and pulseless. The cardiac monitor will show a cardiac arrest rhythm: asystole, PEA, VT, or VF. Asystole is the most frequent rhythm; VF and VT are rare causes of cardiac arrest.

Asystole reflects profound hypoxia and ischemia. PEA may represent a variety of ischemic, hypoxic, hypothermic, and traumatic insults. Some PEAs may arise from low-flow states with blood pressures too low to record in the prehospital setting. VF occurs in children usually older than 2 years from a variety of conditions, including myocarditis, **congenital anomalies**, poisoning, electrocution, or hypoxia.

Chest Compressions

Chest compressions have become the focus of care in a patient in cardiac arrest. AHA guidelines implemented the CAB (circulation–airway–breathing) sequence, which places emphasis on starting compressions more quickly and ensuring that compressions are the primary focus of a patient in cardiac arrest. Compression techniques differ for a child and infant. For a child, the hand(s) should be placed on the lower half of the sternum, rate should be at least 100–120 per minute, and compression depth should be at least 2 inches (5 cm) with complete recoil (to ensure adequate preload). For an infant, as a single rescuer, one places two fingers at the nipple line and compresses at a rate of at least 100–120 per minute with a depth of at least 1.5 inches (4 cm) with complete recoil. When performing two-rescuer CPR for an infant, the recommended technique is the two fingers encircling the chest technique. For the child and infant, when performing single-rescuer CPR, the ratio is 30:2 and changes to 15:2 when there are two rescuers. For a step-by-step explanation of this procedure, see **FIGURE 5-5**.

Length-Based Drug Dosage

Treatment of infants and children in the prehospital setting is difficult because children of different ages require different sizes of equipment, different doses of medications, and different amounts of fluids (**FIGURE 5-6**). Length is a good index for drug dosing and equipment sizing during resuscitations. From a measured patient length, either a computerized resuscitation software program or a color-coded tape can provide correct doses and equipment sizes. Computerized programs offer a wider range of drugs and additional safety features. For a step-by-step explanation of this procedure, see **length-based resuscitation tapes, Procedure 2**.

Presenting Cardiac Arrest Rhythm and Treatment

The top priorities in the management of a patient in cardiac arrest are circulation (emphasis on high-quality compressions), airway and breathing (bag-mask ventilation with an airway adjunct is adequate; consider endotracheal intubation as a priority if the cause of arrest is asphyxial in nature), and defibrillation (if indicated). The presenting cardiac rhythm is a major determinant of the treatment of cardiac arrest. When the child is pulseless and apneic, the treatment of asystole and PEA is the same.

Pediatric Basic Life Support Algorithm for Healthcare Providers—Single Rescuer

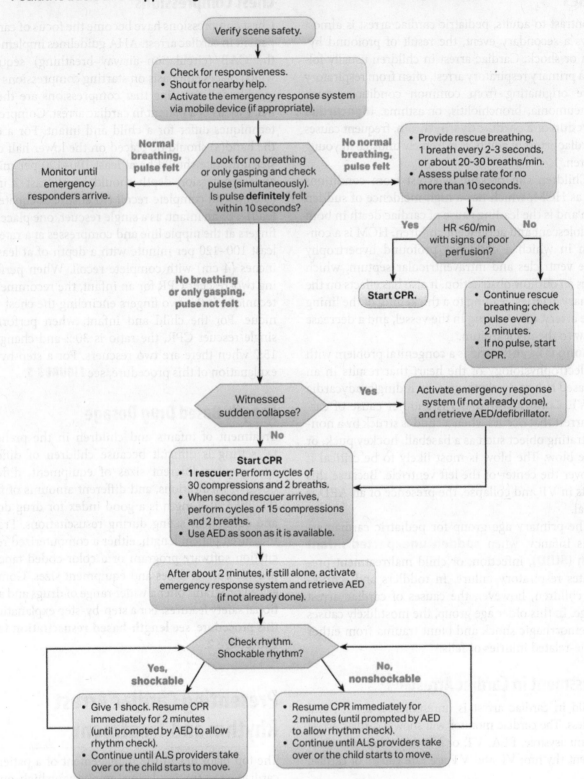

FIGURE 5-5 2020 AHA Guidelines criteria showing the pediatric BLS algorithm.

Pediatric Basic Life Support Algorithm for Healthcare Providers—2 or More Rescuers

FIGURE 5-5 2020 AHA Guidelines criteria showing the pediatric BLS algorithm. (*continued*)

© 2020 American Heart Association.

FIGURE 5-6 Resuscitation tape.
© Jones & Bartlett Learning. Courtesy of MIEMSS.

TABLE 5-5 Six Hs and Five Ts	
Hypovolemia	Tension pneumothorax
Hypoxia	Tamponade, cardiac
Hypoglycemia	Toxins
Hydrogen ion (acidosis)	Thrombosis (cardiac or pulmonary)
Hypo/hyperkalemia	Trauma
Hypothermia	

ALS

Asystole/PEA. Resuscitation efforts for nonshockable rhythms begin with high-quality CPR with an emphasis on chest compressions without interruption. Management of airway and breathing may be taken care of with bag-mask ventilation and an airway adjunct as the primary intervention as long as chest rise and compliance are noted. If the arrest is caused by asphyxia, then an endotracheal tube becomes a priority. An uncuffed endotracheal tube should be sized with the following equation: (age in years divided by 4) + 4. Cuffed endotracheal tubes are sized a half-size smaller.

Venous access can be accomplished by IV or IO. All medications, fluids, and blood products that are administered IV can be administered IO.

Epinephrine is the drug of choice, administered, as soon as possible, at 0.01 mg/kg (0.1 mL/kg of 0.1 mg/mL concentration) IV/IO. High-quality BLS with adequate airway management is continued throughout the resuscitation, with pulse checks every 2 minutes and epinephrine administered every 3–5 minutes.

An important component to the treatment of asystole/PEA is rapidly working to identify the cause; therefore, it is imperative the provider considers the Hs and Ts (**TABLE 5-5**) while providing care.

Survival from pediatric cardiac arrest requires good BLS. IV or IO needle insertion and medication delivery are helpful, but not primary determinants of survival. Endotracheal tube insertion offers no known benefit to survival. In addition, high-dose epinephrine has shown no increased survival when used in cardiac arrest. It may be considered in exceptional circumstances, such as β-blocker overdose.

ALS

VF/Pulseless VT. VF/VT management should start with high-quality CPR while attaching the AED and identifying a shockable rhythm. The initial energy setting for the child should be at 2 J/kg, followed by 2 minutes of excellent CPR. During this time, IV access should be gained. Initial airway management should be maintained with a bag-mask device and oropharyngeal airway as long as there is adequate chest rise and good compliance (an advanced airway may be considered further down the algorithm). When an airway is not maintainable with a bag-mask ventilation or the arrest is caused by a hypoxic event, an endotracheal tube should be considered as soon as possible.

After 2 minutes of high-quality CPR, the patient is reassessed. If a pulse is not present, a shock is administered at 4 J/kg. CPR is continued, and the patient is given 0.01 mg/kg of epinephrine (0.1 mL/kg), 0.1 mg/mL concentration IV/IO, repeated every 3–5 minutes. CPR is continued with pulse/rhythm checks every 2 minutes. Subsequent shocks are delivered at 4 J/kg, but can be increased to 10 J/kg, not to exceed the adult dose. Amiodarone may be given for refractory VF/pulseless VT at 5 mg/kg, repeated up to two times to a total of 15 mg/kg. Lidocaine, 1 mg/kg as a loading dose with maintenance of 20–50 mcg/kg/min by infusion, may also be given; repeat bolus if infusion is begun >15 minutes after initial loading dose.

The Transport Decision: Stay or Go

Deciding which pediatric cardiac arrest patients require hospital transport is another important controversy. Of all children in out-of-hospital cardiac arrest, only 6% will survive. Predictors of survival include type of presenting rhythm and early return of spontaneous circulation

(<5 minutes) after BLS arrives on scene. Survival from pulseless VT/VF is approximately 15%, versus about 3% for asystole. If children in cardiac arrest fail out-of-hospital resuscitation with BLS and ALS, survival is low. Patients who have ingested massive amounts of sedative-hypnotic drugs (e.g., barbiturates) may have a greater chance of survival after prolonged resuscitation and deserve extended treatment prior to a decision to halt CPR.

In some cases, field resuscitation attempts can be stopped before transport if permitted by local EMS death-in-the-field policies. Although survival in unwitnessed out-of-hospital cardiac arrest is rare, prehospital professionals may be uncomfortable in discontinuing resuscitative efforts in children. When resuscitation is terminated, skillful communication with the child's caregivers is critical (**FIGURE 5-7**), as explained in Chapter 13. *Never leave a family member on scene with the deceased child without appropriate supportive personnel.* A system to provide supportive care to the caregivers must be in place if EMS policy permits discontinuation of resuscitative efforts in the

TIP

Prehospital cardiac arrest treatment requires good BLS skills.

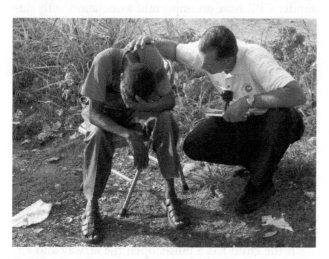

FIGURE 5-7 Skilled communication with the caregivers and family is imperative after the death of a child.
© Glen Ellman.

field. These services might be provided by social services personnel, pastoral care, or grief counselors.

Cardiac arrest in children is associated with high provider stress. Critical incident stress debriefing may be helpful for prehospital professionals after such a tragedy.

CAUTION

Never leave a family member on scene with the deceased child without appropriate supportive care.

Summary of Cardiac Arrest

Pediatric cardiac arrest is an uncommon event. Out-of-hospital arrest survival is low, and asystole has the worst prognosis. VT/VF usually occurs in older children and has higher survival rates. Meticulous attention to chest compressions, airway, oxygenation, ventilation, and early defibrillation, when appropriate, will improve success. In all cases of pediatric cardiac arrest, grief counseling for the caregivers and critical incident stress debriefing for the prehospital professionals are extremely helpful.

Congenital Heart Disease

Children with congenital heart disease are at increased risk for the types of cardiovascular emergencies more commonly seen in the adult population, including dysrhythmias and congestive heart failure. These complications may present in infancy or as late as the teenage years (**TABLE 5-6**). Advances in cardiovascular surgery have allowed the medical community to prolong the lives of children who, just decades ago, would have died in infancy. Many of these children are now living productive lives at home. Prehospital professionals must be prepared to treat "adult problems" in this younger population.

The primary assessment and management of any child experiencing a cardiovascular emergency are the same: airway, breathing, and circulation. However, in any child with a possible cardiac pathology, include a "quick look" at the cardiac rhythm. These children may have treatable cardiac dysrhythmias.

CASE STUDY 3

You are dispatched to the location of an unresponsive 2-year-old boy recently removed from a swimming pool. Estimated downtime is unknown, but the parents are on scene and state that the child had been missing for more than 30 minutes. The parents initiated CPR immediately. Upon arrival you find the child to be cool, blue, apneic, and pulseless.

1. What is the most important intervention for this patient to improve his chances of survival?
2. Should the child be actively rewarmed?

TABLE 5-6 Congenital Heart Diseases Causing Congestive Heart Failure at Different Times During Infancy

Age	Type of Congenital Heart Disease
Newborn	Hypoplastic left heart
	Severe pulmonic insufficiency
	Tetralogy of Fallot
	Severe tricuspid insufficiency
	Third-degree atrioventricular block
	Supraventricular tachycardia
	Total anomalous pulmonary venous return
	Transposition of the great vessels
First month	Aortic coarctation with patent ductus arteriosus
	Ventricular septal defect
	Tricuspid atresia
	Truncus arteriosus
First 6 months	Ventricular septal defect
	Patent ductus arteriosus
6–12 months	Ventricular septal defect
	Endocardial fibroelastosis

Drowning

Drowning is suffocation after submersion in water. Drowning is the leading cause of unintentional death in children between the ages of 1 and 4 years, and the third leading cause of death due to unintentional injury in children younger than 14 years. Unfortunately, drowning is not limited to the summer months. In warmer climates it occurs year round, and in cooler climates it may occur due to submersion in lakes, buckets, hot tubs, and bathtubs (**FIGURE 5-8**).

Prevention

The best management for near-drowning is prevention. The installation of four-sided fencing prevents

FIGURE 5-8 Drowning is the leading cause of death due to unintentional injury in children 1–4 years of age and is the third leading cause of death due to unintentional injury in children 5–14 years of age.

up to 90% of childhood residential swimming pool drownings and near-drownings. Eighty-five percent of boating-related drownings are preventable by wearing personal flotation devices.

Treatment

Early recognition of cardiac arrest and immediate bystander CPR have an important association with survival from severe submersion injuries. ALS care has an unproven benefit.

First, remove the patient from the water and quickly assess for responsiveness, breathing, and pulse. If the child is pulseless, begin CPR with chest compressions, then open the airway and provide two ventilations. Get an AED and wipe water from child's chest before applying the pads. Protect the cervical spine if there is potential head or neck trauma. Perform chest compressions, airway management, oxygenation, and ventilation, and follow protocols for drug therapy and defibrillation/cardioversion depending upon presenting cardiac rhythm.

If the child has a pulse, open the airway and ensure appropriate oxygenation and ventilation, usually with a bag-mask device. Obtain IV or IO access and transport. Provide drug therapy, and rarely defibrillation/cardioversion, as indicated for shock or dysrhythmias.

CASE STUDY ANSWERS

CASE STUDY 1

This child could be experiencing VF/pulseless VT, PEA, or asystole. He is in cardiac arrest, and the appropriate first intervention is to provide excellent CPR and BLS care. Treatment for the patient will be based on the type of arrhythmia. It is likely that he suffered commotio cordis, which is ventricular fibrillation due to a blow to the chest.

CASE STUDY 2

This cardiac arrest appears to reflect a primary cardiac event. Begin 30 chest compressions to 2 ventilations and have one provider get an AED. When the AED arrives, attach the pads and let it analyze the rhythm. If it indicates shock advised, deliver a shock and resume CPR for 2 minutes, then reanalyze the rhythm. If shockable, deliver a shock, and resume CPR.

This child was in VF due to a previously undiagnosed disorder known as prolonged QT syndrome. Survivors from this disease often give a history of blackouts associated with exercise and stress. Other family members may also be affected by the same disorder. A look back at the family history can uncover unexplained deaths of relatives at young ages.

The initial treatment for children in VF, as in adults, is rapid defibrillation. With the increasing availability of AEDs, many of these children will receive rapid recognition and defibrillation by bystanders.

CASE STUDY 3

After removal from the water, begin CPR, starting with chest compressions, then provide bag-mask ventilation with 100% oxygen. Rushing to intubate this child, before providing effective bag-mask ventilation with 100% oxygen, may result in worsened hypoxia and hypercarbia. Most drownings cause airway spasm with little or no water entering the lungs, so bag-mask ventilations may be effective. The best anatomic location for palpating a pulse in a 2-year-old child is over the brachial artery, which is located just proximal to the elbow and medially to the biceps muscle.

Although there have been promising results in adult studies of hypothermia after cardiac arrest, pediatric studies have found no benefit. The hypothermic state may be protective of brain function, and rapid rewarming can introduce dysrhythmias. Therefore, remove wet clothing, and provide rapid transport.

SUGGESTED REFERENCES

Textbooks

The American Academy of Pediatrics; Fuchs S, Klein BL, eds. *Pediatric Education for Prehospital Professionals.* 3rd ed revised. Burlington, MA: Jones & Bartlett Learning; 2014.

Hauda WE. II. Resuscitation of children. In: Tintinalli J, Stapczynski S, John Ma O, et al., eds. *Tintinalli's*

Emergency Medicine. 7th ed. New York, NY: McGraw-Hill; 2010:80–90.

Yee LL, Meckler GD. Pediatric heart disease: acquired heart disease. In: Tintinalli J, Stapczynski J, John Ma O, et al., eds. *Tintinalli's Emergency Medicine.* 7th ed. New York, NY: McGraw-Hill; 2010:827–830.

Articles

Atkins DL, Berger S, Duff JP, et al. Part 11: Pediatric Basic Life Support and Cardiopulmonary Resuscitation Quality: 2015 American Heart Association Guidelines Update for Cardiopulmonary Resuscitation and Emergency Cardiovascular Care. *Circulation.* 2015;132(suppl 2):S519–25.

deCaen AR, Maconochie IK, Aickin R, et al. Part 6: Pediatric basic life support and pediatric advanced life

support: 2015 International consensus on Cardiopulmonary Resuscitation and Emergency Cardiovascular Care Science with Treatment Recommendations. *Circulation.* 2015;132(suppl 1):S177–S203.

Perondi M, Reis A, Paiva E. A comparison of high-dose and standard-dose epinephrine in children with cardiac arrest. *N Engl J Med.* 2004;350(17): 1722–1730.

Other Resources

Raghavan SS. Pediatric long QT syndrome. https://emedicine.medscape.com/article/891571-overview. Accessed August 6, 2019.

Shah SN. *Hypertrophic cardiomyopathy*. https://emedicine.medscape.com/article/152913-overview. Accessed August 6, 2019.

Yabek SM. *Commotio cordis*. Available at http://emedicine.medscape.com/article/902504-overview. Accessed September 12, 2012.

CHAPTER 6
Medical Emergencies

Sharon Chiumento, BS, BSN, EMT-P

Sylvia Owusu-Ansah, MD, MPH, FAAP

LEARNING OBJECTIVES

1. Discuss issues of medication dosing in pediatrics, with attention to weight-based dosing and medication safety.

2. Describe the major types of seizures and the management priorities for each.

3. Compare the advantages and disadvantages of various benzodiazepines and their routes of administration in status epilepticus.

4. Distinguish the common causes of altered mental status in infants and children, and outline management priorities.

5. Describe signs and symptoms of hypoglycemia, and outline management priorities.

6. Discuss the association of fever and serious illness.

7. Outline the assessment and management of common environmental emergencies, including temperature emergencies, bites, and stings.

Introduction

A prehospital study revealed that general illness, respiratory distress, pain (nonchest/nonabdomen), and seizures were the leading medical causes for EMS transport of pediatric patients. Calls involving children with pediatric medical complaints tend to be more serious as a whole, and the varied nature of these complaints makes this group especially challenging to assess and treat. This chapter reviews common out-of-hospital pediatric medical emergencies: seizures, altered mental status (AMS), fever, endocrine disorders, gastrointestinal (GI) illness, and environmental emergencies. It also reviews the importance of

medication dosing in children, as many of the above emergencies may require medication.

Respiratory illness (covered in Chapter 3) and seizures are the two most common out-of-hospital pediatric medical emergencies. Fever is a common medical complaint, but is rarely an emergency in isolation; it is usually a symptom of an underlying illness. Although most children with fever have relatively benign, self-limited conditions (e.g., ear infection, croup, viral syndrome), it is important to identify those febrile children with potentially more serious conditions (e.g., meningitis, sepsis) who require immediate prehospital management. Fevers may be associated with seizures in infants and preschool-aged children. AMS is a less common characteristic of pediatric 9-1-1 patients, but the presence of AMS usually means the child has a serious or life-threatening medical emergency. Endocrine emergencies in childhood frequently involve AMS and altered blood glucose levels.

Environmental emergencies occurring during childhood include heat- and cold-related emergencies and envenomation by bites and stings. The young child is at increased risk for these environmental emergencies because of physiologic, behavioral, and developmental characteristics.

Accurately assessing a child with a medical illness requires an age-based approach to history taking and physical examination, as discussed in Chapters 1 and 2. Communicating with the child and family is essential. Effective communication is fundamental to good clinical care, establishment of trust, and development of comfortable interactions with the child.

Medication Dosing

Managing pediatric patients differs from the adult population, as the majority of pediatric emergency interventions are weight based. These interventions include medication doses, IV fluid requirements, defibrillation energy doses, and equipment sizes. It is important to have consistency in pediatric measurement of weight to provide children the right dose of medication, prevent errors, and preserve patient safety and care quality. The kilogram, instead of the pound, is the standard unit of measurement for pediatric patients. Most medications use the metric system, which is compatible with weight measured in kilograms.

There are numerous ways to determine the weight of a pediatric patient in kilograms, which include length-based tapes/systems (e.g., Broselow or Handtevy) and age-based weight formulas. For a step-by-step explanation, see **Length-Based Resuscitation Tapes, Procedure 2**. The original advanced pediatric life support formula tended to underestimate the actual weight, and the margin of error increased with age. There is increasing evidence that methods based on the length of the child are more accurate than age-based formulas; however, this requires accurate physical measurement. The length-based tapes are accurate for equipment sizing, but with increasing childhood obesity, they may underestimate the child's weight, especially in older children; in some impoverished countries with childhood malnutrition, they may, in fact, overestimate the weight. However, for resuscitation medications, the length-based doses should be used. A key factor is to ensure that the concentration of the medication carried is the same as on the tape (e.g., atropine and naloxone come in different concentrations). In addition, while most of the recent tapes have doses in milliliters, some older tapes had doses in milligrams, except for resuscitation drugs.

As with all patients, the right medication should be administered to the right patient for the right reason by the right route and at the right time. It is also important to check the child's history of allergies and medications already taken to prevent potential negative consequences.

Some drugs may be given by standing orders, while others may be given after consultation with a medical control physician. Verbal orders should always be repeated back to the physician to assure that there is no misunderstanding. Orders that are confusing, unclear, or not within an EMS provider's scope of practice or regional protocols should be questioned to avoid misunderstanding or breaches of standards of care. A medication should be checked carefully to assure it is the correct medication, is not expired, is not contaminated or damaged in any way, and is without particulate matter or discoloration.

Medication administration in children is particularly risky because of the potential for incorrect dosages. Most medications given to children in the prehospital setting are weight based. It is important to remember that weight-based dosing references the amount of drug to be given per kilogram (e.g., mg/kg or mL/kg), not per pound. One kilogram equals 2.2 pounds, so if a calculation is inadvertently based on pounds, the dosage will be too high and can lead to an overdose.

In an emergency setting, it is very easy to miscalculate doses, so the use of medication aids is extremely beneficial. There are different types of aids. Some show the calculated dose when figured with a child's known weight in kilograms—these include wheels, cards, or smartphone applications. Others, such as length-based measuring tapes, determine the length of the child and then give the calculated doses based on the average weight of children of that height. Any of these aids help to decrease mathematical errors, especially the misplacement of decimal points in the calculated dose. A misplaced decimal point can cause a calculation 10 times larger or smaller than the dose should be.

Some medications are prepackaged in doses specifically for pediatrics and adults. An example of this is an epinephrine autoinjector. It is essential that the correct package be selected to administer the correct dose. For example, an adult epinephrine autoinjector is typically 0.3 mg, twice the amount of the usual pediatric epinephrine at 0.15 mg.

Because overdoses of medications can occur easily, with potentially serious consequences, it is essential that the EMS provider do everything possible to safely administer any medications in the course of treatment of the child. It is also important that accurate and complete documentation of any medication doses be completed and given verbally during patient report/handoff to prevent potential overdoses due to hospital staff not knowing what was given in the prehospital setting.

Seizures

Seizures are caused by abnormal, sustained electrical discharges from a cluster of nerve cells in the brain. Seizures have varied presentations, depending on the location of the abnormal electrical activity in the brain and the age of the child. Seizures in the infant (0–12 months of age), whose central nervous system (CNS) is immature, can be very subtle, consisting only of abnormal gaze, horizontal nystagmus, sustained muscle contractions, sucking motions, or "bicycling" (pedaling movements of the legs). In the older child, who has a more mature CNS, seizures are usually more obvious and typically manifest as repetitive muscular contractions (tonic-clonic activity) and/or unresponsiveness. Sustained or repetitive muscular contractions may be associated with upper airway obstruction, resulting in poor air exchange, hypercarbia, and hypoxia. As a result, cyanosis is common.

Generalized seizures are the most common type in children. These seizures are divided into convulsive (with motor activity, such as tonic-clonic movements) and nonconvulsive (no motor activity, such as an absence seizure). Partial seizures are classified based on whether consciousness is maintained. Partial seizures with no loss of consciousness are known as simple partial seizures; those associated with a loss of consciousness are known as complex partial seizures.

Partial seizures are further subdivided based on signs and symptoms, such as motor activity (can be focal and then spread), sensory (paresthesias, vertigo, visual or auditory symptoms), or autonomic changes (sweating, pupillary changes). During a complex partial seizure, the child may have motor automatisms, such as chewing or bicycling movements of the legs. There are also epilepsy syndromes, and these infants and children may demonstrate a variety of seizure types. The term epilepsy refers to a chronic disorder that causes recurrent seizures over time, with or without a known underlying cause. Although caregivers of children with epilepsy may be very calm at the scene of a 9-1-1 call, those who are witnessing a first-time seizure are usually very frightened, may fear that the child is dying, and may have initiated cardiopulmonary resuscitation efforts.

Febrile Seizures

The most frequent type of seizure in childhood is the febrile seizure. Approximately 5% of all children have at least one seizure by 6 years of age, and more than one-half of these children never have another seizure. By definition, a simple febrile seizure is a generalized, tonic-clonic seizure of fewer than 15 minutes' duration that occurs in a febrile child between 6 months and 5 years of age with no underlying neurologic abnormalities, and occurs only once in 24 hours. Simple febrile seizures do not cause brain injury, even if the child has repeated febrile seizures. Most simple febrile seizures stop spontaneously before the arrival of prehospital professionals. Risk factors for recurrence include age less than 1 year at the time of the first febrile seizure, a family history of febrile seizure, or complex nature of the seizure.

CASE STUDY 1

You receive a call for a 2-year-old boy who was playing in the living room of his home when he began having a seizure, with jerking of his arms and legs for 10–15 minutes. On arrival at the scene, you find a child who has decreased level of consciousness, only responding to painful stimuli. There are no abnormal airway sounds, work of breathing is not increased, and skin color is normal. Respiratory rate is 12 breaths/min, heart rate is 100 beats/min, blood pressure is 90/58 mm Hg, and the oxygen saturation is 92%. There are no focal neurologic findings nor any current seizure activity. The child's temperature is 38.6°C (101.5°F). His father tells you his son has had seizures before, and he takes medication for it. He also says that because the seizure lasted so long, he gave his son rectal diazepam, as prescribed by his neurologist.

1. What other information would you want about this seizure and the child's medical history?
2. How should you manage this patient?
3. Should the child be transported?

Complex febrile seizures last longer than 15 minutes, are focal rather than generalized, and occur more than once in 24 hours. This type of seizure has a higher association with serious illness. Most children with febrile seizures have relatively benign etiology of the fever (otitis media, viral syndrome). Although there may be a brief postictal period, these children generally have improving level of consciousness and appear to be well. Children with more serious etiologies (meningitis) usually appear ill after the seizure resolves or may have associated symptoms (petechiae, neck stiffness). A child who has a seizure and a fever may not necessarily have had a febrile seizure and requires physician evaluation to exclude a serious disease. *A prehospital professional cannot make a diagnosis of a febrile seizure.*

CAUTION

A prehospital professional cannot make a diagnosis of a febrile seizure.

TIP

If the child begins to have another seizure, ensure ABCs. If the seizure does not stop in 5 minutes, begin medication administration.

Afebrile Seizures

Although childhood seizures are frequently associated with fever, there are many other possible causes of seizures. These include trauma, especially head injury (including child maltreatment); hypoxia; hypoglycemia; infection; toxic ingestion; CNS bleeding; metabolic disorders; and congenital neurologic problems. A common group of children with **afebrile seizures** are those with known epilepsy who have not received therapeutic doses of their anticonvulsant medication and experience breakthrough seizures. In addition, there is a significant group of children who have breakthrough seizures despite medication compliance; in this group, parents call when normal methods of controlling seizure activity are unsuccessful.

TIP

A seizure with a fever is not the same as a febrile seizure.

Status Epilepticus

The classic definition of **status epilepticus** is either a series of two or more seizures without recovery of consciousness between the seizures, or a continuous seizure more than 20 minutes long. A newer "operational" definition of status epilepticus was developed in the late 1990s by a group of neurologists specializing in seizure management. Based on data indicating that most seizures stop spontaneously in fewer than 5 minutes, they redefined the term status epilepticus and set a threshold for initiating pharmacologic treatment as a seizure lasting longer than 5 minutes. Accordingly, consider any child who is actively seizing on arrival of the prehospital professional to be in status epilepticus, and treat with drug therapy to stop the seizure. Such patients inevitably have been seizing for at least 15 minutes, given the average response times in most emergency medical services (EMS) systems.

Status epilepticus may occur as the child's first seizure. The age of the child in status epilepticus helps forecast the likely cause of the seizure. Children younger than 3 years of age tend to have acute, sometimes progressive causes of status epilepticus, such as hypoxia, infection, or toxic ingestion. Children older than 3 years of age who present with status epilepticus tend to have chronic, static causes (e.g., epilepsy, neurologic disorder, an inborn metabolic disorder, or inadequate anticonvulsant treatment). Therefore, be especially vigilant in care of infants and young children with status epilepticus, especially if they do not have a history of fever or epilepsy.

Status epilepticus is a medical emergency. Early treatment in the field is critical because prolonged seizure activity is difficult to control pharmacologically. Stopping the seizure also facilitates airway management, support of oxygenation and ventilation, and transport. However, the risk of long-term neurologic injury is most closely associated with the underlying *cause* and associated complications (hypercarbia, hypoxia) rather than with the *duration* of the seizure. For example, a child who has a 20-minute febrile seizure is unlikely to sustain brain injury, whereas a child with meningitis who has a seizure of the same duration is at high risk for long-term neurologic problems.

TIP

During status epilepticus, the risk of brain injury is most closely related to the cause of the seizure, not the length of the seizure.

CONTROVERSY

When to treat a seizure is a matter of debate. Although most seizures stop spontaneously and do not need any treatment, some untreated children go on to the dangerous condition of status epilepticus. The best practical approach is to treat if the child is seizing on arrival.

Classification of Seizures

The type of abnormal motor activity and the age of the child are factors important to classifying seizures, as shown in **TABLE 6-1**. The main distinction is whether the seizure involves the entire body (generalized seizures affect both hemispheres of the brain) or only one part of the body (focal seizures affect only one hemisphere of the brain). A generalized seizure usually involves abnormal muscle jerking (tonic-clonic or grand mal seizure), but may be nonconvulsive with only a loss of attention or eye blinking (absence or petit mal seizure). When the child has had a partial seizure, establish whether consciousness and verbal interaction are preserved (simple partial seizure) or impaired (complex partial seizure). **Simple partial seizures** can progress to **complex partial seizures** or to **generalized seizures**. When a partial seizure evolves to a generalized seizure, it is called secondary generalization. **Neonatal seizures** tend to be more subtle, because tonic-clonic activity may not occur during the first month of life. Deviated gaze or horizontal nystagmus and myoclonic seizures (a sudden, single muscle jerk) may be the only evidence of seizures in infants.

Complications

Seizures may cause hypoxia from airway obstruction, aspiration, or inadequate respiratory drive. Good prehospital management minimizes these complications. A second concern is brain injury from prolonged seizure activity in a child with a serious underlying condition, such as infection, intoxication (including toxic exposures), hemorrhage, or congenital neurologic problems. Children have fewer energy reserves than adults, and active seizure activity uses those reserves. Hypoglycemia can cause and/or prolong seizure activity.

Support of airway and breathing, control of seizure activity, checking and treating for hypoglycemia, and rapid transport to a facility with pediatric intensive care capability are the best strategies for minimizing morbidity in this population of critically ill children.

TABLE 6-1 Classification of Seizures

Type	Description
Generalized	
Tonic-clonic (*grand mal*)	■ Trunk rigidity and loss of consciousness, with sudden jerking of both arms and/or both legs; may be only tonic (muscle contraction, rigidity), or clonic (muscle relaxation, jerking)
Absence (*petit mal*)	■ Brief loss of awareness without any abnormal body movements; the child may appear to be staring or may be blinking his or her eyes repetitively
Partial	
Simple	■ Focal motor jerking, without loss of consciousness; may be sensory, autonomic, or psychic; may progress to complex seizure activity
Complex	■ Focal motor jerking, with loss of consciousness; sometimes there is secondary generalization to a tonic-clonic seizure
Tonic-clonic	■ Rigid posturing of trunk and extremities; may have fixed eye deviation; rhythmic twitching of muscle groups, particularly the extremities and face
Multifocal	■ Similar to clonic with multiple muscle groups involved
Myoclonic	■ Brief focal or generalized jerks of extremities or distal muscle groups; may occur as a single jerk or series of repetitive jerks
Neonatal	
Subtle	■ Chewing motions, excessive salivation, blinking, eye deviation, swallowing, swimming arms, pedaling legs, apnea, or color change

TIP

Be especially vigilant in the care of infants and young children with status epilepticus if they do not have a history of fever or epilepsy.

CONTROVERSY

The best position in which to place the child during a seizure is controversial. A supine position may increase aspiration risk, but allows easy airway and breathing management. The lateral decubitus position provides some protection against aspiration, but makes it more difficult to give oxygen and aid breathing.

Assessment and Treatment of the Actively Seizing Child

If a child is actively seizing when the prehospital professional arrives, there are several essential steps:

1. *Open the airway.*
   Managing the airway is the most important initial action (**TABLE 6-2**).

   Consider spinal motion restriction as part of airway management in a posttraumatic seizure, although it is not very effective until the seizure activity has stopped.

TABLE 6-2 Initial Airway Management in Seizing Children

Position the head to open the airway.

Clear the mouth with suction.

Consider the lateral decubitus position if the child is actively vomiting and suction is inadequate to control the airway (**FIGURE 6-1**).

Provide high-flow oxygen by nonrebreathing mask or blow-by.

Consider a nasopharyngeal airway, especially if the teeth are clenched.

FIGURE 6-1 Position the head to open the airway, place the child in the lateral decubitus position, and clear the mouth of vomitus with suction.

ALS

Positioning is the easiest method to maintain a clear airway in a young child. For an infant, toddler, or preschool-aged child, perform the chin lift or jaw thrust. If there are a lot of secretions, open the airway while placing the child in the **lateral decubitus position** (recovery position). Suction the mouth of secretions, if possible. The insertion of a nasopharyngeal airway is the most useful tool after doing chin lift or jaw thrust, as it provides an open airway around clenched teeth. Although an oropharyngeal airway can also be used, it is more difficult to insert if the teeth are clenched and may cause vomiting if the patient has a gag reflex.

Without the use of neuromuscular blockade agents, successful endotracheal intubation during a seizure is extremely difficult, and complication rates are high. *Do not attempt to intubate a seizing child.* If the airway cannot be maintained, attempt to stop the seizure through the administration of anticonvulsant medications. After the seizure is stopped, perform airway management as needed.

2. *Ensure adequate breathing.*
   Many seizures are associated with some degree of hypoventilation. Attempt to assist ventilation if the child is cyanotic or has an oxygen saturation less than 90% on supplemental oxygen. Be aware, however, that it is difficult to obtain an accurate pulse oximetry reading in a child who is having a seizure. Again, stopping the seizure is the key to successful ventilation. Opening the airway, coordinating positive-pressure ventilations with the patient's spontaneous respiratory effort, and expanding a rigid chest wall are technically difficult

procedures during a generalized seizure. Often, the result of **assisted ventilation** is stomach inflation with air. Advanced life support (ALS) providers should consider a nasogastric tube to decompress the stomach if bag-mask ventilation visibly distends the abdomen.

3. *Safeguard circulation.*

   Unless a child has seizures associated with sepsis or trauma, fluid resuscitation in the field or in transport is not necessary. Signs of poor perfusion are most likely associated with prolonged seizure activity, hypoxia, and metabolic acidosis. Once again, treating the seizure addresses these problems.

4. *Manage any disability.*

   Check the bedside glucose level and treat documented hypoglycemia, as described in **TABLE 6-3**.

ALS

Although most seizures stop before the arrival of prehospital professionals, the child who is still actively seizing usually benefits from pharmacologic treatment. Consider options for anticonvulsant administration, in terms of medications approved in the EMS system and available routes of administration. The goal is to stop the seizure while minimizing medication side effects.

Benzodiazepine drugs are excellent first-line anticonvulsants. Common drugs in this class are **lorazepam**, **diazepam**, and **midazolam**. **TABLE 6-4** provides doses and routes of administration.

Although each of the benzodiazepines has the same mechanism of action, differences in specific agent and route of administration lead to significant clinical differences in the time to peak effect and the duration of action.

TABLE 6-3 Dextrose Administration Guidelines During Seizures

Indications
- Infant or child with glucose level <60 mg/dL
- Newborn with glucose level <40 mg/dL

Treatment
- Newly born: give $D_{10}W$, 2 mL/kg IV or IO
- Neonate: give $D_{10}W$, 5 mL/kg IV or IO bolus
- Child <2 years old: give $D_{10}W$, 5 mL/kg IV or IO
- Child ≥2 years old: give $D_{25}W$, 2 mL/kg or $D_{50}W$, 1 mL/kg IV or IO bolus

If above forms of concentrated dextrose are not available, 5 mL/kg of D_{10} IV solution may be drawn up and given by syringe.

IO, intraosseous; IV, intravenous.

TABLE 6-4 Benzodiazepine Administration During Seizures

Generic Name	Initial Dose	Route	Pros	Cons
Diazepam	0.1 mg/kg	IV, IO	Rapid onset Inexpensive No refrigeration	Sedating Respiratory depression Short duration of action for seizure control (15 min)
Diazepam	0.5 mg/kg	PR	Rapid onset No IV access required	Sedating Respiratory depression
Lorazepam	0.05–0.1 mg/kg	IV, IO	Rapid onset Long duration of action for seizure control (12–24 hr)	Must be stored away from heat and extreme temperature
Midazolam	0.1 mg/kg	IV/IO	Rapid onset	Medium duration of action for seizure control (30–120 min)
	0.15 mg/kg	IM		
	0.2 mg/kg	Intranasal		

IM, intramuscular; IO, intraosseous; IV, intravenous; PR, per rectum.

Diazepam. Diazepam is a time-honored drug for status epilepticus. Intravenous (IV) or intraosseous (IO) diazepam, at 0.1 mg/kg, is an effective treatment for status epilepticus or prolonged seizures, but rapid IV administration may cause respiratory depression. Do not give diazepam intramuscularly (IM) because it is not well absorbed and is irritating to muscle tissue. Sublingual and intranasal administrations have been described, although there is little prehospital experience.

The task of cannulating a peripheral vein in a seizing child often slows down delivery of essential ALS drugs, especially in infants and toddlers. *The rectum is an effective alternative route for emergency diazepam administration.* Per rectum (PR) diazepam is effective, causes less respiratory depression, and is easy to administer. Use a higher dose of 0.5 mg/kg.

Rates of respiratory depression associated with PR diazepam are lower than for IV diazepam; however, onset of action is longer, with time to clinical effect in the range of 5 minutes. For a step-by-step explanation of the rectal diazepam administration procedure, see **Rectal Administration of Benzodiazepines, Procedure 21.**

A common home medication is Diastat, a form of rectal diazepam. Caregivers may have already administered Diastat to the child and called for assistance when the seizure did not stop. Administering an additional IV, IO, or IM dose of a benzodiazepine to stop the seizure may be necessary.

Diazepam begins to work quickly but its anticonvulsant action does not last long, a serious limitation in long field or transport times. Another dose of diazepam (or another anticonvulsant medication, if available) may be necessary within 10–20 minutes if the drug is given. If the child is on phenobarbital or has received other benzodiazepines in the previous few hours, consider one-half the normal dose of diazepam to minimize the risk of respiratory depression.

Lorazepam. Of the benzodiazepines, lorazepam, 0.05–0.1 mg/kg, probably has the best pharmacologic profile for seizure management. It has a rapid onset of action, can be given IV or IO, and has a long half-life. Lorazepam is used to stop a seizure and can help to prevent further seizure activity for up to 8 hours, depending on dose. There is little experience with prehospital PR lorazepam administration in children, and drug doses are not well established. In general, this drug has not been widely used by prehospital professionals because of the manufacturer's recommendation regarding refrigeration. Lorazepam may be stocked unrefrigerated on prehospital ALS units if it is replaced every 30 days.

Midazolam. Midazolam is another benzodiazepine that can be given to a patient without IV access and is a potent anticonvulsant, with a fast onset of action. Midazolam can be given IM at a dose of 0.15 mg/kg. Because of its water solubility, midazolam is rapidly absorbed from the injection site and has excellent local tolerability. The pharmacodynamic effects of midazolam can be seen within minutes of its administration, and the seizure usually stops within 10 minutes. Although onset of action is delayed compared to IV diazepam, the time to cessation of seizure activity may be less, when comparing time to start an IV. Midazolam can also be administered IV and IO (dose is 0.1 mg/kg) and also works intranasally. The intranasal dose is 0.2 mg/kg with a maximum dose of 10 mg, best administered by a nasal mucosal atomizer. The buccal route may actually be the best route for midazolam administration, but is not commonly used in the United States. Midazolam has been shown to have minimal respiratory compromise in prehospital pediatric patients given via both IV and IM.

When administering any benzodiazepine by any route, watch closely for respiratory depression, a common side effect of this class of drugs, and be prepared to provide bag-mask ventilatory support. Even in the case of apnea after benzodiazepine administration, a bag-mask device usually suffices because the respiratory depressant effects of the drugs are transitory. Endotracheal intubation is rarely necessary.

If the seizure does not stop after two doses of a benzodiazepine, further doses are unlikely to terminate the seizure. Consider a second drug if the local EMS system permits. Common choices for second-line anticonvulsants include phenytoin, fosphenytoin, and phenobarbital, the dosing and administration of which are described in **TABLE 6-5.**

Phenobarbital is preferred as the first-line drug in neonates at a dose of 20 mg/kg and is a second-line drug for infants and children.

TABLE 6-5 Second-Line Anticonvulsant Drug Administration

Generic Name	Initial Dose	Route	Rate of Infusion	Maximum Rate of Infusion
Phenytoin	20 mg/kg	IV, IO	1 mg/kg/min	50 mg/min
Fosphenytoin	20 mg/kg (PE)	IV, IO, IM	3 mg (PE)/kg/min	150 mg (PE)/min
Phenobarbital	20 mg/kg	IV, IO	1 mg/kg/min	50 mg/min

IM, intramuscular; IO, intraosseous; IV, intravenous; PE, phenytoin equivalents.

ALS

Fosphenytoin, a "prodrug" or metabolic precursor to phenytoin, is a second-line option. Although fosphenytoin can be administered more quickly than phenytoin IV or IO and can also be given IM, it then takes about 15 minutes to metabolize to phenytoin, the active metabolite. *Hence, the total time it takes to get an effective drug level in the blood and brain to stop the seizure is approximately the same with phenytoin and fosphenytoin.* A disadvantage of fosphenytoin is that the drug is much more expensive than phenytoin.

Phenytoin is another second-line drug in neonates, infants, and children. Phenytoin should be administered in normal saline only at a rate no faster than 1 mg/kg/min in children to a maximum of 50 mg/min. The child should be placed on a cardiac monitor and watched carefully for bradycardia and hypotension, the most common serious complications of IV or IO phenytoin. Complications are caused by the diluent or mixing solution, propylene glycol.

Neither fosphenytoin nor phenytoin are indicated for drug-induced seizures.

TIP

Always give oxygen to a child who is having a seizure or who is postictal. For a known drug-induced seizure, first-line anticonvulsants are benzodiazepines, followed by phenobarbital. There is no indication for use of fosphenytoin or phenytoin.

CAUTION

When phenytoin comes in contact with glucose, a gel forms that occludes the IV.

Transport

After providing airway and breathing support and administering a benzodiazepine, transport should be initiated. Some EMS regions allow second-line anticonvulsant medications during transport. Perform history taking and physical examination and the detailed physical examination (trauma patients), if possible, on the way to the hospital. During transport, ongoing assessments should be performed using continuous cardiac monitoring and pulse oximetry, if available. If a patient has not stopped seizing after administration of two doses of a benzodiazepine and a second-line drug (e.g., fosphenytoin, phenytoin, or phenobarbital), the risk for a prolonged seizure is high. Consider options in terms of transport destination because this subset of children is likely to require intensive care.

Assessment of the Postictal Child

Usually the child's seizure is already over when the prehospital professional arrives. This postictal state is characterized by abnormal appearance with sleepiness, confusion, irritability, and decreased interactivity that may last from minutes to hours.

If the child is physiologically stable, perform a complete assessment in the field, including history taking and physical examination, observing particularly for any rash or discoloration of the skin, and the detailed physical examination (trauma patients). Check blood glucose levels and correct hypoglycemia if present.

An example of a stable postictal patient is the child with a previous diagnosis of epilepsy who experiences a brief grand mal seizure, or the child younger than 6 years of age with fever and a possible febrile seizure. Most children who have had a brief seizure show steady improvement in level of alertness, muscle tone, and interactivity within 15–30 minutes. Failure to reach normal mental status over a 30- to 60-minute period after the seizure may reflect a serious underlying problem and trigger early transport with completion of the assessment en route to the hospital. **TABLE 6-6** lists some of the conditions that might lead to a prolonged post-ictal state that require urgent treatment in the emergency department (ED). If the child has had a seizure after head injury, provide spinal motion restriction, as discussed in Chapter 7.

If the postictal patient has a previous diagnosis of epilepsy, include the name and dosage of anticonvulsant medications and when the last dose was given in the history. Inquire when the last blood levels were obtained and whether the levels were adequate. Determine the duration of the seizure, and ask for a description of the motor activity, including where it started, how it progressed, and how long the child was unconscious. From this information, determine the type of seizure (e.g., generalized, partial, or partial with secondary generalization). Ask carefully about head trauma, either before or secondary to the seizure. Consider the possibility of ingestion or overdose, especially in toddlers and adolescents. Keep in mind that overdose of many nonprescription medications (e.g., antihistamines) can cause seizures.

CAUTION

Calm parents' fears about the seizure, but do not diagnose or provide them uncertain information about the cause of the seizure or the chance of recurrence.

TABLE 6-6 Worrisome Circumstances With the Postictal Child

Post-traumatic seizure

Post-ingestion seizure

Seizure and sustained hypoxia

Seizure in a neonate (<4 weeks of age)

First seizure in a child >6 years

More than one seizure

Seizure time >5 minutes

Low glucose level

Attempt to allay the caregiver's fears. If this was the child's first seizure, the caregiver may be extremely frightened.

Summary of Seizures

Seizures are common in children, and frightened caregivers frequently call 9-1-1 to assist in managing this problem. Usually the seizure has stopped before ambulance arrival, in which case the tasks include only assessment of the postictal child and transport to the hospital with supportive care.

Sometimes the child is seizing on arrival and requires medical management. The treatment includes opening and clearing the airway; giving oxygen; and then administering a benzodiazepine medication, usually diazepam, midazolam, or lorazepam. Rectal diazepam stops most seizures in children. Effective alternatives are IV or IO lorazepam; IV, IO, IM, or intranasal midazolam; or IV or IO diazepam. The benzodiazepine medications often cause temporary respiratory depression, which requires bag-mask ventilation support without endotracheal intubation in most cases. If treatment with a benzodiazepine is unsuccessful, second-line drugs, such as phenobarbital, phenytoin, and fosphenytoin, are good options, based on local EMS protocol.

Altered Mental Status (AMS)

AMS is an abnormal neurologic state in which the child is less alert and interactive than is age appropriate. The term AMS refers to a range of abnormal appearances, from irritability to total unresponsiveness. Sometimes the concern of the caretaker is vague, and the complaint is simply that the child is "not acting right." Understanding normal developmental or age-related changes in behavior and listening carefully to the caregiver's opinion about alterations from an individual's normal state are key features in the assessment. A mnemonic recalls many of the severe causes of AMS (**TABLE 6-7**). The mnemonic is the five vowels in the alphabet (AEIOU), followed by tips (TIPPS), and reflects the major causes of AMS.

Assessment

Use the Pediatric Assessment Triangle (PAT) and the disability component of the hands-on ABCDEs to quickly assess neurologic status. These two parts of the primary assessment work in concert to evaluate both **cortical** and **brainstem functions**, as described in Chapter 1. There is a difference between abnormal

CASE STUDY 2

You respond to a call about an unresponsive child. The caregiver states that the 3-year-old boy could not be awakened from his nap. The child is "sleeping" on your arrival, with no abnormal airway sounds or retractions. He is pale. Respiratory rate is 24 breaths/min, cardiac monitor shows a narrow complex with a rate of 160 beats/min, and his blood pressure is 72/50 mm Hg. Pupils are small and slow to constrict to light, and the child withdraws to pain. There is no sign of trauma. The caregiver states that the child has had a viral illness the past few days with vomiting and diarrhea.

1. What other assessment steps might be helpful in evaluating this child?
2. What are the immediate treatment priorities for this child?
3. What additional history may be helpful?

TABLE 6-7 AEIOU TIPPS: Possible Causes of AMS

Alcohol

Epilepsy, endocrine, electrolytes

Insulin

Opiates and other drugs

Uremia

Trauma, temperature

Infection, intussusception

Psychogenic

Poison

Shock, stroke, space-occupying lesion, subarachnoid hemorrhage

FIGURE 6-2 In a child with AMS, look for a bracelet with his or her medical history.
Courtesy of Rhonda Hunt.

appearance and AMS. Abnormal appearance is a more subtle measure of brain function and is evaluated using the TICLS mnemonic (Table 1-1). AMS is a more severe signal of mental status alteration and is evaluated with the alert-verbal-painful-unresponsive (**AVPU**) scale. Although AMS is always associated with an abnormal appearance, some children with more subtle abnormalities in appearance would not have AMS using the AVPU. For example, a child who is irritable or listless and has an abnormal appearance on the PAT may be alert on the AVPU scale of disability during the ABCDE hands-on evaluation.

The AVPU system is a quick way to determine level of consciousness and to assess major changes in mental status during transport. A child with sepsis or brain hemorrhage from inflicted injury, for example, has a serious degree of brain dysfunction and may score verbal or lower on the AVPU.

Finally, observe **motor activity**, and check the pupils. In the assessment of motor activity, watch for purposeful and symmetric movement of extremities, **ataxia**, seizures, **posturing** (**decorticate** or **decerebrate**), or **flaccidity** (**hypotonia**). In the assessment of pupils, check size (small or large), equality, and response to light. Pupils may have abnormal size or reactivity in the presence of drugs, ongoing seizures, hypoxia, or impending **brainstem herniation**. The presence of a deviated gaze is abnormal and should be noted and reported.

Look for a Medical Alert bracelet, and ask about important medical history that may account for the child's AMS, such as diabetes or a seizure disorder (**FIGURE 6-2**).

Management

Regardless of the cause of AMS, focus on the ABCs.

1. *Open the airway.*
   In the poorly responsive patient with compromised airway reflexes, suction the mouth to relieve potential obstruction from secretions or vomitus. If there is no **gag reflex** or if the patient is totally unresponsive, position the head and insert an oropharyngeal or nasopharyngeal airway. Consider spinal motion restriction if there is a suspicion of head or neck injury.
2. *Ensure adequate breathing.*
   Patients with AMS may have inadequate breathing, despite spontaneous respiratory effort, based on inadequate respiratory rate or inadequate tidal volume. Administer high-flow oxygen by nonrebreathing mask. Start bag-mask ventilation with 100% oxygen if the patient is cyanotic, has oxygen saturation less than 90% on high-flow oxygen by nonrebreathing mask, is breathing at a rate too slow for age, or has shallow or irregular respiratory effort.

ALS

Consider endotracheal intubation to protect the airway and to avoid aspiration. Ventilate the patient with suspected brain injury, but do not hyperventilate the patient (see Chapter 3). Use end-tidal CO_2 ($EtCO_2$) or waveform capnography to guide ventilations. Place the patient on a cardiac monitor and a pulse oximeter.

3. *Safeguard circulation.*
   Establish vascular access. Always start isotonic fluids at a to-keep-open (TKO) rate, unless the child is in shock. Reassess the child's level of consciousness.

4. *Perform a bedside blood glucose test* (**FIGURE 6-3**). Obtain blood for **serum glucose** measurement. Administer glucose only to children with documented hypoglycemia. Neurologic outcome in patients with diffuse brain injury is worse when the child also has hyperglycemia. If a bedside glucose test shows hypoglycemia (<40 mg/dL in a newborn, <60 mg/dL in a child), give an IV glucose bolus, diluted as directed, or IM **glucagon** as outlined in Table 6-3. Administer **oral glucose** to a child with diabetes and hypoglycemia who is conscious and has a gag reflex.
5. *In the child with AMS and depressed respirations, consider naloxone administration.*
   The naloxone dose is 0.1 mg/kg, with a usual maximum dose up to 2 mg. However, more is often required with synthetic opioid overdose. Naloxone may be given by a variety of routes: IV, IM, IO, subcutaneous, intranasal, or endotracheal tube. Caution must be exercised when giving naloxone to a depressed newborn of a **narcotic**-addicted mother, because it may induce acute withdrawal symptoms and seizures. Instead of giving naloxone, consider supporting ventilation and transporting the newborn to the hospital. Outside of the newly born, narcotic overdose is an unlikely cause of AMS in children, but is an important consideration in teenagers. Constricted pupils are a universal finding in pure opiate overdoses. This is not necessarily the case with *synthetic* narcotics, such as oxycodone.

FIGURE 6-3 Perform a bedside blood glucose test.
Accu-Chek® Aviva used with permission of Roche Diagnostics.

ENDOCRINE DISORDERS

In children, endocrine disorders include diabetes, congenital adrenal hyperplasia (CAH), panhypopituitarism, and cortisol deficiency. Of these disorders, diabetes is the most common.

Diabetes Mellitus

Diabetes is a disorder of the hormone insulin. Insulin, produced by the pancreas, helps regulate blood glucose levels. Glucose is needed in the production of energy by the cells in the body. Without adequate amounts of insulin, muscle cells cannot access circulating glucose and thus cannot create energy. The disease called diabetes mellitus is a result of a lack of functioning insulin.

Diabetes mellitus is a disease of children and adults. Of the two types, type 1 (insulin-dependent diabetes mellitus, IDDM) and type 2 (non-insulin-dependent diabetes mellitus, NIDDM), younger children are more likely to have type 1 diabetes. These children are more prone to develop antibodies to the cells in the pancreas that produce insulin. The underlying cause is unknown.

There is an increasing prevalence of type 2 diabetes (NIDDM) in childhood. Such children are usually adolescents, often with associated obesity. The child may be on oral hypoglycemic agents, rather than insulin.

Regardless of the type of diabetes, the onset of symptoms is relatively slow, over days (as in type 1 diabetes) to weeks (as in type 2 diabetes). The disease process begins as insulin production is diminished. Diminished amounts of insulin increasingly impair the availability of glucose to the muscle cells. The diminished amounts of glucose available for energy production stimulate the release of fat stores. As fat stores are mobilized, they are converted to ketones and other metabolic acids. Together, the accumulation of glucose and metabolic acids causes the symptoms of diabetic ketoacidosis (DKA).

If the blood glucose level exceeds the renal threshold for reabsorption, an osmotic diuresis is created. This results in frequent urination (**polyuria**) with corresponding loss of body water. The higher the blood glucose level, the higher amounts of body water are lost in the urine. Loss of body water causes intense thirst (**polydipsia**), and fat breakdown leads to increased hunger (**polyphagia**). The hallmark sign of Kussmaul respirations may occur. These respirations are rapid and deep and have the odor of ketones or rotten fruit. These children may fall asleep in school, begin wetting the bed, and have abnormal thirst, and the odor of ketones is often prevalent.

EMS may be called for a child with AMS with a history of abdominal pain, vomiting, and excessive thirst. The child is often severely dehydrated. In the presence of abdominal pain, nausea, and vomiting, sepsis may be suspected. The presence of a blood glucose level higher than 300 mg/dL, or hyperglycemia, may lead one to suspect the presence of DKA.

Assessment

Signs and symptoms of hyperglycemia can be hard to detect, especially because the onset is relatively slow. A key finding in hyperglycemia is dehydration. Depending on the blood sugar level, signs and symptoms may range from mild to severe hypoperfusion. Tachycardia, rapid/deep respirations, and dry skin are all signs of volume depletion. In general, the higher the blood glucose level, the more extreme the dehydration.

Management

After general treatment measures are implemented, initiate an IV and administer isotonic fluid at 10-20 mL/kg over 30 - 60 minutes. Repeat boluses only if the child is hypotensive. If not hypotensive, keep IV fluids at maintenance rate. **Cerebral edema** is a complication of DKA, with warning signs of headache, or a change in mental status. Monitor GCS and reassess patient frequently enroute.

Hypoglycemia

Hypoglycemia is defined as a serum glucose concentration of less than 40 mg/dL in a newborn, or less than 60 mg/dL in a child. The most frequent scenario for out-of-hospital hypoglycemia is a child with known diabetes who uses too much insulin, exerts himself or herself excessively, or delays a meal or begins to vomit after taking insulin. Hypoglycemia may also occur in children with a history of almost any endocrine problem.

In nondiabetic infants, hypoglycemia may occur when the child has been working so hard that glycogen reserves become depleted (e.g., when compensating for a cardiac defect or for an extreme respiratory rate). This is more common in infants and toddlers.

Hypoglycemia may also occur in children with sepsis. Check a bedside glucose level in any acutely ill appearing child, especially in the presence of abnormal appearance or AMS. Other causes of hypoglycemia in children are poor food intake in the face of an acute illness, such as gastroenteritis, especially in infants and toddlers with limited glycogen reserves.

TABLE 6-8 Signs and Symptoms of Hypoglycemia		
Mild	**Moderate**	**Severe**
Hunger, irritability, weakness, agitation, tachypnea, tachycardia	Anxiety, blurred vision, stomachache, headache, dizziness, sweating, pallor, tremors, confusion	Seizure, coma

Assessment

Signs and symptoms of hypoglycemia can be hard to detect, especially in younger infants who have mild hypoglycemia. The changing signs and symptoms are noted in **TABLE 6-8**. Tachycardia, tachypnea, sweating, agitation, and tremor all reflect increased catecholamine release as the body responds to inadequate sugar supplies to support cellular metabolism. When blood sugar is dangerously low, seizures, coma, and death can occur.

Management of Hypoglycemia in Diabetes Mellitus

Children with type 1 IDDM are often well aware of the signs and symptoms of hypoglycemia, based on past experiences with insulin. If a patient with diabetes is at least physiologically stable and cooperative, but is hypoglycemic by blood sugar testing, allow him or her to attempt oral glucose replacement. Give 0.5–1.0 g/kg of sugar. There are 20 g of glucose in 8 oz of regular (not dietetic) soda, as well as orange or apple juice. Milk may be the preferred replacement with a balance of 12 g glucose, 8 g protein, and 8 g fat in 8 oz of whole milk.

Children taking oral hypoglycemic agents (type 2 diabetes) are also prone to hypoglycemia, although not as frequently. When present in the child with type 2 diabetes, hypoglycemia can be more difficult to stabilize. Give the child oral glucose replacement if signs and symptoms of hypoglycemia occur and the child is physiologically stable and cooperative, or treat with IV dextrose or IV or IM glucagon if the child has AMS.

Treatment of Hypoglycemia

Treat hypoglycemia if the child has AMS and measured serum glucose of less than 40 mg/dL in a newborn or less than 60 mg/dL in a child, as outlined in Table 6-3. Children have different tolerances to hypoglycemia, so a child may be alert and cooperative with a blood sugar level between 40 and 50 mg/dL. A child

in this condition can take oral glucose, or an infant can breastfeed.

TIP
Signs and symptoms of hypoglycemia can be nonspecific.

For the physiologically unstable patient with hypoglycemia and AMS, IV or IO dextrose should be administered immediately. Recheck the serum glucose if scene time or transport is prolonged, and repeat glucose doses as needed. Use 10% dextrose for infants, neonates, and those under 2 years of age. Use 10%, 25%, or 50% dextrose for those 2 years and older (see Table 6-3 for dose).

If there is no IV access, glucagon should be administered (0.02–0.03 mg/kg IO or IM, up to 1 mg). Repeat in 20 minutes as needed. Glucagon stimulates a transient increase of the blood glucose level as long as there are liver stores of glycogen (long chains of stored glucose molecules). It is important to note that the incidence of vomiting is increased in children when glucagon is administered. Take care to position the child to ensure airway patency within the first 15–20 minutes after administration.

Congenital Adrenal Hyperplasia

CAH is another endocrine disorder. This disorder involves the hormones of the adrenal glands. The adrenal glands help keep the body in balance by making the right amounts of cortisol, aldosterone, and androgens. Although there are many different types of CAH, the most common type (95%) results in a deficiency of cortisol and sometimes aldosterone. As a result, the body cannot adjust to illness or injury. Hypotension, hypoglycemia, and dehydration may be severe and a threat to life.

Most children with this disorder carry emergency medication with them at all times. Usually, the medication includes hydrocortisone. Parents should be asked if they have given the needed medication, such as hydrocortisone. If not, have them administer the medication if possible. If they have not given steroids, administer hydrocortisone (1 mg/kg) IV, IO, or IM per local protocol. Because the body is unable to adjust to a stress, checking blood glucose level and administering dextrose as needed, monitoring blood pressure, and replacing fluids as necessary are all part of assessment and treatment.

Cortisol Deficiency

This deficiency occurs when the adrenal glands do not produce enough cortisol. This may occur for a variety of reasons, including CAH, pituitary gland malfunction, failure of the adrenal gland itself, or long-term steroid use. When children are prescribed steroids for a period of time, they must be gradually withdrawn to give the adrenal glands a chance to resume function. Normal management includes oral hydrocortisone or IM injections. In certain circumstances, the amount of hydrocortisone should be increased quickly. This is done by administering either oral or IM hydrocortisone.

In any case, when a child with cortisol deficiency becomes sick, many body systems are affected, including the ability to balance blood glucose and regulate body water. These children should always have a blood glucose check. Asking the parent or caregiver if the child's normal medication has been administered is appropriate. If the medication has not been administered, give hydrocortisone (1 mg/kg) IV, IO, or IM per local protocol, call the receiving facility, or follow the care plan (found with the rescue medication).

> **TIP**
>
> In a child with impaired adrenal gland function, administration of steroids (hydrocortisone) can be lifesaving.

Panhypopituitarism

This condition affects the pituitary gland, particularly the anterior pituitary, where thyroid-stimulating hormone, adrenocorticotropic hormone, growth hormone, and others are produced. As a result, many other glands of the child's endocrine system are also affected. These children are usually diagnosed in infancy, or they can develop the condition after removal of certain brain tumors. Parents or other caregivers are well educated in their child's condition. When a child suffering this condition becomes ill, hypoglycemia is common, and dehydration may also be present. These children also need hydrocortisone (1 mg/Kg) IV, IO, or IM.

Transport

With any child having an endocrine issue, transport is important. If the child is suffering from hyperglycemia, do not delay transport for administration of fluid. The child needs to be transported, so IV/IO starts en route are appropriate.

However, if a low blood glucose level is present, treatment should be initiated immediately. After giving IV or IO dextrose or IM glucagon, reassess. Watch for a return to normal appearance and behavior. If the child with AMS does not return to normal in a few minutes after IV or IO administration or within 15–20 minutes after IM glucagon, transport immediately and conduct additional assessment on the way to the ED. If the child returns to normal, consider doing additional assessment on scene. If the child has no history of diabetes or other endocrine problems and has either hyperglycemia or hypoglycemia, transport is indicated.

Additional Assessment

Perform history taking when possible. Ask key questions, such as the following:

- How quickly did the symptoms progress?
- Does the patient have diabetes or any other known illness?
- If the patient is a diabetic, or has another endocrine problem, has there been a recent change in medication or meals?
- Is the child on insulin, an oral hypoglycemia drug, or any other replacement medication?
- Is this the first episode? If not, how often does this happen?
- Is it possible that the child was exposed to drugs or alcohol?
- When was the last time the child had medication?
- How many caregivers are giving medications? Are they doubling up doses?

For newborns, ask the following questions:

- If the patient is a newborn, has the mother received prenatal care?
- Has the mother had any medical problems with the pregnancy?
- Is the mother a diabetic?
- What is the newborn being fed and how often?

After the history, a physical examination should be performed. It is important to continually reassess the patient's status. If the child has diabetes and received too much **insulin** and there are no physiologic or anatomic abnormalities on reassessment, or if the child has another endocrine problem, consider contacting medical control. In some EMS systems, the child with type 1 diabetes, who is not in DKA, may be left at the scene with management directed by the primary care physician in consultation with the caregiver. However, the circumstances with type 2 diabetes are somewhat different, because the oral drugs that are taken for this condition have a longer duration of action than most insulin and the child may need ongoing administration of glucose to maintain blood sugar. *Patients with type 2 diabetes on oral agents who have experienced hypoglycemia should not be left on the scene.* If the child has an emergency medication that needs to be administered, or if the child is a type 2 diabetic with an episode of hypoglycemia, transport the child to the ED.

> **TIP**
>
> Do not leave patients with type 2 diabetes on oral agents who have experienced hypoglycemia on the scene.

Summary of Altered Mental Status and Endocrine Disorders

There are many causes of AMS in children. The caregiver may be the best judge of AMS, especially in the infant or toddler, where developmental assessment is more challenging. Appearance and the AVPU scale work in concert to help assess AMS. Address the ABCs first and especially consider causes of dehydration, such as hyperglycemia, and reversible causes, such as hypoglycemia. Transport the child with hyperglycemia immediately.

Fever

Fever is a sign of infection or inflammation, rather than a problem itself, and is often misunderstood. Most infections in childhood are systemic and result in fevers. Children can run high fevers in response to either bacterial or viral infections. High fever (>40°C [104°F]) can be caused by minor illness, such as a cold, or serious problems, such as pneumonia, meningitis, or sepsis. Fever of any cause leads to an increase in basal metabolic rate, causing a more rapid respiratory rate, tachycardia, increased cardiac output, higher oxygen consumption, and a greater need for fluids and calories. The ill child frequently is not interested in eating or drinking and, with the increased metabolic demands of fever, may be at risk for volume depletion and hypoglycemia. A body temperature less than 41.1°C (106°F) is not itself harmful. However, body temperatures greater than 41.1°C (106°F) may have the potential to be harmful, and the child should be carefully evaluated. In general, fevers are a common cause of concern for most parents, and high temperatures are a cause of concern to caregivers who fear

brain damage as a result of a high fever despite the fact that there is no evidence to support that concern.

Determine the presence of fever by history and field evaluation. Knowing the temperature, however, usually does not change field management.

> **TIP**
>
> Fever less than 41.1°C (106°F) by itself does not cause brain damage.

Assessment

The primary assessment helps determine the severity of the child's illness and the urgency for treatment. If the primary assessment is normal, take a history and perform a physical examination. Ask about important signs and symptoms of infection, such as chills, malaise, poor feeding, lethargy, pulling of ears, vomiting, diarrhea, abdominal pain, presence of a rash or skin discoloration, stiff neck, headache, and irritability.

Ask about exposure to known childhood communicable diseases. Many childhood illnesses begin with a fever before any other symptoms are present. Determine if the child has any significant medical history, because febrile children who may be immunodeficient (e.g., patients with sickle cell disease, cancer, human immunodeficiency virus [HIV], or post-organ transplantation) are at higher risk for serious infection as the cause of fever.

Febrile respiratory infections are very common in children and are characterized by fever, tachycardia, tachypnea, nasal congestion, cough, and respiratory distress. Fever may make a child with a minor illness appear sicker than he or she really is, and parents often report a marked improvement in symptoms after administration of antipyretics, such as acetaminophen or ibuprofen. After the history, if the child has no physiologic abnormalities, a physical examination should be performed to look for possible sources of infection.

Although the height of fever is not reflective of the degree of illness, certain findings suggest a serious underlying illness and must prompt rapid transport. These include a bulging fontanelle (if <12 months of age, palpate with the child sitting up), photophobia (sensitivity to light), nuchal rigidity (stiff neck), paradoxical irritability (an infant who is crankier when picked up and held than when left alone) (FIGURE 6-4), seizures, prolonged capillary refill time, or a petechial or purpuric rash.

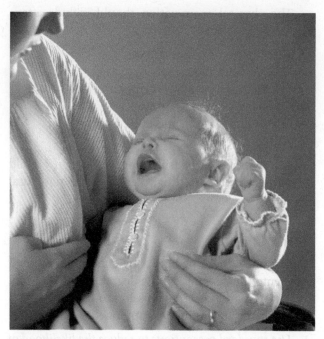

FIGURE 6-4 An infant suffering from paradoxical irritability.
© Stock Connection Blue/Alamy Stock Photo.

Age and Fever

In addition to signs and symptoms, the age of a child is important in assessing the significance of fever. A fever in an infant younger than 3 months may be the only indication of serious infection, but the degree of temperature may be lower in comparison to the severity of illness or in comparison to older children with the same problem. The symptoms of serious bacterial infection in a young infant may be nonspecific, such as fussiness, poor feeding, and sleepiness. Because these very young infants have an immature immune system and are difficult to assess because of their limited range of behaviors and activities, any infant younger than 4 weeks with fever greater than or equal to 38°C (100.4°F) requires blood, urine, and spinal fluid cultures and empiric **antibiotics** in the ED. In the first few days of life, **jaundice** may be a sign of serious bacterial infection. Infants 28 days to 2 months of age usually require a full evaluation, but may be discharged from the ED if the physical examination and laboratory evaluation are normal. A seizure in the presence of a fever in a child younger than 6 months of age also warrants transport.

Management

Management of fever in the child who has a normal primary assessment includes the following:

1. *Prevent transmission of disease to the prehospital professional.*
   Use standard precautions for infection control.

2. *In a febrile child who is older than 6 months, consider administration of antipyretics if none has been administered in the past 4 hours.*
   Give acetaminophen at a dose of 15 mg/kg orally or rectally. Another option for the alert pediatric patient is ibuprofen at 10 mg/kg orally if awake. Ibuprofen is not recommended by the manufacturer for infants younger than 6 months of age and should not be given to a child of any age with kidney problems. A pediatric patient's level of consciousness or history of recent vomiting should be considered before administering anything by mouth. **Aspirin** should be avoided in a febrile infant or child because prior studies suggest that there is an increased incidence of Reye syndrome in children who receive aspirin for a viral illness. Parents may need explanation that overbundling a febrile child retains heat and may increase fever.

3. *Cool the feverish child by undressing him or her, but avoid hypothermia.*
   Do not use cold water, fans, ice, or alcohol baths to lower temperature.

4. *Transport with ongoing reassessment for deterioration.*

5. *Explain to the caregiver that fever alone is not dangerous to the child.*

CAUTION

Never use ice, cold water, fans, or alcohol baths to cool a feverish child.

Summary of Fever

Fever is usually a response to any type of infection. It is rarely a problem in and of itself. However, the longer the child has sustained a fever, the more likely the child is dehydrated. The age of the child and other associated signs and symptoms are important in determining probability of serious illness. The presence of a petechial or purpuric rash, stiff neck, light sensitivity, and/or AMS in a child with a fever is highly suspicious for a more serious problem. In most cases, simple cooling measures and transport are the primary actions for the prehospital professional.

COMMUNICABLE DISEASES

Many communicable diseases are common during childhood. Although most are viral in origin, and mild in terms of severity, infectious diseases on occasion cause significant compromise in the pediatric patient, resulting in the need for prehospital transport. Many childhood diseases have a respiratory component, a GI component, or both. Respiratory diseases are addressed in Chapter 3. This chapter concentrates on the GI signs and symptoms of nausea, vomiting, and diarrhea.

Nausea, Vomiting, and Diarrhea (Gastroenteritis)

Collectively, nausea, vomiting, and diarrhea are termed gastroenteritis. **Gastroenteritis** is an inflammation of the GI tract that presents as vomiting and diarrhea in the pediatric patient. There are numerous causes of gastroenteritis, ranging from food and waterborne diseases, viruses, and bacteria, to a side effect of antibiotics and parasites, many carried by animals, especially pets. Of all the causes, viral agents are most common, with the Norwalk virus being especially contagious. No matter the cause, this infectious illness can result in volume depletion, particularly in younger children. Beware that signs and symptoms most commonly associated with gastroenteritis, such as fever, abdominal pain, or vomiting, can also herald more serious abdominal emergencies, such as appendicitis and bowel obstruction.

It is important to determine the presence and sequence of nausea, vomiting, diarrhea, and/or fever. Conditions of malrotation of the gut (in newborns) and pyloric stenosis (vomiting shortly after nursing but no diarrhea or fever) are conditions more common in young infants. Food poisoning, such as salmonella, usually occurs after eating (sometimes as much as 6–8 hours) and causes vomiting and diarrhea, in that order, then followed by a fever. The diagnosis of gastroenteritis requires exclusion of more serious causes, and this determination is not possible in the field.

Assessment

Focus the assessment of a child with presumed gastroenteritis on the child's state of hydration.

The history should include questions regarding the following:

- The onset, sequence of events, and frequency of vomiting or diarrhea
- Relationship to eating
- Amount of oral intake
- Number of wet diapers or frequency of urination in the past 8 hours
- Character of stool, including the presence of blood
- Last urination or wet diaper

The physical examination should include attention to the following:

- Presence or absence of fever
- Level of consciousness
- Hydration of mucous membranes (moist or dry)
- Presence or absence of tears
- Extremity warmth and pulse quality
- Abdominal tenderness or distention

Always check a bedside glucose level in a child with a history of vomiting, diarrhea, and poor oral intake.

Management

Management of the pediatric patient with presumed gastroenteritis depends on the degree of dehydration. Prevention of disease transmission to the prehospital professional is an additional component of care.

1. *Use standard precautions to reduce the likelihood of disease transmission.*

   Gastroenteritis, whether bacterial, viral, or parasitic in origin, is transmitted by the fecal–oral route. Ingestion of even a few pathogenic organisms can lead to disease in some cases. Some organisms can survive on examination instruments and surfaces for hours, so special care of clothes and instruments and careful hand washing are essential.

2. *Provide supplemental oxygen and airway management for the unstable pediatric patient.*

ALS

3. *Provide fluid replacement for severe clinical dehydration.*

   Establish vascular access, IV or IO, and initiate fluid replacement using crystalloid fluid at 20 mL/kg initial bolus if the child has severe clinical dehydration, as evidenced by elevated heart rate, poor pulses, delayed capillary refill time, cool extremities, and abnormal coloration. Repeat the bolus to a total of 60 mL/kg until perfusion is stabilized.

4. *Treat documented hypoglycemia.*
5. *Reassess vital signs.*
6. *Transport.*

   Transport decisions depend on the degree of dehydration and local resources. A child with mild to moderate dehydration and ongoing vomiting and diarrhea may require transport alone without treatment. Provide oral fluids in the field to children with dehydration, if permitted by the EMS system. The child with signs of severe dehydration or shock benefits from immediate fluid replacement before hospital transport.

Sepsis and Meningitis

Sepsis in children is a clinical syndrome that results in **systemic inflammatory response syndrome (SIRS)** in the presence of, or as a result of, a suspected or proven infection. SIRS is the presence of at least 2 of the following characteristics (1 of which must be an abnormal temperature or abnormal white blood cell count): (1) core temperature >38.5°C (101.3°F) or <36°C (96.8°F); (2) tachycardia, HR >2 standard deviations (SD) for age over a 0.5–4 hour period, or for infants <1 year, bradycardia (mean HR below 10th percentile for age for 0.5 hr); (3) mean respiratory rate >2 SD for age; (4) **leukocyte (white blood cell) count** elevated or depressed for age, or >10% immature neutrophils. While not all of this information is available to the prehospital care provider, the presence of fever and tachycardia and/or tachypnea should make one think about sepsis. Septic shock, which is sepsis and cardiovascular and other organ dysfunction, is covered in Chapter 4.

Some children with sepsis also have **meningitis**, resulting from infection and inflammation of the meninges, the membranes that cover the brain and spinal cord. Other children present with sepsis or meningitis alone. The causative agent of meningitis may be aseptic (nonbacterial) or bacterial. Although children with viral or aseptic meningitis may appear quite ill, the infection is not often life threatening. However, bacterial meningitis is rapidly progressive, with death sometimes following the onset of symptoms within hours to days. Although fever is usually present, except occasionally in the neonatal period, other symptoms may vary from stiff neck and headache to impending brainstem herniation.

Infants in the first 3 months of life are at highest risk for sepsis and bacterial meningitis, and the organisms vary with age. Since the introduction of the *Haemophilus influenzae* type B vaccine in the late 1980s, this previously common cause of childhood illness has almost disappeared. Bacterial sepsis and meningitis in the first month of age are most commonly caused by bacteria acquired from the maternal vaginal area during delivery. These include *Escherichia coli*, group B streptococcus, and *Listeria monocytogenes*.

Outside of the youngest age group, community-acquired infection is the source of sepsis and meningitis, with common bacterial causes in immune-competent children including *Streptococcus pneumoniae* (also the most common cause of bacterial ear infections, sinusitis, and pneumonia in children) and *Neisseria meningitidis* (meningococcus). The pneumococcal vaccine, available throughout the United States, is significantly reducing the incidence of childhood bacteremia and sepsis from the pneumococcal organism. *H. influenzae* type B meningitis has also decreased significantly because of widespread vaccine use. The **enteroviruses** are also common causes of viral meningitis, especially during summer and fall months.

Another group of children who are at risk for sepsis are those who are immunodeficient (e.g., cancer, post-organ transplantation), especially if they have an indwelling central line.

Meningococcal sepsis or meningitis is a life-threatening emergency that presents acutely with high fever, AMS, and a characteristic **petechial rash** or **purpura**. The presence of such a rash should always trigger rapid transport by the highest level of provider to the highest level of care available, because these children can deteriorate very quickly, requiring aggressive life support.

Assessment

In a physiologically unstable child with presumed sepsis or meningitis, limit the scene assessment. Perform the focused history and physical examination during transport, if possible. The focused history should include the following:

- Known exposure to illness
- Perinatal history for infants <1 month of age
- Onset of symptoms and rapidity of progression
- Presence or absence of fever
- Associated symptoms and signs, such as irritability, vomiting, nuchal rigidity, and rash (petechiae or purpura)
- Immunization history

The physical examination should include attention to the following:

- Fever
- Level of consciousness
- Adequacy of perfusion
- Nuchal rigidity
- Presence of a rash (petechiae or purpura)
- Photophobia

Because children with sepsis and meningitis are in a hypermetabolic state, they can develop hypoglycemia and dehydration. Check a bedside glucose level on any patient with presumed sepsis or meningitis.

Management

Management of the pediatric patient with sepsis or meningitis must include infection control precautions. Interventions vary based on the patient's clinical presentation.

1. *Prevent disease transmission.*
   The prehospital professional should use standard and respiratory precautions, including gowns, gloves, and masks, to avoid contact with patient secretions.
2. *Provide supplemental oxygen.*
   Unstable patients may need assisted ventilation or airway management.
3. *Establish vascular access.*

`ALS`

4. *For inadequate perfusion, initiate fluid replacement.*
   For the pediatric patient with inadequate perfusion, initiate fluid replacement using crystalloid fluid at 20 mL/kg initial bolus as fast as possible. Because of the effects of fever, dehydration may be present; in addition, because of the effects of bacterial toxins on the blood vessels, children with sepsis may develop distributive shock requiring aggressive fluid resuscitation. Therefore, repeat fluid boluses of 20 mL/kg up to 60 mL/kg of crystalloid fluid may be required.

5. *Treat hypoglycemia.*
6. *Reassess vital signs frequently.*
   Use continuous cardiorespiratory monitoring and pulse oximetry, if available. Anticipate deterioration in transport.
7. *Transport.*
   Because these children are at risk for rapid deterioration and may need ALS intervention, transport by the highest level of service available. Children with sepsis or meningitis generally require intensive care. Consider this when determining a transport destination.

ENVIRONMENTAL EMERGENCIES

Common pediatric environmental emergencies include temperature-related problems, bites, and stings. Each of these emergencies can range from mild to severe. Match the intensity of the intervention to the severity of the illness or injury.

Heat-Related Emergencies

Heat-related emergencies involve two separate and distinct processes leading to three main heat-related emergencies: (1) heat cramps, (2) heat exhaustion, and (3) heat stroke. Heat cramps and heat exhaustion are caused by a combination of fluid deficit and electrolyte imbalance. Heat stroke, however, is a result of a resetting of the heat-regulating mechanism in the hypothalamus of the brain, resulting in **hyperthermia**.

Heat cramps are a combination of electrolyte imbalance and dehydration where the electrolyte imbalance precipitates spasms of the muscle, typically of the long bones. These children complain of pain in their legs, arms, and sometimes abdomen. Because this has usually occurred during activity, the skin is warm and sweaty. Tachycardia may be present and may be caused by pain.

Heat exhaustion is a combination of electrolyte imbalance and dehydration where the dehydration precipitates dizziness and/or syncope. Because a volume deficit is present, the skin is often pale, cool, and diaphoretic. Tachycardia and tachypnea are also common. Hypoglycemia is not common, but should be assessed for and treated as necessary.

Heat stroke occurs when the temperature-regulating mechanism is reset to a higher set point, usually higher than 40.6°C (105°F). As a result, the basal metabolic rate is greatly increased and every body organ is affected. Because the enzymes within the organs and body systems are designed to work within a relatively narrow temperature range, organ failure occurs. AMS, heart failure with pulmonary edema, kidney and liver failure, and profound hypotension are evident. Because of the increased metabolic rate, hypoglycemia is common. The skin is usually dry and red, tachycardia is extreme (usually >150 beats/min), and tachypnea is present.

Heat-related emergencies, however, are rarely as clear cut as they are described. The child with heat exhaustion may have AMS, or the child with heat stroke may be sweating. Regardless of the type of heat-related emergency, it is very important that a heat-related emergency is recognized and treatment implemented. In the pediatric population, heat-related emergencies occur most commonly when young children are left in a closed car or older children who are not heat acclimated participate in sports during periods of high environmental temperatures and do not hydrate adequately. Because of the difficulty of obtaining temperature readings in the field, the assessment of such patients often occurs without the benefit of an objective temperature.

Physiologic considerations in infants and toddlers with heat-related emergencies include immature thermoregulatory systems, greater body surface area–to-mass ratio, and a reduced ability to dissipate heat (TABLE 6-9). These characteristics predispose infants and toddlers to heat-related emergencies, particularly heat stroke, much more quickly than in older children.

Assessment

The history should include the following:

- Environmental temperature
- Duration of environmental exposure
- Activities and events before symptom development
- Preexisting medical conditions

Management

The management of heat-related illness depends on the severity of symptoms, especially the patient's level of consciousness and cardiovascular status. Because the mechanism is different, use of antipyretics is not effective.

TABLE 6-9 Typical Clinical Presentation of Heat-Related Emergencies

Clinical Presentation	Signs and Symptoms
Heat cramps	<ul><li>Normal level of consciousness</li><li>Slightly elevated body temperature</li><li>Painful muscle spasms</li></ul>
Heat exhaustion	<ul><li>Mild AMS</li><li>Tachycardia, tachypnea, hypotension</li><li>Core temperature 38–40°C (100.4–104°F)</li><li>Fatigue</li><li>Headache</li><li>Diaphoresis</li></ul>
Heat stroke	<ul><li>Severe AMS; confusion to coma</li><li>Tachycardia, hypotension</li><li>Core temperature >40.6°C (105°F)</li><li>Flushed, dry skin</li><li>Nausea and vomiting</li></ul>

AMS, altered mental status.

Heat Cramps

- Cool environment
- Remove excess clothing
- Oral rehydration with an electrolyte-containing solution
- Establish vascular access with normal saline at TKO rate

Heat Exhaustion

- Cool environment
- Cool misting or light sponging with tepid water and allowing moisture to evaporate
- Establish vascular access and initiate fluid replacement with crystalloid fluid at 20 mL/kg for treatment of shock

Heat Stroke

- Airway management, assist ventilations, intubate if indicated
- Establish vascular access and fluid replacement with crystalloid fluid at 20 mL/kg
- Cool misting or light sponging with tepid water and allowing moisture to evaporate
- Aggressive cooling measures: ice bags to axilla, groin, and neck; cold water immersion if immediate transport is delayed
- Frequent remeasurement of core temperature
- Treat hypoglycemia
- Avoid shivering
- Treat for shock

> **TIP**
>
> Early recognition and frequent reassessment of a heat-related emergency are important, because the patient's temperature may continue to rise despite initial management techniques.

Summary of Heat-Related Emergencies

Rapid recognition of heat-related emergencies is essential to effective management. Reassess vital signs frequently to evaluate the patient's response to treatment. Aggressive cooling measures are required for heat stroke.

Cold-Related Emergencies

Hypothermia is a core temperature of less than 35°C (95°F). Infants and toddlers are at especially high risk for hypothermia because of their greater body surface area–to-mass ratio, decreased body fat, increased permeability of thin skin, and limited ability to shiver and produce heat. Extended exposure to a cold environment and immersion in cold water are the two most common causes of hypothermia in young children. Children with severe illness or injury may also develop hypothermia. Finally, infants and young children may become hypothermic while being exposed for medical evaluation, especially in cold environments. The presence of hypothermia may precipitate or extend shock and complicate resuscitation, regardless of the underlying condition.

Assessment

History taking should include recent illness or injury and circumstances of exposure. The physical examination should include special attention to airway and breathing. Because hypothermia leads to a slowing of metabolism, the child may hypoventilate, with slow or shallow respirations.

Circulation

Bradycardia and hypotension may be present because of hypothermia itself, or because of a concurrent hypoxic insult. Hypothermia may also lead to cardiac dysrhythmias. The skin is often pale and cool.

Disability

Mental status may range from confusion to coma, depending on the degree of hypothermia. Again, hypoxia may be the underlying cause of AMS, especially in submersion victims, so ensure the adequacy of oxygenation and ventilation. Depending on the circumstances, hypoglycemia may also be present.

Core Body Temperature

Obtain core body temperature, when possible, with a thermometer that registers less than 34°C (94°F).

Determine degree of hypothermia:

- Mild: 35–36°C (93–95°F)
- Moderate: 30–34°C (86–93°F)
- Severe: less than 30°C (<86°F)

Loss of the compensatory mechanism of shivering to generate heat is characteristic of moderate to severe hypothermia.

Management

Management of the patient with hypothermia depends on the core temperature.

1. *Support airway, breathing, and circulation as indicated.*
2. *Prevent heat loss.*
   It is crucial to prevent further heat loss. Remove wet clothing, dry the skin, and cover the patient after the examination is completed (**FIGURE 6-5**). Apply a hat or head wrap, because a high proportion of heat is lost through the head.
3. *Rewarm.*
   External, passive rewarming is appropriate for mild to moderate hypothermia. In the case of severe hypothermia, external rewarming may shunt cold blood to the core, leading to further complications. Core rewarming in the ED is the appropriate therapy for these patients.
   a. Mild hypothermia: apply warm blankets, increase ambient temperature of the ambulance. Prehospital professionals should be uncomfortably warm!
   b. Moderate hypothermia: warm blankets, heat packs to axilla and groin.

ALS

   c. Severe hypothermia: cautious movement with gentle handling; warmed, humidified oxygen; warmed IV solution; treat hypoglycemia if present; rapid transport to a definitive care facility for core rewarming.

FIGURE 6-5 Cover patient after examination.
© Rawpixel.com/Shutterstock.

Summary of Cold-Related Emergencies

Pediatric patients' physiologic and developmental characteristics place them at risk for the development of cold-related emergencies. Accurate assessment of the degree of hypothermia is essential to effective management of children in the prehospital environment.

> **TIP**
>
> Use caution when rewarming the severely hypothermic pediatric patient in the prehospital environment, because cold acidemic blood from the periphery could lead to further deterioration. Focus instead on preventing further heat loss and supporting the ABCs.

Bites and Stings

Bites and stings typically result in a puncture-type wound or laceration. Most of these injuries are minor. However, some stings, such as from a bumblebee or fire ant, may produce a severe allergic or **anaphylactic reaction**. Some bites, such as from a rattlesnake, spider, or scorpion, can cause life-threatening **envenomation** or bleeding problems. Bites and stings may pose a greater risk to the pediatric patient because of his or her smaller body weight and higher metabolic rate.

Assessment

History taking should include the following:

- Time and type of bite or sting
- Activities since the injury
- Known allergies to bites or stings
- Immunization history

The physical examination should include special attention to the following:

- Clinical presentation varies depending on the type of bite, the presence or absence of envenomation, and the time since the bite occurred.
- Assess airway, breathing, and circulation; respiratory distress and **anaphylaxis** may be the initial signs of a bite envenomation.
- Inspect for type, anatomic location, and number of punctures or wounds.
- Assess for swelling, discoloration, and pain at or around the site.

Management: Bites

Management depends on the type of insect, snake, or animal involved in the envenomation.

General Management

- Support airway, breathing, and circulation; establish vascular access.
- Treat anaphylaxis if present (see Chapter 4, page 88).

Local Management

- Stop bleeding, and perform wound care.
- If an envenomation is suspected, rinse area with water; for spider bites, consider cool compresses to the affected area to reduce swelling and pain. Cool compresses or ice are not recommended for snakebites.
- Minimize the activity level of the pediatric patient. Keep him or her in a supine position. Most venom is transported through the lymphatic system, and increased physical activity increases the rate of spread throughout the body.
- Immobilize an affected extremity at or below the level of the heart. It may be beneficial to keep the patient supine.
- Transport rapidly to evaluate for possible **antivenin** administration and for definitive care.
- Remove any clothing or jewelry on the affected area or limb.

Management: Stings

General Management

- Support airway, breathing, and circulation; establish vascular access.
- Treat anaphylaxis if present (see Chapter 4, page 88).

Local Management

- Remove stinger if visible (swipe away with credit card).
- Apply cold compresses.
- Consider medications based on clinical presentation: epinephrine in the case of anaphylaxis;

CASE STUDY **3**

A 6-year-old girl was playing outside in the garden. The caregiver called 9-1-1 when the child started to have difficulty breathing. On arrival at the scene, the PAT reveals a pale, irritable child with audible wheezing and significant supraclavicular and subcostal retractions. Respiratory rate is 32 breaths/min, heart rate is 140 beats/min, and her blood pressure is 90 mm Hg by palpation. During the physical exam, you note a red, swollen area on the side of her neck.

1. What are the possible causes of respiratory distress in this child?
2. What are the immediate management priorities?

albuterol in the case of wheezing; or diphenhydramine in the case of hives, itching, or swelling. Hydrocortisone administration may also be useful.

Summary of Bites and Stings

Insect bites are common in children and may result in complications ranging from mild local reaction to life-threatening anaphylaxis. Other types of envenomation, such as snake or scorpion stings, are more regionally specific. Early recognition of the nature of

the injury is important. Field treatment of anaphylaxis may be lifesaving. Prompt transport to a definitive care facility is crucial if antivenin treatment is needed.

TIP

Abnormal behavior may be the first clue that the pediatric patient has been bitten or stung. A thorough inspection of the patient's skin, particularly around the waist, distal extremities, axillae, and neck, may reveal the location of the bite or sting.

CASE STUDY ANSWERS

CASE STUDY **1**

It is important to determine if there was a possibility of poisoning, head trauma, or other potential causes of seizures. In addition, the possibility of head trauma during the seizure should be determined. It may also be helpful to determine if this seizure was similar to previous seizures, when the last seizure occurred, and if the child has been taking his regular medication correctly.

All children with a history of seizure activity should be transported to the hospital because it is impossible to diagnose a febrile seizure in the field. There are many causes of seizures, including serious infections, such as meningitis. This child also has a history of seizures, and there are factors, such as adequacy of current treatments, that need evaluation.

Continuous, careful monitoring during transport is especially important if drug therapy has been given, because administration of benzodiazepines, especially in combination with other seizure medications such as phenobarbital, can result in apnea or respiratory depression. Because this child is still not breathing adequately and his oxygen saturation is only 92%, airway maneuvers, 100% oxygen, and bag-mask ventilation are needed. If the child is still febrile, simple cooling methods, such as a cool towel to the forehead, may be useful. There is no need to apply ice packs to the body unless the child has heat stroke. Reassess the patient frequently, and be prepared for repeat seizures.

ALS

If multiple seizures occur or an additional seizure lasts longer than 5 minutes, consider treating with a benzodiazepine (rectal or IV diazepam; IV lorazepam; or IV, intranasal, or IM midazolam) and be prepared to manage airway and ventilation during transport. Although brief seizures do not require pharmacologic treatment, prompt treatment of seizures lasting longer than 5 minutes has the greatest success in terms of seizure cessation. Continuous, careful monitoring of airway and ventilation during transport is especially important if drug therapy has been given, because administration of benzodiazepines and phenobarbital can result in apnea or respiratory depression.

CASE STUDY 2

Oxygen saturation, temperature assessment, and blood glucose measurement can provide additional clues as to the cause of this child's AMS.

The possible etiology of the child's AMS is variable and includes head trauma, toxins, sepsis, hypovolemia, hypoglycemia, or postictal period after a seizure, yet the initial treatment is the same: Open and manage the airway with positioning and administer 100% oxygen by nonrebreathing mask. If there is no trauma, place the patient in the sniffing position and use the jaw-thrust maneuver to maintain the airway. If respirations are shallow or irregular, or if oxygen saturation is less than 90% on supplemental oxygen, assist ventilation with the appropriate-sized bag-mask device. Insert an oropharyngeal or nasopharyngeal airway as needed to maintain a patent airway.

ALS

Because the patient's blood pressure is low (calculated blood pressure for a 3-year-old would be 76 [70 + (2 × age in years)], while measured blood pressure is 72), fluid boluses of 20 mL/kg should be administered. If the glucose level is less than 60 mg/dL, more likely due to the vomiting and diarrhea, give 25% dextrose (2 mL/kg) by IV bolus. If there is no IV access, give glucagon IM. If bedside glucose determination is normal, consider other causes of AMS and consider administering naloxone, 0.1 mg/kg (maximum 2 mg), if appropriate. Use a length-based resuscitation tape or computer software program, as described in **Length-Based Resuscitation Tapes, Procedure 2**, to determine drug doses.

Additional history questions to help determine the possible causes of the AMS may include whether the child has had fever or other symptoms besides the vomiting and diarrhea already reported; whether the child has been taking anything orally, especially fluids; whether urination has been adequate; if the child has any ongoing medical problems; whether there has been any possibility of trauma (especially head trauma) today or in the recent past; and whether there is any possibility of drug or poison ingestion.

CASE STUDY 3

A previously healthy child playing outdoors with an acute onset of respiratory distress should be assessed for bites or stings and for exposure to possible environmental allergens or toxins, such as gardening-related chemicals. Also, it would be useful to determine if the child has a history of asthma or environmental allergies, including to bee stings. In this case, the presence of a swollen, reddened area suggests the possibility of an insect bite, most likely a hymenoptera (bee) sting, and the sudden onset of significant symptoms all suggest anaphylaxis.

Supplemental oxygen and inhaled bronchodilators for wheezing should be provided. In addition, IM epinephrine should be administered because of the possibility of anaphylaxis.

ALS

If possible, establish vascular access and give IV diphenhydramine.

IV hydrocortisone administration may also be beneficial, if included in treatment protocols. Watch for signs of shock and treat with IV fluids as appropriate. Even if the child shows marked improvement with these treatments, transport urgently because symptoms may recur as the medication effect wears off. Monitor carefully during transport.

SUGGESTED REFERENCES

Textbooks

Advanced Life Support Group. *Advanced Paediatric Life Support: The Practical Approach.* 5th ed. Chichester, UK: John Wiley & Sons Ltd.; 2011.

American Academy of Orthopaedic Surgeons. *Emergency Care and Transportation of the Sick and Injured.* 11th ed. Burlington, MA: Jones and Bartlett Learning; 2017.

American Academy of Orthopaedic Surgeons. *Nancy Caroline's Emergency Care in the Streets.* 8th ed. Burlington, MA: Jones and Bartlett Learning; 2018.

American Academy of Pediatrics and the American College of Emergency Physicians. *APLS: The Pediatric Emergency Medicine Resource.* 5th ed. Burlington, MA: Jones and Bartlett Learning; 2012.

Baram T, Shinnar S. *Febrile Seizures*. San Diego: Academic Press; 2002.

Baren JM, Rothrock SG, Brennan JA, et al. *Pediatric Emergency Medicine*. Philadelphia: Saunders/Elsevier; 2008.

Bledsoe B, Porter R, Cherry R. *Essentials of Paramedic Care*. Upper Saddle River, NJ: Prentice Hall; 2003.

Bledsoe B, Porter R, Cherry R. *Paramedic Care: Principles and Practice*. 5th ed. London, UK: Pearson; 2017.

McCance KL, Heuther SE, Brashers VL, et al., eds. *Pathophysiology: The Biologic Basis for Disease in Adults and Children*. 6th ed. St. Louis: Mosby Elsevier; 2010.

Articles

Argall JA, Wright N, Mackway-Jones K, et al. A comparison of two commonly used methods of weight estimation. *Arch Dis Child*. 2003;88:789–790.

Black K, Barnett P, Wolfe R, et al. Are methods used to estimate weight in children accurate? *Emerg Med*. 2002;14:160–165.

Freedman S, Powell E. Pediatric seizures and their management in the emergency department. *Clin Pediatr Emerg Med*. 2003;4;195–206.

Geduld H, Hodkinson PW, Wallis LA. Validation of weight estimation by age and length based methods in the Western Cape: South Africa population. *Emerg Med J*. 2011;28:856–860.

Goldstein B, Giroir B, Randolph A, et al. International pediatric consensus conference: definitions for sepsis and organ dysfunction in pediatrics. *Pediatr Crit Care Med*. 2005;6:2–8.

Holsti M, Sill BL, Firth SD, et al. Prehospital intranasal midazolam for the treatment of pediatric seizures. *Pediatr Emerg Care*. 2007;23;148–153.

Kuppermann N, Ghetti S, Schunk JE, et al. Clinical trial of fluid infusion rates for pediatric diabetic ketoacidosis. *NEJM*. 2018;378:2275-2287.

Lerner EB, Dayan PS, Brown K, et al. Characteristics of pediatric patients treated by the Pediatric Emergency Care Applied Research Network's affiliated EMS agencies. *Prehosp Emerg Care*. 2014;18:52–59.

Lubitz DS, Seidel JS, Chameides L. A rapid method for estimating weight and resuscitation drug dosages from length in the pediatric age group. *Ann Emerg Med*. 1988;17:576–581.

Luscombe M. 'Kids aren't like what they used to be': a study of paediatric patient's weights and their relationship to current weight estimation formulae. *Brit J Anaesth*. 2005;95:578P–579P.

Luscombe M, Owens B. Weight estimation in resuscitation: is the current formula still valid? *Arch Dis Child*. 2007;92:412–415.

Reuter D. Common emergent pediatric neurologic problems. *Emerg Med Clin North Am*. 2002;20(1):155–176.

Shah MI, Macias CG, Dayan PS, et al. An evidence-based guideline for pediatric prehospital seizure management using the GRADE method. *Prehosp Emer Care*. 2014;18;(Supple 1):15–24.

Tinning K, Acworth J. Make your best guess: An updated method for paediatric weight estimation in emergencies. *Emerg Med Australas*. 2007;19:528–534.

Warden CR. Evaluation and management of febrile seizures in the out-of-hospital and emergency department settings. *Ann Emerg Med*. 2003;41(2):215–222.

Wolfsdorf JI, Glaser N, Agus M, et al. ISPAD Clinical Practice Consensus Guidelines 2018: Diabetic ketoacidosis and the hyperglycemic hyperosmolar state. *Pediatric Diabetes*. 2018;19(Suppl 27):155-177.

© blakE+/Getty Images.

CHAPTER 7

Trauma

Kathleen M. Brown, MD, FACEP, FAAP

LEARNING OBJECTIVES

1. Explain the unique anatomic features of children that predispose them to injuries.
2. Sequence the primary assessment of the injured child.
3. Integrate the essential trauma interventions into the hands-on ABCDEs.
4. Distinguish different approaches in airway management of injured children.
5. Discuss assessment and treatment of pediatric burn patients.
6. Explain spinal motion restriction and the methods to achieve it.
7. Assess sports concussions and return-to-play guidelines.

Introduction

One-half of the children transported by emergency medical services (EMS) have an acute injury. Fortunately, the most common injuries are minor such as lacerations, minor or superficial burns, mild closed-head injuries, and extremity fractures. In minor trauma, the role of the prehospital professional is straightforward: Perform a scene size-up, assess for physiologic or anatomic problems, and transport to the emergency department (ED). Treatment usually entails wound care, spinal motion restriction, and splinting when necessary.

Multisystem trauma, in contrast, provides the prehospital professional with a great challenge and demands a disciplined assessment and a child-specific approach to treatment. Most principles of adult trauma management can be effectively and safely applied to children. Important modifications in assessment are related to differences in mechanisms of injury, anatomy, and physiologic responses. Modifications in treatment are related to differences in equipment sizes and emergency procedures.

Between infancy and adulthood, injuries are the most common cause of death. Intentional injuries, primarily nonaccidental trauma in infants and homicide and suicide in adolescents, are the leading mechanisms of traumatic death. Approximately 80% to 90% of pediatric trauma involves a blunt mechanism. This differs from the adult population, where there is a higher incidence of penetrating injuries. Handgun injuries, however, are on the rise in children and are now the most common cause of penetrating injuries in adolescents.

Most injuries are preventable. Child restraint devices in automobiles, bicycle helmets, swimming pool fences, and window barriers have significantly reduced the incidence of blunt injuries and drowning.

CASE STUDY 1

Your unit is dispatched to a call where a child has had a fall. You are greeted in the street by a neighbor who leads you to a 7-year-old boy who is lying face up on the grass next to a tall tree. The neighbor indicates that she observed the child fall about 20 feet out of the tree. No one has moved him. Your primary assessment reveals a child who is only responsive to painful stimuli. His breathing is shallow, with audible snoring sounds. His color is pale with slight cyanosis. Respiratory rate is 10 breaths/min, heart rate is 130 beats/min, and blood pressure is 76 mm Hg/palp. His skin is cool, the radial pulse is weak, and capillary refill time is greater than 3 seconds. Pupils are equal and reactive. The oxygen saturation is 90%. He has a hematoma on the right side of his head. His right upper leg is swollen, with an obvious deformity of the right femur.

1. Based on the primary assessment and mechanism of injury, what are the child's most likely injuries?
2. Discuss the initial stabilization and prehospital management of this child.

Stricter building codes have reduced the incidence of fires, although burns continue to be a cause of death in children younger than 12 years of age. Pediatric trauma challenges the prehospital professional to manage not just the injury and related physiologic abnormalities, but also to treat the child's pain and communicate with and support the injured child and the "injured family."

Death or serious injury of a child from trauma causes tremendous emotional stress on prehospital professionals, who may project feelings and fears about their own children's vulnerability onto the situation. This common provider response may lead to difficulty in maintaining an appropriate emotional distance, and it may compromise objective performance. Experience and education in the care of ill and injured children help the prehospital professional have a greater sense of confidence, competency, and control in these stressful situations. Critical incident stress management or employee assistance programs may be valuable to the prehospital professional after treating a seriously injured child.

Fatal Injury Mechanisms

TABLE 7-1 summarizes the most frequent fatal mechanisms of injury in children and adolescents.

Unique Anatomic Features of Children: Effect on Injury Patterns

Head

Head injury is the most common serious traumatic injury in children. Even in multisystem trauma, the severity of **traumatic brain injury (TBI)** usually defines the patient's medical and functional outcome. Many of the essential interventions in managing pediatric trauma are directed at preserving brain function.

Until early school age (5–6 years old), the child's head is disproportionately large in relationship to overall body mass and surface area compared to adults.

TABLE 7-1 Leading Mechanisms of Injury-Related Death			
Age <1 Year	**Age 1–4 Years**	**Age 5–9 Years**	**Age 10–14 Years**
Suffocation	Drowning	Vehicular trauma	Suicide
Vehicular trauma	Vehicular trauma	Homicide	Vehicular trauma
Drowning	Homicide	Drowning	Homicide
Natural/Environmental	Suffocation	Fire/Burn	Drowning
Fire/Burn	Fire/Burn	Suffocation	Other Land Transport

Data from: 10 Leading Mechanisms of Injury Deaths by Age Group Highlighting Unintentional Injury Deaths, United States – 2017. https://www.cdc.gov/injury/wisqars/LeadingCauses.html

Because of this anatomic feature, in a fall or in an **acceleration-deceleration event**, such as a motor vehicle crash, the head functions like the heavy end of a lawn dart, becoming the lead point (**FIGURE 7-1**). Consequently, the head and brain of a child are more commonly injured in blunt trauma compared to adults.

Spinal Column

As a group, children do not suffer many vertebral fractures or dislocations. When vertebral fractures do occur, the event typically involves a high-energy mechanism (e.g., motor vehicle crash or diving incident) with extreme **flexion** or extension or axial loading of the **spine**. Traumatic spinal cord injury, or disruption of the central nerve pathways, is also rare in children.

The most common cervical spine injuries in children occur at the level of the high cervical spine. Weaker neck muscles and spinal ligaments, in conjunction with a "heavy" head, create greater vulnerability to acceleration-deceleration forces common in motor vehicle crashes and falls. In reality, most children with high cervical injury are in full arrest on the scene and die despite all medical interventions.

The most common lower spine injuries occur in the mid to lower **thoracic** spine. Mechanisms include direct blows, falls, or spinal **compression** during a motor vehicle crash from improper seat belt use. The use of booster seats in vehicles reduces these types of injuries by allowing proper fitting of the lap and shoulder belt.

> **CAUTION**
>
> It is difficult to find a cervical collar that really fits an infant or toddler. When a properly sized collar is not available, use padding around the head and neck and stabilize the child's spine with padding to protect the spinal cord.

> **TIP**
>
> Injuries cause almost one-half the deaths among children from 1–4 years of age and outrank all other causes of death combined among older children and adolescents.

Chest

The ribs of the child are more pliable and compressible than those of the adult because they are composed mainly of **cartilage**. For this reason, rib fractures and **flail chest** are uncommon in younger children, even with high-energy transfers. However, this bony compressibility in conjunction with a **chest wall** that is poorly protected by fat or muscle leads to direct transfer of energy to the lungs and heart on impact (**FIGURE 7-2**). Serious injuries of the thoracic organs can be present with or without external signs of injury, such as **abrasions**, bruises, or tenderness.

Pulmonary contusion, or bruising of the lung tissue itself, is the most common form of serious lung

FIGURE 7-1 A disproportionately large head size in children explains their tendency to fall "head first," leading to a high rate of TBI.

FIGURE 7-2 The child's chest wall is not well muscularized, so it lacks the soft tissue protection from injury that is present in adolescents and adults.

injury in children. You may suspect this condition in a child who sustains blunt chest trauma and has hypoxia or respiratory distress; however, pulmonary contusions may take time to fully develop and can only be diagnosed by X-ray, which makes the distinction between pulmonary contusion and pneumothorax difficult in the field.

If a child has a blunt injury mechanism, be careful about placing a needle in the pleural space because a contusion is more likely than a tension pneumothorax. In contrast, a child with progressive hypoxia and respiratory distress after a penetrating injury probably does have a tension pneumothorax, and needle decompression is indicated.

Penetrating chest trauma may cause serious problems in oxygenation and ventilation. When the chest wall, back, or high abdomen is penetrated, look for **tension pneumothorax** and **sucking chest wounds**. These injuries are unusual in children but, if present, require specific immediate lifesaving treatment in the field. **Needle decompression** may save the life of a child with a tension pneumothorax. The procedure is similar for a child and adult, the major difference being the size of the catheter. The procedure is illustrated in **Needle Thoracostomy, Procedure 23**.

TIP

Because the child's chest wall is smaller, thinner, and less muscular than an adult's, lung sounds may be transmitted throughout the chest cavity, making it difficult to appreciate asymmetric breath sounds. Listening along the lateral sides of the chest wall under the axillae (armpits) may improve the ability to distinguish sound variability between the right and left lungs.

TIP

If there is penetration of the chest wall below the nipples, or below the scapula, anticipate abdominal injury as well as tension pneumothorax.

CAUTION

Remember that young children rely on their diaphragm to breathe, but also use abdominal muscles. Do not restrict the abdomen when protecting the patient's spine or restraining for transport.

The diaphragm of a child can rise as high as the nipple line during full expiration. When there is blunt or penetrating trauma to the chest below the nipple line or below the scapula, internal injury may include both chest and abdominal organs (**FIGURE 7-3**).

Abdomen

The **abdomen** is often the site of serious blood loss in pediatric patients and is the most common site of injury causing shock. The solid organs of the upper

A

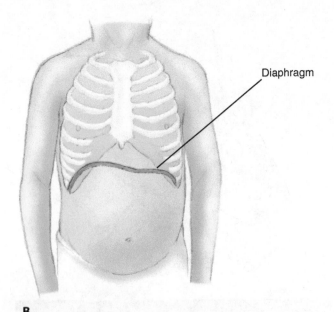

B

FIGURE 7-3 The diaphragm can rise as high as the nipple line during full expiration **(A)** and can flatten to the level of the lowest ribs during full inspiration **(B)**. Therefore, injuries to the abdominal organs may occur after chest trauma.

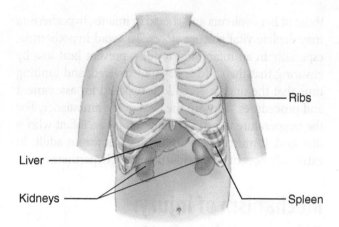

FIGURE 7-4 The solid organs of the upper abdominal cavity are disproportionately large and more exposed in children than in adults. They are poorly protected by the thin chest wall and undeveloped abdominal muscles.

abdominal cavity are the liver, **spleen**, and kidneys. These organs are disproportionately larger and more exposed than in adults and are poorly protected by the child's softer ribs and relatively undeveloped abdominal muscles (**FIGURE 7-4**). The liver is the largest abdominal organ, located in the right upper quadrant of the abdomen, and extends below the rib cage in infants, toddlers, and preschool-aged children. It is the most commonly injured abdominal organ in young children. The spleen, located in the left upper quadrant, is also commonly injured. Injuries to the hollow organs of the abdomen—the stomach, small bowel, and bladder—are less common than solid organ injuries. Although **pelvic fractures** are uncommon in children, they become more frequent in adolescents.

Assume that every child with a serious trauma has a life-threatening abdominal injury. Many children with abdominal injury have no localizing signs and may not complain of pain. Fear, young age, or distracting injuries may hide signs and symptoms. When present, signs include progressive abdominal distention, rigidity, tenderness, abdominal wall contusions or abrasions, and hemodynamic instability. **Serial examinations** in timed intervals (5–10 minutes) may improve the accuracy of abdominal assessment.

TIP

The abdomen is the most frequent site of injury causing shock. Serial examinations greatly improve the accuracy of assessment of abdominal injury. In the injured child with multisystem blunt trauma, the prehospital provider should always have a high index of suspicion for intra-abdominal bleeding if shock presents.

CAUTION

Never overlook the possibility of solid organ injury when there has been blunt injury because fear, inability to speak, or distracting injuries may mask signs and symptoms.

Extremities

Children's bones are more flexible, and their muscles are not as well developed as those of adults. They are especially vulnerable to fractures at the weak, cartilaginous growth plates near the ends of the bones (**FIGURE 7-5**). Fractures that disrupt the **periosteum** on only one side of the bone (often called **greenstick fractures**) are common, as are "**buckle fractures**" in which the pliant bone is compressed with **axial loading**. These fractures may be present in the absence of significant swelling, bruising, or deformity. *Suspect a fracture whenever there is point tenderness or limited range of motion, especially around a joint.*

ALS

Pain is frequently underestimated and undertreated in children. Consider analgesia for pain management in children with isolated extremity fractures. **Morphine** sulfate or fentanyl are the medications of choice for severe pain. Fentanyl can be given via the intranasal (IN) route with an atomizer (**Intranasal Medication Administration, Procedure 15**). Repeat with half doses as needed for pain control. **Fentanyl** is faster acting than morphine and also has a shorter duration of action. Be extremely careful with morphine administration in children with a serious injury mechanism or signs of compensated or decompensated shock. Morphine can drop the child's blood pressure and critical perfusion when it is administered to a hypovolemic patient. Always be alert for signs of respiratory depression, especially if multiple doses of a narcotic are administered.

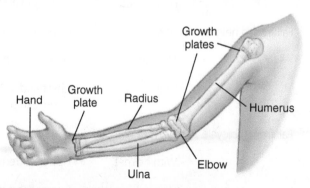

FIGURE 7-5 The physeal (growth) plates at the ends of children's bones are easily fractured.

The most serious complications of extremity injuries are **neurovascular** problems and blood loss into the soft tissues at the fracture site. Blood loss may be severe in long-bone fractures (e.g., fractures of the femur) or in pelvic fractures. The symptom usually associated with serious extremity injuries is pain.

> **TIP**
>
> Suspect an extremity fracture whenever findings include point tenderness or limited range of motion.

> **TIP**
>
> Injuries to the **physeal plate** or growth plate of a long bone can be permanently damaging to the limb.

Skin

The skin provides temperature regulation. Children's skin is thinner and has a greater surface area in relation to their overall size and weight than does the skin of adults. Because of this, heat transfer (loss or gain) from the skin can be rapid. Even without injuries that damage the skin, such as burns, injured children are at increased risk for hypothermia, which can in turn compromise core organ function. The signs and symptoms of hypothermia can mimic those of hypovolemia and shock. In infants, hypothermia may deplete vital glucose stores. To avoid hypothermia, especially in an infant and toddler, prevent heat loss by ensuring that the child is dry and covered, and limiting time that the undressed child is exposed for assessment and procedures. Turn up the heat in the ambulance. For the temperature to be warm enough for an infant who is disrobed, it must be uncomfortably hot for an adult. In extremely hot environments, beware of hyperthermia.

Mechanism of Injury: Effect on Injury Patterns

The different mechanisms of injury in children in combination with their unique anatomic features lead to predictable patterns of injury. Head injury caused by blunt trauma is very common in children. Although there are many cases of minor closed-head injuries associated with play that do not have neurologic consequences, high-energy impacts are often associated with TBI. Because of a child's small size, high-energy blunt impacts can lead to **multisystem trauma**, including the head, chest, abdomen, and long bones.

TABLE 7-2 lists the common mechanisms of pediatric injury and the associated patterns of injury. **FIGURE 7-6** illustrates several typical injury sequences in children.

TABLE 7-2 Common Mechanisms and Associated Patterns of Pediatric Injury

Mechanism of Injury		Associated Patterns of Injury
Motor vehicle crash (child is passenger)	Unrestrained	Multiple trauma, head and neck injuries, scalp and facial lacerations
	Air bag	Head and neck, facial and eye injuries
	Restrained	Chest and abdominal injuries, cervical and lower-spine fractures
Motor vehicle crash (child is pedestrian)	Low speed	Lower-extremity fractures
	High speed	Chest and abdominal injuries, head and neck injuries, lower-extremity fractures
Fall from a height	Low	Upper-extremity fractures
	Medium	Head and neck injuries, upper- and lower-extremity fractures
	High	Chest and abdominal injuries, head and neck injuries, upper- and lower-extremity fractures
Fall from a bicycle	Without helmet	Head and neck injuries, scalp and facial lacerations, upper-extremity fractures
	With helmet	Upper-extremity fractures
	Hitting handlebar	Internal abdominal injuries

FIGURE 7-6 **A.** A restrained child in a motor vehicle crash may have a lap belt injury involving solid organs, bowel, and spine. **B.** Children frequently sustain multisystem injuries involving the head, chest, abdomen, and long bones. **C.** A fall from height frequently involves injuries to the head and neck, chest, abdomen, and the extremities. **D.** A fall over the handlebars of a bike may result in injuries to the abdomen and extremities.

Assessment of the Injured Child

The initial steps in assessing the injured child follow the generic approach for all children outlined in Chapters 1 and 2. This includes prearrival mental preparation based on dispatch information and a scene size-up on arrival. Always use **universal precautions** or personal protective measures and equipment to prevent potentially harmful or infectious exposures to bodily fluids.

The on-scene trauma evaluation includes (1) general assessment using the Pediatric Assessment Triangle (PAT), (2) the primary assessment with the hands-on ABCDEs, and then (3) additional assessment consisting of a focused history and physical examination and a detailed physical examination (trauma). A child with multisystem injuries needs a prioritized, efficient on-scene approach to assessment and treatment and rapid transport to the appropriate regional trauma center. Typically, the prehospital professional gets no further than the primary assessment of a child with multisystem trauma, because the recognition and management of life-threatening physiologic problems are the focus of field care. The anatomic problems identified in the additional assessment are generally not life threatening and can be treated in the hospital when the child is physiologically stable.

The General Assessment

The PAT

The PAT is the first part of the primary assessment of trauma as well as medical patients, and allows rapid determination of the type of physiologic disturbance, severity of injury, and urgency of treatment.

Appearance

Appearance reflects brain function, which may be abnormal in injured children because of **primary brain injury** (caused by direct trauma to the brain tissue itself) or **secondary brain injury** (caused by an indirect insult to the brain tissue by hypoxia or ischemia). The most likely causes of abnormal appearance in a pediatric trauma patient are closed-head injury; hypoxia; hemorrhage; and pain from fractures, burns, and **soft-tissue injuries**.

TIP

There are many potential causes of abnormal appearance in a pediatric trauma patient, including closed-head injury; hypoxia; hemorrhage; and pain from fractures, burns, and soft-tissue injuries.

Toxins may also cause an abnormal appearance, but are uncommon causes of poor responsiveness in the preschool- and school-aged trauma patient. However, toxins (most often recreational drugs) are an important contributor to trauma in the adolescent, who may incur injuries caused by high-risk behaviors while "under the influence." **TABLE 7-3** lists common causes of abnormal appearance in injured children.

Work of Breathing

Work of breathing is increased by injuries that affect the airway, lungs, pleura, or chest wall. **TABLE 7-4** summarizes the causes of increased work of breathing in pediatric trauma patients. Effortless tachypnea, or a rapid respiratory rate in the absence of increased work of breathing, may be seen in a child with traumatic shock. This is a reflexive mechanism to compensate for **metabolic acidosis**, caused by **hypoperfusion**, by "blowing-off" carbon dioxide.

Listen for abnormal airway sounds, such as stridor or change of speech, which may reflect tracheal injury or obstruction. Wheezing reflects lower airway irritation and bronchospasm. This may occur from inhalation of vaporized toxins. When children are confined

TABLE 7-3 Common Causes of Abnormal Appearance in Injured Children

Category of Injury	Examples
Primary brain injuries	Closed-head injury Cerebral edema Concussion Contusion Intracranial hematoma (subdural, epidural) Intracranial hemorrhage Penetrating brain injuries

Secondary brain injuries (ischemia and hypoxia)	Hemorrhage with hypoperfusion/shock due to:
	    Solid organ abdominal injury
	    Hemothorax
	    Pelvic fracture
	Hypoxia due to:
	    Aspiration of gastric contents
	    Failure of central respiratory drive
	    Pulmonary contusion
	    Smoke inhalation
	    Tension pneumothorax

Pain	Burns Fractures Soft-tissue injuries
Toxins	Alcohol Recreational drugs Carbon monoxide

in a house fire, this type of inhalation should always be suspected.

Grunting, an infant's method of positive end-expiratory pressure, indicates decreased gas exchange at the level of the alveoli and may be seen with pulmonary contusion. After listening, look for retractions and nasal flaring to further assess for hypoxia.

Circulation to Skin

Circulation to skin reflects the blood flow to the skin and mucous membranes. If skin color and skin temperature are abnormal in an injured child who is not in a cold environment, it suggests hypovolemia and poor perfusion. Hemorrhage from abdominal solid organ injury is the most common cause of hypoperfusion and shock in pediatric trauma patients. The use of tourniquets in children with exsanguinating

TABLE 7-4 Injury Causes of Increased Work of Breathing in Injured Children

Cause	Examples
Airway injuries	Hematomas or lacerations of the tongue, mouth, or neck
	Smoke and hot gas inhalation
	Penetrations into the upper airway
Chest injuries	Pulmonary contusion
	Sucking chest wound
	Tension pneumothorax/ hemothorax
Abdominal injuries	Diaphragmatic injury
	Solid or hollow viscus injury with pain and "splinting"

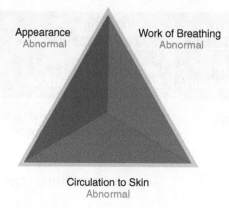

FIGURE 7-8 A patient with multiple system injury has an abnormal appearance, abnormal work of breathing, and abnormal circulation to skin.

The Primary Assessment

Hands-On ABCDEs

The ABCDEs are the hands-on primary assessment. The trauma ABCDEs have a special focus on spinal motion restriction and control of blood loss. The pediatric assessment, including the PAT and ABCDEs, does not require any specialized equipment. Potentially life-threatening problems should be treated as they are identified in the ABCDE sequence. **TABLE 7-5** lists the key features of the pediatric trauma ABCDEs and interventions specific to the trauma patient.

Airway

Airway maintenance is always the first priority. Trauma victims are at risk for airway obstruction from bleeding, **emesis**, edema, or foreign objects. TBI may cause loss of protective airway reflexes or impair central respiratory drive.

Consider spinal injury in a child with any of the following:

- Mechanism of injury involving high-velocity forces transmitted to the head or spine (e.g., fall from a height, ejection from a motor vehicle, diving, axial loading
- Altered mental status (AMS)
- Neck or spine pain/tenderness
- Inability to move neck
- Neurologic deficit (e.g., acute weakness or loss of sensation after an injury)
- Deformity to the neck or spine

If the child has any of these findings, care should be taken to protect the spine to minimize risk of secondary injury. The current term for this practice is **spinal motion restriction (SMR)**.

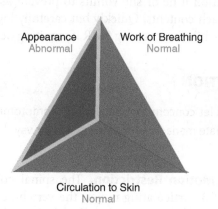

FIGURE 7-7 A patient with closed-head injury has an abnormal appearance, but normal work of breathing and normal circulation to skin.

hemorrhage from an extremity to prevent blood loss should be considered. An isolated closed-head injury cannot account for signs of hypoperfusion or shock in children outside of infancy, because the closed space of the skull cannot accommodate a significant volume of blood. However, infants can lose large volumes of blood based on intracranial bleeding; because the plates of their skull (sutures) are not yet fused, and the skull can expand under pressure.

FIGURE 7-7 and **FIGURE 7-8** show the PAT findings for the two most common patterns of major pediatric trauma: closed-head injury and multisystem injury.

TABLE 7-5 Pediatric Trauma ABCDEs

Element of Assessment	Special Interventions
Airway	Jaw-thrust maneuver while maintaining cervical spinal motion restriction
	Suction airway of fluid or blood
	Consider airway adjunct
Breathing	Needle thoracostomy
	Dressing to sucking chest wound
Circulation	External hemorrhage control
	Tourniquet application
	Splinting of fractured extremity
Disability	Elevated intracranial pressure management (head midline, head of stretcher raised, assisted ventilation to maintain normal CO$_2$ levels)
Exposure	Prevent heat loss

FIGURE 7-9 If airway obstruction is suspected in a child with possible spine injuries, use the modified jaw-thrust maneuver combined with manual spinal motion restriction.

Insert an oral **airway adjunct** if unable to maintain an open airway and the child has no gag reflex. Use suction to clear any fluid or Magill forceps to remove foreign bodies from the mouth, nose, or upper airway. Be prepared to turn the child on his or her side and suction if he or she vomits to prevent aspiration of stomach contents. Quickly but carefully logroll the patient while maintaining SMR if vomiting occurs.

CAUTION

Never let concern for spinal injury compromise appropriate management of the child's airway.

Spinal Motion Restriction. The spinal column is made of 33 articulating bones, the vertebrae, and its structure changes significantly during childhood growth. The incidence and type of spinal injuries depend on the age of the child and the mechanism of injury, and in turn are influenced by the child's developmental level and activity. Cervical spine trauma can lead to **quadriplegia**, the most devastating type of spinal injury. If cervical spine injury is suspected, an appropriately sized cervical collar should be applied. The use of a backboard should follow local protocols (**FIGURE 7-10**). Spinal cord injuries and lifelong paralysis may follow thoracic or lumbar trauma. For a step-by-step explanation of this procedure, see **Spinal Motion Restriction, Procedure 22.**

SMR may involve placing a cervical spine collar and/or securing patient to a stretcher and taking care to minimize movement of the neck, especially when transferring the patient from scene to stretcher or into an ambulance. Use of a rigid backboard to immobilize the patient is now thought to cause potential harm. If a backboard or other rigid device is used to extricate a child or transfer him or her to a stretcher, the child should be removed from the rigid board as soon as possible. An injured child should be transported secured to a stretcher or appropriate-size car seat.

Although great care must be taken to prevent further injury in the unlikely event of an unstable spine injury, these concerns must not take precedence over appropriate management of the child's airway. *An injured child is far more likely to die from untreated hypoxia or shock than spinal trauma.*

Actions. If airway obstruction is present, use a jaw-thrust maneuver combined with manual SMR (**FIGURE 7-9**) to establish and maintain airway patency.

Breathing

Breathing is the second priority in the ABCDEs. Injuries to the airway, chest wall, lungs, or abdomen, as

FIGURE 7-10 Spinal motion restriction may involve securing the body to a stretcher to minimize motion of the spine.
© Kzenon/Shutterstock.

well as gastric distention caused by air swallowing, may compromise oxygenation and ventilation. Head and cervical spine injuries sometimes depress central respiratory drive mechanisms or diminish protective airway reflexes. Pulmonary aspiration of gastric contents is a common and potentially serious complication of head injuries that results in hypoxia and increased work of breathing.

Look for soft-tissue or penetrating injuries of the chest or back. Watch for the adequacy and symmetry of chest rise, and then listen with a stethoscope to assess air entry and equality of breath sounds. Feel the chest wall for **crepitus**, pain, or instability. Apply a pulse oximeter to assess for hypoxia, because pallor and cyanosis can be late findings. A normal pulse oximetry reading does not, however, rule out respiratory distress. A child with profound tachypnea or increased work of breathing may need **assisted ventilation** regardless of the reading on the oximeter, before he or she exhausts compensatory mechanisms.

Actions. If breathing is inadequate, position the child and assist ventilation. Lift the jaw into the mask; pushing the mask onto the face to make a seal may cause cervical spine flexion and exacerbate airway obstruction. The E-C clamp technique (**FIGURE 7-11**) helps with proper hand placement for good mask-to-face seal. Consider inserting an airway adjunct to help maintain an open airway, although an oral airway is not tolerated by a child with an intact gag reflex.

Give 100% oxygen by nonrebreathing mask or bag-mask ventilation. Use a properly fitted oxygen mask. Provide assisted ventilation with a bag-mask device if the child's respiratory effort is inadequate or if he or she has deteriorating cardiopulmonary or mental status. Use the "squeeze-release-release" timing technique, because the tendency is to bag too fast. Allow a brief pause between each breath to minimize the chance of gastric distention. If the child has signs of increased intracranial pressure or signs of impending brainstem herniation, such as fixed and dilated pupils, unequal pupils, and/or posturing, use waveform or digital capnography to keep $EtCO_2$ between 30 and 35 mm Hg (usual between 35 and 45 mm Hg). Be extremely careful, because hyperventilation may decrease perfusion to the brain. In each breath, provide only enough tidal volume to achieve chest rise.

Treating penetrating chest injuries, sucking chest wounds, impaled objects, and tension pneumothorax in pediatrics is the same as in adults. Cover sucking chest wounds with an **occlusive dressing**, such as petrolatum gauze, taped on three or four sides (depending upon local protocol) (**FIGURE 7-12**) or a specially

> **TIP**
>
> Pulmonary aspiration of gastric contents is a common and potentially serious complication of head injuries. Therefore, an orogastric tube should be inserted.

CASE STUDY 2

You are dispatched to a local recreation field where a 6-year-old boy was struck in the head by a baseball bat that flew out of another player's hands while batting. The child has a large hematoma on his forehead and is crying in his coach's arms. The child did not lose consciousness, but is not making eye contact with you or his coach. Other than his altered appearance, the PAT is normal and the hands-on ABCDEs reveal normal vital signs and no other apparent injuries. The child becomes increasingly somnolent during your assessment and is difficult to arouse.

1. What is the child's greatest threat to life?
2. What interventions are required?

A

B

C

FIGURE 7-11 The E-C clamp technique facilitates proper hand placement for good mask-to-face seal. **A.** Hand displaying E-C shape. **B.** Fingers resting on bony ridge of jaw. **C.** Bag-mask ventilation in place.

© Jones & Bartlett Learning.

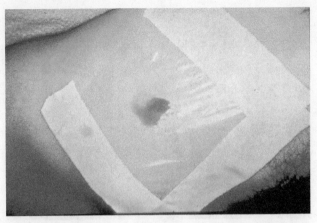

FIGURE 7-12 Management of a sucking chest wound. Cover sucking chest wounds with an occlusive dressing, such as a petrolatum gauze, taped on three or four sides. A defibrillator pad can also be used.

Courtesy of the State of North Carolina EMSC.

TIP

If a patient with penetrating chest trauma also has respiratory distress, hypoxia, and shock, perform needle decompression on the affected side to treat possible tension pneumothorax.

ALS

Management of Tension Pneumothorax. If a patient with penetrating chest trauma has increasing respiratory distress, hypoxia, and shock, perform needle decompression on the affected side to treat possible tension pneumothorax.

Needle decompression may also be necessary in the child with blunt chest injury if the child has serious blunt chest-wall injury and respiratory distress, especially if he or she worsens with assisted ventilation. In this situation, when there is a closed pneumothorax, positive-pressure ventilation quickly increases the air pressure in the **pleural space**, creating a dangerous level of "tension." Tension pneumothorax not only compromises ventilation of the affected lung, but impairs venous return to the heart. This can lead to shock unresponsive to fluid resuscitation. Needle decompression of the tension pneumothorax improves oxygenation, ventilation, and perfusion. For a step-by-step explanation of this procedure, see **Needle Thoracostomy, Procedure 23.**

Management of Gastric Distention With a Nasogastric/Orogastric Tube. Assisted ventilation or prolonged crying can cause air swallowing and gastric distention. Nasogastric (NG) or orogastric (OG) tube placement may improve ventilation by

---

designed bandage/seal for sucking chest wounds. This technique allows trapped air to escape while helping to prevent the entrance of air and development of tension pneumothorax. Do not remove impaled objects. Instead, stabilize them in place.

decreasing the upward pressure on the diaphragm caused by the distended stomach, and reduce the risk of vomiting. If possible, insert an OG tube after endotracheal intubation of a comatose patient, because positive-pressure ventilation can cause gastric inflation even in an intubated child. **Contraindications** for NG insertion include midfacial trauma and suspected **basilar skull fracture** (raccoon eyes, Battle sign, or suspected cerebrospinal fluid rhinorrhea or otorrhea) because of the risk of passing the tube through the disrupted cribriform plate into the cranial vault. In these cases, perform OG insertion. Weigh the benefits of **gastric decompression** against the possible complications of vomiting and aspiration during passage of the tube or tube misplacement into the trachea. For a step-by-step explanation of this procedure, see **Orogastric and Nasogastric Tube Insertion, Procedure 10.**

Circulation

Multisystem pediatric trauma more often involves respiratory failure than shock. Sometimes, however, shock develops because of external or internal bleeding, pneumothorax, spinal injury, or pump failure caused by cardiac contusion or **tamponade**. The combination of the PAT and the hands-on ABCDEs allows ongoing perfusion evaluation. Measure heart rate continuously with a cardiac monitor or with frequent pulse checks. Tachycardia may be caused by pain, fear, cold, or anxiety, but a trend of rising heart rate suggests ongoing blood loss. Blood pressure measurement is not a good indicator of hypovolemia because a child can be in compensated shock with a normal blood pressure. When there is frank hypotension, assume the child is in hypotensive (decompensated) shock. If blood pressure is significantly higher than normal in a child with possible TBI, consider possible **intracranial hypertension/increased intracranial pressure**.

Because of the technical challenges of obtaining a reliable blood pressure, and because skin signs, capillary refill time, and pulse quality are good signs of perfusion, make only one attempt at obtaining a blood pressure in children older than 3 years of age. Make sure the blood pressure cuff size is correct, or the measurement is inaccurate. In children younger than 3 years of age, taking the time on scene to get a blood pressure is of limited value.

Actions. Stop any visible external bleeding with direct pressure on the wound. Use sterile gauze compresses, and use gloves and personal protective equipment. Splint any extremities with obvious deformity. Apply oxygen, and place the child in a supine position for

TIP
Frequently reassess heart rate, preferably with an electronic monitor. Tachycardia may be a response to pain, fear, cold, or anxiety, but a trend of rising heart rate suggests ongoing blood loss.

TIP
Remember, the systolic blood pressure for a child 1–10 years of age should be greater than 70 + 2 × age in years. If not, the child is in hypotensive (decompensated) shock.

transport. Consider tourniquet application if there is uncontrolled hemorrhage (see **Tourniquet Application, Procedure 25**).

Begin transport when the airway is properly secured, ventilation is adequate, and the child's spine is appropriately stabilized. In a poorly perfused, or hypotensive, patient, administer 20 mL/kg of isotonic saline as rapidly as possible.

ALS

Volume Resuscitation. If the child has signs of shock or significant ongoing blood loss, obtain vascular access and start **volume resuscitation** on the way to the ED. Look first for peripheral intravenous (IV) sites in the upper extremities. Attempt to secure two lines. Insert an intraosseous (IO) needle if IV access cannot be obtained immediately and the child has signs of hypotensive shock. Then give 20 mL/kg isotonic fluid as rapidly as possible.

Disability

Disability in the context of trauma care relates to TBI or spinal cord trauma. Injuries may be open or closed. Children may have primary or secondary brain injuries, or both.

Primary brain injury is the direct result of the traumatic insult and may include brain hemorrhage, **cerebral edema** (brain swelling), or **diffuse axonal injury**. Increased intracranial pressure may develop quickly after primary brain injury. Untreated, the downward spiral of increased intracranial pressure can lead to **brainstem herniation**, cardiopulmonary arrest, and **brain death**. By the time the prehospital professional reaches the scene, any damage incurred from the primary brain injury is complete.

Secondary brain injury results from central nervous system (CNS) hypoxia or ischemia and disorders of blood glucose. The prehospital professional has a key role in preventing secondary brain injury. Hypoxia may be the result of airway or chest injury, or of compromised central respiratory drive caused by the primary brain injury. Brain ischemia may result from hemorrhage, usually in the abdomen or chest. CNS cells cannot survive without sufficient blood glucose levels.

Ensuring adequate oxygenation, ventilation, perfusion, and normal blood glucose are the keys to preventing secondary brain injury.

A 9-1-1 call sometimes involves an infant with AMS, apnea, or seizures with no report of preceding trauma. Assessment of these infants may not reveal any physical examination findings suggestive of head trauma or TBI, despite the fact that they have sustained severe TBI. This is a typical scenario in **abusive head trauma**, where the infant is forcibly shaken by a caregiver, sometimes with impact of the baby's head against a fixed object. This mechanism involves severe acceleration-deceleration forces to the infant's brain and consequent diffuse axonal injury or intracranial hemorrhage. Abusive head trauma is further discussed in Chapter 11.

Assess the injured child's degree of neurologic disability with the AVPU scale (see Table 1-8). Disability, as categorized in the AVPU scale, is not the same as "abnormal appearance" in the PAT. An injured child may have an abnormal appearance for many reasons other than brain or spinal cord injury, such as pain, fear, shock, hypoxia, or intoxication. Appearance may be quite abnormal in a child who is "alert" on the AVPU scale. Appearance is a more subtle indicator of overall physiologic function in children than AVPU. The AVPU scale is more helpful in categorizing children with severe neurologic insults, including critical primary or secondary brain injuries.

Some EMS systems use the Pediatric Glasgow Coma Scale (PGCS) to assess neurologic injury (**TABLE 7-6**). Neither the AVPU score nor the PGCS has been validated in young children. Although both systems attempt to objectively assess neurologic function, the AVPU is less complex and easier to remember. When using the PGCS, pay special attention to the motor component of the score, which has the highest value in predicting neurologic outcome from TBI.

After evaluating the level of consciousness with AVPU or the PGCS, note abnormal positioning (including posturing) and seizures, and check for pupil size, symmetry, and **reactivity**. Seizures are common with head injury in children. Beware of persistent horizontal nystagmus, which may indicate persistent seizure activity.

TABLE 7-6 Pediatric Glasgow Coma Scale

Score	Child	Infant
Eyes		
4	Opens eyes spontaneously	Opens eyes spontaneously
3	Opens eyes to speech	Opens eyes to speech
2	Opens eyes to pain	Opens eyes to pain
1	No response	No response
_____ = Score (Eyes)		
Motor		
6	Obeys commands	Spontaneous movements
5	Localizes	Withdraws to touch
4	Withdraws	Withdraws to pain
3	Flexion	Flexion (decorticate)
2	Extension	Extension (decerebrate)
1	No response	No response
_____ = Score (Motor)		
Verbal		
5	Oriented	Coos and babbles
4	Confused	Irritable cry
3	Inappropriate words	Cries to pain
2	Incomprehensible words	Moans to pain
1	No response	No response
_____ = Score (Verbal)		
_____ = **Total Score (Eyes, Motor, Verbal). Scores will range from 3 to 15.**		

Modified from James HE, Anas NG, Perkin RM. *Brain Insults in Infants and Children*. Orlando, FL: Grune & Stratton; 1985.

The pupils provide important information about brainstem function, and the pupillary examination helps determine the need for hyperventilation in patients who are at risk of brainstem herniation.

Concussion. Concussion, a mild form of TBI, occurs after a bump or blow to the head or due to a fall onto the head. These rotational and acceleration forces on the brain result in chemical changes and sometimes damage to the brain cells. Frequently sports related, loss of consciousness is seen in only 10% to 15% of concussed patients. Symptoms include headache, nausea or vomiting, double or blurry vision, confusion, dizziness, sensitivity to light (photophobia), sensitivity to noise (phonophobia), and concentration or memory problems. While some of these may occur shortly after the injury, others may occur a few hours to days later. While the child/adolescent may say that he or she does not feel well, if the child appears dazed or stunned, is confused, answers questions slowly, moves clumsily, or cannot recall events prior to the injury, he or she has suffered a concussion. If a child is involved in a sports activity, he or she should be removed from play. Recovery may require physical and cognitive rest and may take weeks to months. A second impact during the recovery phase may lead to rapid brain swelling and death. Patients who experience a concussion should be evaluated by a medical professional and should not return to play until they have been cleared to do so.

Actions. In pediatric trauma patients with AVPU scores of P or U, provide assisted ventilation to maintain good oxygenation and adequate ventilation. Hypoxia is an important cause of secondary brain injury in these children with TBI. Hypoxia may be associated with increased intracranial pressure, a situation that may occur rapidly and sometimes deceptively in a child with a primary brain injury.

Children with TBI require oxygenation and ventilation, but the rate of ventilation is controversial. Although hyperventilation was widely recommended in the past as a way of rapidly decreasing intracranial pressure, extreme hyperventilation can itself cause decreased brain perfusion and secondary brain injury. Reserve hyperventilation for patients with TBI who have signs of increased intracranial pressure or signs of impending brainstem herniation, and use waveform or digital capnography to keep $EtCO_2$ between 30 and 35 mm Hg.

Consider this intervention if the child has a severe neurologic disability, as defined by a rating of P or U on the AVPU scale; a score of less than 9 on the PGCS; or a fixed and dilated pupil, asymmetric pupils, or posturing (decerebrate or decorticate).

TIP

A child with head trauma has impending brainstem herniation if the AVPU score is P or U; if the PGCS is less than 9; or there is a fixed dilated pupil, asymmetric pupils, or active posturing.

ALS

Management of Elevated Intracranial Pressure. If the child has AMS (not alert on AVPU or <15 on the PGCS), anticipate elevated intracranial pressure. Cushing's triad of bradycardia, elevated blood pressure, and irregular respirations occur with elevated intracranial pressure. Take a graded approach to intracranial pressure management, always balancing risks and benefits of treatment.

- Support the patient's head in a midline position to facilitate jugular venous return to the heart.
- If the patient is not in shock, elevate the head of the backboard or stretcher. Ensure adequate oxygenation and ventilation.
- Consider hyperventilation only in patients with signs of impending herniation syndrome. Use waveform or digital capnography to keep $EtCO_2$ above 30 mm Hg, preferably in a range of 30–35 mm Hg (normal is 35–45 mm Hg).
- If there is head injury and hypovolemia, administer fluid to maintain brain perfusion. The injured brain hates ischemia.
- Mannitol or 3% hypertonic saline may be useful to acutely decrease intracranial pressure in the child with asymmetric pupils or posturing, but must be used with caution in a child with associated injuries who is at risk for hemorrhagic shock.

Exposure

Exposure is the last step in the primary assessment. Good exposure allows full assessment of the child's entire anatomy, including the extremities. Quickly examine the back during the spinal stabilization procedure for soft-tissue or penetrating injuries. Assess circulation and neurologic function distal to obvious or suspected extremity injuries. Although not usually life threatening, complicated extremity injuries (e.g., open fractures of the humerus or femur) may cause significant blood loss and pain. Remember to cover the patient after the examination to prevent heat loss and hypothermia.

> **CAUTION**
>
> Administration of mannitol can acutely decrease intracranial pressure through changes in CNS fluid distribution and diuresis. Do not administer mannitol to patients with hypovolemic shock.

Summary of Primary Assessment

The assessment of the injured child requires knowledge of anatomic and developmental differences that lead to pediatric-specific patterns of injury. The child's airway is small and easily obstructed, the lungs are vulnerable to contusion, and the solid organs and long bones are poorly protected. The prehospital professional's primary role in multisystem trauma is to ensure an open airway, assist ventilation, and minimize secondary brain injury. Treatment goals are to avoid hypoxia and hypotension. Short time on scene and rapid transport to the ED are overriding priorities for all children who are physiologically unstable or have concerning mechanisms of injury. Vascular access and volume resuscitation are secondary tasks to be considered on the way to the hospital.

> **CAUTION**
>
> Mannitol is temperature sensitive. Do not store in temperatures less than 45°F.

> **TIP**
>
> Use assisted ventilation to maintain oxygenation and to avoid carbon dioxide retention in pediatric trauma patients with AVPU scale scores of P or U.

> **TIP**
>
> In the prehospital environment, endotracheal intubation is not always the optimal airway management tool.

Special Airway Considerations in Pediatric Trauma

Children with severe head injuries with neurologic disability and impending herniation often require field interventions for the following reasons:

- Protect the airway and prevent aspiration
- Improve or control ventilation
- Improve or control oxygenation

Optimal airway management balances the potential risks of the procedure against the potential benefits to the patient. Although endotracheal intubation has long been considered the best method for airway management in a critically injured patient, the procedural risks are significant. These risks may include prolonged scene time, worsened hypoxia, vomiting and aspiration, elevation of intracranial pressure during laryngoscopy, or a misplaced tube. The decision to support ventilation using a bag-mask device versus an endotracheal tube (ET) is a complex one and must take into consideration the following factors:

- Risk of increasing intracranial pressure (by increasing the child's combativeness or inducing gagging during intubation procedure)
- Ability to access the airway
- Length of on-scene and transport times
- Personnel availability and experience
- Availability of a drug-assisted intubation protocol and training on its use

TABLE 7-7 lists the factors that the prehospital professional must consider to choose the optimal airway management approach for each patient.

TABLE 7-7 Factors Influencing Optimal Airway Management Decisions
Factors Favoring Basic Life Support (bag-mask ventilation)
Combativeness, strong gag reflex
Presence of **trismus** (spasm of jaw muscles)
Short on-scene and transport times
Factors Favoring Advanced Life Support (endotracheal intubation)
Inability to ventilate with a bag-mask device
Unresponsive child
Absent gag reflex
Apnea, poor muscle tone
Long extrication or transport times
Limited personnel to assist during transport
Availability of a drug-assisted intubation protocol and training

Advanced Airway Management of the Pediatric Trauma Patient

If a severely injured child needs endotracheal intubation, the preferred path is orotracheal, with manual neutral stabilization of the cervical spine (see **Endotracheal Intubation, Procedure 11**).

Although blind nasotracheal intubation may cause less cervical spine motion in the adult than the orotracheal technique, the procedure is not applicable to children because of the anterior location of the larynx and the increased risk of adenoidal bleeding. *Do not attempt blind nasotracheal intubation in a child.*

Drug-assisted intubation (often called rapid sequence intubation) for pediatric endotracheal intubation, with sedatives and paralyzing drugs, is standard practice in many EDs and in a number of EMS regions. Its effectiveness, safety, and feasibility in the prehospital setting are controversial, and its use requires specialized training. See **Advanced Airway Techniques, Procedure 13**, for a detailed explanation of this procedure.

CAUTION

Do not attempt blind nasotracheal intubation in children.

CONTROVERSY

The use of sedative and paralytic drugs to facilitate pediatric endotracheal intubation is standard practice in EDs and in a number of EMS regions. Its effectiveness and safety in the field are controversial, and its use requires specialized training.

The Primary Assessment

The Transport Decision: Stay or Go?

After the primary assessment and initiation of life support, consider the timing for transport. *Immediately transport every pediatric trauma patient who has any abnormal physiologic or anatomic findings, or a serious mechanism of injury.* Stable trauma patients with apparently minor injuries may undergo further evaluation and treatment on scene. If the scene size-up suggests circumstances that could be dangerous to the child or prehospital professional, transport immediately. Potentially dangerous conditions that warrant immediate transport and completion of assessment in the ambulance include proximity to fire or hazardous materials, threatened violence, angry bystanders or caregivers, and suspected nonaccidental trauma.

Additional Assessment

The additional assessment consists of the focused history and physical examination and the detailed physical examination (trauma patient). This part of the assessment is directed at anatomic problems. Perform the focused history and physical examination and the detailed physical examination in the field only if the patient is physiologically normal and the conditions are safe. Otherwise, address these components of the assessment in the ambulance while on the way to the ED. In physiologically unstable patients, defer the additional assessment and do en route, if possible.

When obtaining the focused history, use the SAMPLE template, as outlined in Chapter 1. Focus only on points likely to affect primary trauma assessment and interventions. **TABLE 7-8** provides a SAMPLE template oriented to pediatric trauma patients.

TABLE 7-8 SAMPLE History in Pediatric Trauma

Component	Explanation
Signs/symptoms	Time of event
	Nature of symptoms or pain
	Age-appropriate signs of distress
Allergies	Known drug reactions or other allergies
Medications	Chronic medications—timing and dose of last dose
	Timing and dose of analgesic/antipyretic medications
Past medical problems	Prior surgeries
	Immunizations
Last food or liquid	Time of the child's last food or drink, including bottle or breastfeeding
Events leading to the injury	Key events leading to the current incident
	Mechanism of injury
	Hazards at the scene

The focused physical examination includes a careful look at the anatomy in the suspected areas of injury. This may involve a conscientious examination by exploration and palpation of the head and scalp for a child with closed-head injury, observation and palpation of the back and axillae in a child with a penetrating chest injury, or inspection and palpation of the neck in a child with a strangulation injury.

The detailed physical examination (trauma) is a head-to-toe (in infants, toddlers, and preschool-aged children, toe-to-head), then front-to-back complete physical examination of the patient. This examination uses the traditional assessment tools of observation, palpation, and auscultation, as outlined in Chapter 1. After the child is on the way to the ED, perform ongoing reassessments, especially with patients with abnormal physiology. This includes serial evaluations of the PAT, ABCDEs, pulse oximetry, vital signs (including heart rate and rhythm on the cardiac monitor), anatomic problems, and response to treatment. Be sure to monitor and treat pain, if possible. When the child arrives in the ED, diagnostic testing with blood tests and imaging studies may assist with continued assessment.

Summary of Additional Assessment

After the primary assessment, determine the timing of transport and the appropriate destination. Do an additional assessment, or on-scene focused history and physical examination and detailed physical examination, only on stable patients in safe scene circumstances. All other patients require immediate transport with continuation of assessment on the way to the ED. Frequent reassessment is important in all injured patients. Transport severely injured pediatric patients to trauma centers rather than community hospitals when possible. Many state trauma programs have algorithms for directing patients, including children, to the appropriate level of care.

Spinal Motion Restriction and Splinting for Transport

Indications for SMR of children are the same as for adults and are indicated for any child with a concerning mechanism of injury, signs of significant head injury, or multisystem trauma. When a cervical spine injury is suspected (discussed earlier), stabilize the

FIGURE 7-13 Keep the airway and spine in a neutral position by placing a layer of padding beneath the child's body from shoulders to hips before securing the child to the stretcher.

neck using a properly sized pediatric extrication collar and/or a head immobilizer, when available. Otherwise, use properly secured towel rolls and tape. For a step-by-step description of this procedure, see **Spinal Motion Restriction, Procedure 22**.

Preschool-aged children may not be able to localize or communicate the presence of neck or back pain. Anatomic differences, specifically the large size of an infant's or toddler's head, require modification of SMR procedures. For example, placing a thin (1-inch) layer of padding beneath a child's body from shoulders to hips before securing the child to the stretcher (**FIGURE 7-13**) helps to properly align the airway and the spinal column.

The spine does not stop at C-7, and SMR precautions should be used if a spine injury is suspected. *Secure the patient against all axes of motion on the spine board or extrication device during extrication.* Near-vertical positioning may be necessary during extrication. Secure the patient against lateral movement by padding along the sides of the body to eliminate all space between the patient and the straps.

Avoid chin straps and other SMR aids that might impair ventilation. Leave room for chest expansion during breathing when tightening chest straps or flaps. Make sure cervical collars fit properly, or use manual spinal stabilization until the child can be secured to the stretcher if a properly sized collar is not available. Ensure that spinal stabilization equipment does not interfere with assessment and access to the patient. A child who does not have severe injuries, and there is no concern of c-spine or spinal injury, may not require SMR, based on local protocol.

FIGURE 7-14 Splinting.

Splinting deformed or painful extremities is also an important prehospital intervention. Splinting has several important functions: pain control, hemorrhage reduction, and preservation of neurovascular function. Unless the extremity shows signs of neurovascular compromise or there is severe pain, splint bones that may be fractured or dislocated in an "as is" position (**FIGURE 7-14**). An open femur fracture should be reduced by traction ONLY if the traction can be maintained. This controls the bleeding at the fracture site and helps to control pain. Otherwise, unless circulation is compromised, leave exposed bone out to avoid introducing further contamination by forcing fractured bone fragments back under the broken skin.

Restraint of Children During Transport

Make sure all persons riding in an ambulance are appropriately restrained. Secure children with possible spinal injury in a supine position on a stretcher. If the child has mild to moderate trauma without suggestion of spinal injury, use EMS system guidelines for age-appropriate restraint. All states have well-defined regulations on proper child restraint in a passenger vehicle. However, these regulations may not extend to ambulance transport. The appropriate use of a child restraint seat in an ambulance is controversial. When car seats are used for EMS transport, both the device and the method of securing the seat to the gurney must conform to industry standards and meet local requirements. If EMS local policy allows, have the child's caregiver remain within view or speaking distance of the child, if the caregiver's presence does not compromise the child's treatment or crew safety. This is comforting for the conscious and **hemodynamically stable** child.

Pediatric Burn Patients

The assessment and management priorities for the burn patient are the same as for any other trauma patient. Make sure the scene is safe before approaching the child. Always anticipate exposure to hazardous materials and carbon monoxide, and use protective measures. Get technical help, if needed, from authorities on hazardous materials.

Assessment

Assess the scene for risk factors for airway and breathing. Important considerations in patients with fire and smoke exposures include the following:

- Enclosed space
- Heavy smoke
- Fumes
- Steam
- Hot vapors
- Chemical hazards
- Explosions with blunt or penetrating injury

Assess the patient for signs of smoke or particle inhalation and thermal burns of the airway. Give 100% oxygen for suspected carbon monoxide poisoning in children with abnormal appearance or AMS or in children exposed to fire or smoke in an enclosed space. Anticipate hidden injuries (especially abdominal) from a fall or a blast injury.

Make a quick estimation of burned body surface area. A modified anatomic diagram of children of different ages gives an approximation of burned body surface area, as shown in **FIGURE 7-15**. If such a diagram is not available, use the "rule of palms," which states that the patient's palm plus fingers equals 1% of body surface area (**FIGURE 7-16**). The percentage of burned body surface area is therefore roughly equal to

FIGURE 7-15 Modified anatomic diagrams of children of different ages give an approximation of involved body surface area for calculation of extent of burn in **(A)** an infant, **(B)** a child, and **(C)** an adolescent.

FIGURE 7-16 The palm plus fingers is approximately 1% of the body surface area.

the number of patient palm plus fingers–sized areas burned. Electronic apps that facilitate the calculation of percent body surface area burned are available.

Although most burns are unintentional, assess all burn patients for risk factors for intentional injury. **Scald** and **contact burns** are common in children and are frequent findings in nonaccidental trauma, as explained in Chapter 11. A "pattern" burn (where there is a clear demarcation of an object in the burned skin), "glove" or "stocking" distribution of a scald burn (**FIGURE 7-17**), or a history that is inconsistent with the injury are suspicious circumstances for intentional injury.

Management

Remove any burning clothes. Give 100% oxygen to all patients with flame or blast burns. High-flow oxygen therapy is the only field treatment for suspected carbon monoxide poisoning. Because of the risk of hypothermia, do not flush or wet burned areas unless necessary to decontaminate or stop the burning process. Cover burned areas with clean dry sheets or burn **dressings**. Covering helps to reduce pain by minimizing exposure to air currents. *Do not apply ointments or creams to burn areas.*

Pain Management and Sedation. Fear and pain in children are frequently ignored or misinterpreted.

FIGURE 7-17 Consider intentional injury with a suspicious pattern of the burn, especially a "stocking" or "glove" distribution.

Pain management is an important prehospital priority, especially in trauma and burn patients with long transport times. Infants and young children experience the same degree of pain as older children and adults; they just cannot express it in words.

Pain and anxiety are different things and require different treatments. Treat pain with a narcotic analgesic drug, such as morphine or fentanyl. Treat anxiety with a sedative drug, such as a benzodiazepine (e.g., **diazepam** or **midazolam**). For example, a child with continued pain after a burn needs morphine or fentanyl to control the principal problem, which is pain. Narcotics, such as morphine or fentanyl, are pain killers, but also provide some sedation. However, a child who is anxious or a child who has been intubated and is fighting the endotracheal tube needs a medication such as diazepam or midazolam because anxiety is the problem, not pain.

CAUTION

Do not apply ointments or creams to burn areas.

ALS

Advanced Airway Management of the Pediatric Burn Patient. Consider early (before edema starts) endotracheal intubation in any patient exposed to a fire in an enclosed space with a suspected inhalation injury to the airway. Such patients may have abnormal airway sounds, abnormal positioning, and respiratory distress or failure. Singed or burned nasal hairs and carbonaceous sputum may also indicate airway injury. Smoke inhalation may cause bronchospasm. If wheezing is present, give a

bronchodilator, such as albuterol or give intramuscular (IM) **epinephrine**.

Fluid Management of the Pediatric Burn Patient. Try to establish at least one IV line in patients with partial or full-thickness burns greater than 5% body surface area. Insert IV catheters through a burn site, if necessary. If indicated, initiate fluid resuscitation with 20-mL/kg boluses of isotonic crystalloid fluid. Fluid and heat are rapidly lost through disrupted skin, with the rate of loss proportionate to the percentage body surface area burned. Provide early analgesia and sedation, and titrate to effect. For longer transports, contact the medical control to determine IV infusion rates.

TIP

The Parkland formula is the most common method of determining fluid resuscitation after a burn. It is intended only as a guide for fluid resuscitation. Based on this formula, the patient receives 2–4 mL/kg of crystalloid multiplied by the percentage body surface area burned of crystalloid for the first 24 hours. Therefore, it is useful in the field only for prolonged transport times.

IV narcotic analgesics are appropriate in hemodynamically stable trauma patients with burns or with isolated long-bone fractures or dislocations. If serious blood loss or bleeding is suspected, or if assessment suggests shock, avoid the use of narcotics because of the tendency to contribute to hypotension. Compared to morphine, fentanyl may cause less hypotension.

Consider sedative drugs when transporting an awake, intubated child or a child who has received neuromuscular blocking agents (paralytics) to help with endotracheal intubation. Benzodiazepine drugs can also contribute to hypotension, so titrate the dose carefully.

TABLE 7-9 lists common medications to treat pain or anxiety in a hemodynamically stable child after consultation with medical control as per local EMS protocol.

All IV sedatives and narcotics cause respiratory depression. Give by slow IV push over 3–5 minutes. Another option is to give intranasal fentanyl. Give supplemental oxygen to all children receiving these medications. Place the child on a cardiac monitor and use pulse oximetry and waveform or digital capnography. Be ready to begin positive-pressure ventilation

TABLE 7-9 ALS: Pharmacologic Management of Pain and Anxiety

Pain	
Morphine sulfate	*Neonates*: 0.05 mg/kg IM, IV, IO, or SQ
	Infants and children: 0.05–0.1 mg/kg IM, IV, IO, or SQ
	Adolescents: 3–4 mg IV or IO
Fentanyl	1–2 mcg/kg/dose every 30–60 minutes IV, IO, intranasal
Anxiety	
Diazepam	0.1 mg/kg IV (max 5 mg/dose)
Midazolam	0.05–0.1 mg/kg IV, IM, or IO; 0.2 mg/kg intranasal

IM, intramuscular; IO, intraosseous; IV, intravenous; SQ, subcutaneous.

with a bag-mask device if the child develops respiratory depression. **Naloxone** (0.1 mg/kg/dose to a maximum single dose 2 mg IV/IO/intranasal/ET tube) may temporarily reverse respiratory depression caused by narcotic administration. Keep in mind that use of naloxone also negates any analgesic effect and prevents further positive effects of narcotics until the naloxone has been metabolized by the child's body.

Treat circulatory compromise with IV fluid boluses of 20 mL/kg.

CAUTION

Avoid narcotics in unstable multiple trauma patients, because they may contribute to hypotension.

TIP

Pain and anxiety are different things and require different treatments.

Transport Decisions. The American Burn Association criteria for transfer to a burn center include the following: partial thickness burns >10% body surface area; burns involving the face, hands, feet, genitals, perineum, and major joints; and full-thickness burns. If there is a burn center in close proximity that can handle pediatric burns, transport to this location would be ideal. If there is no facility available, transport the child to the hospital based on local protocol. If needed, they can then be transferred to a burn center.

Summary of Burns

Burns are common pediatric injuries but usually are small and require only first aid. Burns involving the airway, that cover more than 5% of body surface area, or are full-thickness burns require important field interventions, including possible airway protection and fluid administration. Burns from fires in enclosed spaces raise the possibility of carbon monoxide and cyanide poisoning. Pain is a universal feature of burns, and analgesia is usually a primary intervention.

CASE STUDY 3

You are dispatched to a child who has been run over by a vehicle. On your arrival you notice a full-sized SUV parked in the middle of the road, and a 6-year-old girl, conscious and alert, lying on the ground. She has no abnormal airway sounds or increased work of breathing, and her skin is pale. According to bystanders, the child was walking behind the car when her dad backed up. The patient is cool and clammy to the touch. Respiratory rate is 40 breaths/min, heart rate is 146 beats/min, and you are unable to obtain a blood pressure. Lung sounds are decreased in lower fields. While exposing the child, you notice a tire track impression across the abdomen and sternum area. Pulse oximetry is 87% on room air.

1. What critical injuries do you suspect?
2. What are your treatment and transport priorities?

CASE STUDY ANSWERS

CASE STUDY 1

This patient requires immediate treatment and transport. The patient has sustained multisystem trauma to the head and lower extremities, and the primary assessment confirms respiratory failure and shock. Snoring respirations are likely caused by airway obstruction by soft tissues or blood. Positioning the airway and suctioning may alleviate the problem. Perform rapid SMR.

The patient is hypoxic with a slow respiratory rate due to his altered level of consciousness.

Do a jaw thrust and provide oxygen at 100% by positive-pressure ventilation. Consider endotracheal intubation if the oxygenation does not improve with less-invasive airway management.

Stabilize the femur with a splint. Start IVs en route to the hospital and initiate fluid resuscitation. Transport rapidly to a trauma center with pediatric expertise.

CASE STUDY 2

This child appears to have an isolated head injury and TBI. The child's rapid deterioration suggests an expanding intracranial hematoma, which may be life threatening. Provide SMR, and be prepared for vomiting. Apply 100% oxygen. Rapidly transport.

Establish an IV en route for the administration of medications and leave at a keep-vein-open rate. Consider use of an OG tube to relieve gastric distention from crying and limit possibility of aspiration.

Transport to a facility with pediatric neurosurgical capability, or consider rendezvous with an air ambulance service if such care is not available in your community. This is a surgical emergency, and immediate access to operative care may make the difference between the life and death of this child.

CASE STUDY 3

The injuries to this child are life threatening and she appears to be in shock. Transport immediately after spinal stabilization and 100% oxygen. Consider the use of a pelvic binder or sheet.

Do not prolong scene time with IV attempts. Give fluid resuscitation during transport.

This child is at risk for massive internal injury, including abdominal solid organ hemorrhage (liver, spleen, and kidneys); viscus rupture of the stomach, small bowel, and large bowel; and pelvic fracture. The source of bleeding is not relevant to field care, but the recognition and treatment of hypotensive (decompensated) shock are critical.

Transport to the highest level of trauma care available in your community, based on local trauma triage protocol. This child requires rapid radiologic assessment of the extent of injury and possibly early operative intervention.

SUGGESTED REFERENCES

Textbooks

American Academy of Pediatrics and the American College of Emergency Physicians. *APLS: The Pediatric Emergency Medicine Resource.* 5th ed. Burlington, MA: Jones and Bartlett Learning; 2012.

American College of Surgeons, Committee on Trauma. *ATLS Advanced Traumas Life Support.* 10th ed. Chicago, IL: American College of Surgeons; 2018.

Bledsoe B, Porter R, Cherry R. *Essentials of Paramedic Care.* Upper Saddle River, NJ: Prentice Hall; 2003.

Campbell J. *BTLS for Paramedics and Other Advanced Providers.* 5th ed. Upper Saddle River, NJ: Pearson-Prentice Hall; 2004.

National Association of Emergency Medical Technicians. *PHTLS: Prehospital Trauma Life Support.* 9th ed. Burlington, MA: Jones and Bartlett Learning; 2018.

Articles

Adelgais KM, Brown K. Pediatric prehospital pain management: Impact of advocacy and research. *Clin Pediatr Emerg Med*. 2014;15(1):49–58.

Adelson PD. Guidelines for the acute medical management of severe traumatic brain injury in infants, children, and adolescents. Chapter 4. Resuscitation of blood pressure and oxygenation and prehospital brain-specific therapies for the severe pediatric traumatic brain injury patient. *Pediatr Crit Care Med*. 2012;13(suppl 1):S1-82.

Atabaki SM. Prehospital evaluation and management of traumatic brain injury in children. *Clin Pediatr Emerg Med*. 2006;7(2):94–104.

Fischer PE, Perina DG, Delbridge TR, et al. Spinal motion restriction in the trauma patient – a joint position statement. *Prehosp Emerg Care*. 2018; 22(6):659–661.

Leonard JC, Browne LR, Ahmad FA, et al. Cervical spine injury risk factors in children with blunt trauma. *Pediatrics*. 2019;144(1):e20183221.

Lerner EB, Dayan PS, Brown K, et al. Characteristics of the pediatric patients treated by the Pediatric Emergency Care Applied Research Network's affiliated EMS agencies. *Prehosp Emerg Care*. 2014;18(1):52–59.

Sadow KB. Prehospital intravenous fluid therapy in the pediatric trauma patient. *Clin Pediatr Emerg Med*. 2001;2(1):23–27.

Shah MI. Prehospital management of pediatric trauma. *Clin Pediatr Emerg Med*. 2010;11:10.

Other Resources

Centers for Disease Control and Prevention. Heads up concussion. http://www.CDC.gov/concussions. Accessed April 8, 2019.

Centers for Disease Control and Prevention. Leading causes of death and unintentional injuries, 2017 United States. https://www.cdc.gov/injury/wisqars/fatal.html. Accessed July 2, 2019.

© LaRVI.+/Getty Images.

CHAPTER 8

Toxic Emergencies

J. Hudson Garrett Jr., PhD, MSN, MPH, FNP-BC, PLNC, IP-BC, AS-BC, NREMT, VA-BC, FACDONA, FAAPM, FNAP
Mary Otting, RN, BSN, CEN

LEARNING OBJECTIVES

1. Identify the age groups at risk for toxic exposures and the substance and management issues unique to each group.
2. Describe the physical assessment of the child with a suspected toxic exposure.
3. Explain the risks and the benefits of different forms of gastric decontamination.
4. Discuss the use of antidotes in a child with a toxic exposure.
5. Identify situations where online contact with the regional poison center might influence the assessment and treatment of toxic exposures.

Introduction

A toxic exposure is an ingestion, inhalation, injection, absorption, or application of any substance that causes illness or injury. There are a myriad of reasons that children experience such exposures, including unintentional ingestions of poisons, environmental exposures, and deliberate intoxications. An example of an unintentional exposure is a toddler who ingests a caregiver's medication. An environmental exposure might be a child who inhales carbon monoxide during a house fire, or a child with a systemic reaction to a skin contact with an insecticide or other chemical. Deliberate intoxications include recreational drug or alcohol exposures and attempted suicides.

Age-Related Differences

Toxic exposures are a common pediatric prehospital complaint. Although children younger than 6 years of age account for most of the total exposures for all age groups, according to 2017 data from the American Association of Poison Control Centers, the percentage of fatalities in this age group remains low at 0.9%, similar to statistics from previous years (**TABLE 8-1**). Although the number of reported exposures for the adolescent population (13–19 years) is relatively low at 8.1%, the mortality rate is much higher at 5.1% of fatalities and is usually caused by intentional exposure.

Most toxic exposures in infants and preschool children younger than 6 years of age are asymptomatic.

TABLE 8-1 Toxicological Cases 2017, American Association of Poison Control Centers Toxic Exposure Surveillance System

Total reported cases	2,115,186
Patients <3 years	711,011 (33.6%)
Patients <6 years	956,871 (45.2%)
Total patients <20 years	1,265,052 (59.8%)

Data from 2017 Annual Report of the American Association of Poison Control Centers' National Poison Data System (NPDS): 35th Annual Report. *Clinical Toxicology*. 2018; 56(12): 1213–1415.

FIGURE 8-1 Toddlers are "oral explorers"; they will try to taste or swallow almost any substance.
© Antonio_Diaz/iStock/Getty Images Plus/Getty Images.

The toddler is a fearless, curious individual who explores the world by placing objects in his or her mouth (**FIGURE 8-1**). Because toddler ingestions are unintentional, and most nonfood items ingested are not very palatable, poisonings in this age group often involve small volumes of a single substance. The most common ingestions in young children include cosmetics and personal care products, cleaning substances, and analgesics. The great majority of toddlers are initially asymptomatic; however, toddlers may also present with significant symptoms without a known history or witnessed ingestion. It is important that providers consider this possibility and survey the scene to better understand possible causes. In addition, it is important to keep in mind that the initially asymptomatic child may have dangerously high levels of a toxin in his or her body that may not become apparent until much later. In the absence of any apparent life threats, obtaining a thorough history before making a transportation decision is absolutely imperative. In this age group, analgesics, button batteries, and hydrocarbons cause the most fatalities.

Button (disk) batteries usually pass through the digestive tract without a problem, but can get stuck in the esophagus or anywhere else in the body. If there is suspicion that a child has ingested a battery (or one is stuck in the nose, ear, or elsewhere), attempt to find out exactly what kind of battery it is and bring the child to the emergency department (ED). More than one-third of patients with disk batteries lodged in the esophagus are initially asymptomatic. Symptoms develop when the battery begins to erode and damages surrounding tissues. Although battery ingestion can be fatal, most pass through the gastrointestinal tract in 1–4 days.

Children 6–12 years of age are less likely to ingest nonfood articles or nonprescribed medications (**TABLE 8-2**). Although most exposures continue to be unintentional in this age group, intentional exposure begins to play a role, particularly among the middle school–age group. Unintentional fatal exposures are mostly caused by smoke inhalation and carbon monoxide poisoning. Intentional exposure, nonfatal and fatal, is seen with "huffing," the intentional inhalation of volatile chemicals.

Among adolescents (13–19 years), toxic exposures are usually intentional, either as recreational abuse or as a suicide gesture or attempt. Intentional exposures lead to more ED visits and hospital admissions than unintentional exposures. In suicide attempts, adolescents usually ingest two or more substances, often

CASE STUDY 1

A mother calls 9-1-1 because her 3-year-old toddler is drooling and having trouble breathing. On arrival at the home, you find a young boy coughing. He has no abnormal airway sounds, no flaring, and no retractions. His skin is pink. The respiratory rate is 32 breaths/min, the pulse oximetry is 98%, and the heart rate is 120 beats/min. His lungs are clear. On further assessment, you note that the child has a brightly colored laundry pod in his hand that has been bitten into. His mother states that she was doing the laundry when she received a telephone call and left her son briefly.

1. What are key aspects of the scene size-up?
2. Outline transport and management priorities.

TABLE 8-2 Top Ten Substances Involved in Toxic Exposures

Children (<6 years)	Children and Adolescents (<19 years)
Cosmetics/personal care products	Analgesics
Cleaning substances (household)	Sedatives/hypnotics/antipsychotics
Analgesics	Antidepressants
Foreign bodies/toys/miscellaneous	Cardiovascular drugs
Topical preparations	Cleaning products (household)

Note: Analgesics include aspirin, acetaminophen, ibuprofen, and narcotic analgesics such as methadone and morphine.

Modified with permission from 2014 Annual Report of the American Association of Poison Control Centers, National Poison Data System. To locate your local poison center call 1 (800) 222-1222 or visit aapcc.org.

in large quantities. Recreational abuse often involves alcohol in addition to another recreational drug. The number of fatalities in this age group is increasing. Statistics represent an underestimation of the true incidence, because statistics only include those cases reported to the poison control database. Many adolescents would have difficulty getting the resources to purchase illicit drugs, which leads to the ever-evolving creative ways they find to get high. Huffing usually involves common household products, such as markers, glue, aerosol air freshener or hair spray, spray paint, correction fluid, gasoline, and other products. These substances are inexpensive, easy to find in many homes, and give the teenager an easy-to-hide substance because it would not normally seem out of place to have these items in one's home. Botanical substances including salvia and jimsonweed (hallucinogenics) are also easy to grow or obtain. Other drugs, often sold inexpensively and legally on the Internet and in convenience stores, include what are commonly known as "bath salts," a group of synthetic cathinones that mimic the symptoms of methamphetamine and can cause agitation, tachycardia, violent behavior, and hallucinations. "K2" or "spice" is synthetic marijuana; symptoms include mood elevation and altered perception, but can also cause tachycardia, palpitations, elevated blood pressure, and nausea. Another popular synthetic drug is "ecstasy" or "Molly." This is 3,4 methylenedioxy-methamphetamine (MDMA), and it has stimulant and hallucinogenic properties. It causes

an elated mood, euphoria, and increased energy, but it also causes tachycardia and hypertension. Because this drug can affect the body's ability to regulate temperature, it can lead to hyperthermia resulting in dehydration; heart, kidney, and liver failure; and seizures.

It is important to remember crew member safety first, because some of these substances can cause delusional and violent behavior in the teenage patient. Restraints may be necessary if approved by local medical protocol.

Another problem continues to be the exposure of young children to the chemicals used in methamphetamine laboratories and the use of methamphetamines. Crew safety in these situations is critical because of explosion and fire hazards.

An unusual form of abuse involves deliberate intoxication of infants or young children, a condition called Munchausen syndrome by proxy. This condition is a complex form of deliberate poisoning of a child by a caregiver. In these cases, the caregiver frequently possesses more than average medical information and is trying to induce a state of illness in the child in an attempt to bring attention to himself or herself. Children with such exposures may be especially difficult to identify because the intoxication is secretive and often chronic. It is important to also alert child protective services and the receiving ED as required by local laws and regulations, as well as department policy.

Common Substances Responsible for Serious Poisonings in Children

Most poisonings occur in the home. Table 8-2 lists common substances responsible for poisonings by age.

Summary of Age-Related Differences

Most toxic exposures in children are minor and involve household products. The most common patient is the toddler who unintentionally ingests a single agent in small quantity and is asymptomatic. The second most common patient is the adolescent who uses recreational drugs or who is making a suicide attempt or gesture. Adolescent exposures often consist of more than one drug and often involve large quantities. Common serious exposures in young children involve analgesics, whereas those in adolescents involve analgesics, alcohol, and recreational drugs. An unusual form of intoxication in young children involves a condition called Munchausen syndrome by proxy, a complex form of deliberate poisoning or abuse of a child by a caregiver.

Prearrival Preparation and Scene Size-Up

Sometimes, at the time of dispatch, the toxin has already been identified by the caregiver, the poison center, or another healthcare professional. In such cases, immediately contact medical control or the poison center, depending on local emergency medical services (EMS) protocol. They help clarify the toxicity of the agent and priorities in assessment and treatment. In other cases, where the dispatch involves a toddler or adolescent with a sudden change in behavior, consider a toxic exposure. Poison center resources can be substantial and provide great insight into the appropriate treatment needed for the ingested substance.

On arrival, first perform the scene size-up. Note if there are potentially hazardous toxins in the area or on the patient's clothes or skin. If so, assess the scene and whether immediate patient decontamination is safe to perform. The poison center or other public health agency may assist in defining risk and the need to mobilize other personnel (e.g., hazardous materials team). Pay close attention to scene safety when dealing with adolescents with sudden behavioral changes, because some common substances of abuse can lead to paranoia and sudden violent actions.

If there is a possible toxin or hazardous material, secure the scene and minimize the risk of toxic exposures to the EMS crew through the skin, eyes, or lungs by use of personal protective equipment. Use all your senses to gather information at the scene. Pay particular attention to your initial impression with smell on the scene. Some dangerous toxins quickly overwhelm the sense of smell, rendering it useless after just a few sniffs ("olfactory fatigue"). Other toxins have an odor only at low levels, such as hydrogen sulfide. The "rotten egg" smell given off by this chemical overwhelms the sense of smell and one cannot smell it at the high toxic levels. Other key smells include bitter almonds (cyanide) and garlic (organophosphates, arsenic). Pay attention to confined spaces, and remember that some toxic gases are heavier than air and may affect children first or may only be in low-lying areas, such as cesspools or ditches.

Be aware of the possibility of a mass exposure to a toxic substance, either because of unintentional or deliberate action (e.g., bioterrorism). If a disaster or mass-casualty event is suspected, implement disaster response preparedness (see Chapter 14).

Next, look over the surrounding area. Bring any bottles, containers, or plastic bags containing possible toxins and samples of ingested plants or syringes to the ED along with the patient (**FIGURE 8-2**). If the caregiver refuses to let a poisoned child be transported to the hospital, ask medical control to talk to the caregiver over the telephone or radio. If this strategy does not work, then request assistance from law enforcement personnel.

A

B

FIGURE 8-2 Bring any bottles or plant samples to the ED. **A.** Bottles and containers. **B.** The poisonous plant jimson-weed.

TIP

Have caregivers look around (e.g., in purses, under child's bed) to help determine what could have been ingested.

TIP

The adolescent who makes a suicide attempt or gesture must be transported to the ED for medical and psychological assessment, even if the child refuses. This is true even if the injury or immediate medical risk is assessed as trivial.

CAUTION

Never forget about toxic hazards on scene. Watch out for absorbable toxins and protect the skin and eyes by using gloves and other personal protective equipment.

Role of the Poison Center

Almost every state in the United States has at least one regional poison center. The telephone number within the state is usually toll-free. For ease of access, there is also a national toll-free number (1-800-222-1222) that forwards calls to the state poison center, when available. At the other end of the telephone are specialists who can provide information about the potential toxicity of an item or adverse effects and can recommend home or hospital management. Caregivers often call the poison center for advice before or while awaiting the arrival of the prehospital professional.

TIP

The poison center has a key role in individual and community prevention and treatment of toxic exposures. Have the toll-free number (1-800-222-1222) posted near or on your telephone.

The regional poison center can also be a valuable resource to the prehospital professional when managing children with a toxic exposure. Local EMS system protocol should define the circumstances when contact with the poison center must be made by medical control and when the call can be made directly.

TIP

Poison centers have the capability to follow up with continuing reassessment by telephone.

Assessment of the Child With a Possible Toxic Exposure

General Assessment

After the rapid scene size-up and environmental evaluation for toxins, assess the child. Use age-appropriate techniques to approach the patient, as outlined in Chapters 1 and 2, and conduct a general assessment (pediatric assessment triangle [PAT]), a primary assessment, and then an additional assessment when appropriate. If the child is unstable, treat the physiologic abnormalities detected in the general (PAT) and primary assessments, and then transport. En route, do a reassessment and the additional assessment, if possible.

A detailed history is the best tool for overall assessment of risk and for determining urgency for treatment in pediatric poisoning. It is usually more accurate than a physical evaluation in determining the specific type of toxic exposure. In the first few minutes, the important questions are as follows: (1) the identity of the agent, (2) the route of exposure (ingestion, inhalation, injection, absorption), (3) the time since the exposure occurred, and (4) the amount of the agent involved in the exposure; if unknown, assume the worst-case scenario. Using the acronym TART can help one to remember: T = Toxin, A = Amount, R = Route, T = Time. See **TABLE 8-3**.

Special Considerations in the Primary Assessment

After the PAT, do the hands-on ABCDEs to complete the primary assessment, and then immediately treat any physiologic abnormalities. Special elements of the physical assessment that may help identify the type of poison include breath odor, vital signs, pupillary size, skin temperature, and skin condition. An odor of bitter almonds may be caused by cyanide, a sweet smell by ethylene glycol, or garlic odor may be caused by organophosphates. Also, look for stains and powders on the skin or clothes. Use assessment information to match the patient's signs and symptoms with possible "toxidromes," identifiable clinical patterns of single-agent intoxications. **TABLE 8-4** outlines the signs and symptoms of important toxidromes in pediatrics.

TABLE 8-3 TART Chart

Toxin	Amount	Route	Time
Name of substance Type (pill, capsule, liquid, seed, root, flower, suppository, patch, etc.)	Milligrams or other amount if known. Include approximate number of pills or seeds, amount of liquid, and so forth (note if any spilled on floor or clothes). Any vomitus? Take with you if possible.	By mouth, snorted, smoked, injected, rectal, skin absorption, eyes, nose, etc.	Approximate time of first exposure or ingestion. Include duration and whether confined space, if applicable.

TABLE 8-4 Common Toxidromes

Toxidrome	Agents	Signs and Symptoms
Anticholinergics	Antihistamines, cyclic antidepressants	"Hot as a hare, red as a beet (hot, dry skin; hyperthermia), blind as a bat (dilated pupils), mad as a hatter (delirium, hallucinations)"
Cholinergics	Organophosphates	DUMBELS: diarrhea/diaphoresis, urination, miosis, bradycardia/bronchoconstriction, emesis, lacrimation, salivation
Narcotics	Morphine, methadone	Hypoventilation, bradycardia, hypotension, miosis
Sympathomimetics	Cocaine, amphetamines	Tachycardia, hypertension, hyperthermia, mydriasis (dilated pupils), diaphoresis (sweating)

Airway

Clear, maintain, and control the airway in the child with a suspected toxic exposure who has altered mental status (AMS). This may happen in a child exposed to a sedative or hypnotic drug, such as a benzodiazepine or a barbiturate. Beware of the child who has ingested a caustic agent, such as lye. This child may have severe burns of the esophagus and present with drooling, dysphagia, and signs of upper airway obstruction. Have a suction unit on hand; if using it becomes necessary, do so gently.

Breathing

Give 100% supplemental oxygen by a nonrebreathing mask if there is AMS, respiratory distress, or a history of exposure to a toxic substance known to cause breathing problems. One example of this type of toxic exposure is hydrocarbon inhalation. Obtain pulse oximetry, but be aware that the reading is not accurate for some toxic exposures, notably carbon monoxide poisoning. Sedative or hypnotic drugs, opiates, and γ-hydroxybutyrate may decrease the respiratory rate, whereas sympathomimetic agents (cocaine, amphetamines), phencyclidine (PCP), and aspirin may increase the respiratory rate.

Close monitoring of the airway is essential to evaluate the adequacy of breathing so that intervention with a bag-mask device with supplemental oxygen can be started without delay should breathing become inadequate. End-tidal capnography is very helpful to monitor respiratory status.

Circulation

If the child has eaten or swallowed a possible cardiopulmonary toxin, place him or her on a cardiac monitor to watch for dysrhythmias. Such drugs as β-blockers, digoxin, or calcium channel blockers may decrease the heart rate, whereas sympathomimetic agents and anticholinergic agents (scopolamine, antihistamines, and jimson weed) may increase heart rate. Skin can be warm and dry because of such drugs as antihistamines

TABLE 8-5 Specific Agents

Agent	Alternate Names	Signs and Symptoms
γ-Hydroxybutyrate	GHB, "date rape drug"	Initially drowsiness, dizziness, and disorientation; high doses result in bradycardia, hypoventilation, and apnea
Ecstasy, MDMA	3,4 methylenedioxy-methamphetamine, mephedrone and/or methylenedioxypyrovalerone (MDPV), "Molly"	Euphoria, increased energy, intense visual perceptions Complications: hyperthermia, hypertension, tachycardia, seizures, dehydration, myocardial infarction, intracerebral hemorrhage
Rohypnol	Flunitrazepam, "roachies," "roofies"	Drowsiness, sedation, amnesia, blackout
Synthetic cannabinoids	Spice, "synthetic marijuana," K2, fake weed	Elevated mood, relaxation, and altered perception Complications: agitation, hallucinations, severe paranoia, seizures, vomiting, tachycardia, hypertension, myocardial ischemia
Synthetic cathinones	"Bath salts"	Tachycardia, hypertension, euphoria, paranoia, agitation, hallucinations, violent behavior, sweating, nausea, vomiting, dizziness, panic attacks
Second generation (atypical) antipsychotics	Olanzapine (Zyprexa), risperidone (Risperdal), aripiprazole (Abilify), ziprasidone (Geodon), quetiapine (Seraquel)	Drowsiness, QT prolongation, stomach pain; can also cause neuroleptic malignant syndrome (NMS), a rare, but life-threatening, idiosyncratic reaction to these antipsychotics/neuroleptic medications characterized by fever, muscular rigidity, hypertonicity, altered mental status, and autonomic dysfunction. NMS often occurs shortly after the initiation of neuroleptic treatment or after dose increases.
Selective serotonin reuptake inhibitors (SSRI)	Sertraline (Zoloft), fluoxetine (Prozac), paroxetine (Paxil), fluvoxamine (Luvox)	Restlessness, hallucinations, shivering, diaphoresis, nausea, diarrhea, headache. These medications can also cause serotonin syndrome, which is characterized by agitated delirium, high fever, elevated blood pressure, tachycardia, and diaphoresis. It can occur within minutes of exposure to the precipitating agent and can deteriorate to shock and muscle rigidity

and anticholinergics, whereas the skin may be hot and sweaty from sympathomimetics, organophosphates, aspirin, and PCP.

Disability

AMS is a common effect of many different chemical exposures. Recreational drug use with sedatives or hypnotics depresses the central nervous system (CNS). Sympathomimetic drugs may stimulate the CNS and cause excitement, agitation, paranoia, or hallucinations. Cyclic antidepressants may cause seizures or coma. In

the comatose or unresponsive patient, always consider the other common causes of AMS, such as a head injury, seizure, or hypoglycemia (which may accompany alcohol or β-blocker ingestion). Check the bedside glucose level in any patient with AMS, even if toxins are suspected, and treat as needed. **TABLE 8-5** outlines the signs and symptoms of specific agents in pediatrics.

Exposure

Undress the child and look for evidence of toxic exposure to the eyes and skin. Many substances, such as hydrocarbons, irritate the eyes. Other toxic substances, such as **hydrochloric acid**, are caustic to skin. **Organophosphate insecticides** can be inhaled and also enter through the skin and can cause a severe **cholinergic crisis** with diaphoresis (sweating), diarrhea, urination, **miosis** (small pupils), bradycardia, bronchoconstriction, emesis, tearing, and **salivation**. The mnemonic DUMBELS helps identify signs of cholinergic drug intoxication. In some systems, the mnemonic SLUDGEM is used: Salivation, Lacrimation, Urination, Defecation, Gastrointestinal pain, Emesis, and Muscle twitching (seizures or coma). These signs, coupled with agitation and respiratory distress, signal a severe exposure, as you will read in Chapter 14.

Initial Management of Toxic Exposures

After the primary assessment, determine the need for treatment and transport of the poisoned child by combining the physical assessment with a risk assessment. The physical assessment is a way to determine the child's physiologic stability and the overall urgency for treatment and transport. The risk assessment evaluates the probability of serious toxicity (early and delayed) from the exposure. *Perform the risk assessment with knowledge of the identity of the drug involved, time since ingestion or exposure, and amount of poison involved. The child's weight should also be considered* (see **TABLE 8-6**). Contact with the poison center can provide much of this information.

CONTROVERSY

If the child is stable and has a history of a single, small ingestion of a low-risk agent, some EMS systems allow non-transport in consultation with medical control. Although this approach may be medically sound, it eliminates an opportunity for ED assessment of psychosocial risk factors.

TIP

In suspected toxic exposures, perform risk assessment to determine the chances of serious toxicity.

Common toxic agents, such as aspirin, **acetaminophen**, or iron, have predictable physiologic effects that are determined by how much of the drug was taken, time since exposure, and amount of drug per kilogram. By collecting information and evidence at the scene, the prehospital professional serves

---

TABLE 8-6 Risk Assessment

Assess the chances of serious toxicity from the following five pieces of information:

1. The agent involved and its lethality, usually identified through consultation with medical control or the poison center
2. Amount of the toxin, in milligrams when possible
3. Child's weight
4. Route of exposure
5. Time since the exposure

---

an important role in later ED testing and treatment. Be sure to ask about *all* medications (prescription and over-the-counter), preparations, and other substances to which the child may have been exposed. Caregivers may not realize that some topical preparations (e.g., Bengay or wart treatments) contain salicylate and can contribute to the potential salicylate toxicity when a child ingests aspirin or some common herbal preparations and oils, many of which also contain salicylates.

Sometimes the prehospital professional's risk assessment determines that a child has had a potentially lethal exposure, although the child is physiologically stable. Indeed, in a small child, one ingested pill or teaspoon of some common medications can kill. **TABLE 8-7** lists potentially dangerous agents where a tiny toxic exposure (e.g., one pill) may be fatal to a toddler.

Iron poisoning is one of the leading causes of fatal poisonings in young children. Tasty chewable children's vitamins have, on average, 17 mg of iron, and the tempting new chewable gummy prenatal vitamins have 27 mg each. A young child can easily mistake either of these for candy and eat excessive amounts. Consider that seriously toxic doses begin at 60 mg/kg of iron and as the ingestion climbs toward 120 mg/kg and higher, the poisoning can easily be lethal without prompt treatment. Gather up all bottles, and assume that when pills are missing, the child has eaten them until proven otherwise.

TIP

Nicotine in any form (e.g., gum, patch, lozenge, e-cigarettes) can be toxic if ingested. Signs and symptoms include vomiting, sweating, drowsiness/tiredness, shaking, confusion, seizures, and death.

CASE STUDY 2

You respond to a call for a 3-year-old who just ingested all of her mother's prenatal iron gummies (approximately 30). On your arrival, the child is active and running around the room, but complaining that her "tummy hurts." She has no increased work of breathing, and her skin is pink. Her respiratory rate is 22 breaths/min, heart rate is 110 beats/min, and blood pressure is 90/60 mm Hg. Her physical examination reveals no abnormalities. The mother hands you the empty bottle of fruit-flavored chewable prenatal gummy vitamins. Reading the label, you learn that each vitamin contains 27 mg of iron.

1. Do you need to transport this child to the hospital?
2. Should you give activated charcoal?

TABLE 8-7 One Sip or Pill Can Kill: Potentially Lethal Toddler Ingestions

Medicine	Lethal Dose
Camphor	One teaspoon of oil
Chloroquine	One 500-mg tablet
Clonidine	One 0.3-mg tablet
Glyburide	Two 5-mg tablets
Imipramine	One 150-mg tablet
Lindane (lice removal—not available in the United States)	Two teaspoons of 1% lotion
Diphenoxylate/atropine (Lomotil Rx)	Two 2.5-mg tablets
Liquid nicotine (vaping liquids/e-cigarettes)	One teaspoon
Oil of wintergreen (methyl salicylate)	One teaspoon
Propranolol	One or two 160-mg tablets
Theophylline	One 500-mg tablet
Verapamil	One or two 240-mg tablets

The Transport Decision: Stay or Go?

After the primary assessment, initial treatment, and risk assessment, consider whether to transport immediately, performing additional assessment and treatment on the way to the ED, or to stay on the scene. If the results of the physical assessment and the risk assessment reveal an asymptomatic child and the ingestion of a small amount of a single low-risk agent, consider non-transport after appropriate consultation with medical oversight or the poison center. This is controversial, however, because some EMS systems consider hospital transport necessary in all toxic exposure cases. Other systems allow the poison center to manage minor ingestions exclusively over the telephone. Always follow the advice of your local medical control.

If the physical assessment indicates that the child has any physiologic abnormality, or if the risk assessment indicates that the toxic exposure is potentially harmful, transport and perform additional assessment on the way to the ED, if possible. The onset of symptoms varies with the substance involved. A child without symptoms on arrival of EMS may still have ingested a lethal dose of a substance. For example, ingestions of acetaminophen, a common household over-the-counter medicine, may be extremely dangerous but cause no early symptoms. History from the scene is critical to the management in the ED.

TIP

Most pre-adolescent pediatric poisonings do not require any treatment in the field.

Additional Assessment

If the child has no physical abnormalities and is asymptomatic, and if the risk assessment indicates no serious toxicity, perform a complete assessment on scene. Additional assessment includes the focused history and physical examination and the detailed physical examination (trauma). Sometimes it is more appropriate to perform this additional assessment on the way to the ED. **TABLE 8-8** lists important history in a suspected toxic exposure, presented in the standard SAMPLE format. During the primary assessment and

TABLE 8-8 The Pediatric SAMPLE for Toxic Exposures

Component	Explanation
Signs and symptoms	Time of suspected exposure Behavior changes in child Emesis and content of vomitus
Allergies	Known drug reactions or other allergies
Medications	Identity of suspected toxin Amount of toxin exposure (count pills or measure volume) Pill or chemical containers on scene Exact names and doses of prescribed medications
Past medical problems	Previous illnesses or injuries
Last food or liquid	Timing of the child's last food or drink Type and time of home treatment
Events leading to the exposure	Key events leading to the exposure Type of exposure (inhaled, injected, ingested, or absorbed through the skin) Poison center contact

the risk assessment, the prehospital professional will have already obtained some of the SAMPLE history.

Summary of Assessment of the Child With a Possible Toxic Exposure

Every child with a toxic exposure needs a careful physical assessment and risk assessment. The physical assessment includes all of the features of the standard assessment, with an emphasis on the history, which is usually the most important part of the toxicologic evaluation. Preparation begins on the way to the scene with dispatch information about the age of the patient, the type and potential toxicity of exposure, and the need for personal protective equipment. Preparation then continues with the scene size-up and environmental assessment. If multiple patients are involved, consider disaster plan activation to ensure adequate resources are available to respond.

After the physical assessment, the risk assessment helps determine if there might be serious toxicity based on the type of toxin involved, the amount of the toxin, the weight of the child, the route of exposure, and the time since the exposure. The risk assessment gives important information about expected physiologic effects, need for treatment, and timing of transport. The poison center often plays a key role in helping decide about treatment and transport.

Toxicologic Management

The prehospital professional has three possible options for toxicologic management of serious or potentially lethal exposures: (1) decontamination to reduce local or systemic exposure to the toxin, (2) enhancement of natural elimination or increasing the speed of removal of the toxin, or (3) antidote administration to reverse the actions of the poison directly. In most cases, documenting a thorough history, evaluating the risk assessment, and appropriate transport supporting the ABCs are usually the best treatment.

Decontamination

After the treatment and transport decision, consider decontamination. There are several ways to decontaminate, depending on the toxin and the type of exposure.

Skin

If there is a chance that the poison was **absorbed** through the skin, remove the child's clothing. The prehospital professional must protect his or her own skin and eyes by using gloves and protective gear. Flood the skin with large amounts of warm water for 15–20 minutes (if time allows and no apparent life threats take priority), and then wash it well with mild soap and water, avoiding harsh scrubbing.

Eyes

Immediately wash out the eyes if there has been direct eye contact (**FIGURE 8-3**). **Alkali** burns with caustic agents, such as lye, are the most dangerous. Flush the eyes for 20 minutes using normal saline or water. Attach intravenous (IV) tubing to the bag of normal saline and flush the eye with the end of the IV tubing. If this is not possible, hold the patient's head under the

FIGURE 8-3 Immediately wash out the eyes if there has been direct eye contact.
© Jones & Bartlett Learning.

FIGURE 8-4 Ipecac has no role in prehospital professional treatment of pediatric poisoning.
© Jones & Bartlett Learning.

TABLE 8-9 Toxins Poorly Adsorbed by Activated Charcoal
"PHAILS"
Pesticides, potassium
Hydrocarbons
Acid, alkali, alcohol
Iron
Lithium
Solvents

sink and pour water into the eye from a pitcher or cup. When the eyes are the main point of exposure, continue flushing during transport if possible.

Gastrointestinal Decontamination

Before any **gastrointestinal (GI) decontamination**, contact medical control or the poison center, depending on EMS protocol. In some cases, it may be beneficial to dilute mild **acid** or alkali ingestions by asking the alert patient to drink an 8-ounce glass of milk or water. Dilution is contraindicated when there is absent gag reflex, airway compromise, diminished level of consciousness, or ingestion of a hydrocarbon corrosive or caustics (strong alkalis and acids).

Ipecac, an old-time remedy for ingestions, although *no longer recommended for home, EMS, or hospital use*, may have been given in the home by the caregiver (**FIGURE 8-4**). Make note of this and the time it was given. The vomiting induced by ipecac does not remove significant amounts of ingested toxins from the stomach and may cause prolonged emesis, delaying the administration of activated charcoal.

Activated Charcoal. Most high-risk ingestions in toddlers and preschool children do not require any prehospital treatment. In cases where GI decontamination is necessary, consider using activated charcoal. **Activated charcoal** is made from burned wood products. Its surfaces are "activated" by steam or chemical treatment, so the material can irreversibly **adsorb** ingested toxins in the stomach and small bowel, reducing bloodstream absorption of the toxins. Charcoal itself is not absorbed from the GI tract, nor is it metabolized. Activated charcoal has no odor or taste, but has a granular consistency that makes many children unwilling to drink it. Charcoal administration is messy,

even with a cooperative child. In a child with altered or deteriorating mental status, aspiration of charcoal can lead to serious pulmonary consequences. There are limited data on the use of activated charcoal in the prehospital setting, and the risks of prolonged scene time must be weighed against the potential benefits of rapid transport and early ED management. Some agents are not adsorbed by activated charcoal, as noted in **TABLE 8-9**.

Administration of Activated Charcoal. The activated charcoal dose is 10 times the mass of the ingested substance. However, because the actual amount of ingested material is usually not known, use 1–2 g/kg of the child's body weight. Activated charcoal begins working immediately, and it is most effective when given within 1 hour of ingestion (**FIGURE 8-5**).

FIGURE 8-5 Activated charcoal is a treatment option for potentially serious ingestions of bindable toxins.

Never force a child to take activated charcoal, because this may lead to aspiration and pulmonary complications. If local EMS policy allows, consider adding a flavoring agent (e.g., cola, juice, milk) to make the mixture more acceptable to drink, then transport the child. Some formulations of activated charcoal also contain sorbitol. **Do not use charcoal and sorbitol formulations in children younger than 1 year of age** due to a risk of causing electrolyte abnormalities and dehydration from diarrhea. **TABLE 8-10** summarizes activated charcoal and guidelines for use.

ALS

The child must be stable and cooperative to receive activated charcoal. Because young children or adolescents may not want to drink the activated charcoal, some EMS systems use a nasogastric tube as an alternative method of delivery if the ingestion is potentially serious or lethal. Delivery of activated charcoal by nasogastric tube can be dangerous and must be reserved for highly unusual circumstances where transport time is long and risk assessment indicates severe toxicity.

TIP

The biggest problem with field use of activated charcoal is the difficulty getting children to take it.

TABLE 8-10 Activated Charcoal: Guidelines for Use

Product Information	■ A highly adsorbent, harmless, tasteless material made from wood pulp.
Indication	■ To limit amount of drug absorbed by the body in most toxic ingestions (i.e., intestinal decontamination). ■ Repeated doses may enhance the elimination process.
Technique	■ Mix 1–2 g/kg patient weight with water to form a **slurry**. If the quantity of ingested substance is known, give 10 times the ingested dose of toxin by weight (maximum dose, 100 g). ■ Administer orally (or by nasogastric tube in rare situations). ■ Consider adding a flavoring agent to make the slurry more acceptable.
Contraindications	■ Loss of gag reflex. ■ Altered mental status. ■ Unwillingness voluntarily to take the drug. ■ **Corrosive** substance ingestion. ■ Drugs not adsorbed by charcoal.
Adverse effects	■ **Constipation** or intestinal **bezoar** (large foreign-body mass in gut). ■ Pulmonary aspiration. ■ Diarrhea and dehydration may occur in children younger than 1 year given a combined **cathartic** (e.g., sorbitol) and activated charcoal.

CONTROVERSY

The value of activated charcoal for prehospital treatment of ingestions is unproven. Although the drug has a possible advantage of early binding of toxins in the gut, there are potential complications, such as aspiration and bowel obstruction.

Enhancement of Elimination

Sorbitol is a cathartic medication that is mixed with many commercial activated charcoal preparations. Cathartics have been promoted to clear the bound toxin from the gut and help speed up elimination. The effectiveness of cathartics has not been proved, and sorbitol is not an approved drug in most EMS systems. Prehospital professionals may think they are giving pure activated charcoal when the preparation actually is a mixture of activated charcoal and sorbitol. Sorbitol may cause nausea, vomiting, abdominal discomfort, diarrhea, and electrolyte disturbances in young children. *Therefore, never use a cathartic in children in the prehospital setting.*

Antidotes

Antidotes are medications that reverse or treat the side effects of toxic ingestions. Prehospital providers carry several antidotes (**TABLE 8-11**) that may be life-saving for poisoned patients. Use these medications with knowledge of the type of ingestion or exposure, patient's clinical status, and possible adverse effects associated with the antidote.

Naloxone is an antidote used frequently in adult patients with suspected opioid overdose. It can have a therapeutic and diagnostic effect in selected pediatric patients. If the child has signs of an opioid ingestion or overdose (respiratory depression, bradycardia, coma, small pupils), administer 0.1 mg/kg. Maximum dose is

TABLE 8-11 Commonly Available Prehospital Antidotes

Poison	Antidote
Carbon monoxide	Oxygen
Organophosphate	Atropine/2-PAM
Tricyclic antidepressants	Sodium bicarbonate
Opiates	Naloxone
β-Blockers	Glucagon
Calcium channel blockers	Calcium, glucagon
Benzodiazepine	Flumazenil
Oral hypoglycemics	Glucose, glucagon

2 mg. Although IV is the preferred route, it can be given intramuscularly (IM), intraosseously, intranasally, endotracheally, or nebulized. The child may then awaken slightly or fully, with improvement in vital signs. The duration of action of naloxone is 20–60 minutes, so repeat doses may be necessary if a longer-acting narcotic (e.g., methadone, Lomotil) is involved. When administering naloxone, as with adults, give the lowest effective dose and administer slowly. In adolescents chronically addicted to opioids, too rapid administration may induce undesired acute withdrawal symptoms. Have suction on hand in case vomiting should occur. It is also important to prepare for the patient to awake violently to prevent danger to the EMS crew.

Although flumazenil is an effective benzodiazepine antagonist, do not use this antidote routinely for patients with AMS of unknown cause. One of the most common causes of AMS in children is the postictal state after a seizure. If flumazenil is given and the child has further seizures, benzodiazepines are not effective. Also, flumazenil may precipitate seizures if administered to the patient who is on chronic therapeutic doses of a benzodiazepine.

Sodium bicarbonate helps reverse the adverse cardiac effects seen with cyclic antidepressant overdoses, including conduction abnormalities. It alkalinizes the blood to reverse the sodium channel blockade caused by the drugs. The dose is 1–2 mEq/kg IV slowly.

Glucagon, a familiar drug to prehospital professionals because of its role in treatment of hypoglycemia, helps reverse toxicity from β-blocker overdose. β-blockers are drugs commonly used for treatment of hypertension and adult cardiac disease. Overdose in children can cause bradycardia and hypotension. Although there are no good pediatric studies, the suggested dosage of glucagon is 0.03–0.15 mg/kg followed by 0.07 mg/kg/hr (maximum 5 mg/hr) given IV. β-blocker overdose can also cause hypoglycemia in young children, so check the bedside glucose level and treat hypoglycemia if present.

Calcium channel blockers are another frequently prescribed medication for hypertension in adults. Pediatric ingestions may result in severe toxicity that is similar to β-blocker overdose, including bradycardia and hypotension. There also can be secondary respiratory and neurologic effects (respiratory depression, decreased level of consciousness). IV fluids are the first line of therapy, and calcium can be beneficial. Give either IV calcium chloride 10% (20 mg/kg = 0.2 mL/kg) or IV calcium gluconate 10% (60 mg/kg = 0.6 mL/kg) slowly. The patient needs to be on a cardiac monitor during administration of these drugs and during transport. Glucagon is another potential therapy for refractory hypotension in such patients.

Organophosphates

DUMBELS is the mnemonic that summarizes the clinical hallmarks of organophosphate poisoning toxidrome. Treatment involves several steps:

1. Ensure your personal protection (use protective gloves and other protective clothing to prevent exposure).
2. Remove contaminated clothing, and place them in a bag.
3. Perform the primary assessment, and ensure adequate oxygenation and ventilation.
4. Decontaminate the patient (flush the skin with large amounts of water; wash the skin, hair, and under the nails well with soap and water).
5. Flush exposed eyes with large amounts of warm water or saline.
6. If the child has refractory bradycardia, consider treatment with the antidote, **atropine**. The drug helps reverse the "muscarinic" organophosphate effects (salivation, bronchorrhea, bronchospasm, bradycardia, respiratory depression, seizures, coma). The initial pediatric atropine dose is 0.05 mg/kg IV (higher than usual atropine dose). Repeat doses until the airway is dry and the child has adequate perfusion. If no response to atropine, administer **pralidoxime (2-PAM)**.

With the advent of possible chemical terrorism incidents, there has been much attention to the side effects of organophosphates, which are the same as those for such nerve agents as sarin gas. Because some EMS agencies have distributed MARK 1 or MARK 2 kits to their providers for management of chemical terrorism, it is important to realize that the medication doses in these autoinjector kits are for adults. However, in severe, life-threatening pediatric cases, administer the contents of these kits to children 3 years or older by IM injection. Keep in mind that the likelihood of responding to a child involved in an event of weapons of mass destruction is far less likely than responding on a sunny afternoon to a backyard for a child poisoned by one of the many household and commercial pesticide preparations containing organophosphates.

Summary of Toxicologic Management

Most children with toxic exposures do not require treatment of any kind in the field. Consider non-transport after consultation with medical control or the poison center only if the child is asymptomatic, has ingested a small amount of a single low-risk substance, and there are no "red flags" for child neglect or maltreatment. In other circumstances, when physical assessment and risk assessment together show physiologic instability or possible toxicity, treatment is indicated. After managing the ABCDEs, consider toxicologic management by decontamination or, in special situations, administering an antidote. Perform skin and eye decontamination when indicated. Attempt GI decontamination for serious or potentially fatal ingestions based on local protocol. Activated charcoal is a useful binding agent for many types of toxic ingestions, but can be safely administered only to a cooperative child. Sorbitol is contraindicated in children. Several antidotes carried by prehospital professionals may be diagnostic, therapeutic, and even lifesaving. More advanced antidote therapies are best performed in the ED or hospital setting. Remember to educate the family or caregiver on poisoning prevention if circumstances allow, as discussed in Chapter 1.

Medicolegal Issues

There are several scenarios where medicolegal issues play an important role in the management of toxicologic emergencies in children. If the caregiver refuses therapy and transport to the hospital, ask medical control to talk to him or her over the telephone. If this strategy does not work, then request assistance from law enforcement personnel.

The adolescent who makes any suicide attempt or gesture must be transported to the ED. An individual who has attempted suicide is legally incompetent to make treatment decisions and cannot refuse transport. In some cases, law enforcement must become involved in scene management. Place the patient in temporary protective custody and transport to the hospital (see Chapter 15).

The adolescent can also present legal problems because of such issues as the ability of a dependent minor to **consent for care** and illegal use of alcohol or recreational drugs. If an adolescent has taken a potentially toxic dose of medication, or has life-threatening complications of drug use or overdose, treat based on the emergency exception rule (the doctrine of implied consent), as explained in Chapter 15. Leave the legal issues of alcohol or drug use to law enforcement officials.

CASE STUDY 3

You respond to a call about a seizing female at a park. On arrival, you find a group of high-school students surrounding a female who is lying on the ground having a tonic-clonic seizure. She is unresponsive and is cyanotic. Her heart rate is 90 beats/min, respiratory rate is 6 breaths/min, and you are unable to get a blood pressure.

They tell you she is 16 years old and that they were partying after a football game, smoking some "spice" and drinking beer. She was happy, dancing one minute, then she became agitated then started to seize. They deny any head trauma. She has been seizing for 10 minutes.

1. What are your initial treatment management priorities?
2. Can you treat and transport this patient without parental consent?

CASE STUDY ANSWERS

CASE STUDY 1

Scene size-up should include assuring your safety with gloves and other personal protective equipment as needed. Note if there has been skin or eye involvement in addition to ingestion. If present, remove the child's clothes and undertake skin and eye decontamination.

The emergence of brightly colored laundry pods has resulted in numerous pediatric ingestions. The toddler will usually bite into the pod, and the liquid is swallowed. The main issue is the components of these pods. They often contain a detergent and surfactant, but some contain alkaline substances.

The most likely symptoms from these ingestions are vomiting, coughing, and drowsiness, but if an alkali is present, mouth burns, drooling, and airway compromise can occur.

Rapidly transport this child to the hospital, frequently reassessing his airway. Bring the bitten pod as well as an intact one to the ED. Allow the child to sit upright in a position of comfort. Administer blow-by oxygen because a face mask will not likely be tolerated. Contact with medical control or the regional poison center can provide information on potential complications to anticipate in transport, such as airway edema, stridor, or wheezing. Do not give anything by mouth, including charcoal or fluids, due to the risk of vomiting.

CASE STUDY 2

Although this child appears well, this is a potentially dangerous ingestion. Iron is one of the most common fatal ingestions in children. There are four phases to an iron ingestion. The initial phase begins with the ingestion and lasts 6 hours. Common signs and symptoms in mild ingestion include nausea and vomiting. Stage 2 (at 6–12 hours) is the quiet phase, during which the child appears well. It is not until stage 3 (12–24 hours after ingestion) that the child begins to show signs of toxicity, including GI hemorrhage, hypotension, AMS, and renal and hepatic failure. Stage 4 is the postrecovery phase, during which GI strictures can still occur. Because the extent of toxicity cannot be predicted from early symptoms, a cautious approach is warranted. Transport any child who has ingested iron-containing pills to the hospital for further evaluation unless the regional poison center has been contacted and has determined that this is a nontoxic ingestion based on the nature and number of pills taken. This is commonly the case with ingestion of children's multivitamins, where the concentration of iron is low; however, because children's vitamins are often manufactured to look and taste a lot like candy, it is not unheard of for a toddler to ingest a full bottle of 60 colorful character vitamins, many of which can contain up to 17 mg of iron each. The ingestion of prenatal vitamins, however, can be very serious, especially now that the more palatable fruit-flavored chewable vitamins and gummies are becoming more and more popular for women with morning sickness and who are unable to swallow the larger traditional prenatal vitamins with iron. (The prenatal formulations often contain 27 mg of iron each.) Bring any pill bottles to the ED to ensure proper identification and risk assessment. Because iron is not absorbed by activated charcoal, do not attempt GI decontamination.

CASE STUDY 3

The first priority is to establish an effective airway and begin bag-mask ventilation with 100% oxygen, because respiratory failure is present. Based on local protocols, you can provide medications such as intranasal or IV midazolam or rectal diazepam.

Some questions to ask her friends include a SAMPLE history:

- Signs and symptoms: Did anyone see her before she started to seize? Was she acting normally?
- Allergies: Any known drug reactions or other allergies?
- Medications: Does she take any medications (both prescription and non-prescription, such as herbs/vitamins)? Was she drinking any alcohol? Does she use illicit drugs? Did anyone see other drugs being passed around?
- Past medical problems: Does she have any medical problems?
- Last food or liquid: When was the last time anyone saw her with something to eat or drink?
- Events: What was she doing before she began to seize?

Because they admit to smoking "spice," the real question is, besides synthetic marijuana, were there any other drugs in the mixture? The key finding of a seizure can be caused by this drug, but also think of hypoglycemia due to alcohol ingestion. Once the seizure has stopped, reassess vital signs and transport to the hospital with bag-mask ventilation and IV fluids.

Even without the girl's assent or her parents' consent, you are legally bound to treat and transport this patient because she has a life-threatening condition.

SUGGESTED REFERENCES

Textbooks

American Academy of Pediatrics and the American College of Emergency Physicians. *APLS: The Pediatric Emergency Medicine Resource*, 5th ed. Burlington, MA: Jones and Bartlett Learning; 2012.

Dieckmann R. Toxic exposures. In: Seidel J, Henderson D, eds. *Prehospital Care of Pediatric Emergencies*, 2nd ed. Burlington, MA: Jones and Bartlett Learning; 1997:122–129.

Olson K. *Poisoning & Drug Overdose*, 7th ed. New York, NY: McGraw-Hill Education; 2018.

Tenenbein M, Macias CG, Sharieff GQ, Yamamoto LG, Schafermeyer RW, eds. *Strange and Schafermeyer's Pediatric Emergency Medicine*. 5th ed. New York, NY: McGraw-Hill; 2019.

Articles

Bar-Oz B, Levichek Z, Koren G. Medications that can be fatal for a toddler with one tablet or teaspoonful: a 2004 update. *Pediatr Drugs*. 2004;6(2):123–126.

Bassett RA, Osterhoudt K, Brabazon T. Nicotine poisoning in an infant. *N Engl J Med*. 2014;370:2249–2250.

Bonney AG, Mazor S, Goldman RD. Laundry detergent capsules and pediatric poisoning. *Can Fam Physician*. 2013;59:1295–1296.

Gummin, DD, Mowry JB, Spyker DA, et al. 2017 Annual Report of the American Association of Poison Control Centers' National Poison Data System (NPDS): 35th Annual Report. *Clin Toxicol*. 2018;56(12):1213–1415.

Kim JW, Baum CR. Liquid nicotine toxicity. *Pediatr Emerg Care*. 2015;31(7):517–521.

Lowry JA, Leeder JS. Over-the-counter medications: update on cough and cold preparations. *Pediatr Rev*. 2015;36(7):286–297.

Stromber PE, Burt MH, Rose SR, et al. Airway compromise in children exposed to single-use laundry detergent pods: a poison center observational case series. *Am J Emerg Med*. 2014;33(3):349–351.

Wang GS, Hall K, Vigil D, et al. Marijuana and acute health care contacts in Colorado. *Preventive Med*. 2017;104:24–30.

Other Resources

American Addiction Centers. The dangers of inhalants. https://americanaddictioncenters.org /inhalant-abuse. Accessed May 3, 2019.

Karb R. One pill (or sip) can kill. https://www .acep.org/how-we-serve/sections/toxicology/news /march-2016/one-pill-or-sip-can-kill. Accessed May 3, 2019.

National Capitol Poison Center. Button batteries. https://www.poison.org/battery. Accessed May 9, 2019.

National Institute on Drug Abuse. Commonly abused drugs charts. https://www.drugabuse.gov/drugs -abuse/commonly-abused-drugs-charts. Accessed July 5, 2019.

New York State Bureau of Emergency Medical Services, Department of Health. Prehospital treatment protocols https://www.health.ny.gov /professionals/ems/pdf/statewide_prehospital _treatment_protocols_ver16-04.pdf. Accessed May 3, 2019.

© iStock/E+/Getty Images.

CHAPTER 9

Behavioral Emergencies

Victoria Barnes, RN, BSN, EMT

Saranya Srinivasan, MD, FAAP

LEARNING OBJECTIVES

1. Describe psychiatric conditions in children and adolescents, including autism spectrum disorder (ASD), attention-deficit/hyperactivity disorder (ADHD), behavior or conduct disorders, anxiety, and depression.
2. Discuss the management of behavioral emergencies in children.
3. Explain suicidal ideation and proper evaluation of suicidal patients.
4. Review management of common suicidal intentional ingestions.
5. Discuss de-escalation methods for agitated patients.
6. Provide information on chemical restraint.
7. Review issues that may arise during patient restraint.

Introduction

Behavioral emergencies in children and adolescents are a significant public health issue, resulting in numerous emergency department (ED) visits and prehospital patient encounters (**FIGURE 9-1**). The most common disorders diagnosed in childhood include attention-deficit/hyperactivity disorder (ADHD), behavior disorders (includes oppositional defiant disorder [ODD] and conduct disorder), anxiety, and depression. One in six U.S. children between 2 and 8 years of age have been diagnosed with a mental, behavioral, or developmental disorder (the latter includes autism spectrum disorder [ASD]). Behavior problems are more common in those 6–11 years old, while diagnoses of anxiety and depression increase with age. Often, those with ASD and ADHD are included as a subset of children with special health care needs (CSHCN).

Behavioral health emergencies may present alone, as part of, or together with other special health care needs. There are many barriers to effective treatment, including few resources for inpatient and outpatient treatment of mental health problems and a shortage of mental health providers. Additionally, identifying and treating behavioral health emergencies are challenging because they may present at nearly any age, from toddlers to adolescence, and can occur in a variety of settings, including the school and home environment. Onset may occur gradually or suddenly.

Examples of behavioral emergencies in children include suicidal behavioral, such as self-harm or intentional ingestions; depression with suicidal ideation; and ODD with aggressive behavior. Behavioral emergencies may also present in children without a previous formal diagnosis. It is up to prehospital providers and ED health care professionals to be aware of

CASE STUDY 1

You are called to the scene of a 6-year-old boy who was stung by a bee while playing outside at a summer barbecue. Upon your arrival, the child's mother states that the boy began crying uncontrollably and pointing at his arm. The mother noted a visible welt with surrounding redness along with swelling of the child's lips. She also states that her son has been inconsolable since the sting. The mother reports no allergies and a history of mild asthma, with an albuterol inhaler as needed. She also reports that her son has been diagnosed with autism spectrum disorder. As a result of this, he can be very difficult to calm when upset and becomes very anxious around medical providers.

Your assessment reveals an agitated child seated near his mother, crying and kicking his legs. He appears anxious. His actual work of breathing is difficult to obtain due to his crying; his skin is pink. You note swelling of his lips and around the eyes and urticaria on his neck and arms. The child is initially pulling away and will not make eye contact with prehospital providers; however, you are now able to hear expiratory wheezes between cries. The child is uncooperative with your exam, and you are unable to obtain vital signs, but respirations appear to be fast and the hives are spreading. The mother sent another family member to retrieve the child's favorite blanket and stuffed animal.

1. What are the key principles in assessing this child?
2. Describe treatment and transport approaches.

FIGURE 9-1 Behavioral health emergencies in children and adolescents are a significant public health issue, resulting in numerous emergency department visits and prehospital patient encounters.

© Jacqueline Watson/Shutterstock.

behaviors that should be brought to the attention of mental health experts.

The frequency of these encounters and the burden on the prehospital care system are overwhelming both for initial and repeat encounters.

Common Pediatric Psychiatric and Behavioral Conditions

To fully understand the types of behavioral emergencies faced by prehospital providers, it is important to define and describe common pediatric psychiatric conditions, including ASD, ADHD, ODD, depression, bipolar disorder, and schizophrenia.

Autism Spectrum Disorder

Of the aforementioned conditions, ASD presents at the earliest age. Autism spectrum disorder is defined in the *Diagnostic and Statistical Manual of Mental Disorders,* Fifth Edition (DSM-5), as a neurodevelopmental disorder characterized by two primary features: (1) persistent deficits in social communication or interaction with others and (2) repetitive, restrictive patterns of behavior or actions. Because this is a spectrum disorder, the outward signs of a child with autism can range from mild to severe. Most children on the autism spectrum will have sensory sensitivities, which includes hypersensitivity to environmental stimuli such as light, sound, touch, and activity. These symptoms typically present early in development, sometimes as early as 18 months of age (see **TABLE 9-1**). As such, according to the American Academy of Pediatrics, all children should be screened at 18 and 24 months of age so that early diagnosis and therapeutic interventions can be provided. Unfortunately, many children do not receive a diagnosis until they are older. In fact, most children are not diagnosed until after 4 years of age. According to the Centers for Disease Control and Prevention, autism affects an estimated 1 in 59 children in the United States today. It is four times more common in boys than girls and affects all races, ethnicities, and socioeconomic groups. There has been a significant increase in the diagnosis of this disorder in recent years.

Treatment of children with autism spectrum disorders often consists of a multidisciplinary team consisting of psychiatrists, pediatricians, behavioral therapists, psychologists, teachers, and social workers, along with many others (**FIGURE 9-2**). For some patients

TABLE 9-1 Signs and Symptoms of Autism Spectrum Disorder

Age	Clinical Manifestations
6 months	▪ Few or no big smiles or other engaging expressions ▪ Limited or no eye contact
9 months	▪ Little or no back-and-forth sharing of sounds, smiles, or other facial expressions
12 months	▪ Little or no babbling ▪ Little or no back-and-forth gestures such as pointing, showing, reaching, or waving ▪ Little or no response to name
16 months	▪ Very few or no words
24 months	▪ Very few or no meaningful, two-word phrases (not including imitating or repeating)

FIGURE 9-2 Treatment of children with autism spectrum disorders often consists of a multidisciplinary team consisting of psychiatrists, pediatricians, behavioral therapists, psychologists, teachers, and social workers, along with many others.
© Oksana Kuzmina/Shutterstock.

with significant agitation or severe and frequent behavioral outbursts, medications, such as alpha-2-adrenergic agonists (e.g., guanfacine [Intuniv, Tenex] and clonidine [Catapres]) may be prescribed. Rarely, atypical antipsychotics such as risperidone are required if initial pharmacotherapy fails.

Prehospital providers may be called to care for an individual with autism who is experiencing a medical, trauma, or behavioral emergency, and the approach taken to scene size-up, history taking, assessment, intervention, and transport will require special attention to ensure the best outcome for the child and family. Children with ASD are at risk for wandering or running away from help, drowning, or other accidental injuries. They also have difficulty understanding and communicating when stress levels are increased, such as in an emergency, and may be frightened or scared by strangers or medical providers. As a result, they may present with aggression, agitation, or outbursts that may make it difficult for prehospital providers to care for them. In such situations, children with ASD who may normally communicate with minimal difficulty may suddenly become nonverbal, repeat words or movements, or take increased time to respond to questions or requests. There are adjustments that can be made when responding to, caring for, and transporting a child with known ASD. For example, avoiding lights and sirens, loud noises, and quick sudden movements, when possible, can help alleviate some of the sensory sensitivities that can heighten during an emergency in a child with ASD.

Additionally, it is often helpful to have a discussion with the parent or caregiver regarding successful calming or de-escalation techniques that have worked in the past. While many children with ASD will present similarly to other children, as with any pediatric patient, prehospital providers will need to rely on information provided by family members or other caregivers to ascertain what may be normal or baseline for a child. Caregiver participation is also necessary in helping to keep the patient calm and cooperative during an assessment. Keep instructions simple, explain what you are going to be doing to the child before you do it, have family available as a resource, and minimize portions of the exam that may be overstimulating. It is also best to limit the number of prehospital providers involved in the assessment, preferably just yourself and your partner, to help reduce anxiety in the children with ASD unless it is necessary to have additional assistance on scene. It is helpful to work slowly, avoid any sudden movements, and perform your exam distal to proximal. Be aware that dressings or bandages may cause tactile sensory sensitivities. Other strategies for ensuring a successful patient encounter include conducting your assessment in a quiet area whenever possible; avoiding any unnecessary physical contact with the patient; and, when physical assessment is necessary, offering simple explanations before and during the assessment. Throughout treatment and transport, continue to reassure the child and parent and utilize any special comfort adjuncts, such as stuffed animals or blankets, which may help calm and soothe the child

FIGURE 9-3 Children with ASD may have sensory aids that assist them in self-soothing.
© ChrisSteer/iStock/Getty Images Plus/Getty Images.

during times of increased stress (**FIGURE 9-3**). If a legal caretaker of the child tells you that a formal medical diagnosis of ASD had been made, be sure to include the diagnosis of ASD in your radio and in-person report, along with any approaches that proved successful in your providing care. Otherwise, report only the behavior that is witnessed, such as "child is hypersensitive to touch" or "child rocked rhythmically back and forth during the assessment." By modifying your usual pediatric care to include best practices for the patient with presumed or diagnosed ASD, the best possible outcome can be achieved.

> ### TIP
>
> Enlist the parent or caretaker when caring for a patient with ASD. He or she will know ways to approach the child, calming mechanisms for the child, and what may cause agitation in the child.

Attention-Deficit/Hyperactivity Disorder

ADHD is the most common behavioral condition in children. It is defined in the DSM-5 as a constellation of symptoms that are present in more than one setting for at least 6 months and have an onset before 12 years of age (median age of onset: 6 years). Symptoms such as inattentiveness, hyperactivity, and impulsiveness should be inconsistent with the expected developmental findings of the child's chronologic age and need to be significantly impairing function at home or in school for this diagnosis to be made by a mental health professional.

Treatment of ADHD may consist of behavioral modification therapy, pharmacotherapy, or a combination of the two. Behavioral modification therapy includes interventions aimed at changing behaviors using nonpunitive consequences and reward systems. Examples of such interventions are time-outs, positive reinforcements, or withdrawal of privileges. One behavioral intervention that combines all these strategies is a "token economy." In a token economy, children receive tokens in response to desired behaviors and are later able to exchange those tokens for rewards or privileges.

While behavioral modification therapies are preferred in younger patients, pharmacotherapy is considered first-line treatment for children aged 6 years or older to treat symptoms of inattention, impulsivity, and hyperactivity. Stimulants such as methylphenidate (Ritalin, Concerta) or dextroamphetamine (Adderall) are the usual first-line pharmacotherapy agents offered to patients. Stimulants are preferred to other agents given their rapid onset of action and tolerable side effect profile. Other medications such as atomoxetine (Strattera, a selective norepinephrine reuptake inhibitor [SNRI]) and alpha-2 agonists such as guanfacine (Intuniv, Tenex) or clonidine (Catapres) may also be considered.

Both in the prehospital and in-hospital settings, children with ADHD have difficulty following directions and may be frightened or agitated by medical encounters. Because the parent–child relationship is crucial in children in ADHD, engaging the parent in the interaction with the child will result in a far more productive patient encounter. Children with ADHD respond well to positive reinforcement, minimal distractions, and using calming disciplinary techniques. Children with ADHD should be encouraged to participate in their own care by being provided with limited choices (for example, "Which arm do you want me to put the blood pressure cuff on?") and encouraging them with positive reinforcement (**FIGURE 9-4**).

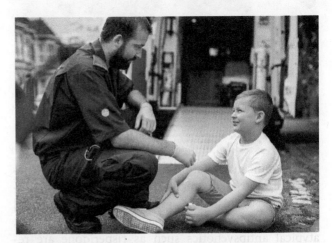

FIGURE 9-4 Children with ADHD should be encouraged to participate in their own care by being provided with limited choices.
© Rawpixel.com/Shutterstock.

Behavior Disorders: Oppositional Defiant Disorder and Conduct Disorder

ODD and conduct disorder are two mental disorders of childhood and adolescence both defined in DSM-5. Children who are diagnosed with ODD must have at least four symptoms in the following categories: vindictiveness, argumentative behavior, defiance, or angry mood. These symptoms must persist for at least 6 months and must be negatively impacting the child's functioning for the diagnosis to be made. Patients with ODD typically present with defiant, argumentative, and hostile behavior. These children are often vindictive and frequently disobey rules, argue with authority figures, and blame others for their mistakes or behaviors. ODD usually starts before age 8 years, but no later than age 12 years.

Conduct disorder is a separate disorder that is comorbid with ODD in 42% of patients. Conduct disorder is characterized by behavioral abnormalities that manifest as ongoing aggression or violence toward other people or animals, and serious violation of rules such as destruction of property, thieving, or deceitful behaviors.

Both ODD and conduct disorder are difficult to treat and require a multidisciplinary approach, with behavioral therapy considered as first-line treatment for these disorders. Examples of such therapies include parent management therapy, which teaches parents and caregivers how to manage disruptive behaviors and to utilize collaborative problem solving, in which children and their parents are taught to work together to solve problematic behavior. Pharmacologic therapy may be used as an adjunct to behavioral therapy, but is not considered the first-line treatment. It has been shown that treatment of comorbid disorders, such as ADHD, diminishes symptoms of ODD and may also help in patients with conduct disorder.

From the prehospital perspective, you may be called to transport a patient due to his or her aggressive behavior. It is important to enlist the parent or caregiver, if possible, to calm the patient. While performing your assessment and physical exam is important, do not get injured in the process. In some cases, law enforcement assistance may be needed. To transport the aggressive patient, if the above methods fail, chemical or even physical restraint may be necessary, based on your local protocols (see Assessment and Transport of the Child with a Behavioral Emergency).

> **CAUTION**
>
> The use of restraints is a last resort when transporting an aggressive child.

Anxiety

When children do not outgrow fears and worries typical of children, or there are so many worries that they interfere with home, school, or daily activities, a child may be diagnosed with an anxiety disorder. Such fears can include being separated from parents while at school (separation anxiety), fears of a specific situation (phobias), being afraid of places where there are other people (social anxiety), or worried about the future and bad things happening (general anxiety). Anxiety affects 7.1% of children ages 3–17 years. Therapy includes behavior therapy, family therapy, or both. In many cases, medication is prescribed, the most common being selective serotonin reuptake inhibitors (SSRIs) such as fluoxetine (Prozac), sertraline (Zoloft), fluvoxamine (Luvox), and paroxetine (Paxil), or venlafaxine (Effexor), an SNRI.

The most common reason emergency medical services (EMS) is called is due to a panic disorder. This can make the child feel like his or her heart is beating too fast; he or she may be dizzy or sweaty, have trouble breathing, or even pass out. Check vital signs, pulse oximeter readings, and bedside glucose. Ask if this has happened before. Have the child seated or supine, apply a nonrebreathing mask, and tell him or her to breathe slowly, and speak to the child calmly. Transport decisions should be made based on exam findings and discussion with the parents.

> **TIP**
>
> Lights and sirens are not needed for transporting a patient with a panic attack. This can lead to increased anxiety.

Depression

Major depression, also known as major depressive disorder, is defined as a period of at least 2 weeks in which a person experiences a depressed mood or loss of interest or pleasure in daily activities. He or she must also have a specified symptom such as problems with eating, energy, sleep, concentration, or feeling worthless. Approximately 3.2% of children aged 3–17 years have been diagnosed with depression.

Patients with depression typically present in the prehospital setting with evidence of self-harm, suicidal ideation or behaviors, or suicide attempts. These presentations may be physical in nature, such as cutting behaviors or attempts at strangulation, or pharmacologic (deliberately ingesting potentially lethal quantities of various substances).

Treatment of major depressive disorder in children and adolescents consists of behavioral therapy and possibly pharmacotherapy. The most commonly used pharmacotherapeutic agents for treatment of major depressive disorder in children and adolescents are SSRIs such as fluoxetine (Prozac), sertraline (Zoloft), escitalopram (Lexapro®), and citalopram (Celexa). Abrupt discontinuation of these agents may result in withdrawal symptoms such as worsening anxiety, fatigue, nausea, myalgias, or chills. As such, these medications should be gradually decreased over time.

Unlike some of the other mental health conditions that have been discussed, while suicidal ideation and/or attempt is a medical emergency, a child or adolescent simply saying they are depressed is not. It is important to see if the patient has thought about suicide or has a plan. It is important that any child with depression seek a mental health evaluation. The primary focus of prehospital providers is to keep themselves and their patients safe from harm using de-escalation techniques whenever possible. Patients who have attempted to harm themselves should be thoroughly assessed for physical injuries, and such injuries should be addressed and treated during transport.

> ### CAUTION
>
> When transporting patients who have expressed suicidal ideation or a plan, ensure that they cannot harm you or themselves during transport.

Bipolar Disorder

Bipolar disorder is classified as a mood disorder and was previously known as manic-depressive disorder. It is thought to be caused by a chemical imbalance in the brain, usually between dopamine and norepinephrine levels. Adverse childhood experiences can also contribute to the development of bipolar disorder. Bipolar disorder usually has an onset in adolescence or young adulthood and affects males and females equally. A person cannot be diagnosed with bipolar disorder until they exhibit an episode of both mania (increased mood and energy, overconfidence, decreased need for sleep, increased talk and ideas) and depression (unusually sad, sleeping and eating issues, feeling worthless, thoughts of death, irritability, and withdrawal). Children with bipolar disorder may fluctuate among periods of mania, depression, and balanced moods.

Prehospital providers may encounter children in either state of bipolar disorder. The lack of insight, inhibitions, and feelings of grandeur in the manic phase can often lead to common traumatic injuries seen in children. During the depressive phase, children may present with nonspecific medical complaints, have exacerbations of chronic medical issues, present as suicidal, or even attempt suicide.

Bipolar disorder is treated with psychotherapy and medications. Mood stabilizers such as lithium (Lithobid) or valproate (Depakote, Depacon, Depakene) are often prescribed. Even patients without a comorbid seizure disorder may also be prescribed anticonvulsant medications, as these have been found to help treat bipolar disorder effectively.

CASE STUDY 2

You are called to the scene of a 14-year-old-girl for an assault. On your arrival, the school nurse reports that the adolescent got into an altercation with another female student that led to hair pulling, but no reported or visible injuries. The adolescent is screaming expletives and telling you to get away. She is picking up books and equipment and threatening to throw them at you. She is also yelling, "Get away from me, don't even think about touching me." The nurse tells you privately that the child is in the custody of the state and being fostered by a local family. She was recently placed there due to behavioral issues in a prior school. The patient takes methylphenidate (Concerta) 18 mg, fluoxetine (Prozac) 10 mg, and aripiprazole (Abilify) 5 mg daily for ADHD, conduct disorder, and posttraumatic stress disorder.

Your assessment shows an adolescent female, visibly agitated, pacing around the nurse's office threatening to harm others and yelling. You observe the patient from a safe distance initially and note that she is very agitated and appears to be hyperventilating. You are unable to obtain vital signs due to her agitation.

1. What are the key principles in assessing this adolescent?
2. Describe treatment and transport approaches.

Schizophrenia

Schizophrenia is a complex mental health disorder that can be disabling to those affected. It is believed to start with a chemical imbalance in the brain; however, it is considered to be a multifactorial condition, in that genetic, behavioral, and environmental factors may also play a role. It is uncommon for children younger than 12 years to be diagnosed with schizophrenia. Schizophrenia can be severe and disabling and can cause distorted thinking, changes in behavior, and unusual use of language and words. Schizophrenia is not a split-personality disorder as once thought. Due to its similarities to other behavioral health disorders, schizophrenia is commonly misdiagnosed, especially in children and young adults.

Children may develop schizophrenia slowly, or it can be a sudden onset. Prehospital providers may be called when a child has a psychotic episode. Children may present with confused thinking, paranoia, distorted perception of reality, hallucinations (auditory, visual, tactile), delusions, moodiness, anxiety, agitation, withdrawal, catatonia, or odd behaviors.

Treatment for schizophrenia can be as complex as the illness itself. Pharmacologic management may include antipsychotics and mood stabilizers, which are designed to help minimize the severity of delusions and hallucinations and treat the intrusive and disturbing thoughts seen in schizophrenia. Although these medications do not cure the disease, they can help control the symptoms. Psychotherapy, structured activity programs, and support groups can help children and their families cope with this illness.

Suicide Attempt/Intentional Ingestions or Exposures

Suicide is the second leading cause of death in those 10–14 years of age. Firearms, suffocation, and poisoning are the most common methods used. Among males, firearms is the most common method, while in females it is poisoning.

Ingestions or exposures may either be pharmacologic or chemical. Common pharmacologic ingestions include acetaminophen, aspirin, ibuprofen, antidepressants, ethanol, and illegal drugs. Common chemical ingestions or exposures include bleach, household cleaning products, or industrial adhesives (e.g., glue). In this section, common pharmacologic ingestions and their presentations will be discussed. Additional information about toxic ingestions is presented in Chapter 8.

> **TIP**
>
> The Poison Control Center is available 24/7 and is an invaluable resource regarding treatment for poisonous ingestions or exposures. To reach the Poison Control Center, dial **1-800-222-1222**.

History Taking

When obtaining a medical history on a patient with a suspected harmful ingestion or exposure, there are several questions that are very important to ask:

- When did the ingestion/exposure occur?
- Which medication/substance was taken?
- Were multiple medications taken?
- How much of each medication/substance was taken? Has the patient used this substance before?

These questions will need to be tailored to the specific circumstances and ingestions.

> **TIP**
>
> Contact the Poison Control Center if you need help identifying the medication(s) involved in an ingestion, as well as for prehospital treatment.

Medications

Acetaminophen

Acetaminophen or paracetamol is an antipyretic (fever reducer) and analgesic that is readily available over the counter. Its easy accessibility makes it a frequently used medication in intentional ingestions, as teenagers can easily obtain the medication. Additionally, adolescents may not perceive it as being as dangerous or lethal as other medications. Acetaminophen overdoses are often asymptomatic initially and can remain so for up to 24 hours after the ingestion. After that, patients typically develop abdominal pain, nausea, and vomiting. Lethargy may be noted. Laboratory studies typically demonstrate elevated liver function tests, abnormal coagulation studies, and even renal damage. Acetaminophen overdoses may be fatal due to end-organ damage, usually more than 24 hours after the overdose. Treatment consists of *N*-acetyl cysteine and serial monitoring of laboratory studies and hospital admission.

Aspirin

Aspirin (acetylsalicylic acid) is a common anticoagulant and analgesic used primarily in the adult population.

Because this product is available over the counter, it is readily available to children and adolescents. When taken as an intentional overdose, it produces a compensatory respiratory alkalosis and metabolic acidosis. A patient with an aspirin overdose will present with tachypnea (fast breathing), hyperpnea (deep breathing), and tachycardia. Symptoms that may appear early in the presentation include nausea, vomiting, diarrhea, and tinnitus (ringing in the ears). In severe cases, altered mental status and coma may occur. Treatment of an aspirin overdose is primarily supportive, but may also include **sodium bicarbonate** to induce alkaline diuresis.

Tricyclic Antidepressants

Tricyclic antidepressants (TCAs) were initially developed in the 1950s to treat depression. They work by inhibiting the uptake of serotonin and norepinephrine at the presynaptic junction. Although they have largely been replaced by SSRIs, TCAs, such as amitriptyline (Elavil®) and nortriptyline (Pamelor®), are still used in some patients. Overdoses of TCAs are still relatively common and can be extremely dangerous and even fatal.

Overdoses of TCAs present with tachycardia, altered mental status, and signs of anticholinergic toxicity (e.g., dilated pupils, flushing, and hyperthermia). In severe cases, TCA overdoses can result in seizure activity and cardiac arrythmias secondary to QRS prolongation. Treatment of TCA overdoses includes supportive management and, in some cases, activated charcoal. Care must be taken with oral administration of medications due to the potential sudden onset of unconsciousness and seizures. Seizure activity should be treated with benzodiazepines, while cardiac arrythmias such as QRS prolongation may respond to sodium bicarbonate.

Selective Serotonin Reuptake Inhibitors. SSRIs are the preferred agent for the treatment of depression in children, although only fluoxetine (Prozac) and escitalopram (Lexapro) are approved for pediatric patients. Many others, such as sertraline (Zoloft), bupropion (Wellbutrin), paroxetine (Paxil), and fluvoxamine (Luvox), are also used. As such, SSRIs are one of the more common intentional ingestions, though they are generally less toxic than TCAs. SSRIs function by inhibiting the uptake of serotonin into neurons, both centrally and peripherally, and act by stimulating serotonin receptors.

Overdoses of SSRIs are typically mild. Patients may be asymptomatic even after ingesting 30 times the usual dose. When symptoms do appear, they consist of tachycardia, hypertension, vomiting, and drowsiness/lethargy, but seizures, respiratory failure, and even death have occurred, especially with bupropion (Wellbutrin®). Treatment of SSRI overdoses is primarily supportive, but activated charcoal may be used.

TABLE 9-2 Signs and Symptoms of Serotonin Syndrome	
Neurologic	Agitated delirium (agitation, hypervigilance, easy startle reflex)*
Neuromuscular	Myoclonus (most common finding) Hyperreflexia* Muscle rigidity (more in legs)* Clonus* Tremor* Akathisia
Autonomic	Tachycardia Hyperthermia* Hypertension that progresses to hypotension Diaphoresis (sweating)* Shivering Diarrhea Dilated pupils

*Used to meet some diagnostic criteria.

A potentially life-threatening form of an SSRI overdose is serotonin syndrome, which occurs because of increased serotonergic activity in the central nervous system. Serotonin syndrome most commonly occurs when SSRIs are combined with other serotonergic agents such as TCAs, lithium, migraine medications such as triptans, some anticonvulsants (carbamazepine, valproic acid), opioids, and drugs of abuse (cocaine, LSD, methamphetamine). Therefore, it can also occur in the absence of an overdose. Serotonin syndrome typically presents with severe altered mental status, symptoms of neuromuscular hyperreflexia, and autonomic symptoms as illustrated in **TABLE 9-2**.

Treatment of serotonin syndrome requires prompt recognition and aggressive intervention. All serotonergic agents should be discontinued immediately. Sedation with benzodiazepines is often necessary, with intravenous (IV) fluids for autonomic instability; both can be performed in the prehospital setting. In-hospital, treatment with serotonin antagonists such as cyproheptadine may be required. Rarely, patients with severe hyperthermia (>41°C) may require endotracheal intubation, sedation, and paralysis.

Adverse Reactions of Psychiatric Medications

Although many antipsychotics are well tolerated, adverse reactions can occur. Examples of serious adverse reactions include acute dystonic reactions, tardive dyskinesia, and neuroleptic malignant syndrome.

Acute Dystonic Reactions

Acute dystonic reactions primarily occur in patients who are taking antipsychotics. Dystonic reactions are more common with first-generation (typical) antipsychotics rather than second-generation (atypical) antipsychotics. Acute dystonic reactions are characterized by involuntary muscle tics or spasms that generally affect the head and neck and are most prominent in the tongue and jaw. They can occur even at therapeutic doses of the medications. Although dystonic reactions are rarely life threatening, symptoms can be very distressing to patients and their families and should be treated whenever possible. One life-threatening adverse effect is laryngeal dystonia, which presents as a choking sensation, difficulty breathing, or stridor. Diphenhydramine is the first-line treatment for patients with dystonic reactions and should be administered as soon as possible. If the patient does not experience any relief with diphenhydramine, benzodiazepines may be administered.

Neuroleptic Malignant Syndrome

Neuroleptic malignant syndrome (NMS) is a rare, but life-threatening, complication of antipsychotic medications such as haloperidol and risperidone; mortality rates range from 5% to 20%. NMS typically presents over the course of 3 days, and symptoms include altered mental status, hyperthermia (temp >41°C), extreme muscular rigidity, and autonomic instability, which generally presents as tachycardia. Altered mental status, which can vary from delirium to agitation to coma, is often the initial presenting symptom, but other findings include blood pressure instability, diaphoresis, cardiac dysrhythmias, normal pupils, dysphagia, and drooling. The most common neurologic finding is lead-pipe rigidity. Unfortunately the signs and symptoms of NMS are similar to those of serotonin syndrome so the history of which drugs have been taken is important. Treatment requires aggressive management of complications and may include pharmacologic agents such as dantrolene and bromocriptine (neither of which is carried by EMS). Patients with NMS require close monitoring in the intensive care unit and often require mechanical ventilation, cooling measures, IV fluids, antihypertensive agents, and benzodiazepines to control agitation.

Assessment and Transport of the Child With a Behavioral Emergency

When transporting a child with a behavioral emergency, provider safety is of the utmost importance. Prehospital providers should attempt to establish a rapport with the child while assessing the likelihood for violence. If the child seems cooperative and gives permission to be touched for examination purposes, take a thorough history and perform a physical examination. Next, assess mental status. Is this child a risk to him- or herself or others? Lastly, determine the need to transport the child. Consider chemical or physical restraints only if the patient is a danger to him- or herself or others. A caregiver should either ride in the ambulance or follow the ambulance to the hospital. In cases of self-harm, it is necessary to check for potential sources of injury to the patient or providers, such as removing knives, blades, or pills from the patient from his or her clothing.

Before considering restraint, it is important to maximize the safety of yourself and the patient and

---

CASE STUDY 3

You are dispatched to a high school where a 13-year-old student has just admitted to her guidance counselor that she wants to kill herself. On your arrival, she is awake but tearful; she has no increased work of breathing, and her color is pink. Her heart rate is 76 beats/min, respiratory rate is 16 breaths/min, and blood pressure 106/70 mm Hg. When you take her blood pressure, you note numerous healing horizontal cuts on her left forearm. She has no other injuries. She states she wants to kill herself because she broke up with her boyfriend 2 weeks ago, which is when she cut herself. She denies taking any medication.

1. Do you need to take her to the hospital?
2. What additional assessment may be helpful en route?

assist the patient in managing his or her emotions or regaining control of his or her behavior. If these do not work, use the least-restrictive age-appropriate methods of restraint possible and minimize coercive interventions that may exacerbate agitation.

Restraint

Restraint refers to methods of restricting a person's freedom of movement, physical activity, or normal access to his or her body due to a concern of self-harm or harming others. Restraint can be verbal, chemical, or physical.

Verbal Restraint

Verbal restraint is preferable to the other methods of restraint. Children may experience emotional distress for a variety of reasons, including a mental health issue, substance abuse, trauma, or everyday childhood and adolescent issues. At times, this behavior can escalate into aggression. Children voicing threats or warnings should be taken seriously. You can prepare for aggressive behavior by being aware of and trained in de-escalation techniques, while being sure to maintain your safety and that of other responding individuals.

De-escalation techniques from the Youth Mental Health First Aid USA program from the National Council of Behavioral Health provide practical strategies, such as the following:

- Speak slowly and confidently with a gentle, caring tone of voice.
- Avoid raising your voice or talking too fast.
- Do not respond in a hostile, disciplinary, or challenging manner.
- Do not argue with or threaten the young person, because it may increase fear or prompt aggressive behavior.
- Use positive words (such as "Stay calm") instead of negative words (such as "Don't fight"). Ask, "What happened? rather than "What's wrong with you?"
- Avoid nervous behavior (e.g., shuffling your feet, fidgeting, or making abrupt movement).
- Do not restrict the young person's movement (e.g., if he or she wants to pace up and down the room, allow him or her to do so).
- Keep your distance from the youth, calculated for his or her cultural comfort.
- Remain aware that certain acts, such as involving the police, might exacerbate the situation.
- Consider taking a break from the conversation to allow the young person a chance to calm down.

- Invite the young person to sit down if he or she is standing.
- If the young person is responsive, ask him or her if he or she has a safety or crisis plan in place, and work with him or her to follow the plan as well as you can.

As a prehospital professional, your behavior can set the tone for not only how a call goes, but future interactions the child may have. By remaining calm with relaxed body language and offering a safe personal space, you are modeling behavior you hope the child can achieve. Take time to learn about resources in your community that are available to assist youth before, during, and after a crisis.

Chemical Restraint

Chemical restraint with medications such as midazolam or diphenhydramine has been used by some EMS agencies in adults. The use of chemical restraint in children may be considered if local protocols exist, with medical direction.

Physical Restraint

Physical restraint involves the use of mechanical devices to limit physical activity. It should be reserved for those times when the patient is in acute danger to harm him- or herself or others and when other, less-restrictive methods have failed.

A method that can be used in younger children includes therapeutic holding, in which the caregivers or health care providers hold the child to control the agitated behavior (**FIGURE 9-5**).

If physical restraint is necessary, explain to the patient's caregivers what you are doing and why you are

FIGURE 9-5 A method that can be used in younger children includes therapeutic holding, in which the caregivers or health care providers hold the child to control the agitated behavior.

© interstid/Shutterstock.

restraining their child. Enlist their assistance. Talk to the patient. Explain what you are doing and why, but do not negotiate. Do not attempt restraint placement alone—this often requires 3–5 people. If the child is young enough, securing the child in his or her car seat provides enough restraint and may be preferable to the child, as he or she is already familiar with the seat. Before restraining a child, consider calling law enforcement officials. Do not allow the child to become positioned near an escape route. Should this happen, the child may injure the provider who has lost the ability to quickly escape, or the child can escape. If placed on a stretcher, the patient should be positioned supine with the head of stretcher elevated. Apply restraints to each extremity first, then secure the restraints to the stretcher frame, not the side rails. Do not cover the patient's face or head except with a spit mask or other appropriate device to control spitting and/or biting. Document carefully the reasons for and the types of restraints in the run sheet. Perform periodic assessments.

There may be conflict between parental wishes and the needs of the child. If the child is in immediate danger of self-harm or is an immediate danger to others, notify law enforcement officials to help restrain the patient so he or she can be transported to the closest appropriate facility.

Your Emotional Well-Being

Calls involving children in emotional distress can be especially draining and difficult to deal with. Be sure to process your own emotions with peers or any employee assistance program that may be available in your agency. Take time to care for yourself by getting plenty of sleep, eating properly, and allowing time for reflection and healing.

CASE STUDY ANSWERS

CASE STUDY 1

Assessment of the airway, breathing, and circulation suggests an anaphylactic reaction related to a bee sting. You should ask the child's mother about any past history of insect bites and if the child's inhaler is available. It would be beneficial to utilize the child's comfort items to try to calm the child, as intramuscular epinephrine administration is indicated for anaphylaxis and will further agitate the child.

You should approach the child calmly and utilize the mother to help answer any questions you need to ask of the child. Have your partner administer high-flow oxygen while you explain to the mother that, based on symptoms and presentation, her son is going to need an intramuscular epinephrine injection. Suggest that the mother hold the child in his position of comfort, preferably on her lap, and have her use the blanket and stuffed animal to comfort the child while administering epinephrine. Use proper temporary restraint techniques per your agency guidelines and protocol if necessary. Calmly vocalize to the child each intervention you will take and allow extra time, as symptoms allow, for the child to respond.

An albuterol inhaler can be used to help open the child's airways and alleviate respiratory distress. In this case, the parent states that the child's inhaler is available. The child has begun to calm down, but is now rocking back and forth on his mother lap and is repetitively saying "ouch." The child's father is now at your side with the albuterol inhaler and spacer. The child is agreeable to assisted administration by you and his parents.

You decide to transport this child to the hospital for further evaluation and workup. Appropriate advanced life support modalities may include IV access, diphenhydramine, and solumedrol. The child is now calm, breathing is at a normal rate and rhythm, and the facial swelling is beginning to dissipate. He is now asking questions about the equipment in the bag you have at your side. You are now able to spend some time allowing the child to touch and try out your stethoscope and blood pressure cuff. After doing so, the child now lets you obtain his vital signs, which are blood pressure 90/56 mm Hg, heart rate 130 beats/min, respiratory rate 22 breaths/min, and oxygen saturation of 100% on nasal cannula. You now trial the patient on room air; the child maintains an oxygen saturation of 98%. The child is currently stable, and you can begin your transport to the hospital without lights and sirens, as this can aggravate children with ASD. You should continue to monitor and assess the patient every 5 minutes during transport for any change in condition and allow his mother to accompany him, in the back of the ambulance if possible, to assist in keeping the child calm and cooperative. Be sure to give a full report to the receiving facility, including the diagnosis of ASD, as the sensory stimulation of an ED can cause negative escalation of behavior. A quiet, private room is recommended, as availability allows.

Children with autism cannot always be identified by appearance alone, and it is important to remember that some may be nonverbal at baseline or may become nonverbal when stressed. A 3- to 4-second delay from question to answer is not uncommon. If the child does not answer a question, oftentimes it is because he or she does not understand, so you should continue to explain interventions calmly. It is common for children with ASD to have tactile sensory issues. When assessing these patients, try to avoid any unnecessary or repetitive touching, restrictive bandaging, or other confining equipment. These children may also have difficulty with lights and sirens, so use of lights and sirens should be limited whenever possible as per local protocol.

CASE STUDY 2

While this adolescent clearly needs assistance, scene safety must be paramount throughout the call. Remain vigilant, know your egress routes, and enlist the help of law enforcement or additional EMS personnel as needed to ensure the safety of the patient, yourself, your crew, the school staff, faculty, and other students. At times, less may be more and additional personnel may further aggravate the patient, but this will vary from situation to situation.

You should remain calm and attempt to verbally de-escalate the situation. Do not try to talk above or over the patient. Speak calmly and confidently in a caring manner. Do not argue with or challenge the patient.

Do not restrict the patient's pacing, but invite her to sit down. Give clear, calm instructions, such as "Please put that item down so we may talk," or "Please tell me what happened." Explain that the throwing of objects is not safe for the patient or those around her. Try to gain the patient's trust by stating that you are there to help *her* and you would like to hear what happened. If the patient is able to calm down, you may be able to gather information about events leading up to the altercation and any potential injuries. You may also be able to obtain a health history and vital signs.

If the patient does not calm down with verbal de-escalation techniques and continues to pose a threat to herself and others, physical and/or chemical restraint and transport to the ED is indicated. Physical and/or chemical restraint should be a secondary intervention and used per local agency guidelines only.

You should also attempt to ascertain whether she is an immediate threat to herself or others and requires immediate transport to the ED. If ED transport is chosen and patient is calm and able, allow her to walk to the stretcher and maintain as much independence and control as you deem safe.

ADHD, ODD, and conduct disorder are all classified as behavioral disorders. Children with conduct disorder have difficulty following rules and social norms, which causes them to have difficulty interacting with family and peers; symptoms may be particularly disruptive in the school setting. Physically aggressive behaviors such as theft, vandalism, substance use and abuse, harm to animals, and sexual promiscuity may also be seen in conduct disorder. The cause of conduct disorder is not fully known, but some potential risk factors include early maternal rejection, separation, and neglect; abuse; and domestic violence. Early and continued intervention is important in these children and, many times, the hormonal changes that routinely occur during puberty can exacerbate symptoms.

CASE STUDY 3

Because this adolescent is expressing suicidal ideation and has signs of hurting herself, she does need to have a mental health evaluation. If she is already seeing a mental health professional who can see her now, her parents should be called; if they are able to take her, she can be released to her parents to seek care. If this is the first time, and she has no mental health follow-up, she should be transported to the ED where a physical exam and mental health evaluation can occur.

En route, assure that the adolescent has no other injuries or signs of an ingestion (see toxidromes in Chapter 8). You can engage her in a conversation about how she is doing at school and home, or whether there are any other stressors in her life, but if she does not want to answer you, that is OK. Just explain that she will need to be on the stretcher and basic safety measures (straps) are needed for the transport.

SUGGESTED REFERENCES

Textbooks

Adirim T, Smith E. *Special Children's Outreach and Prehospital Education (SCOPE)*. Burlington, MA: Jones and Bartlett Learning; 2006.

American Academy of Pediatrics and the American College of Emergency Physicians. *APLS: The Pediatric Emergency Medicine Resource*. 5th ed. Burlington, MA: Jones and Bartlett Learning; 2012.

American Psychiatric Association. *Diagnostic and Statistical Manual of Mental Disorders*. 5th edition. Washington, DC: American Psychiatric Association; 2013.

Articles

Chun TH, Mace SE, Katz ER. American Academy of Pediatrics Committee on Pediatric Emergency Medicine. Evaluation and management of children and adolescents with acute mental health or behavioral problems. Part I: Common clinical challenges of patients with mental health and/or behavioral emergencies. *Pediatrics*. 2016;138(3):e20161570.

Chun TH, Mace SE, Katz ER. American Academy of Pediatrics Committee on Pediatric Emergency Medicine. Evaluation and management of children and adolescents with acute mental health or behavioral problems. Part II: Recognition of clinically challenging mental health related conditions presenting with medical or uncertain symptoms. *Pediatrics*. 2016;138(3):e20161573.

Fishe JN, Lynch S. Pediatric behavioral health-related EMS encounters: a statewide analysis. *Prehosp Emerg Care*. 2019;23(5):654–662.

Floet AM, Scheiner C, Grossman L. Attention-deficit/hyperactivity disorder. *Pediatr Rev*. 2010;31(2):56–69.

Graudins A, Stearman A, Chan B. Treatment of the serotonin syndrome with cyproheptadine. *J Emerg Med*. 1998;16(4):615–619.

Hyman SL, Levy SE, Myers SM; American Academy of Pediatrics Council on Children with Disabilities, Section on Developmental and Behavioral Pediatrics. Executive summary: identification, evaluation, and management of children with autism spectrum disorder. *Pediatrics*. 2020;145(1):e20193448.

Kennedy SP, Baraff LJ, Suddath RL, Asarnow JR. Emergency department management of suicidal adolescents. *Ann Emerg Med*. 2004;43(4):452–460.

Knowlton AR, Weir B, Fields J, et al. Pediatric use of emergency medical services: the role of chronic illnesses and behavioral health problems. *Prehosp Emerg Care*. 2016;20(3):362–368.

Mason PJ, Morris VA, Balcezak TJ. Serotonin syndrome. Presentation of 2 cases and review of the literature. *Medicine*. 2000;79(4):201–209.

Michelson D, Faries D, Wernicke J, Kelsey D, et al. Atomoxetine in the treatment of children and adolescents with attention-deficit/hyperactivity disorder: a randomized, placebo-controlled, dose-response study. *Pediatrics*. 2001;108(5):E83.

Myers SM. Management of autism spectrum disorders in primary care. *Pediatr Ann*. 2009;38(1):42–49. PubMed PMID: 19213293.

Overburg A, Morton S, Wagner E, Froberg B. Toxicity of buproprion overdose compared to selective serotonin inhibitors. *Pediatrics*. 2019;144(2):e20183295.

Riley M, Ahmed S, Locke A. Common questions about oppositional defiant disorder. *Am Fam Physician*. 2016;93(7):586–591.

Varigonda AL, Jakubovski E, Taylor MJ, Freemantle N, et al. Systematic review and meta-analysis: early treatment responses of selective serotonin reuptake inhibitors in pediatric major depressive disorder. *J Am Acad Child Adolesc Psychiatry*. 2015;54(7):557–564.

Wolraich ML, Chan E, Froelich T, et al. ADHD diagnosis and treatment guidelines: a historical perspective. *Pediatrics*. 2019;144(4):e20191682.

Zwaigenbaum L, Bryson S, Lord C, Rogers S, et al. Clinical assessment and management of toddlers with suspected autism spectrum disorder: insights from studies of high-risk infants. *Pediatrics*. 2009;123(5):1383–1391.

Other Resources

Centers for Disease Control and Prevention. Anxiety and depression in children. https://www.cdc.gov /childrensmentalhealth/depression.html. Accessed September 5, 2019.

Centers for Disease Control and Prevention. Anxiety and depression in children: Get the Facts. https://www .cdc.gov/childrensmentalhealth/features/anxiety -depression-children.html. Accessed September 5, 2019.

Centers for Disease Control and Prevention. Behavior or conduct problems in children. https://www.cdc .gov/childrensmentalhealth/behavior.html. Accessed September 5, 2019.

Centers for Disease Control and Prevention. Children's mental disorders. https://www.cdc.gov /childrensmentalhealth/symptoms.html. Accessed September 5, 2019.

Centers for Disease Control and Prevention. Data and statistics on children's mental health. https:// www.cdc.gov/childrensmentalhealth/data.html. Accessed September 5, 2019.

Centers for Disease Control and Prevention. What is autism spectrum disorder? https://www.cdc.gov /ncbddd/autism/facts.html. Accessed September 3, 2019.

Autism Spectrum Disorder (ASD). Data & Statistics on Autism Spectrum Disorder. https://www.cdc.gov /ncbddd/autism/data.html. Accessed September 3, 2019.

Autism Spectrum Disorder (ASD). New Data on Autism Spectrum Disorder in 4-Year Old Children. https://www.cdc.gov/ncbddd/autism/features/asd -data-four-year-old-children.html. Accessed September 3, 2019.

Attention-Deficit/Hyperactivity Disorder (ADHD). https://www.nimh.nih.gov/health/topics/attention -deficit-hyperactivity-disorder-adhd/index.shtm. Accessed September 3, 2019.

Leonte KG, Puliafico A, Na P, Ryan MA. Pharmo-cotherapy for anxiety disorders in children and ad-olescents. *UpToDate*. Waltham, MA: UpToDate, Inc, 2019. Accessed September 5, 2019.

National Institute of Mental Health. Autism Spec-trum Disorder (ASD). https://www.nimh.nih.gov /health/statistics/autism-spectrum-disorder-asd .shtml. Accessed September 3, 2019.

National Institute of Mental Health. Bipolar disorder. https://www.nimh.nih.gov/health/statistics/bipolar -disorder.shtml. Accessed September 3, 2019.

National Institute of Mental Health. Major depres-sion. https://www.nimh.nih.gov/health/statistics /major-depression.shtml. Accessed September 3, 2019.

National Institute of Mental Health. Mental illness. https://www.nimh.nih.gov/health/statistics/mental -illness.shtml. Accessed September 3, 2019.

National Institute of Mental Health. Personality dis-orders. https://www.nimh.nih.gov/health/statistics /personality-disorders.shtml. Accessed September 3, 2019.

National Institute of Mental Health. Suicide. https:// www.nimh.nih.gov/health/statistics/suicide.shtml. Accessed September 3, 2019.

© Mike Powell/Stone/Getty Images Plus/Getty Images.

CHAPTER 10

Children With Special Health Care Needs

S. Heath Ackley, MD, MPH, FAAP

Mary Otting, RN, BSN, CEN

LEARNING OBJECTIVES

1. Define and describe two examples of cognitive disabilities, physical disabilities, and chronic conditions seen in children.

2. List important modifications of field assessment techniques for children with special health care needs (CSHCN).

3. Outline common transport considerations for CSHCN.

4. Describe the most common complications associated with assistive devices (tracheostomy tubes, central venous lines, gastrostomy tubes or gastric feeding tubes, cerebrospinal fluid [CSF] shunts, ostomies, implantable pacemakers and defibrillators) and the emergency management of those complications.

5. Describe the use of health information technology (HIT), including an interoperable emergency information form (EIF), for CSHCN.

Introduction

According to an article by McPherson in *Pediatrics*, children with special health care needs (CSHCN) are defined as "those who have or are at an increased risk for a chronic physical, developmental, or emotional condition and who also require health and related services of a type or amount beyond that required by children generally."

The conditions can be either acquired or congenital. These children are a diverse group of patients who frequently need prehospital emergency assessment and treatment. This high-user group includes but is not limited to children who were born prematurely; have suffered closed-head injury and/or have central nervous system (CNS) injuries; or have chronic problems of the lungs, brain, or kidneys. Examples of acquired conditions include cerebral palsy or bronchopulmonary dysplasia. Examples of **congenital** problems are **cyanotic heart disease** or **spina bifida**.

Children assisted by or dependent on technology are a subgroup of CSHCN who need medical devices for their survival. Common devices include tracheostomy tubes, home ventilators, indwelling central venous lines, feeding tubes, pacemakers, and cerebrospinal fluid (CSF) shunts.

Today, CSHCN are surviving longer and often live at home. They need emergency medical care more frequently than children without special health care needs. Because of their unique baseline status, CSHCN pose unique challenges in field assessment and treatment. Therefore, prehospital professionals should recognize common types of CSHCN, incorporate modifications during assessment, and understand management of frequent problems.

Cognitive and Physical Disabilities

According to the American Association on Intellectual and Developmental Disabilities, an intellectual disability is defined as a "disability characterized by significant limitations both in intellectual functioning (reasoning, learning, problem solving) and in adaptive behavior, which covers a range of everyday social and practical skills." The terms "intellectual disability" and "mental retardation" mean the same thing, yet intellectual disability is less offensive and is the preferred term.

Mental processes, such as judgment, reasoning, memory, and comprehension, are cognitive in nature and develop as the child acquires knowledge. Cognitive impairments are present when there is an alteration in the child's ability to think, reason, learn, and abstract. Several examples include autism spectrum disorder (ASD), attention-deficit/hyperactivity disorder (ADHD), which are covered in Chapter 9, as well as intellectual disability which is limited mental function in areas such as communication, social skills, and self-care.

Physical disabilities may alter the child's ability to be mobile or to accomplish activities of daily living independently. Medical and traumatic emergencies may occur that have nothing to do with the actual physical impairment. This includes physical conditions such as hearing impairment and visual impairment.

Chronic conditions are present when the child receives ongoing treatment for an injury or illness. Even if the child seems to be healthy, he or she may be on maintenance medications or treatments to prevent complications. Examples of chronic conditions include asthma, cancer, post-transplant patients, and congenital heart disease. Additional chronic conditions include:

- **Bronchopulmonary dysplasia (BPD)** which is a chronic lung condition that develops in premature infants who require respiratory support after birth. These infants are at risk for deterioration with any respiratory illnesses, can have constant wheezing, may require supplemental oxygen at home, and may have pulmonary hypertension and decreased pulmonary function.
- **Cerebral palsy** is a disorder of movement and tone that results from brain injury during fetal development or at birth. These children may have increased motor tone, leading to trouble walking, or with coordination. They may wear orthotics on their legs to assist with ambulation or they may be wheelchair bound. They may have intellectual disability, but many do not.
- **Cystic fibrosis** is a congenital disorder that results in lung and digestive disorders due to improper functioning of mucus producing or exocrine glands. This results in frequent lung infections and pneumothoraces and impaired

CASE STUDY 1

You are called to the scene of a 9-month-old girl with multiple underlying medical problems, including ventilator dependence at night through a tracheostomy tube.

On your arrival, her caregiver states that the girl has had difficulty breathing all day, with a fever and increased tracheostomy secretions. The child has cerebral palsy with spasticity and a seizure disorder. She depends on a ventilator because of chronic lung disease as a result of prematurity at birth and respiratory distress syndrome. The child receives carbamazepine for her seizures and received her morning dose. Currently, she is receiving her feedings through her gastrostomy tube, which is connected to a pump.

Your assessment shows a child who is in bed and connected to a home ventilator. She does not engage visually and has subcostal retractions and nasal flaring. Her skin is pink. She has wheezing and crackles on lung examination. Her heart rate is 130 beats/min, respiratory rate is 60 breaths/min, blood pressure is 85 mm Hg/palp, and pulse oximetry is 90%. Her ventilator is set at 20 breaths/min.

1. What are the key principles in assessing this child?
2. Describe treatment and transport approaches.

digestion and absorption of nutrients resulting in poor growth.

- **Down syndrome** is a congenital disorder in which the child is born with 3 copies of the X chromosome, so it is also called trisomy 21. They have typical facial features and are at risk for congenital heart defects and cervical spine injuries due to C-spine abnormalities. They also have varying levels of cognitive delay.
- **Hemophilia** is a congenital condition that results in abnormalities in blood clotting. This can lead to prolonged bleeding, so there is risk of intracranial bleeding even with minor head trauma.
- **Muscular dystrophy** is a genetic muscle disorder that results in muscle weakness and wasting. These children are at risk for aspiration and pneumonia.
- **Spina bifida** is a congenital anomaly in which the spine has failed to fuse, resulting in protrusion of the spinal cord and meninges at birth, usually in the lumbar region, but can occur anywhere along the spinal column. While these lesions can be repaired, the children may have hydrocephalus, impaired lower extremity strength and feeling, and bowel and bladder problems.

Assessment of CSHCN

Modifications

The most important resource for the prehospital provider is the child's caregiver. He or she usually knows how to care for the child's particular condition and understands the child's equipment. Often, caregivers have forms or cards that outline the child's medical history; medications; and **baseline** general appearance, oxygen saturation, and vital signs.

Begin evaluation of CSHCN with emergency pediatric assessment techniques adjusted to the child's developmental level, rather than his or her chronologic age. Caregivers can usually provide the child's developmental age, weight, and baseline vital signs. *With children assisted by technology, do not become distracted by their specialized equipment.* Care for the child, not the machinery. Caregivers are often extremely helpful in figuring out the baseline status of CSHCN or in operating or troubleshooting the equipment. *Ask for assistance from the caregiver!*

The assessment of CSHCN has the following important modifications:

1. Baseline status: Ask the caregivers what is usual for the child. Most likely, they will know the child's baseline better than anyone.

2. Rely on the caregivers' opinions: What do they think is wrong? In what ways is the child "acting differently"?

3. If the child is physiologically stable, take a full history on scene. Caregivers usually know the child's medical history, health problems, medications, medical devices, and current complaints. They are also aware of what approaches work best.

4. The child may be slow to answer questions or may be unable to talk. Use a patient approach to the stable child and begin by talking directly to the child, rather than to his or her caregiver.

5. Seemingly minor illnesses can be life threatening in some CSHCN. An example is a cold in a child with chronic lung disease who is dependent on a ventilator. The child may have little reserve and may easily become hypoxic.

6. Communicate with the child using developmentally appropriate language, gestures, and techniques, as discussed in Chapter 2.

7. If a caregiver is not present, find out if the child has a form or card with information about his or her medical problem, normal vital signs, medications, and other important medical data. An emergency information form (EIF) is also available from the American Academy of Pediatrics (AAP) and the American College of Emergency Physicians (ACEP). Several states recommend that CSHCN carry information cards, such as New Mexico's Children's Updated Medical Summary (ChUMS) and the District of Columbia's EMS Outreach program.

8. Look for a bracelet or necklace that might describe the child's condition.

9. The usual baseline vital signs for a CSHCN may be "out of the normal range" compared to a child of the same age who does not have special health care needs. Standard vital signs may have limited value in assessment of these children. Pay more attention to the Pediatric Assessment Triangle (PAT) and observations from the caregiver.

10. Do not assume that a child with a physical disability is cognitively impaired. Many children with cerebral palsy, for example, have **spasticity** but do not have cognitive limitations. Discreetly ask the caregiver about the child's typical level of functioning, understanding, and interactions.

11. Be polite and professional. Listen to the caregiver and take his or her concerns seriously. Families of CSHCN often have had a lot of experience with the medical system. If most of their experience has been positive, they view the prehospital professional as an ally. However, if they have had bad experiences with the medical system, they may be suspicious or aggressive.

12. Keep in mind the amount of stress caregivers of a CSHCN may be experiencing.

13. Ask the caregivers what therapies or interventions have been already undertaken in response to their child's emergency.

14. If possible, try to transport CSHCN to their "medical home" facility. Always follow local protocol.

> **CAUTION**
>
> Do not become distracted by the specialized equipment used by children assisted by technology. Care for the child, not the machinery.

Pediatric Assessment Triangle

The PAT is a good way to look and listen for signs that help determine the type of physiologic problem and the urgency for treatment of a CSHCN. However, because CSHCN often have altered baseline physiology, there are several limitations and modifications to the PAT.

Appearance

Although the child's overall appearance reflects the adequacy of oxygenation, ventilation, perfusion, and CNS status, this is the part of the PAT that may differ the most in CSHCN. The underlying medical problem may cause abnormal muscle tone, such as the increased tone and spasticity in a child with cerebral palsy or the decreased tone seen in children with Down syndrome. There may be decreased interactiveness, a common behavioral state in a child with brain damage or an intellectual disability. Look or gaze is helpful because many CSHCN can recognize their caregiver by looking or by hearing their voice. A CSHCN may be unable to speak, but the strength and quality of his or her cry or facial expressions may be a useful sign of health or distress. For example, a high-pitched cry in a child with a CSF shunt may mean obstruction.

Work of Breathing

Many CSHCN have respiratory problems. Children with chronic pulmonary disease, such as bronchopulmonary dysplasia (BPD), have rapid respiratory rates and increased work of breathing. When such children have a fever or experience an added respiratory illness or injury, such as pneumonia or chest trauma, they have less reserve. Therefore, work of breathing in these patients increases rapidly with any acute illness or injury.

> **TIP**
>
> Assess appearance by asking the caregiver about the child's baseline.

> **CAUTION**
>
> Do not assume that a child with a physical disability is mentally impaired. Many children with cerebral palsy, for example, have spasticity, but not cognitive limitations.

Assess abnormal breath sounds (stridor, wheezing, or grunting) from across the room. Some "abnormal" airway sounds may be usual for a CSHCN. For example, a child with a tracheostomy tube usually has noisy breathing, and an infant with BPD may have slight expiratory wheezing. Children with BPD or congenital heart disease are much more likely to develop respiratory infections, especially from **respiratory syncytial virus (RSV)**, in the winter. They can decompensate quickly. CSHCN who have an intellectual disability and neurologic problems are at high risk for aspiration, pneumonia, and respiratory failure.

Unusual positioning, such as tripoding and head bobbing, is an important visual sign of increased work of breathing and hypoxia, and usually indicates serious breathing problems. For the child who usually has mild retractions, the degree or location of retractions provides clues to increased work of breathing. For example, the baseline retractions may be mild and only **subcostal**, but are now severe and also **suprasternal**. Nasal flaring is an indication of increased work of breathing, especially when associated with tachypnea, grunting, or retractions.

Circulation to Skin

The skin color may appear different in CSHCN, such as in infants with cyanotic congenital heart disease, chronic lung disease, cancer, or liver failure. A child with cyanotic congenital heart disease or chronic lung disease may have bluish lips and mucous membranes, nail beds, and extremities at baseline. A child with cancer may appear pale, whereas the skin of a child with liver disease may appear yellow. Ask a caregiver to describe the child's baseline color.

Adaptations in the Hands-On ABCDEs

After performing the PAT, complete the primary assessment by adjusting the evaluation of the ABCDEs to the child's baseline.

Airway

Open and maintain the airway. Keeping an open airway may be more difficult with CSHCN. The child may have poor muscle tone and head control, or copious secretions. In children with Down syndrome, the large, protruding tongue may make airway procedures difficult. Getting, and then keeping, the right head position may require several maneuvers: a shoulder roll to correctly position the head in a neutral axis with the airway, and a chin lift or jaw thrust to open the airway. Always have suction available.

Many children with spina bifida have an Arnold-Chiari malformation, in which the base of the brain pushes down through a large foramen magnum. Do NOT hyperextend the neck of a child with spina bifida because any pressure on the herniated brain may cause the child to stop breathing. For these children, use in-line stabilization for any airway maneuvers even if no trauma is suspected.

Special Management in CSHCN: Tracheostomy Care. A child with a tracheostomy has an artificial airway that is easily blocked by secretions or by dislodgment of the device. The tracheostomy section of this chapter addresses specific management techniques for these children.

Breathing

Count the respiratory rate. Listen to the lungs for bilateral air movement and abnormal chest sounds. Listening may not give accurate results in the CSHCN who cannot sit still or who has noisy breathing. Also, obtain pulse oximetry and compare to baseline. Keep the child in a position of comfort. Give supplemental oxygen to any CSHCN with increased work of breathing or increased respiratory rate by blow-by, face mask, or bag-mask device. If the caregiver knows the usual baseline oxygen saturation, only give oxygen to achieve baseline levels. Children with chronic lung disease or some forms of congenital heart disease can get worse if too much oxygen is given. For CSHCN, the caregiver may know the best way to give oxygen to the child. For infants or children already on home oxygen, increase the flow rate. For a patient with a tracheostomy tube, place the oxygen directly over the tube or stoma.

Special Management in CSHCN: Bronchodilator Administration. If a CSHCN has a history of breathing problems or uses bronchodilators at home, give a nebulized bronchodilator when wheezing is present.

Circulation

Assess heart rate, pulse quality, skin temperature, and capillary refill time. These are not usually different in

CSHCN and require no modifications in clinical interpretation. If the child's age is 3 years or younger, you can consider obtaining a blood pressure; however, the value may be hard to obtain and interpret in this age group. You should attempt to measure blood pressure at least once in all children older than 3 years of age. Tachycardia is a common baseline finding in some CSHCN and by itself does not indicate shock. This is diagnosis dependent, so asking the child's caregiver about the child's usual heart rate can be helpful. To evaluate heart rate and blood pressure, assess with the other key characteristics of circulation, as outlined in Chapters 1 and 4.

In some CSHCN, management of shock may be no different than for children without disabilities. Standard management includes oxygen, positioning, and bag-mask ventilatory support as needed. Some CSHCN may need volume replacement, unless the child has a congenital heart defect and possible heart failure. CSHCN have the same fluid requirements as any other child. If the patient is injured, transport immediately and attempt vascular access. Give 20-mL/kg boluses of crystalloid fluid on the way to the emergency department (ED). If the child is ill and has compensated shock, transport and attempt access and fluid administration on the way. If the ill child has hypotensive (decompensated) shock, make one attempt at vascular access on scene, if possible. In extreme cases, intraosseous access may be necessary. When a child has a vertical chest scar or a history of congenital heart disease, consider cardiogenic shock as an explanation for poor perfusion. Because CSHCN may be more difficult to assess accurately, and because vascular access is often troublesome, always transport a child with suspected shock as soon as possible.

Some children with severe, uncontrolled epilepsy may be on the ketogenic diet. This regimen

---

CAUTION

Do not give glucose or glucose-containing fluids to children on a ketogenic diet.

ALS

Special Management in CSHCN. Bradycardia is not usual for CSHCN. It is a sign of hypoxia or inadequate brain perfusion. Suspect hypoxia in a child with BPD or other chronic cardiopulmonary condition who has a heart rate below normal for chronologic age. Suspect increased intracranial pressure in a child with a CSF shunt.

eliminates foods with glucose and keeps the child in a state of ketosis to control the seizures. For these children, do NOT use any fluids containing **dextrose**.

Disability

Many CSHCN often have a compromised baseline neurologic status. Assess neurologic status by looking at appearance as part of the PAT, and establish level of consciousness with the Alert, Verbal, Painful, Unresponsive (AVPU) mnemonic. Compare the findings to the child's baseline. In the assessment of motor activity, assess purposeful movement, symmetric movement of extremities, seizures, posturing, or flaccidity. Treat altered mental status if it is a change from baseline. The Glasgow Coma Scale may not be applicable for assessment of CSHCN because many CSHCN have baseline cognitive and physical challenges that would affect the score. It is better to describe the child as being different from baseline.

> **TIP**
>
> The usual baseline vital signs for CSHCN may be different or "out of the normal range" for the child's chronologic age.

> **TIP**
>
> Bradycardia is not usual for CSHCN.

Exposure

Be sure to inspect the child's entire body, but respect his or her modesty. Do not allow the child to become cold. Many CSHCN have minimal body fat and can become hypothermic quickly.

Summary of Assessment of CSHCN

Listen carefully to the caregiver when assessing CSHCN. Ask about the child's baseline status. What is typical for this child? Such children may present a confusing picture, with unexpected behaviors, communication difficulties, extensive medical histories, and complicated equipment. The child's neurologic status is often compromised. If the caregiver is not present, look for sources of baseline information, such as a medical information form or a bracelet. Use standard assessment techniques and developmentally appropriate approaches modified by baseline comparisons to evaluate and manage acute problems. Transport early.

> **CAUTION**
>
> The Glasgow Coma Scale may not be applicable for assessment of CSHCN because many CSHCN have baseline cognitive and physical challenges that affect the score.

Transport

TABLE 10-1 lists key principles of transport of CSHCN. *Always restrain children in the ambulance.* The best type of restraint device and the best method for securing the device in the ambulance are controversial issues.

In general, if the child is critically ill or injured, restrain the child on his or her back secured on a gurney. Try to use a device for spinal motion restriction if the child has suffered an injury to the head or has a suspected spinal injury. Be careful if the child has any contractures or rigid posturing, such as scissoring of the legs or an exaggerated arching of the back seen in children with cerebral palsy. Pad any open areas and

TABLE 10-1 Principles of Transport for CSHCN
1. Transport CSHCN who are on home oxygen with the oxygen (except for liquid oxygen). If the child has no respiratory distress, continue the same rate of oxygen flow.
2. Transport a child on a home ventilator with the ventilator if there are no equipment problems. If there is a concern about the ventilator, manually assist ventilation. Regardless of the method of ventilation, always secure the child's home ventilator in the ambulance and transport with the child, so that it can be assessed by hospital personnel for potential problems and appropriate settings.
3. If the child has poor muscle control or increased muscle tone, immobilize the child as needed in a position that is comfortable for him or her. If the child has a special seat, wheelchair, or other equipment (e.g., feeding pump or suctioning device), transport these items to the ED if these items can be safely secured in the ambulance while still allowing enough room to safely care for the child during transport.
4. If the child has any contractures or rigid postures, such as scissoring of the legs or an arched back, pad around any open areas when the child is on the stretcher or during spinal motion restriction. Do NOT force the child to conform to the equipment.

do not force the child to conform to the equipment. Check with the caregiver about positioning and the availability of any special car seat. In some children, the supine position may compromise the airway because of an abundance of secretions, poor tone, or anatomic differences. The child's specially designed child restraint system or car seat may be the best option if it can be safely secured in the ambulance.

Many CSHCN have supplemental oxygen and oxygen delivery equipment. It is unsafe to transport liquid oxygen in an ambulance. Consider transporting nonliquid (or gaseous) oxygen and the child's personal devices or equipment to the ED.

Summary of Transport

CSHCN often have special transport considerations. Make sure the child is safely restrained in the ambulance. An appropriately sized child safety seat can be used, always facing the rear of the ambulance, if it can be secured appropriately. Parents may have an adaptive restraint, travel vest, or harness that can be used with the car seat. Ensure that no belts or harnesses make contact with tracheostomies or gastrostomy feeding tubes. Do not use rigid cervical collars to restrain a child's head if he or she has poor head control, unless deemed necessary due to trauma. Address the issue of transport with the caregiver, and consider bringing ancillary medical equipment (e.g., ventilators, feeding pumps) to the ED if it can be safely secured in the ambulance. If a child in a wheelchair cannot be removed from the wheelchair, ideally a transit option chair should be used. If this is not available, the wheelchair should have a metal frame to which tie down straps and hooks can be attached at frame junctions, and it should be secured in a forward-facing direction.

Children Assisted by Technology

Children assisted by technology have devices that may malfunction at home. The most common devices are **tracheostomy tubes**, **cerebrospinal fluid (CSF) shunts**, **indwelling central venous catheters**, and **feeding tubes** (buttons). Equipment malfunction can cause a range of problems. Some malfunctions may have minor or no immediate effects, such as loss of a feeding tube or clotting of an indwelling central venous catheter. Other malfunctions may cause serious physiologic effects, such as respiratory distress from loss of a tracheostomy tube or intracranial pressure elevation from obstruction of a CSF shunt.

Tracheostomy Tubes

A tracheostomy is a surgical opening (stoma) in the front of the neck into the trachea. A tracheostomy tube (sometimes called a "trach tube") is an artificial airway passed through this opening that allows the child to breathe (**FIGURE 10-1**). Infants and children may have a tracheostomy for several reasons, as noted in **TABLE 10-2**.

There are several types of tracheostomy tubes, and they come in many sizes. The size is written on the wings or flanges of the tube. The size and name (indicating type of tube) are also on the box. The inner and outer diameters are often on the wings (**FIGURE 10-2**). The most common pediatric tube sizes are 2.5–10 mm (sizes 000–10). A 3.0 tracheostomy tube is the same diameter as a 3.0 endotracheal tube. Tracheostomy tubes have a standard outer opening or hub outside the neck so a bag-mask device can be attached. For some tubes, an adapter may be needed to make this connection.

Types of Tracheostomy Tubes

The main types of tracheostomy tubes are fenestrated, double lumen, and single lumen (**FIGURE 10-3**). Tubes can also come with or without a cuff. These cuffs can

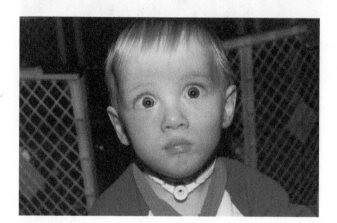

FIGURE 10-1 A tracheostomy.
Courtesy of Cindy Bissell.

TABLE 10-2 Indications for a Tracheostomy
1. To bypass an obstruction in the upper airway caused by trauma, surgery, or a birth defect
2. To allow clearance of secretions
3. To provide long-term mechanical ventilation of children with chronic respiratory problems, injuries to the lungs, major CNS deficits, or severe muscle weakness

CNS, central nervous system.

FIGURE 10-2 Sizes and inner and outer diameters are often written on the wings of tracheostomy tubes.

FIGURE 10-3 Fenestrated, double-lumen, and single-lumen tracheostomy tubes (top to bottom).

be filled with air or foam. All tubes have an **obturator**, which is a solid plastic guide placed inside the tube to make insertion easier. Use the obturator to clear the tube of secretions in an emergency if a suction catheter is not available.

A single-lumen tracheostomy tube has one hollow tube or cannula for airflow and suctioning of secretions. Uncuffed, single-lumen tubes are usually used for neonates, infants, and young children. A double-lumen tube has a hollow outer cannula and a removable (also hollow) inner cannula. Remove the inner cannula for cleaning, and keep it in place to provide mechanical ventilation. Never remove the outer cannula unless the entire tube must be replaced.

A fenestrated tube has holes (fenestrations) for air to flow upward through the vocal cords and mouth. This structure lets the child talk and breathe naturally. Fenestrated tubes have a decannulation plug attached to the outer cannula that blocks airflow through the stoma. If the child cannot breathe through the nose or mouth, remove this plug so breathing is possible through the stoma. In addition, many fenestrated tubes also have a hollow inner cannula that must be in place for mechanical ventilation.

> **TIP**
>
> If the inner cannula of a double-lumen tracheostomy tube has been removed, a bag-mask device will not secure to the outer lumen of the tube. To ventilate a tracheostomy tube with the inner cannula removed, secure an infant face mask onto the bag, and then cover the tracheostomy tube's opening and seal the face mask on the neck.

Oxygen Delivery and Assisted Ventilation Through a Tracheostomy Tube

A child with a functioning tracheostomy tube can receive oxygen from the blow-by method, by a face mask or tracheostomy mask placed directly over the tube opening, or by manual ventilation with a bag-mask device.

1. Provide blow-by oxygen. Place a stoma mask or pediatric face mask a short distance above the tracheostomy tube or stoma and give oxygen at 10–15 L/min.
2. Secure a face or tracheostomy mask directly over the tracheostomy tube opening and secure the straps around the neck.
3. Attach a bag-mask device to a tracheostomy tube adapter. Attach a bag-mask device directly to the outer end of the tracheostomy tube (**FIGURE 10-4**).

For a child who has a stoma (surgical opening in the neck) but no tracheostomy tube, or when a tube cannot be reinserted, apply a seal with a mask over the stoma and ventilate through the stoma; or cover the stoma with a **sterile gauze**, and ventilate with a mask to the mouth or mask to the mouth and nose technique. Begin bag-mask ventilation as needed.

Tracheostomy Complications: Obstruction

Obstruction of the tracheostomy tube is a life-threatening emergency. Obstruction can be caused by secretions, incorrect insertion (tube malposition), improper positioning of the child's head, or mechanical problems with the tube. Obstruction causes respiratory distress and failure.

FIGURE 10-4 Bag-mask device attached directly to the external end of the tracheostomy tube.

FIGURE 10-5 Suctioning a tracheostomy tube.

Assessment. When a child has an obstructed tracheostomy tube, the chest is not rising and the child cannot breathe on his or her own. The PAT shows poor appearance, increased work of breathing, and cyanosis in cases of respiratory failure. The ABCDEs further indicate poor air movement and bradycardia.

> ### TIP
>
> The most common complication of a child with a tracheostomy tube is respiratory distress caused by obstruction of the tube.

Treatment: Clearing an Obstructed Tube. To clear an obstructed tracheostomy tube, follow these steps:

1. Position the child's head with a towel roll under the shoulders. Ensure that the outer opening of the tube is clear.
2. Check that the tube is in the proper location. The wings or flange should be against the neck, and the obturator should not be in place.
3. If the child has a fenestrated tube, remove the decannulation plug.
4. If the child has a double-lumen tracheostomy tube, remove the inner lumen to clear secretions.
5. If none of these maneuvers works, suction the tube with a suction catheter.

Treatment: Suctioning a Tracheostomy Tube. If efforts to clear the obstruction are unsuccessful, suction the tracheostomy tube using the following procedure (**FIGURES 10-5** and **10-6**):

1. Ask the caregiver if he or she has suction catheters, equipment, and supplies. If so, use these. Otherwise, choose a suction catheter small enough to pass through the tube. (A size 1.0 [or 3.0-mm]

A

B

FIGURE 10-6 A. Insertion of suction catheter to proper depth; suction port remains open. **B.** Suctioning airway in circular motion as catheter is removed; suction port is closed.

tube will take a size 6 to 8 French catheter.) The caregiver may know the right size catheter. If equipment is not immediately available, insert the obturator to try to clear the obstruction.

2. If using a portable suction machine, set it to –100 mm Hg or less.

3. Give oxygen via a ventilation bag with a mask, and then loosen secretions by placing up to 1.0 to 2.0 mL of normal saline into the tube.

4. Insert the suction catheter approximately 2 inches (5 cm) into the tube. If the child begins to cough, the catheter is through the tube and into the trachea, and the depth of insertion is too deep. Do not use suction while inserting the catheter, and never force the catheter.

5. Cover the suction port (hole on the tubing) and suction for 3 to 5 seconds, while slowly removing the catheter. Never suction for longer than 5 seconds. Always monitor the child's heart rate and color during this procedure. Stop suctioning immediately if the heart rate begins to drop or the child becomes blue.

6. If the obstruction is removed, and the child can breathe on his or her own, do not suction further. If additional suctioning is needed, apply oxygen (by blow-by or direct ventilation) and repeat steps 3–5.

7. Always provide supplemental oxygen after suctioning by using the blow-by method or with manual ventilations.

Replacing a Tracheostomy Tube

Treatment of a tracheostomy problem usually requires simple techniques to establish a patent airway, such as suctioning or removal of the old tracheostomy tube and replacement with a new tube (**FIGURE 10-7**). Occasionally, it is impossible to ventilate a child through an existing tracheostomy tube because of decannulation or complete obstruction. Under these conditions,

FIGURE 10-7 Replacing a tracheostomy tube.

the prehospital professional must place a new tracheostomy tube to save the child's life. For a step-by-step explanation of this procedure, see **Removing and Replacing a Tracheostomy Tube, Procedure 24**.

Central Venous Catheters

Many children receive nutritional support or medications at home through a **central venous catheter**. This includes children with poor weight gain caused by gastrointestinal or liver problems, children with cancer who require chemotherapy, and children with infections who are receiving antibiotics at home.

Many central venous catheters require a surgical incision, but some can be placed percutaneously or through intact skin (often called **PICC lines [peripherally inserted central catheter]**). They can enter through the skin of the chest, neck, or arm, and the internal end usually lies in or near the **superior vena cava** or right **atrium**. Some are single-lumen lines. Others are double lumen, with two separate external openings, but only one internal opening or port.

CASE STUDY 2

You are called to the home of a 6-year-old boy whose central venous catheter has bleeding around the insertion site. His mother panicked because it is a new catheter and she is not used to taking care of it. She tells you that he has a history of short-gut syndrome caused by an infarcted bowel sustained 6 months ago. He also has a gastrostomy tube through which he receives some medications, but it was just pulled out. He is totally reliant on his central venous catheter for his nutrition.

On arrival, you note a thin 6-year-old boy sitting quietly on the family's couch. He has no increased work of breathing. His skin is yellowish. His respiratory rate is 22 breaths/min, his heart rate is 95 beats/min, and his blood pressure is 90/50 mm Hg. Pulse oximetry is 98%. There is a tiny ooze of blood from the insertion site of the catheter in the right neck.

1. What are the key historical points?
2. Outline the assessment and management priorities.

Types of Catheters

Central venous catheters may be inserted into the femoral, internal jugular, and subclavian veins (**FIGURE 10-8**). The skin entry site for the catheter is usually on the chest or arm. This is called a peripherally inserted central catheter (PICC).

Totally implanted devices (ports) are catheters attached to totally implanted injection ports or reservoirs. The catheter is in a central vein, such as the superior vena cava. Instead of coming out of the skin, as in partially implanted catheters, the end is attached to a reservoir (dome or port) that is in a subcutaneous pocket, usually on the chest. Therefore, there are no external parts visible, just a bulge or bump where the device rests.

TIP

The most common complication in a child assisted by technology with a partially implanted central venous catheter is a broken or dislodged catheter. If the bleeding is from the catheter and the catheter is in place, inspect the catheter and its end. Apply direct pressure to the bleeding site with a sterile gauze. If a cap is missing, replace the cap, if possible.

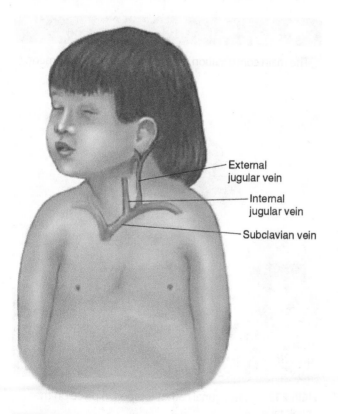

- External jugular vein
- Internal jugular vein
- Subclavian vein

FIGURE 10-8 Possible insertion sites for a central venous catheter. Subclavian, internal jugular, and external jugular sites.

Complications of Central Venous Catheters

TABLE 10-3 lists common complications of central venous catheters. The most common problem with partially implanted devices is a broken or dislodged catheter. Check the site for bleeding. If the catheter is in place, but there is bleeding from the entry site, apply direct pressure with sterile gauze. Likewise, if the catheter has been completely pulled out, and there is bleeding, apply direct pressure with sterile gauze.

ALS

Clamping a Leaking Central Venous Catheter. If the child is bleeding through a hole or cut in the catheter, clamp the exposed end. The caregiver usually has a clamp available, but if this has been misplaced, wrap the tips of a hemostat with gauze and apply to the catheter. If no **hemostat** is available, open the emergency delivery kit, wrap the sharp edges of the umbilical clamp with gauze, then apply to the catheter. If there has been bleeding, estimate the amount of blood loss.

Provide appropriate fluid therapy if there are signs of poor perfusion or shock. Do not use the central venous catheter.

Infection at Catheter Site. Infection can occur at the site where a partially implanted catheter enters the skin or in the pocket where a totally implanted device is placed. Signs of infection are redness, tenderness, swelling, warmth, or yellow discharge (pus) from the site.

The child can also have a blood infection with fever, chills, and shock. In this case, treat for **septic shock**, as described in Chapter 4. If the line is possibly infected, do not use it for vascular access.

TABLE 10-3 Common Central Venous Catheter Complications

Dislodged or broken catheter
Infection at catheter site
Problems with accessing or flushing the catheter (obstruction)
Air embolism
Medical problems related to **infusion**

Obstruction. A problem with accessing or flushing the catheter usually means obstruction. This complication can occur with all types of catheters. All that is required is patient assessment and transport. The major concern is a child who depends on **hyperalimentation** (intravenous [IV] nutrition) for calories and glucose. If the line is malfunctioning, and the child has not received any nutrition, their blood glucose may be low, so perform a fingerstick check of the blood sugar.

> **CAUTION**
>
> If the indwelling central venous catheter seems infected, do not use it for vascular access.

> **TIP**
>
> In a child who depends on hyperalimentation for calories and glucose, if the line is malfunctioning and the child has not received any nutrition, his or her blood glucose may be low.

Treatment of Hypoglycemia. Perform a quick fingerstick check of the blood sugar if there are signs or symptoms of hypoglycemia. For low blood sugar, basic life support providers can give oral glucose per local protocol or advanced life support (ALS) providers can treat with IV dextrose or intramuscular (IM) **glucagon** as described in Chapter 6.

Air Embolism. This complication can occur if air accidentally gets into a central venous catheter when the line is being flushed or if the catheter breaks. Symptoms of air embolism include shortness of breath, chest pain, and coughing. Sometimes there is cardiovascular collapse and cardiopulmonary arrest.

Treatment of Suspected Air Embolism. Clamp the catheter or ask the caregiver to clamp the catheter, provide the child with oxygen, place the child on his or her left side in the head-down position, and transport to the ED.

Medical Problems Related to Infusion. Because of the various fluids and medications delivered through central venous catheters, several medical problems can develop, such as allergic reactions, abnormal heart rate or rhythms, or respiratory problems. Treat the appropriate problem, and bring the fluids that were being infused to the ED for analysis.

Feeding Devices

A feeding device provides an avenue for nutrition and medications to CSHCN who are unable to take food or fluids by mouth. This device allows the child to take in enough calories for adequate growth and nutrition and may be used to administer medications.

Types of Feeding Tubes

Some feeding tubes go through the nose (nasogastric [NG]) or, occasionally, through the mouth (orogastric [OG]) and into the stomach or small intestine (nasojejunal, orojejunal) (**FIGURE 10-9**). These tubes are usually long catheters that are taped in place on the child's face.

Another type of feeding tube goes directly into the stomach from an external site on the abdomen (**gastrostomy tube** or **G-tube** or "**button**") (**FIGURE 10-10**). It has a balloon on the end inserted into the stomach that is similar to the balloon on an endotracheal tube. It is inflated to keep the button in place. There is also a small cap with a valve on the outside to allow access. It can be replaced by the child's caregivers. Another device is called a percutaneous **endoscopic gastrostomy (PEG)**, which is a longer tube. Many caregivers prefer a button because there is no tube hanging from the abdomen that could be dislodged during physical activity.

> **TIP**
>
> The main complication of feeding tubes is dislodgment.

FIGURE 10-9 Nasojejunal catheter taped in place on the child's face.

FIGURE 10-10 A G-tube (button) with a connector attached.

Courtesy of Cindy Bissell.

Complications of Feeding Tubes

The main complication of a feeding tube is dislodgment. The child may have aspirated fluid if a nasal or oral feeding tube has come out. For tubes inserted into the abdomen, there may be bleeding or leakage of fluid. For a button, a replacement button may not fit into the stoma on the abdomen if it is the wrong size or there was a delay in replacing it. Perform an assessment, paying special attention to the work of breathing, chest auscultation, and pulse oximetry.

Treatment

If an implanted tube (G-tube) comes out, check the site for bleeding and apply direct pressure with a sterile dressing. If the insertion site around the implanted tube seems irritated or infected (the skin seems red, warm, or swollen), apply a sterile dressing to the site.

Whenever a tube dislodges or there is evidence of infection, transport the child to the ED. Ask the caregiver to bring the tube that fell out with the child to the hospital for sizing purposes. If the child was on an infusion of fluid or medication, ask the caregiver to disconnect the pump (infusion device) and transport it with the child. If the child has received fluid through a feeding catheter within 30 minutes of EMS arrival, consider transporting the child in a sitting position to prevent reflux, vomiting, and possible aspiration.

Removing a Feeding Tube. If the NG or OG tube seems to be in place but the child is having respiratory difficulty, ask the caregiver to check its position. If position cannot be confirmed, remove the tube.

CSF Shunts

A CSF shunt is a device that drains excess CSF from the brain. It is usually inserted from a ventricle (in the brain) under the skin, then down the neck into the **peritoneum** of the abdomen (ventriculoperitoneal or VP shunt), the **pleura** of the chest (ventriculopleural or VP shunt), or the heart (ventriculoatrial or VA shunt) (**FIGURE 10-11**). Its path (or track) can usually be felt on one side of the head and down the neck until the track reaches a scar on the chest wall or abdomen. A CSF shunt helps a child with **hydrocephalus** maintain normal brain pressure. The hydrocephalus may be caused by a congenital problem or by an acquired condition, such as bleeding, trauma, tumor, or infection.

Complications of CSF Shunts

The major complications with a CSF shunt are obstruction and infection. The most common complication is a shunt obstruction/malfunction. **TABLE 10-4** lists key questions to ask during assessment to evaluate the severity of the complaint and the urgency for treatment.

Assessment of a Child With a Possible CSF Shunt Obstruction or Infection

Symptoms of a CSF shunt obstruction are the same as those of increased intracranial pressure and include headache, lethargy, sleepiness, irritability, nausea or vomiting, or trouble walking. Fever is usually a sign of a shunt infection or an **intercurrent** illness, but can occur with a shunt malfunction alone. Signs of a shunt

Point where shunt dips into ventricles

Reservoir/pump

Point where shunt dips into abdomen

FIGURE 10-11 A CSF shunt directs CSF from a ventricle in the brain to either the abdomen or the heart.

TABLE 10-4 Key Questions for Suspected CSF Shunt Malfunction

When was the CSF shunt placed?

Is the child acting the same as the last time there was a shunt problem (obstruction)?

Has the child had a fever?

Has the child complained of a headache, vomiting, or nausea?

CSF, cerebrospinal fluid.

obstruction are abnormal appearance, high-pitched cry, seizures, or altered mental status. A very worrisome finding is **Cushing triad** (bradycardia, elevated blood pressure, and irregular respirations), which indicates increased intracranial pressure caused by an obstructed shunt.

TIP

Many CSHCN, especially those with spina bifida, have a sensitivity or allergy to latex. Always use latex precautions with these patients. Reactions to latex can range from a localized skin reaction to anaphylaxis.

A child with a shunt infection may have a fever, headache, feeding difficulty, or altered behavior. Signs of a shunt infection include abnormal appearance, altered mental status, and shock.

Treatment

Make sure the child has a clear airway and effective breathing. Supply supplemental oxygen, and transport the patient. Keep the head in midline position and elevate 30 to 45 degrees whenever possible. If the child has bradycardia, irregular respirations, and elevated blood pressure (Cushing triad), there is increased intracranial pressure and herniation is imminent. Begin bag-mask ventilation and rapidly transport.

ALS

Hyperventilation for Suspected Increased Intracranial Pressure. Hyperventilation is a treatment for children with impending or frank herniation. However, the role of hyperventilation in treating prehospital intracranial pressure elevation from hydrocephalus is not well understood. Hyperventilation, through carbon dioxide reduction and cerebral vasoconstriction, reduces brain perfusion. However, overly aggressive ventilation may dangerously decrease perfusion and cause brain ischemia. If a child with a CSF shunt has signs of impending or frank herniation, use capnography to keep end-tidal carbon dioxide levels at 30 to 35 mm Hg. This is the same treatment as outlined for traumatic brain injury in Chapter 7.

Ostomies

Some conditions, such as Crohn's disease, spinal cord injury, distal ureter or bladder defects, and necrotizing enterocolitis in an infant, interfere with regular elimination of urine and feces. Several types of **ostomies** are created to accomplish this bodily function. With a **colostomy** or **ileostomy**, an opening in the abdomen is formed when the large or small intestine is surgically brought out to the surface and sutured in place, creating a stoma. This procedure allows the digestive system to continue functioning while bypassing any inflamed or damaged bowel. An external pouch is placed over the stoma to collect digestive waste matter. The intestines below the ileostomy site may not have been removed if there is a possibility of reconnecting the bowel at a later time. Colostomies can also be temporary or permanent. With a **urostomy**, a stoma is surgically created to allow the elimination of urine.

Complications of Ostomies

Complications of ostomies include infection and pouch displacement. Because of an increased risk for dehydration, a child with a colostomy needs to be assessed carefully for clinical signs and symptoms of dehydration and shock, particularly if there is a history of diarrhea or decreased oral intake.

Signs of infection at the ostomy site include red, warm, tender skin spreading away from the stoma site. Ask the child or caregiver if the area is more tender than usual. If the child has signs of infection, transport the child for further evaluation.

Replacing a Pouch

Ask the caregiver to empty the pouch before transport, especially if the pouch is full. Before the pouch is emptied, document that amount of fluid in the pouch. Be sure the pouch is resealed after emptying to prevent leakage. In some instances, the pouch breaks or is torn off. If another pouch is not available, circle the stoma with moist gauze and then attach anything available that can serve as a substitute collection device. If no pouch is available, place several thicknesses of moist gauze over the stoma until a proper replacement is found. Another option is to secure a nonrebreather face mask over the stoma. Remove the valve leaflet, so the reservoir in the mask collects the excreted stool or urine.

Lastly, be respectful of the child's privacy. Keep the site, and pouch if in place, covered in public.

Internal Pacemakers and Defibrillators

Pacemakers are implanted medical devices that regulate the heart rate. Indications include bradycardia that does not maintain adequate perfusion; a previous cardiac arrest; and heart block, especially after open heart surgery. They usually include a generator and leads. The generator houses the software and battery and supplies the electrical impulse. The leads are insulated wires that carry the electrical impulse to the heart and carry information about the heart's natural rhythm back to the pulse generator.

Complications of Internal Pacemakers

Several complications can occur for children with pacemakers. Some devices do not allow the child's heart rhythm to go above a certain rate. If that child is in shock or shock is impending, the body cannot compensate by increasing the heart rate. Begin treatment, and transport immediately. Another complication is pacemaker failure. The child's heart rate drops and becomes too slow to maintain perfusion. Again, begin treatment and transport immediately. A third complication is pacemaker malfunction. The child may experience bradycardia if the pacemaker is not firing. In another instance, the leads may become dislodged and cause the child's diaphragm to contract instead of the heart muscle every time the pacemaker fires. The respiratory rate will equal the preset pacemaker rate. One unusual problem may be dislodgement of the leads after some type of chest trauma. Monitor the heart rate closely and transport.

Internal Cardiac Defibrillators

An **implantable cardioverter-defibrillator (ICD)** or **automated internal cardiac defibrillator (AICD)** is an electronic device implanted under the skin. Its purpose is to monitor the heart rhythm and slow down or stop excessively fast heart rates that originate in the ventricles. Such rhythms include ventricular tachycardia and ventricular fibrillation.

The mechanical parts of an ICD include a generator and a lead. This generator is a tiny battery-operated electronic device located inside a case that monitors and records the heart rhythm. It sends out shocks or uses bursts of pacing to convert excessively fast heart rates when needed. The computer also records any shocks that it sends to the heart. A lead (or wire) is attached to the generator and is connected to the heart muscle to monitor the heart rhythm and carry shocks to the heart.

For any child with a pacemaker, ICD, or AICD, prehospital professionals should ask the caregivers the following questions:

- What type of heart problem does the child have?
- What rate is the child's underlying rhythm?
- What type of pacemaker, ICD, or AICD does the child have?
  - If a pacemaker, is the child dependent on the pacemaker? What are the settings?
  - If an ICD or AICD, what are the settings, at what heart rate does the ICD fire, and how many shocks has the child felt? In addition, has the child experienced any of the following:
    - More than three shocks in a row?
    - Continuation of unusual symptoms after experiencing a shock?
    - Sensations of dizziness, lightheadedness, palpitations, and so forth for a period of time yet has felt no shock?

> **TIP**
>
> The internal pacemaker can easily be felt near the clavicle or in small children in the abdomen. Never place defibrillator paddles, "hands off" defibrillating-pacing patches, or automated external defibrillator patches directly over the internal pacemaker or defibrillator generator. The battery life for implanted pacemakers and defibrillators is 6–12 years.

Vagal Nerve Stimulator

The **vagal nerve stimulator (VNS)** was approved by the Federal Drug Administration in 1997 for those patients with intractable epilepsy. Some children continue to have seizures despite conventional medication, surgical procedures, and diet. The VNS provides hope for better seizure control.

The VNS is an implantable device that looks like a pacemaker and is surgically placed by a neurosurgeon just under the skin in the left upper chest. It is programmed to provide baseline intermittent stimulation of the left vagus nerve, which leads directly to the brain. The patient or caretaker activates the device by placing a handheld magnet over it.

When responding to a call involving a CSHCN with an implanted VNS who is seizing, first assist the caregiver with activation of the VNS. Alternatively, contact medical control for guidance. Children with VNS devices should otherwise be treated as any other patient who is seizing, with attention to airway, breathing, and circulation.

Dialysis Shunts

Chronic renal failure is progressive and irreversible inadequate kidney function caused by permanent loss of nephrons. This disease develops over months or years and causes scarring in the kidneys, leading to diminished kidney function and the buildup of waste products and fluid in the blood. **Renal dialysis** is a technique for filtering toxic wastes from the blood, removing excess fluid, and restoring the normal balance of electrolytes. There are two types: **peritoneal dialysis** and **hemodialysis**.

In peritoneal dialysis, large amounts of specially formulated dialysis fluid are infused into and back out of the abdominal cavity. This fluid stays in the cavity for 1–2 hours, allowing equilibrium to occur. It is very effective, yet carries a high risk of peritonitis. Many patients undergo peritoneal dialysis at home after the caregivers have received appropriate training. Prehospital professionals are not usually involved in this process.

In hemodialysis, the patient's blood circulates through a machine that functions much like a kidney and requires the use of some type of shunt or surgically created connection between a vein and an artery. External shunts may be located near the wrist, in the upper arm, or on the proximal anterior thigh. Some patients have an internal shunt also known as an arteriovenous (AV) fistula that is usually located in the forearm or upper arm (**FIGURE 10-12**).

When moving and transporting the patient, make sure the external shunt is protected and is not compromised by any straps. For all blood pressure measurements, use the arm **without** the device. If the patient has an internal shunt or AV fistula, do NOT attempt to access the fistula to draw blood or to infuse any fluids.

> **CAUTION**
>
> Never use an AV fistula for vascular access.

Summary of Children Assisted by Technology

Children assisted by technology may encounter many challenging problems with their equipment. The prehospital professional must be familiar with the basic purpose, design, and common complications of tracheostomy tubes, central venous catheters, feeding tubes, CSF shunts, pacemakers, and implantable defibrillators. Always ask the caregiver about the equipment, and transport all devices and infusions with the child to the ED. Ask whether the current problem has ever happened before and how the situation was handled previously. Finally, remember that the child may be well versed on the medical device that he or she uses. Consider asking the child your questions about the device; in doing so, you may gain his or her trust, which ultimately leads to better patient care.

FIGURE 10-12 A. Hemodialysis access by an AV fistula or graft that creates a bulge in the skin. **B.** An AV graft creates a raised area that looks like a large vessel.

A: © Terrapanthera/Shutterstock.

The Medical Home for CSHCN

Care coordination for CSHCN who often have involvement of multiple organ systems is quite complex. A specialist or general pediatrician's office can provide compassionate, comprehensive, continuous care in a culturally sensitive manner by being the child's family-centered medical home. Information is available at www.medicalhomeinfo.org.

CSHCN usually see multiple physicians, therapists, home care personnel, and other health care providers to manage their chronic conditions. To coordinate that care, these clinicians need to communicate with the medical home and one another in an effective manner. Traditionally, communication has occurred on paper, with hospitals and offices faxing reports or sending copies to one another. This system is flawed in that some of these paper reports are lost, are misfiled, or do not arrive at the office or hospital in time for additional visits or procedures. For example, if the child sees the pediatric neurologist who places the child on different medications to manage seizures, the primary care physician may not know about this change and prescribe another medication for an illness, which may cause a dangerous interaction that could be detrimental to the child. In addition to adverse drug reactions, the poor coordination of care may result in unnecessary hospitalizations, duplicate testing, advice from one clinician that contradicts that of another, and poor clinical outcomes.

The Institute of Medicine identified ineffective care coordination as a cause of poor clinical outcomes and recommended electronic health records (EHRs) as one way to improve the quality of care for patients with chronic conditions. By documenting care and treatment in an EHR, the child's past medical and surgical histories, medications, allergies, contact information for multiple providers, schedule of preventive services, baseline neurologic status, and other information can be immediately available.

Electronic documentation can be beneficial, but sharing that information across systems of care presents yet another challenge. Some areas of the country have developed **health information exchanges (HIEs)** whereby electronic data are shared among hospitals, physician practices, and other entities where patients may be treated. The presence and use of these HIEs are sporadic at best, and many of them do not involve EMS systems.

In an emergency involving a CSHCN, obtaining accurate medical information is a priority because of the multitude of treatments, medications, and ongoing care. To address this, an electronic version of the EIF, originally developed by the AAP and ACEP is available (see Figure 17-6).

Through websites containing emergency information forms, parents and providers may enter data and then access the data in a secure fashion. This effort is one example of how the care of CSHCN can be enhanced through health information technology and the electronic exchange of data. In addition, contact with the patient's medical home can provide EMS professionals with important information about the patient.

Additional EMS Considerations for CSHCN

1. Many CSHCN, especially those with spina bifida, have a sensitivity or allergy to latex. Always use latex precautions with these patients. Reactions to latex can range from a localized skin reaction to anaphylaxis.
2. Speak quietly and calmly to the child, and explain what he or she can expect by using words

CASE STUDY 3

A distraught mother calls 9-1-1 because her infant son is having difficulty feeding and appears more blue than usual. She tells you that the child is a 2-month-old boy with Down syndrome and a heart defect. He has been home for a few weeks and is being allowed to grow before surgery to repair his heart. His mother confirms that he usually has a pulse oximetry reading in the 80s. She hands you a card with the child's medical history, medications, and hospital information and states that he has been vomiting since the day before and has not kept down any of his medications.

You approach the child and note that he is poorly interactive, has retractions and nasal flaring, and is cyanotic. The chest has crackles, and the pulse oximetry is 75%. His heart rate is 130 beats/min, respiratory rate is 70 breaths/min, and blood pressure is 86 mm Hg/palp.

1. What is the likely physiologic problem?
2. What are your primary interventions?

appropriate for that child's developmental level. This approach decreases the child's anxiety and increases cooperation. Recognize that most CSHCN respond best with slower movements and firm, secure contact.

3. Children with musculoskeletal conditions, such as cerebral palsy or muscular dystrophy, need special care during preparation for transport. Children with cerebral palsy are often stiff and may have contractures. Do not force movements. Secure these children in their natural position, and pad any open areas. Children with paralysis or muscular dystrophy may not have regular sensation, so special care should be taken to ensure that their limbs are secured on the stretcher and do not hang off the edges.

4. Assess pain in CSHCN. If the child cannot communicate, then ask the caregiver if the child is in pain. Position the child for comfort. Use blankets under vulnerable areas of the body. If local protocols allow, administer medications for pain control after ensuring the caregivers did not give the child any pain medication before EMS arrival.

5. When leaving the home of a CSHCN:
   - Ask the parents or caregivers for the child's "go bag." This bag contains all of the supplies necessary (and that are not routinely stocked on ambulances) to manage the child's tracheostomy tube, feeding catheter, or central venous line.
   - Ask the parents for the child's daily medical information form or EIF, which contains pertinent medical information regarding the child's medical condition, baseline vital signs, allergies, doctors' names and numbers, medications, therapies, and necessary home support equipment. Ask how you can make the patient most comfortable.
   - Ensure any compressed air or oxygen in the home is turned off before departure.

6. Request that the child's direct caregiver accompany the child to the hospital to continue assisting with the child's care. The caregiver not only becomes a valuable resource for repeated assessments and interventions, but also provides familiarity and reassurance to the child in the midst of an unfamiliar and potentially chaotic environment.

7. Recognize when the caregiver is overwhelmed with emotion or exhaustion. In these circumstances, it may be best to offer the caregiver a more passive role in the child's care while allowing him or her to continue to be with the child.

CASE STUDY ANSWERS

CASE STUDY 1

Assessment of the airway, breathing, and circulation suggests respiratory distress. Ask the child's caregiver about her baseline vital signs and activity level. Ask if there have been any changes and, if so, what is different.

Take the child off the ventilator and manually ventilate with a bag to the trach. Determine the ease of air entry through the tracheostomy tube and determine if aided respirations help the child's respiratory distress. Ask the caregiver when the last tracheostomy tube change was and the frequency of suctioning. Suction the tracheostomy to determine if this helps the child's breathing. Consider a tracheostomy tube change if there are copious secretions or there is difficulty with air entry during manual ventilations.

Consider an **albuterol** nebulizer treatment. Albuterol can open the child's airways to alleviate distress. In this case, the parent states that he has had to suction more frequently than usual and that he has already changed the tracheostomy tube that day. He states further that he thinks the child is getting sick and that her older sister has had a cold for the last few days. This history makes an exacerbation of the child's chronic lung disease more likely, and a mucous plug obstructing the tube less likely.

You decide to transport this child to her medical home hospital and continue the albuterol nebulizer treatment through her tracheostomy tube en route. You ask the caregiver to disconnect the feed through the gastrostomy tube to prepare for transport.

CASE STUDY 2

This boy is in no distress. The PAT is normal. His vital signs are stable. He is totally dependent on this central venous catheter for his nutrition and hydration. Ask the caregiver how long the catheter site has been bleeding. Check the catheter for dislodgement or breakage. Apply direct pressure to the site to stop the bleeding. Ask the caregiver to disconnect the catheter if it is still connected. Prepare the child for transport, preferably to his medical home hospital, so that the catheter can be repaired or replaced. If the child has not received nutrition for 1–2 hours, check blood glucose.

Another very common problem is dislodgement of a feeding catheter. This is especially true if the child is totally dependent on the gastrostomy tube (G-tube or button) for all nutrition and hydration. Also, the longer the tube is out, the more difficult it is to replace. Ask the family to bring the dislodged tube to the hospital, and if they have a replacement tube, bring that as well. Not all hospitals have the proper size tubes for children, so either call ahead to the local ED or transport the child to his home hospital.

Short-gut syndrome results when a large section of the bowel has been removed. This phenomenon is more likely to occur in premature children, but can also occur in children who experience shock or hypoxemia to the bowel from infections, obstruction of the intestines, or trauma. These children often receive their nutrition through feeding catheters as this child did; however, if they have lost a significant amount of their bowel, they may need their nutrition (hyperalimentation and lipids) delivered through a central venous line. This boy no longer could receive all of his feeds through the gastrostomy tube and needed supplementation through his central venous catheter.

A young child who misses many hours of fluids may be tachycardic and have signs of dehydration, such as dry mucous membranes and no tears, in the early stages of hypoperfusion. Interventions include oxygen supplementation, keeping the child warm, covering the stoma site with a dry gauze, and transporting the G-tube that fell out (along with any special adaptors) for sizing purposes.

ALS interventions include a 20 mL/kg crystalloid fluid by peripheral IV bolus in a child who seems dehydrated with a G-tube out or dislodged or a broken central venous line. If glucose is low, treat with IV dextrose.

CASE STUDY 3

Assess airway, breathing, and circulation. You decide that this child needs assisted ventilations and begin to manually ventilate with a bag-mask device. As your partner is looking for an appropriate IV site, she notes that the child has pedal edema. You then consider that this child is in congestive heart failure and decide not to start this child on IV fluids without advice from medical control. Because blood pressure and perfusion are adequate, do not start a pressor drug. Transport immediately to the ED.

Children with Down syndrome are at increased risk of medical complications. Some of the organ systems affected include the cardiovascular, sensory, endocrine, orthopedic, gastrointestinal, neurologic, and hematologic systems. People with Down syndrome are developmentally delayed and often have intellectual disabilities.

Cardiovascular defects are a leading cause of neonatal death in Down syndrome caused by congenital abnormalities. When an infant is born with a severe cardiac anomaly, interventions are primarily directed toward home health care until definitive surgery can be performed or toward supportive treatment in the home of a child whose defect cannot be surgically repaired.

SUGGESTED REFERENCES

Textbooks

Adirim T, Smith E. *Special Children's Outreach and Prehospital Education (SCOPE)*. Burlington, MA: Jones and Bartlett Learning; 2006.

American Academy of Pediatrics and the American College of Emergency Physicians. *APLS: The Pediatric Emergency Medicine Resource*. 5th ed. Burlington, MA: Jones and Bartlett Learning; 2012.

Wertz E. *Emergency Care for Children*. Albany, NY: Delmar; 2002.

Articles

American Academy of Pediatrics, Committee on Children with Disabilities. Care coordination: integrating health and related systems of care for children with special health care needs. *Pediatrics*. 2005;116:1238–1244.

Bhandari A, Bhandari V. Pitfalls, problems, and progress in bronchopulmonary dysplasia. *Pediatrics.* 2009;123:1562–1573. doi:10.1542/peds.2008-1962.

Burton LC, Anderson GF, Kues IW. Using electronic health records to help coordinate care. *Milbank Quarterly.* 2004;82:457–481. doi: 10.1111/j.0887-378X.2004.00318.x.

Institute of Medicine. Committee on Identifying Priority Areas for Quality Improvement. In: Adams K, Corrigan J, eds. *Priority Areas for National Action: Transforming Health Care Quality.* Washington, DC: National Academies Press; 2003:1–13.

McPherson M. A new definition of children with special health care needs. *Pediatrics.* 1998;102: 137–139.

National Task Force on Children with Special Health Care Needs. EMS for children: recommendations for coordinating care for children with special health care needs. *Ann Emerg Med.* 1997;30:274–280.

O'Neil J, Hoffman B. American Academy of Pediatrics Council on Injury, Violence, and Poison Prevention. Transporting children with special health care needs. *Pediatrics.* 2019;143(5):e20190724.

Spaite DW, Conroy C, Karriker KJ, et al. Improving emergency medical services for children with special health care needs: does training make a difference? *Am J Emerg Med.* 2001;19:474–478.

Spaite DW, Conroy C, Tibbitts M, et al. Use of emergency medical services by children with special health care needs. *Prehosp Emerg Care.* 2000;4:19–23.

Spaite DW, Karriker KJ, Seng M, et al. Training paramedics: emergency care for children with special health care needs. *Prehosp Emerg Care.* 2000;4:178–185.

Other Resources

Center for Pediatric Emergency Medicine (CPEM). *Teaching resource for instructors in prehospital pediatrics (TRIPP), Version 2.0* [CD-ROM]. New York: Center for Pediatric Emergency Medicine; 1998.

National Center for Medical Home Implementation. www.medicalhomeinfo.aap.org. Accessed July 14, 2019.

National Down Syndrome Society. Down syndrome fact sheet. http://www.ndss.org/wp-content /uploads/2017/08/NDSS-Fact-Sheet-Language -Guide-2015.pdf. Accessed July 14, 2019.

American Academy of Pediatrics. Emergency information forms and emergency preparedness for children with special health care needs. https://pediatrics .aappublications.org/content/125/4/829.

American College of Emergency Physicians. Emergency information form for children with special health care needs. https://www.acep.org/globalassets /new-pdfs/policy-statements/emergency-nformation -form-for-children-with-special-health-care-needs/. Accessed October 2, 2019.

CHAPTER 11

Child Maltreatment

Joyce Foresman-Capuzzi, MSN, APRN, CCNS, CEN, CPEN, CTRN, TCRN, CPN, EMT-P, FAEN

Toni M. Petrillo, MD, FAAP

LEARNING OBJECTIVES

1. Discuss the known signs, causes, and complications of child maltreatment.
2. Define the terms physical abuse, emotional abuse, sexual abuse, and child neglect.
3. Explain the role of child protection services (CPS) in management of suspected child maltreatment.
4. Distinguish features in the scene size-up, in the history and physical assessment, and in the caregiver's behaviors that suggest child maltreatment.
5. Describe appropriate communication with caregivers of suspected victims of maltreatment.
6. Outline the prehospital professional's legal responsibility to document and report suspected child maltreatment.
7. Identify clues to human trafficking.

Introduction

Prehospital professionals must know when to suspect **child maltreatment**. Although providing emergency medical care is always the top priority, prehospital professionals also provide valuable scene documentation and are often the first step in the reporting process of suspected cases of maltreatment. All of these actions are critical to protect vulnerable children and to break the cycle. When caring for a pediatric patient who has suffered obvious trauma, prehospital providers need to remain vigilant in looking for potential signs of abuse.

Unfortunately, child maltreatment is common. It is one of the leading causes of death in infants younger than 12 months of age. Physical abuse and neglect are often detectable, but sexual abuse, emotional abuse, and child neglect may not be so obvious. Some children who die from maltreatment are known to local

child protection services (CPS), the legal organizations established in every community to monitor, manage, and prevent child maltreatment. These deaths are sometimes preventable. Abused or neglected children have a high probability of being maltreated again. Early recognition is important to prevent future injury or death.

Background, Cost, and Definition

In 2017, there were 3.5 million referrals reported to CPS organizations in the United States through the National Child Abuse and Neglect Data System. Of those, 674,000 children were determined to have been abused or neglected. The highest prevalence is seen in infants from birth to 1 year (25.3 cases per 1,000). For each case of child maltreatment reported,

9-1-1 is called for an unresponsive infant. On arrival, you find a 10-month-old male infant who is unresponsive, has irregular respirations, and is pale. The mother's boyfriend (mom is at work) tells you that he found the baby in this condition when he went to get him up from his nap. You note that it is 7 PM. The boyfriend is not holding the infant, and when you pick the baby up from the crib, you also note that there is no muscle tone and the infant is flaccid. During your assessment and treatment, you note bruises on both upper arms.

1. What are your initial patient management priorities?
2. What concerns you about the history reported by the boyfriend and the infant's injuries?
3. What do you suspect is the primary injury?

TIP

When adults with poor coping skills are faced with stressful situations, a cycle of child maltreatment may result.

it is estimated that there are one to two cases that go unrecognized. In 2017, an estimated 1,720 children died of abuse or neglect, which is more than four children every day. Many survivors are negatively affected for the rest of their lives. After being physically and psychologically affected, survivors may themselves become abusive or neglectful to children, thus perpetuating the cycle of abuse. The number of children who suffer long-term effects from neglect is not as well documented, but is believed to be substantial. **TABLE 11-1** lists some of these long-term complications.

Younger children are at higher risk for fatal abuse and neglect than older children. Approximately 71.8% of maltreated children who die are younger than 3 years of age, and more than 49% are younger than 1 year of age. Approximately one-half of these deaths occur in children who are known to CPS agencies as current or prior clients. It has been estimated that child maltreatment costs the United States $220 million every day.

Definition of Child Maltreatment

Child maltreatment is a general term that includes all types of abuse and neglect. Yearly, approximately 75% of substantiated maltreatment is classified as neglect, 17% is physical abuse, and 8% is sexual abuse. The remaining types include emotional abuse, medical neglect, or combinations of the different types.

TABLE 11-1 Potential Complications of Maltreatment

Low self-esteem and underachievement
Psychological disorders or psychiatric symptoms
Abnormal growth and development
Permanent physical or neurologic damage
Poor school performance
Teen promiscuity and pregnancy
Social withdrawal
Eating disorders
Substance abuse
Negative learned behavior
Criminal behavior beginning in young adulthood
Vulnerability to further abuse
Suicidal tendencies
Increased survivor health care costs to family and society
Death

Physical Abuse

Physical abuse occurs when a person intentionally inflicts injury, or allows injury to be inflicted, to a child younger than 18 years of age or to a mentally disabled child younger than 21 years of age, which causes or results in risk of death, disfigurement, or distress.

Emotional Abuse

Emotional abuse occurs when there is an ongoing and consistent pattern of behavior that interferes with the normal psychological and social development of a child. This includes unreasonable, excessive, or aggressive demands on the child that are not age appropriate; setting tasks that are beyond the physical ability of the child; or the caregiver not providing the nurturing, guidance, and psychological support critical for the growth and development of a healthy child. Verbal attacks, such as belittling, insults, rejection, and constant criticism, are a few patterns of emotional abuse.

Sexual Abuse

Sexual abuse occurs when an older child or adult engages in sexual activities with a dependent, developmentally immature child or adolescent for the older person's own sexual excitement or for the enjoyment of other persons (e.g., child pornography or prostitution).

In most cases of sexual abuse, the perpetrator is an adult who knows the child and is often living under the same roof. A common misconception is that child sexual abuse is perpetrated by strangers. According to the American Psychological Association, an estimated 60% of sexual abuse perpetrators are known by the child but are NOT a family member, 30% are family members, and only 10% are strangers.

Sexual abuse usually does not occur as a single incident. It does not always involve violence and physical force and commonly leaves no visible sign. The perpetrator may use the power of adult–child authority or the parent–child bond instead of force or violence. The child may be manipulated into thinking that "it's OK" and a normal behavior or that the child is "special" for making the perpetrator feel good. The child may also be made to feel deeply ashamed and powerless or may even be kept silent by threats from the perpetrator. The insidious nature of this abuse makes it difficult to detect unless the child discloses the information to a confidant or the prehospital professional.

Child Neglect

Child neglect occurs when a child's physical, mental, or emotional condition is harmed or endangered because the caregiver has failed to supply basic necessities or engages in child-rearing practices that are inadequate or dangerous. Child neglect may involve a caregiver's misuse of drugs or alcohol, or child abandonment. Neglect is the failure to act on behalf of a child and is an act of omission. Neglect may not have visible signs, and it usually occurs over a period of time rather than as a discrete episode.

Neglect may be physical or emotional. Physical neglect is a failure to meet the requirements basic to a child's physical development and safety, such as supervision, housing, clothing, medical attention, and nutrition. Some social service agencies subdivide this category into more specific acts of omission, such as medical neglect, lack of proper supervision, or educational neglect. Emotional neglect is failure to provide the support or affection necessary for a child's psychological and social development.

Abuse Versus Neglect

The difference between abuse and neglect is that abuse represents an action against a child, whereas neglect represents a lack of action for the child. *Abuse is an act of commission; neglect is an act of omission.* In abuse, a physical or mental injury is inflicted on a child. In neglect, there is a failure to meet the basic needs of the child for adequate food, supervision, shelter, guidance, education, clothing, or medical care.

> **TIP**
>
> Abuse represents an action against a child (commission). Neglect represents a lack of action for the child (omission).

High-Risk Groups

Younger children are more vulnerable and at risk for maltreatment than older children, who have more resources available to them and can better take care of themselves. The National Child Abuse and Neglect Data System reports that children younger than the age of 3 years are at greatest risk for severe injury or death from abuse. Child maltreatment involves risk factors and lapses in child protection at the individual, family, community, and societal levels. No geographic, ethnic, or economic setting is free of child maltreatment. The incidence rates for sexual abuse are similar for urban, suburban, and rural communities. Children from low-income or single-parent families, however, have more reported occurrences of neglect or physical maltreatment than children from higher-income families, and physically maltreated children are less likely to be identified in Caucasian, two-parent families.

TABLE 11-2 Child Maltreatment Victims by Race or Ethnic Group

African-American	20.6%
Caucasian	44.6%
Hispanic	22.3%

U.S. Department of Health & Human Services, Administration for Children and Families, Administration on Children, Youth and Families, Children's Bureau (2017). Child Maltreatment 2017. Available from http://www.acf.hhs.gov/cb/research-data-technology /statistics-research/child-maltreatment.

The 2017 data on child maltreatment show that 88% of the victims are represented by three races or ethnic groups (**TABLE 11-2**).

The prehospital provider must consider maltreatment whenever circumstances suggest it, regardless of the family's socioeconomic status.

Other risk factors for child maltreatment, besides nonverbal toddlers and infants, include factors where there are additional stressors, but insufficient resources are available to the parents or caregivers, such as children with special needs (mental and physical disabilities and developmental issues) and children with chronic medical conditions—all conditions in which there are increased responsibilities to care for the child and a financial impact that may also affect the level of stress in the home.

A perpetrator of child maltreatment can be any person who has care, custody, or control of the child. This can include the child's parents, relatives, teachers, babysitters or child care staff, institution staff, bus drivers, playground attendants, coaches, religious leaders, caregivers, or boyfriends or girlfriends of the caregiver. Abusive head trauma (formerly known as shaken baby syndrome) may lead to seizures or apnea, but the person with the infant at the time emergency medical services (EMS) is called should not be assumed to be the perpetrator. *The caregiver with the child at the time of the 9-1-1 call or EMS arrival may not be the individual who injured the child.* This individual may be unaware of the abuse or in denial and unable to believe that the child has been harmed. He or she may also be a victim of abuse or afraid of the abuser. Maltreatment happens for many different reasons. Often the perpetrators genuinely care for the child, but lack the resources or the parenting skills to deal with frustration and cope with anger. Rarely does the prehospital professional have sufficient information to determine with certainty that maltreatment has occurred. Information gathered in the field can, however, be critical in

TABLE 11-3 Assessment Factors Associated With Maltreatment

Does the history change over time?
Was there a delay in seeking care, or was the closest treatment center bypassed?
Are there injuries of multiple stages of healing?
Does the history fit the child's developmental level?
Do the injuries fit the history?
Does the patient not seek comfort from the caregiver?
Does the caregiver inappropriately respond to the patient's needs?
What are the other siblings' involvements with the patient and caregiver?

the eventual confirmation of maltreatment. **TABLE 11-3** lists assessment factors that are suggestive of maltreatment. Particularly important is the documentation of the exact history given by the caregiver in cases of presumed injury. A changing story is one of the most common hallmarks of maltreatment. Recognizing and reporting suspected child maltreatment is one of the most important ways the prehospital professional can prevent childhood injury.

Duties and Communication by the Prehospital Professional

The prehospital professional has an extremely important role at the scene. CPS and health professionals in the emergency department (ED) rely on the EMS scene assessment and documentation of suspected child maltreatment. **TABLE 11-4** lists the prehospital professional's duties in suspected maltreatment cases.

Mandatory Obligation to Report

In most states, licensed health care professionals, including prehospital professionals, have a legal obligation (mandate) to report suspected child maltreatment and other situations where a crime may have been committed or a vulnerable population is harmed. In other states, the duty of the prehospital professional

TABLE 11-4 Duties of the Prehospital Professional in Suspected Maltreatment
Recognition of suspicious circumstances at the scene
Physical assessment of the child
Assessment of the history given by the caregiver
Communication with the caregiver and family
Careful documentation
Notation of other children living at the scene
Reporting of maltreatment concerns to the proper authority

TABLE 11-5 "Red Flag" Caregiver Behaviors
Apathy
Bizarre or strange conduct
Little or no concern about the child
Overreaction to child misbehavior
Not forthcoming with events surrounding injury
Intoxication
Overreaction to child's condition

is to ensure that a report is filed with the receiving hospital, law enforcement, or a designated state office. States with maltreatment laws may require health care providers to independently report suspected maltreatment to either law enforcement or CPS.

Although no law can forbid the filing of civil or criminal charges, most state laws protect the reporter of suspected child maltreatment from any decision or award in a lawsuit, if the report was made in good faith. *However, failure to report suspicion of child maltreatment may result in legal action against the mandated reporter.*

In small communities, especially when the prehospital professional knows the individuals involved, reporting suspected child maltreatment may have significant social implications. In many states, anonymous reports can be filed, and the identity of the person who reports maltreatment is protected. Remember that a report of suspected child maltreatment is not an attempt to harm or punish a family, but an attempt to help the child. All prehospital personnel should become familiar with the particular obligation to report laws in the state in which they practice.

Assessing the Caregiver's Behavior

Common characteristics among caregivers of maltreated children are drug use, poor self-concept, immaturity, lack of parenting knowledge, and lack of interpersonal skills. Although none of these factors in and of themselves means that an individual has abused the child, be alert for these "red flag" behaviors, as noted in **TABLE 11-5**. Conversely, an "appropriate" caregiver, who does not show any of these characteristics,

may still be maltreating a child. In some cases, a caregiver may appear to be overreacting to the child's condition, such as in cases of **Munchausen syndrome by proxy**, in which a caregiver may intentionally inflict illness or injury on a child to obtain attention for herself or himself.

Never confront a caregiver with suspicions of maltreatment. Such an approach at the scene may delay care, endanger the child, and create a hostile and dangerous situation for the prehospital professional.

Instead, note the presence of alcohol or drugs in the prehospital report, and document any statements from the caregiver that reflect apparent misinformation, inconsistency, or evasiveness. Watch interactions among the caregivers and document them if they seem noteworthy. Be careful, however, to keep the tone of the report objective and neutral. Report what you see and hear, but avoid making judgments or interpreting intent in the written documentation. Particularly note any comments made by the child about how he or she was hurt. However, be aware that young children may attribute injury to an abstract perpetrator, such as a monster or "bad man," rather than identifying the caregivers on whom they depend.

Documentation

There is no difference between basic and advanced level documentation of suspected child maltreatment. Be sure to document your findings of the scene assessment related to possible child maltreatment (e.g., whether there is child-appropriate food available, heat or air conditioning, appropriate clothing, supervision, and any safety concerns). Make a note of the child's position and location when you first encountered him or her. It is also recommended to document who else is at the scene (e.g., caretakers) and their relationship to the child. When documenting the history and physical assessment, be thorough but objective. Interjecting feelings or interpreting the facts may make the documentation inadmissible in court. For example, write, "palms show a 1-cm circular burn" instead of "cigarette burn to hand." Use objective, clear, specific terminology. Place in quotation marks and note in the records any statements from caregivers (e.g., father states that "child climbed into hot bathtub").

FIGURE 11-1 Document scene conditions that might support suspicion of maltreatment.
© sangriana/iStock Editorial/Getty Images.

> **TIP**
>
> Document physical findings objectively. The facts speak for themselves in court.

Communicating With the Child and Caregivers

Communicate with the child in an age-appropriate manner. When assessing a stable child for whom there is concern of maltreatment, transport the child to the safe environment of the ED for full evaluation as soon as possible.

Communication with the caregiver in suspected maltreatment is a challenging task for the prehospital professional. Resist the impulse to "find out what really happened" or express anger at the caregiver. Do not make accusations or assume a judgmental tone. When confronted with suspicions of abuse, caregivers often respond defensively or angrily, whether or not they were the ones who inflicted the injuries.

Sometimes a caregiver may refuse to cooperate in further assessment, decline transport, or attempt to leave the scene with the child. If you believe the child to be in danger, immediately contact law enforcement for assistance. Never attempt to physically restrain a caregiver or to forcibly take possession of a child, because this may put everyone in danger. If the scene is chaotic but not dangerous, consider contacting medical control, who may be able to convince the caregiver to permit treatment and transport.

Patient Assessment

Scene Assessment

First, ensure that the scene is safe for the child and for the prehospital professionals. If you suspect maltreatment, make a mental note of any conditions at the scene, because you need to document the conditions in the patient care report (**FIGURE 11-1**). Record remarks or specific conversations with the caregiver and document specifics about the environment where injuries were reported to occur. For example, note the approximate height of furniture an infant rolled off, the floor surface, or the location and condition of the sink or room where a child was burned.

Consider child maltreatment in every pediatric trauma call and every pediatric cardiac arrest situation in children younger than 1 year of age. Suspicious circumstances in the environment, behavior of the child or caregiver, history, or physical examination may also raise concerns of abuse in responding to calls for unrelated complaints. Look for unsanitary or dangerous home conditions, such as guns, drug paraphernalia, or other unsafe care situations.

If the scene is safe, assess the child and provide appropriate medical care. If an infant with suspected maltreatment has an abnormal appearance (e.g., listlessness, inconsolability, weak cry) or altered mental status (abnormal response to verbal or painful stimuli), assess for a traumatic brain injury.

> **TIP**
>
> Consider child abuse in every injury case, as well as in illness cases with suspicious circumstances in the environment, behavior of the child or caregiver, history, or physical examination.

One cause of traumatic brain injury is **abusive head trauma**, formerly called shaken baby syndrome.

FIGURE 11-2 Human hand and fingertip marks can appear as oval bruises.

Abusive head trauma involves diffuse intracranial hemorrhage, usually from violent shaking of the child with or without impact with another object. The signs, symptoms, and physical findings in abusive head trauma vary depending on the amount of trauma to the brain. These range from lethargy, irritability and vomiting to seizures, coma, apnea, or death. Petechiae or hand grip patterns on the arms or chest (**FIGURE 11-2**) may also be found in abusive head trauma. The incidence of permanent neurologic damage from abusive head trauma is high. Seizures, learning disabilities, blindness, and other handicaps are common. The fatality rate in abusive head trauma is 20%–30%.

If the child with suspected maltreatment is physiologically unstable or has significant injuries, begin transport after the primary assessment. If the scene is unsafe for the child or prehospital professional, call for law enforcement back-up and move to the ambulance to complete the assessment and initiate treatment. Transport every child with suspected maltreatment, even if the injuries are trivial.

CAUTION

Never leave a suspected victim of child maltreatment. Transport every child, even if the injuries are trivial.

Additional Assessment

Stay on scene for additional assessment only if the child is stable and the scene is safe. Take a careful history, using the questions suggested in **TABLE 11-6**. *The history may be more important than the physical assessment.* Ask questions in a nonjudgmental way to maximize the quality of information and to avoid escalating the situation. Pay close attention to and document in detail the caregiver's description of the events leading to the call, noting inconsistencies or evasiveness. Consider the developmental capabilities of the

TABLE 11-6 Focused History: Questions and Considerations in Evaluating Suspected Child Maltreatment

Question	Considerations
How did the injury occur?	Is the caregiver's explanation plausible? For example, is the child developmentally able to roll and fall? Do the physical conditions at the scene support the alleged mechanism of injury? How high was the fall, to what type of surface, etc.?
When did it happen?	Was there a long delay before 9-1-1 was notified? Does the injury appearance match the time frame?
Who witnessed the event?	Do all of the caregivers' or witnesses' stories match? Was there adequate supervision?
What is the child's medical history?	Are there preexisting psychosocial, developmental, or chronic problems?
Does the child have a physician?	When was the last visit? Does the physician know the child?

FIGURE 11-3 A caregiver's history of a child biting his or her tongue is not believable in an infant who has no teeth. This discrepant history suggests an inflicted injury.

Courtesy of Ron Deickmann, MD, FAAP.

TABLE 11-7 Distinguishing Fact From Common Fiction

History	Fact
"He fell off the couch, and then seized."	Fewer than 1 in 1,000 falls of 4 feet (1.2 m) or less result in serious injury.
"My 1-month-old rolled off the bed."	Most infants cannot roll over until 3–4 months of age.
"He must have bruised himself."	Bruises are rare in infants who are not yet pulling to a stand; even those who do, certain places, like the pinna (ear), buttocks, and back, are concerning for abuse.
"I found him with his leg stuck in the crib slat."	Without an external force, either intentional or accidental, infants do not sustain fractures.

child. Be concerned about inflicted trauma when the history does not account for the observed injuries (**FIGURE 11-3**), the caregiver's history changes over the course of the interview, or the mechanism of injury described is not plausible given the developmental level of the child. Note any unusual interactions between child and caregiver or other possible perpetrators. Although a child may seem wary or frightened of the perpetrator, at times a child may cling to or try to appease an abusive caregiver to avoid further abusive behavior.

If the injury is described as an "accident," determine the mechanism. For example, if the caregiver reports that the child fell, determine the distance, the stopping surface, and the initial reactions of the child (**TABLE 11-7**). The information obtained at the scene may be more accurate than that obtained by the ED staff, CPS agency, and law enforcement.

Physical Examination

The prehospital professional may note suspicious findings in the physical examination of the child. Up to 90% of physical maltreatment victims have some kind of skin injury. The physical examination may reveal the suspicious patterns and physical findings of child abuse. In cases of suspected sexual abuse, defer a genital examination to providers with specialized training.

Bruises

Physical findings that suggest inflicted injury include the following:

- Bruises located on soft tissues, such as neck, back, thighs, genitalia, or buttocks

- Bruises on or behind ears
- Bruises in a child younger than 4 months of age
- Facial bruises (**FIGURE 11-4**)

In fact, the TEN-4 bruising rule has been developed in which any bruising of the Torso, Ears, or Neck in any child 4 years or younger, or any bruising in an infant younger than 4 months, are significant indicators of abuse.

Differentiating bruises resulting from maltreatment versus normal wear and tear depends on appearance, location, and developmental age of the child. Bruises over bony prominences, such as the elbow, forehead, or below the knees, are the common result of play injuries in children. However, bruises over soft tissues, such as the thighs, buttocks, cheeks, ears, or on the back, are less common and should raise suspicions of inflicted injury (**FIGURE 11-5**).

ANY bruising in an infant who is not yet mobile may suggest inflicted injury. Most children are able to roll over by 4 months of age and able to pull to a stand and cruise by 9 months of age. A child who is not yet cruising should not have unexplained bruises or fractures—*no cruising means no bruising.* As children become older and increasingly mobile, bruises and lacerations from normal activity become more common.

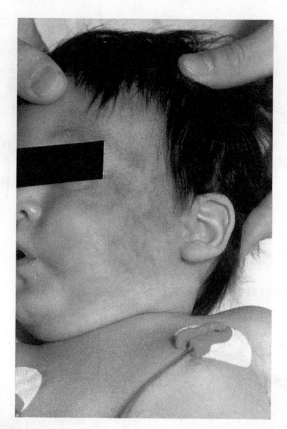

FIGURE 11-4 The face is a common target for physical abuse.

Courtesy of Ron Deickmann, MD, FAAP.

FIGURE 11-5 Bruises on the buttocks are usually inflicted injuries.

Courtesy of Ron Deickmann, MD, FAAP.

Bruising is the most common sentinel event. This is a previous injury reported in the medical history as a poorly explained visible injury or detectable minor injury. Early detection of sentinel injuries may provide the opportunity to identify and intervene before more serious injuries occur.

> **TIP**
>
> "Those who don't cruise rarely bruise." In a child who cannot yet pull up to stand and walk while holding onto furniture (cruise), bruising or injury is rare. Most infants do not start cruising until they are about 9 months of age.

Any bruise with an identifiable pattern is almost certain to have been inflicted. Common items include belts, cords, and hands. When an object hits the skin with high velocity, the edges leave an outline of petechiae. If a very thin object, such as a switch or a cord, hits the skin, parallel **petechial** lines form as an outline of the object.

It was previously thought that the time that a bruise was inflicted could be determined based on its appearance. This is now known to be inaccurate. Bruises resolve at differing rates based on their location and the mechanism of injury, and bruises of different colors can result from injuries sustained in one event. Still, document the location and colors of all bruises to provide a complete description of the injuries sustained.

Burns

Inflicted burns are usually from immersion in hot water (scalds) or from forced contact between the child and a hot object. Adult skin can develop a full-thickness burn from 2 seconds of exposure to 150°F water; children may burn even faster. Accidental scald burns typically have varying depths and irregular borders, with a "flow" pattern evident. They are rarely symmetric (i.e., both hands or both feet) and occur infrequently in the preambulatory child. In contrast, scalds from deliberately dipping a child in hot water are clearly **demarcated**, in a stocking/glove distribution, sparing **flexural creases** (e.g., the creases behind the knees or inside the elbows) because these areas are "protected" when the child reflexively tries to withdraw. "Donut burns" with sparing of the buttocks occur in children who have been dipped into hot water, but whose buttocks are pushed firmly down against the relatively cooler surface of the tub or sink (**FIGURE 11-6**). Children with inflicted burns may also have arm or leg bruises where they were restrained.

Pattern burns that are an even thickness throughout or are repeated are red flags for maltreatment. Remember that any **acute** burn can be extremely

FIGURE 11-6 Donut burn.
Courtesy of Ron Deickmann, MD, FAAP.

painful. Advanced life support (ALS) providers should consider the administration of an analgesic as local protocol allows.

Fractures

Fractures in children who are not yet ambulatory are also suspicious for maltreatment. Although an infant who is being carried and is unintentionally dropped may sustain a fracture, it is not plausible that an infant who is only crawling or cruising could develop sufficient energy on their own to fracture a bone. Infant fractures of abuse have typical patterns on hospital radiographs. A history of **osteogenesis imperfecta** or problems causing decreased bone calcification may increase fracture occurrence in some children. Include these conditions in the documentation of the child's history.

Skin Signs That May Be Mistaken for Abuse

Sometimes, normal physical findings suggest an inflicted injury. For example, "**Mongolian spots**" are birthmarks frequently seen in children of color (e.g., African American, Asian, Latino) that can be easily mistaken for bruises (**FIGURE 11-7**). These birthmarks often take the form of large, flat patches of hyperpigmented skin, most commonly found on the low back or buttocks. Mongolian spots will blanch; bruises will not.

Certain disease states, such as **leukemia**, **vasculitis**, **meningococcemia**, or bleeding disorders (i.e., **hemophilia**), can rarely produce skin findings that appear to be bruises. Infectious processes, such as impetigo, can appear to be burns, but are much less painful. Insect bites in some children can cause redness

FIGURE 11-7 Mongolian spots appear on the buttocks, back, and extremities of many infants.

FIGURE 11-8 Cupping is the cultural practice of placing warm cups on the skin to pull out illness from the body. The red, flat, rounded skin lesions are often more intensely red at the borders.
Courtesy of the American Academy of Pediatrics.

and blistering. Distinguishing intentional injuries with certainty is sometimes impossible in the field.

Another benign skin finding that may be mistaken as abuse is the pattern of lesions produced by cultural rituals/traditional healing practices. The most common of these patterns are associated with Asian practices called **cupping** (**FIGURE 11-8**) and **coin rubbing** (**FIGURE 11-9**). These superficial lesions have distinctive rounded edges. Caregivers of these children can explain the purpose for such practices—information that can help distinguish injuries that are intended to help from inflicted injuries that are intended to harm.

CASE STUDY 2

You respond to an apartment at 3 AM for a baby not breathing. On arrival, an apparently intoxicated female meets you at the door with an unresponsive 6-month-old female, apneic and cyanotic, with no pulse. Your partner begins cardiopulmonary resuscitation, and you are able to determine that the woman is the grandmother who is supposed to be watching her granddaughter while the baby's mother is working an overnight shift. The grandmother tells you that she and the infant must have fallen asleep on the couch, and she woke up "next" to the baby and that she found the baby this way. You also notice several beer cans in the room. There are at least three blankets and a pillow piled up on the couch.

1. What are the red flags for maltreatment?
2. What are your medical and legal responsibilities?

FIGURE 11-9 Rubbing hot coins, often on the back, produces rounded and oblong red, patchy, flat skin lesions.
Courtesy of the American Academy of Pediatrics.

Summary of Duties, Communication, and Assessment in Suspected Maltreatment

When child maltreatment is suspected, the prehospital professional faces a challenging and potentially explosive situation. Communication with the child may be difficult or limited, and interactions with the caregiver may be frustrating and sometimes hostile.

A professional, nonjudgmental approach is necessary. Document conditions in the environment, the child's and caregiver's behaviors, the history, and relevant physical findings that may suggest maltreatment. The prehospital professional has a moral and legal duty to report suspected cases of maltreatment to the proper authorities.

The prehospital professional is in a unique position to recognize signs of possible child maltreatment. The initial principles of field care are the careful scene size-up, history taking, and physical assessment for physiologic abnormalities or anatomic patterns of inflicted injuries. Additional assessment and identification of "red flag" child and caregiver behaviors are sometimes extremely important to maltreatment investigations. The diagnosis of child maltreatment is rarely possible in the field. All cases require a complete investigation by the community CPS agency.

Legislation, Principles, and Protocols

Child Protective Services

The CPS agency is a legal community organization responsible for protection against child maltreatment. CPS has the legal authority to temporarily remove children at risk for injury or neglect from the home and to secure foster care placement. CPS is responsible for initial investigations of suspected maltreatment. They must make complicated and important decisions about the maltreatment accusations, at times remove children from the home and place them into foster care, and provide services for abusive and neglectful families. **TABLE 11-8** lists the initial actions of the CPS when a report is filed. CPS may work in concert with law enforcement to investigate the facts and determine

TABLE 11-8 Initial CPS Actions

When a report of child abuse or neglect is received, either from a health care professional or a law enforcement agency, the protocols of the receiving agency determine the timing and scope of the initial response.

The facts are reviewed to determine if a home visit is appropriate and, if so, which members of the team will be involved.

The CPS caseworker assesses risk to the child, the family's ability to provide safety, and supportive resources available to the family.

After the investigation and assessment, a reported incident is determined to be founded, unfounded, or unable to be determined because of lack of information.

who is responsible for maltreating the child. Ultimately, the judicial system determines if an accused individual is "guilty." Although emotions may run high when the prehospital professional suspects child maltreatment, it is neither appropriate nor safe to confront caregivers with these concerns at the scene.

CAUTION

Judging or confronting caregivers or attempting to intervene in issues of dysfunctional parenting may interfere with patient care or a subsequent maltreatment investigation. The caregiver may in fact not know how the child was injured or by whom. Your interventions may put you at risk, and a confrontation does not help the child.

The prehospital professional can provide scene information that helps CPS determine safe placement of the patient. When maltreatment is suspected, always note the presence of other children in the home. If a determination is made that an environment may be unsafe, contact law enforcement or CPS to evaluate the safety of any other children who are present, based on local EMS protocol. When a patient is transported to a hospital, communicate any concerns of maltreatment to hospital staff, who also have a mandatory obligation to report.

Another resource to know and be familiar with is the Child Abuse Prevention and Treatment Act (CAPTA). CAPTA is a federal law that provides funding, resources, grants, and guidance to states and organizations to protect children from child maltreatment. This law, among many other items, provides for a national clearinghouse to collect data (National Clearinghouse on Child Abuse and Neglect Information), establishes the Office on Abuse and Neglect, and coordinates activities and programs that serve this particular population. Other national resources of note include the Never Shake a Baby Campaign (National Center on Shaken Baby Syndrome; www.dontshake.org) and Healthy Families America (www.healthyfamilies america.org; which provides education and support to expecting and new parents to help with the arrival of a newborn in the family).

TIP

Note and report the presence of other children in situations suggestive of maltreatment.

CAUTION

Never attempt to physically restrain a caregiver or to forcibly take possession of a child. Call law enforcement if the scene is unsafe.

TIP

Even in the face of probable maltreatment, remain nonjudgmental with the caregiver; maintain control of the scene and transport.

CONTROVERSY

The on-scene role of law enforcement in suspected child maltreatment is controversial. In most cases, it is prudent to transport a child to the ED for physician and CPS evaluation. If the scene is not safe or caretakers are refusing transport, the prehospital professional must call law enforcement for protection and assistance.

Pediatric Human Trafficking

Human trafficking, while an international problem, proliferates today in the United States. It is estimated that there are over 40 million victims globally, with almost 30% of them children. Considered modern day slavery affecting both sexes, it is an international crime and is defined by the United Nations as the "recruitment, transfer, harboring or receipt of persons by means of threat or use of force or other forms of coercion, abduction, fraud, deception, the abuse of power or a position of vulnerability to achieve the consent of a person, having control over another person, for the purpose of exploitation."

In the United States, the average age at which the child enters the commercial sex industry is 12–14 years; however, infants and toddlers are not immune from this crime. It is not uncommon for a woman who is trafficked to allow or even sell her children to be trafficked as well. However, this is not the only way infants and children are introduced into the sex industry.

With limited life experience, poor impulse control, and poor critical thinking skills, it is easy to see why children are targeted. Additionally, minors are more easily coerced and controlled and are less likely to recognize they are victims, and thus a preferred population over adults. Very young children may be exploited for prostitution or production of child sexual material, such as videos and Internet sites, and may lack verbal skills to disclose their plight; however, their symptoms of abuse, such as temper tantrums and sleeping problems, may be misinterpreted or missed completely. While physical abuse or restraint may occur, it is not a necessary component of trafficking, as perpetrators prey on the child's vulnerability and use manipulation. Children who experience feelings of worthlessness or low self-esteem may be considered easy targets. This further enhances the trafficker's ability to manipulate the child into feeling they are loved and protected. While children from all walks of life can be affected, perpetrators may prey on those with minimal support systems. These can include, but not be limited to, runaway youth, homeless children, kidnapped children, LGBTQ youth, and those within the foster care system. Additionally, physical, emotional, or sexual abuse is a common precursor. These children may not realize that what they are experiencing is not normal and often are isolated and have threats or actual violence to make escape difficult.

Compounding this, the trafficker, who may be of a different culture or speak a different language, often destroys all forms of identification, drastically changes the appearance of the child, and travels frequently to reduce the ability of the child to get help.

Researchers have found that among adult and adolescent female trafficked survivors, almost 90% of them encountered a health care professional, including EMS providers, during the time they were being exploited. Of those, 63% were seen in the ED. Forty percent of trafficking survivors said that a physician could have done or said something to help them while they were in that situation, but did not. None of these survivors was asked by EMS, nurses, or physicians about their situation or were identified as being trafficked and, thus, they remained unidentified, resulting in a missed opportunity to rescue the individual. It is imperative that the interaction between not just ED staff, but EMS professionals, identify and begin treatment for trafficked children to avoid such a tragic omission in recognition.

Identifying an EMS patient as a victim of trafficking can be challenging, but the red flags of recognition can be helpful. It is unlikely that the child will speak up, so it is incumbent on the EMS professional to separate the child from others they may be with in order to ask questions. This may be the one thing that separates the child from a life of continued trafficking and one of being rescued. The trafficker will likely be very rehearsed, well spoken, and very presentable so as to not arouse suspicion. They also may appear very parental, caring, and sympathetic. The child may not be permitted to answer any questions, and the "friend" or "family member" may not allow the child to be alone with a medical professional. Developmental considerations must be recognized, as the very young child may not know his or her address, for example, but the older child who does not know his or her address, or what city or state he or she is in, should raise a red flag (see **TABLE 11-9**).

Questions must be asked in a developmentally appropriate, culturally sensitive, and child-centered manner. The EMS professional needs to build trust, convey respect in a nonjudgmental and patient manner, ensure the child's safety, and empower the child to participate in his or her care and rescue. Ensure that basic needs are met while in your care; in addition to

TABLE 11-9 Human Trafficking Red Flags

HISTORY

- Trafficker presents with multiple children who may be trafficking victims
- Person with child reluctant to leave him or her alone with medical professional
- Inconsistent or vague history
- Patient or trafficker angry if law enforcement is mentioned
- May not know address or how to get home upon discharge
- May have no identification or personal belongings
- History of suicide, suicide ideation, depression, mental health issues or substance abuse, posttraumatic stress disorder, shame, and guilt
- Unexplained absences from class
- Inappropriate dress for venue or weather conditions
- Sexualized behavior
- Overly tired in class
- Working while sick
- Untreated chronic illness
- Possession of fake identification or with children and hotel keys
- Trauma bonding (Stockholm syndrome: a condition that causes hostages to develop a psychological alliance with their captors as a survival strategy during captivity)
- Expensive items, such as clothing, handbags, or shoes; large amounts of cash; or any cash in the very young child
- Forced drug use
- No use of insurance; pays with cash
- Refers to boyfriend as "Daddy"
- History of running away (especially >3 times over past year), throwaway status (child being told to leave home or forbidden to return), or homelessness
- Child has older boyfriend/girlfriend (>4 years older)

PHYSICAL ASSESSMENT

- Chronic lack of care
- Failure to thrive, malnutrition, eating disorders
- Disheveled appearance
- Sexually transmitted infection
- Urinary tract infection
- Unusually high number of sexual partners
- Use of street slang, refers to "the life" or "the game," signs of gang affiliation (i.e., a preference for specific colors, notebook doodles of gang symbols, etc.)
- Cotton or debris in vagina to stop menstrual flow
- Foreign objects in vagina or rectum
- Pattern injury of causative agent (rope, lighter, electric cord, handprint, etc.)
- Trauma to vagina, scrotum, penis, or rectum
- Cigarette, iron, or acid burns
- Tuberculosis
- Dental caries/rotting teeth/bottle mouth
- Injuries to frenulum (from clapping hand over mouth or forcefully shoving bottle into mouth)
- Jaw and neck pain from strangulation
- History of abortions or miscarriages
- Physical injuries
- Ligature marks on neck, wrists, ankles
- Tattoos, especially with male name, branding, symbol of money, initial, slogan, or barcode, could indicate trafficking; often on back of neck, lower back, groin area, or feet as permanent mark or ownership and of being someone's "property"
- Hyperstartle reflexes
- Self-injury (cutting and scratching, hitting, biting, picking at skin, pulling out hair)

assuring the child that he or she is safe, ask the child if he or she is warm enough, hungry, or thirsty (keeping in mind the potential need for forensic evidence collection). If applicable, allow the child to have a choice to help empower him or her, as he or she likely has not had this right while in captivity. Do not allow anyone other than an official and approved translator to interpret for the child if English is not the native language. Remember the importance of sitting down or getting down to the eye level of the child. It is imperative to remember that play is the world of the child and much of this may be accomplished with the use of stuffed animals or other comfort items, songs or rhymes, and bubbles or other diversion techniques. The EMS professional may discover what is self-soothing to the child, such as thumb sucking, certain music, or positions of comfort, and make every attempt to allow the child to use them.

Just one or two red flags should create enough suspicion to assess further and communicate findings with ED staff. It is important to remember that summoning law enforcement or appearing to collaborate with police might cause the trafficker and/or the patient to refuse treatment or transport, placing the child in further jeopardy. When trafficking is suspected, a helpful question to ask, using age-appropriate language, is "Have you ever been made to do something that you didn't want to do?" Other questions are outlined in **TABLE 11-10**.

Having the distinct advantage of assessing the scene and environment, as well as the persons present during the EMS call, knowing the red flags and asking the right questions puts the EMS professional in the ideal position to identify and begin processes to rescue the child from human trafficking. Every pediatric encounter should provide heightened awareness

TABLE 11-10 Questions to Ask Potential Victims of Human Trafficking

Using age- and developmentally appropriate language, ask the following questions:

- Is it okay for you to be talking to me now? Will there be any problem with so-and-so if you and I are talking alone for a bit?
- Can you tell me what it is that makes it not okay to talk to me alone? Is there something we can do to make it all right, so you can feel comfortable talking to me?
- Can you come and go from your home or job whenever you please?
- Has anyone at home physically harmed you?
- Do you have to ask permission to eat, sleep, or use the bathroom?
- Are there locks on your doors or windows that prevent you from leaving?
- Have you ever been denied food, water, sleep, or medical care?
- Has anyone ever threatened your family?
- Has anyone ever taken away your identification papers or cards?
- Have you ever broken any bones, been knocked unconscious, or had any injuries that required stitches? (If yes, Can you tell me about those times?—determine if abuse, peer violence, dating violence.)
- Some kids have a hard time living at home and feel that they need to run away. Have you ever run away from home? (If yes: Have you stayed out all night, or longer? How many times have you run away? How long is the longest time you've been gone from home? When you were gone, how did you get money for food? Where did you stay?)
- Kids often use drugs or drink alcohol these days, and different kids use different drugs. Do you use drugs or drink alcohol? (Follow up with specifics—frequency of use, type of drug, reason for using drugs/alcohol [recreation, self-medication].)
- Sometimes kids have run-ins with police. Maybe for running away, for breaking curfew, for shoplifting. There can be lots of different reasons. Have you ever had any problems with the police? Do you feel comfortable telling me about them?
- Kids are getting involved with sex at different ages. They start having oral sex, vaginal sex, or anal sex at different times. Have you been sexually active in the past, and by that I mean having oral, vaginal, or anal sex? If child answers yes, then ask: Have you had more than five sexual partners? Have you ever had any sexually transmitted infections?
- Has a boyfriend, a girlfriend, or anyone else ever asked you or forced you to have sex with them or another person?
- Sometimes kids are in a position where they really need money, drugs, food, or a place to stay. They feel they have no option except to exchange sex or some sort of sexual activity for money or other things they need. Have you ever had to exchange sex for money, food, shelter, or something else you wanted?

for child sex trafficking regardless of gender, ethnicity, culture, sexual orientation, residence, health, socio-economic status, appearance, or behavior. As mandated child maltreatment reporters, it is imperative to know your state's law and to follow departmental policy and protocol when reporting child human trafficking suspicions. EMS can be the intersection between the child and the outside world, making this single interaction life changing for the child and his or her family.

See **TABLE 11-11** for helpful resources and phone numbers.

TABLE 11-11 Resources

National Center for Missing & Exploited Children
1-800-843-5678

If you have information about a missing child or suspected child sexual exploitation, call to report it or visit their website (http://www.missingkids.com/).

National Human Trafficking Hotline
1-888-373-7888

The National Human Trafficking Hotline is a national anti-trafficking hotline and resource center serving victims and survivors of human trafficking and the anti-trafficking community in the United States. The toll-free hotline is answered live 24 hours a day, 7 days a week, 365 days a year. For more information, visit www.humantraffickinghotline.org.

The National Runaway Switchboard
1-800-RUNAWAY

The National Runaway Switchboard (NRS) serves as the federally designated national communication system for homeless and runaway youth. NRS, with the support of more than 150 volunteers, handles an average of 100,000 calls annually—more than 3 million calls since the organization's inception. Through hotline and online services, NRS provides crisis intervention, referrals to local resources, and education and prevention services to youth, families and community members throughout the country 24 hours a day, 365 days a year. For more information, visit www.1800RUNAWAY.org.

U.S. Immigration and Customs Enforcement
1-866-347-2423 (United States & Canada)
1-802-872-6199 (International Calls)

ICE's hotline to report suspected child predators and any suspicious activity.
Call or complete an online tip form (www.ice.gov/tips/).

CASE STUDY 3

9-1-1 is called by a babysitter because a child has been burned. On arrival at the scene, the EMS crew finds a teenage girl holding a sobbing 2-year-old boy. The teenager states that the child has been fussy and crying for the 2 hours in her care. On changing the child's diaper, the sitter noted what looked like burns on the buttocks, and on her mother's advice called 9-1-1.

The child is alert but upset and is not easily consolable by the babysitter. There is no increased work of breathing; the skin color is pink. There are areas of denuded skin on the buttocks covered with diaper rash cream, with one unpopped blister near the sacrum. The centers of both buttocks, and the gluteal cleft, do not appear to be injured. Extremity examination shows no bruises or other abnormalities.

1. Is this injury caused from abuse?
2. What interventions are indicated?

CASE STUDY ANSWERS

CASE STUDY 1

Be alert for the signs of abusive head trauma in any infant or small child with a sudden onset of altered mental status and irregular respirations. Remember that grab bruises and marks may be found on the arms of children who are held and shaken, and their presence should be documented. Carefully document the scene, the comments of the caregiver, and the reported events leading to the injury.

Immediate transportation is critical. One common complication of inflicted head injury is Cushing's triad of bradycardia, elevated blood pressure, and irregular respirations, which can lead to respiratory failure or apnea as a result of elevated intracranial pressure and compression of the medulla (respiratory center in the brainstem). Be prepared to provide respiratory support. Ensure that the ED staff will make a report to the CPS agency, or file a report yourself.

CASE STUDY 2

This case may be the result of the grandmother accidently suffocating the infant. Co-sleeping, especially with a caregiver who is under the influence of alcohol or drugs, can have deadly consequences. Adults may roll over on top of infants and not realize it because of their intoxicated state. Infants do not have the strength to push back or to get the adult to notice that he or she is lying on them. Make a note of the scene, and call law enforcement. Your attention needs to be focused on resuscitation efforts for the child.

CASE STUDY 3

This child has obvious signs of an inflicted scald injury. The lack of burn in the creases and the center of the buttocks (donut burn) may indicate the child was forcibly held in hot water. There is no way for the prehospital professional to know who inflicted the injury, nor is establishing responsibility part of his or her role.

Provide analgesia if possible. Large burns can lead to significant fluid losses, so ALS providers should start an intravenous line and begin fluid resuscitation. Document the scene size-up, the child's and caregiver's behaviors, and the history. Transport this child to an ED for burn care as well as an evaluation for inflicted injury. Treatment at a burn center may ultimately be necessary.

SUGGESTED REFERENCES

Textbooks

American Academy of Pediatrics and the American College of Emergency Physicians. *APLS: The Pediatric Emergency Medicine Resource*. 5th ed. Burlington, MA: Jones and Bartlett Learning; 2012.

Bush KM. Human trafficking. In: *Emergency Nurse Pediatric Course*. Burlington MA: Jones & Bartlett; 2018:143–149.

Hazinski M, Zaritsky A, Nadkarni V, et al. *PALS Provider Manual*. Dallas: American Heart Association; 2016.

Lasky A, Sirotnak A. *Child Abuse: Medical Diagnosis and Management*. 4th ed. Itasca, IL: American Academy of Pediatrics; 2019.

Articles

Andrea G, Asnes AG, Leventhal JM. Managing child abuse. *Pediatr Rev*. 2010;31(2):47–55.

Becker H.J, Bechtel K. Recognizing victims of human trafficking in the pediatric emergency department. *Pediatr Emerg Care*. 2015;31(2):144–147.

Donahue S, Schwien M, LaVallee D. Educating emergency department staff on the identification and treatment of human trafficking victims. *J Emerg Nurs*. 2019;45(1):16–23.

Ernewein C, Nieves R. Human sex trafficking: recognition, treatment, and referral of pediatric victims. *J Nurse Pract*, 2015;11(8):797–803.

Escobar MA, Wallenstein KG, Christianson-Lagay ER, et al. Child abuse and the pediatric surgeon: A position statement from the Trauma Committee, the Board of Governors and the Membership of the American pediatric Surgical Association. *J Pediatr Surg*. 2019;54:1277–1285.

Grace AM, Lippert S, Collins K, et al. Educating health care professionals on human trafficking. *Pediatr Emerg Care*. 2014;30(12):856.

Greenbaum VJ, Dodd M, McCracken C. A short screening tool to identify victims of child sex trafficking in the health care setting. *Pediatr Emerg Care*. 2018;34(1):33–37.

Hoehn EF, Wilson PM, Riney LC, et al. Identification and evaluation of physical abuse in children. *Pediatr Ann*. 2018;47(3):e97–e101.

Johnson CF. Child maltreatment 2002: Recognition, reporting and risk. *Pediatr Int*. 2002;44:554–560.

Kairys S. Distinguishing sudden infant death syndrome from child abuse fatalities. American Academy of Pediatrics Committee on Child Abuse and Neglect. *Pediatrics*. 2001;107(2):437–441.

Kempe CH. The battered child syndrome. *JAMA*. 1962;181:17–24.

Krug EG, Dahlberg LL, Mercy JA, et al. World report on violence and health. Geneva: World Health Organization; 2002.

Normandin PA. Child human trafficking: see, pull, cut the threads of abuse. *J Emerg Nurs*. 43(6); 588–590.

Pierce MC, Kaczor K, Aldridge S, et al. Bruising characteristics discriminating physical abuse from accidental trauma. *Pediatrics*. 2010;125:67–74.

Other Resources

American Academy of Pediatrics. *Visual Diagnosis of Child Abuse*. 4th ed. [CD-ROM]. Itasca, IL: American Academy of Pediatrics; 2016.

Child Welfare Information Gateway. What is child abuse and neglect? Recognizing the signs and the symptoms. https://www.childwelfare.gov/pubpdfs/whatiscan.pdf. Accessed July 5, 2019.

Child Welfare Information Gateway. Child maltreatment 2017: summary of key findings. https://www.childwelfare.gov/topics/systemwide/statistics/can/can-stats/. Accessed July 5, 2019.

Children's Healthcare of Atlanta. Clinical Practice Guideline for Assessment and Treatment of Potential Victims of Child Sex Trafficking and Commercial Sexual Exploitation (CSEC) ≥ 11 yrs old. http://aapdc.org/wp-content/uploads/2013/12/Child-Sex-Trafficking-FINAL-published-guideline-may-28-2015.pdf. Accessed July 16, 2019.

Gelles RJ, Perlman S. *Estimated Annual Cost of Child Abuse and Neglect*. Chicago, IL: Prevent Child Abuse America; 2012.

Ford, H. Child, infant sex trafficking; It's like the Wild West. https://www.11alive.com/article/sports/nfl/superbowl/child-infant-sex-trafficking-its-like-the-wild-west/85-f4c0520a-acb7-4370-abbd-be8139caa99d. Accessed July 16, 2019.

Lauridsen J, Levin A, Parrish R, et al. *Shaken Baby Syndrome: A Visual Overview*. Version 3.0. National Center on Shaken Baby Syndrome(CD-ROM).

Polaris. The Facts. https://polarisproject.org/human-trafficking/facts. Accessed July 16, 2019.

US Department of Health & Human Services, Administration for Children and Families, Administration on Children, Youth and Families, Children's Bureau. 2017.Child Maltreatment https://www.acf.hhs.gov/cb/research-data-technology/statistics-research/child-maltreatment. Accessed August 30, 2019.

Hotlines and Websites

National Center for Missing and Exploited Children. 1-800-843-5678

National Human Trafficking Hotline. 1-888-373-7888 www.Humantraffickinghotline.org

National Runaway Switchboard 1-800-RUNAWAY www.RUNAWAY.org

U.S. Immigration and Customs Enforcement. 1-866-347-2423 (United States and Canada) 1-802-872-6199 (international)

© maczkus/iStock/Getty Images.

CHAPTER 12

Emergency Delivery and Newborn Stabilization

Andrew Bartkus, RN, MSN, JD, CEN, CCRN, CFRN, NREMT-P, FP-C

Tabitha Cheng, MD

Joyce Foresman-Capuzzi, MSN, APRN, CCNS, CEN, CPEN, CTRN, TCRN, CPN, EMT-P, FAEN

LEARNING OBJECTIVES

1. Describe the components of the patient history and physical exam that would identify pregnant patients at risk for emergent delivery of a newborn outside of a hospital setting.

2. List potential maternal, fetal, and newborn risk factors that may adversely affect the health of the mother or child during or immediately after delivery.

3. Compare and contrast when it is appropriate to initiate transport of a pregnant patient to a hospital for delivery of a newborn versus when it is appropriate to prepare for imminent delivery of a newborn in the prehospital setting.

4. Describe how to prepare for a delivery, perform a delivery, and provide postdelivery care to the mother and newborn.

5. Recognize the conditions, and identify the correct interventions when complications jeopardize the health of the mother or newborn during childbirth.

6. Explain the indications and technique for assisting ventilations in a newborn infant.

7. Identify situations in which a newborn infant might require vascular access for drug and fluid administration.

Introduction

Emergency medical services (EMS) providers may be called to assess a patient in labor or assist with childbirth in the prehospital setting. In early history, childbirth occurred in the home, often without the presence of trained medical personnel. Gradually, it has evolved into a highly specialized area of medicine, using technology and hospitalization for care of the mother and delivery of the child. Despite the overwhelming trend toward childbirth in a health care setting, a significant number of parents choose to deliver a child at home. Over 1% of childbirths occur each year outside the hospital setting, with the trend steadily increasing since 2004.

Approximately 30% of planned home births involve a certified nurse midwife, while the remainder are attended by "lay midwives" or other non certified attendants. For these patients, EMS providers may become the only trained option when complications develop for the mother or newborn. EMS personnel may encounter pregnant patients in active labor in a variety of prehospital settings. EMS may be called to assist with transport of childbirth when labor or pregnancy is unrecognized or concealed, when a transportation misadventure prevents a patient in labor from reaching a hospital in time, when unexpected complications develop during a planned out-of-hospital delivery, or when labor or precipitous delivery occurs in another prehospital setting.

Obstetric Delivery in the Prehospital Setting

EMS Capabilities, Scope of Practice, and Legal Pitfalls

Newborn delivery is not a common procedure in the prehospital setting, so the level of anxiety for both the laboring patient and the prehospital professional is often high. Most newborns require only minimal assistance to make the transition to life outside the uterus. EMS providers should remain aware that although most obstetric deliveries require minimal resuscitative efforts, complications during delivery have the potential to cause devastating, lifelong neurologic impairment for the child. Limited training, experience, scope of practice, and equipment may prevent EMS providers from recognizing serious complications of pregnancy or delivery until it is too late to prevent injury to the mother or child. Although uncomplicated childbirth is arguably a basic life support (BLS) level skill, many neonatal or maternal complications outlined in this chapter require advanced life support (ALS) interventions. The highest level of prehospital care available should be requested when prehospital childbirth is imminent.

Ethical Considerations and EMS Professionalism

The goal of every obstetric delivery is a healthy mother and child. Not every childbirth performed by EMS providers produces a viable, healthy newborn. Extreme fetal prematurity and latent fetal demise each create situations where full resuscitative efforts may not be appropriate. EMS providers periodically encounter these situations without the benefit of prior diagnosis and often without the opportunity to discuss resuscitation decisions with the child's parents in a controlled environment. When faced with this situation, EMS providers should contact medical control and delicately balance ethical responsibilities to the patient(s) with the professional requirement to adhere to EMS laws and regulations pertaining to initiation and termination of resuscitation.

Complications During Pregnancy

A wide variety of conditions can adversely impact the health of the mother and fetus during pregnancy. These conditions have the potential to create complications for the mother or newborn during or after delivery. EMS providers should consider these conditions when weighing the risks and benefits of performing a delivery in the prehospital setting versus initiating prompt transport to a health care facility for delivery. Many complications, such as certain breech presentations or placenta previa, simply cannot be managed in the prehospital setting. When known complications exist that are beyond the ability of EMS personnel, it is often better to begin transportation immediately.

Preterm Labor

Preterm labor refers to labor beginning before the 37th week of gestation. EMS providers should expect complications roughly proportional to the degree of

---

EMS is requested to respond to a local mall for a 32-year-old woman reported to be in labor. The patient reports that she is 38 weeks pregnant and this is her fourth pregnancy. She has been having contractions for 30 minutes just after her "bag of water broke," but they are now becoming more frequent and intense. She states she was in labor for 3 hours with her last child.

1. What questions will help you determine whether to transport immediately or perform a delivery at the scene?
2. What physical findings would tell you to prepare to deliver on scene?

prematurity. Technologic advances allow newborns as young as 22–24 weeks to survive, although often with severe, lifelong complications. Infants delivered before 22 weeks' gestation have a low chance of survival, although there are isolated case reports of infants between 21 and 22 weeks surviving with minimal or no long-term complications. Between 24 and 37 weeks, each additional week of gestation reduces the impact or severity of complications on a newborn. EMS providers may encounter patients in labor with a gestational age younger than 22–23 weeks; in many instances, the infant will not survive an out-of-hospital delivery. Follow local protocols regarding neonatal resuscitation, but many protocols call for no resuscitation in neonates younger than 24 weeks with no signs of life after delivery. If the gestational age is not known, some findings to identify preterm infants include body hair (lanugo), eyelids fused shut (eyes open at 26–29 weeks), foot <40 mm, transparent skin, low body fat (weight <2 lbs), and low muscle tone. Older preterm infants require immediate assistance from health care providers who specialize in newborn resuscitation. Treatment of a patient in preterm labor is largely supportive until definitive care can be reached.

Postterm Pregnancy

The normal gestational period lasts from 37 to 42 weeks. As a fetus remains in the uterus past 42 weeks, the uterus and placenta are unable to support the physiologic and environmental needs of the growing fetus. The fetus may become distressed and stool (expel meconium) while still within the amniotic sac and uterus. If the fetus inhales the amniotic fluid while in the uterus, the meconium in the fluid may cause respiratory distress after delivery. In a mother who is postterm or has meconium-stained fluid leaking from her vagina, EMS providers should provide supportive care to the mother and expect a difficult labor and delivery and newborn resuscitation.

Multiple Gestations

Most multifetal (more than one fetus) pregnancies are diagnosed during prenatal care. Every maternal assessment should include questions about the possibility of multiple gestations, especially if delivery is believed to be imminent. EMS providers should consider every multifetal pregnancy a high-risk pregnancy. Breech presentation, umbilical cord prolapse, premature labor, and a variety of other maternal and fetal conditions are more common when more than one fetus is present.

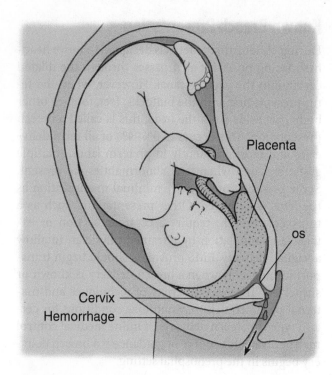

FIGURE 12-1 Placenta previa.

Placenta Previa

During gestation, the placenta may become implanted either partially or completely over the cervical os (opening) at the base of the uterus. This is placenta previa (**FIGURE 12-1**). If placental rupture occurs, either from cervical dilation or mechanical perforation, bleeding can be massive and is usually painless. Patients with a placenta over or close to the cervical os (opening) require a cesarean section for delivery. Profound hemorrhage can be fatal for mother and fetus. These patients cannot safely have childbirth by EMS in the field. Prompt transport of patients with placenta previa or painless vaginal bleeding should begin immediately.

Placental Abruption

Prehospital professionals may also encounter patients with a placental abruption (abruptio placentae). In these patients, the placenta has either partially or completely detached from the uterine wall, causing venous bleeding. In contrast to placenta previa, patients with placental abruption tend to have abdominal pain with darker vaginal bleeding. Other symptoms include uterine contractions, abdominal tenderness, and signs of fetal distress. Prehospital management is focused on restoring circulating fluid volume and immediate transportation to a facility capable of fetal monitoring and definitive management.

Known Breech Presentation

During childbirth, the fetus is designed to move head-first, facing posterior as it passes through the dilated cervix into the vaginal canal. However, when the fetus presents first with the buttocks, feet, foot, or other body part aside from the head, this is called a breech presentation. This occurs in 3%–4% of all term deliveries and more frequently in preterm labor, multiple gestations, and when fetal abnormalities are present. Some presentations require minimal manipulation as the fetus is delivered. Other presentations, such as a transverse breech, require a cesarean section or extensive manipulation by a trained physician to allow a vaginal delivery. EMS providers should begin transport immediately when a breech delivery is known or suspected. There are a variety of techniques and maternal positions that may optimize conditions for certain types of breech deliveries. Online medical control may be a valuable source of guidance if a breech delivery begins in the prehospital setting.

Triage of a Patient in Labor

EMS providers must be capable of deciding whether a patient can safely be transported to a hospital for childbirth or when they must prepare for an imminent delivery outside the hospital. The goal of every EMS response should be to transport the patient in labor to a hospital before childbirth occurs. Physicians and nurses, experienced in labor and delivery, have the training, diagnostic equipment, and procedural skills necessary to intervene in many situations that cannot be adequately managed in the prehospital setting. In instances when labor has progressed or delivery is imminent, EMS providers may be forced to assist with childbirth outside the hospital. Transport time, type of health care facilities available, EMS capabilities, anticipated complications, and ultimately the patient presentation guide the decision regarding whether to transport or assist with childbirth on scene.

Maternal History

EMS providers should obtain a brief, focused patient history when assessing a patient suspected to be in labor. Many factors help determine whether delivery is imminent or if complications should be expected. Ultimately, the answer to three questions helps determine whether EMS should anticipate a prehospital delivery (**TABLE 12-1**):

1. How many times has the patient given birth? Typically, the time in active labor is longer for first-time mothers (primiparas) than for women who

TABLE 12-1 Determining if Delivery is Imminent
Questions
Is this your first delivery?
If you have delivered before, how long was the labor?
Do you feel the "urge to push"?
Physical Findings
Is the child's head crowning?
Is the head or scalp visible at the perineum during contractions?

have had prior deliveries (multiparas). If this is not a first-time delivery, ask the woman the length of her previous labors. A history of short labor with prior pregnancies may repeat itself. Unless there is a long period between pregnancies, expect each successive labor to be shorter than the previous.

2. Does the patient feel the need to push? Most pregnant patients experience this sensation as delivery becomes imminent, usually within 30 minutes, often sooner. Patients with the urge to push require immediate inspection of the perineum and preparation for delivery.

3. Do anatomic conditions allow for a successful prehospital delivery? Such conditions as placenta previa or transverse breech presentation cannot be safely delivered in the prehospital setting. Transportation should begin immediately.

As time permits, prehospital providers should inquire about maternal medical history (including medications and allergies), whether abnormalities were identified during prenatal care, previous complications during delivery, and gestational age of the fetus. The gestational age or the due date may be calculated from the last menstrual period or the expected date of conception. Other factors, such as rupture of membranes, the possibility of multiple gestations, and prior newborn anomalies, should also be included when obtaining a patient history. History may be obtained while simultaneously performing a physical examination or preparing the ambulance and equipment for delivery.

Maternal Physical Assessment

Every patient encountered by EMS requires a primary assessment to identify any immediate threats to life.

This assessment includes airway patency, the quality of respirations and perfusion, and an assessment of level of consciousness. In many instances, immediate threats to life can be excluded if a patient is awake, speaking appropriately in full sentences, and demonstrating good skin color and strong pulses. Any deviation from these findings suggests a potential threat to life and must be further evaluated before proceeding to a more focused assessment related to the pregnancy.

The prehospital provider needs to perform a brief physical assessment of the perineum if an imminent delivery is suspected. Look for **crowning**—the visible appearance of the fetal head at the **vaginal introitus** (**FIGURE 12-2**). Crowning is a sign that delivery is near.

If the child's head is not immediately visible, inspect the mother's perineum during a contraction and note if the head becomes visible. If the infant is crowning or if the head is visible at the perineum with contractions, prepare for delivery unless the transport time is extremely brief (<5 minutes). Assessment of the perineum should be deferred if imminent delivery is unlikely and the patient is able to reliably report the absence of any pressure, unusual sensation (including urge to defecate), or fluid discharge (blood or amniotic fluid) in the vaginal area. The presence or suspicion of any of these items requires a visual inspection of the perineum by the EMS provider.

Amniotic fluid, released from the vagina before delivery, should be examined for meconium (fetal stool), a dark-green viscous substance visible in the normally clear amniotic fluid. Meconium aspiration is a major concern for newborns, and meconium aspiration syndrome may result.

Uterine contractions provide valuable clues regarding the likelihood of a prehospital delivery. Most patients in active labor demonstrate obvious contractions readily identifiable through simple visual observation of a patient. The patient may show periods of discomfort, panting respirations, and often verbalize that a contraction is occurring. Gentle palpation of the abdomen reveals a uterus that becomes noticeably firm during a contraction and relaxes between contractions. When contractions increase in intensity and duration, while becoming closer together (<2 minutes from the start of one until the start of the next), delivery of the newborn is expected within a short period of time. It is always possible for patients to present with subtle contractions, occasionally described as back pain, urge to defecate, or even abdominal or menstrual cramping. The absence of classic, obvious uterine contractions does not exclude the potential for imminent prehospital delivery.

Breech Deliveries

Three to four percent of term deliveries are breech deliveries (**FIGURE 12-3**). Inspection of the perineum does not show a head crowning, but another anatomic part, such as the feet or buttocks, might be visible. In this situation, transport immediately to the nearest emergency department with labor and delivery capabilities. Given the risk of complications and the potential need for an emergency cesarean section to safely deliver the baby, initiate transport to the hospital as soon as a breech presentation is identified, even if delivery

FIGURE 12-2 Use the presence or absence of crowning to help decide whether to transport or prepare for delivery.

FIGURE 12-3 Breech birth.

seems imminent. If the feet are presenting first and the infant is delivering, support the body while the head is delivered; however, if the head fails to deliver, place a gloved hand into the vagina with fingers between infant's face and uterine wall to create an open airway.

Additional Complications

Many of the conditions identified during the prenatal period or through the maternal history and physical examination prompt EMS providers to anticipate complications. Some complications can be mitigated by the skills and experience of EMS providers, but many complications require specialized care, techniques, and equipment not available in the prehospital setting. When potential or certain complications are identified, EMS providers must carefully consider whether the risks and benefits of delivering a newborn on scene (**TABLE 12-2**) exceed the risks and benefits of initiating prompt transportation (**TABLE 12-3**).

TABLE 12-2 Risks and Benefits of Delivery on Scene

Benefits	Risks
▪ At least one additional EMS provider to assist with delivery ▪ Nobody is needed to drive the transport vehicle at this time	▪ No progress toward definitive care if complications develop or additional trained personnel or equipment are needed
▪ Possible helpful assistance from patient's family or bystanders	▪ Bystanders or patient's family may interfere with patient care, disrupt privacy, or otherwise distract EMS providers from providing optimal care
▪ No vehicle movement, noise, or road hazards to undermine patient care	▪ The scene may pose safety hazards to EMS personnel or patient; may not have adequate climate control for newborn care
▪ Possibly more room to assess patient and deliver newborn	▪ Scene may have less room, more obstacles, or poor lighting, which make assessment and newborn delivery more difficult

TABLE 12-3 Risks and Benefits of Initiating Prompt Transportation

Benefits	Risks
▪ Movement toward definitive patient care where trained personnel, specialized equipment, and a controlled environment are available	▪ One less EMS provider to assist with patient care (this may be mitigated in certain situations if an alternate trained driver is available)
▪ Patient may have increased privacy in the transport vehicle, without detrimental interference from bystanders or family members	▪ Limited or no assistance available from family or bystanders
▪ May avoid safety risks and uncontrolled environmental temperature that may have been present on scene	▪ Vehicle movement, noise, and road hazards may undermine patient care efforts
▪ May have more room to assess patient and deliver the newborn than was available on scene ▪ May have better lighting; resuscitation equipment immediately available	▪ May have less room or less access to the patient for assessment and newborn delivery

Transport Considerations for the Patient in Labor

Patients in labor, who have not delivered before transport, may require a wide range of services at the destination hospital. This is also true when a newborn has been delivered and complications are present. The destination decision for EMS providers is based on a combination of patient preference, geographic location, and the type of services required by the mother and child. When complications are expected and delivery is not imminent, it may be much better to bypass a smaller community hospital and transport the patient to a health care facility with high-risk obstetric services or neonatal intensive care unit capabilities. Conversely, it may be in the patient's best interest to transport directly to the closest available facility where the mother or child can be stabilized before a longer transport to a tertiary care center. EMS providers should consult with online medical control when required by protocol or when the appropriate destination choice is not clear. Providers should also make efforts to understand the obstetric capabilities of the various destination hospitals within their coverage area. Not every hospital has labor and delivery services. In many locations, obstetric physicians are not always in the hospital. Early notification provides hospitals the opportunity to activate essential resources when they are not immediately available 24 hours, 7 days a week.

Routine care for patients in labor includes skills frequently performed by EMS. Patients in labor who are hypoxemic should receive supplemental oxygen to prevent or limit the severity of unrecognized fetal hypoxemia. The routine use of oxygen in the absence of maternal hypoxemia is controversial. Consult local guidelines or online medical control regarding oxygen use in these situations. Intravenous (IV) fluids should be administered to patients in active labor to prevent dehydration or hemoconcentration and maintain a favorable fluid volume status.

Vital signs remain a valuable part of any prehospital patient assessment and should be monitored at appropriate intervals during patient care. Patients in active labor may have vital signs temporarily deferred if delivery is imminent, personnel are limited, and the primary assessment does not suggest any likelihood of abnormality.

Because of the position of the vena cava, pregnant patients are at risk of hypotension when placed in a supine position. In the supine position, the uterus can compress the inferior vena cava, which may decrease preload to the heart, resulting in decreased cardiac output. This is primarily a complication during the third trimester. Whether placed on an ambulance stretcher or backboard, the pregnant patient

FIGURE 12-4 A pregnant patient tipped in a left lateral recumbant position.
© Jones & Bartlett Learning. Courtesy of MIEMSS.

should be positioned on an angle to one side or the other to displace the uterus off of her inferior vena cava and promote optimal blood return to her heart (**FIGURE 12-4**). The left lateral recumbent position is preferred, but this may not be possible in certain transport vehicles when continuous airway monitoring is needed. Stretcher and backboard straps should not be placed over the pregnant patient's gravid abdomen. Place straps or seat belts above and below the patient's abdomen instead during transport.

> **TIP**
>
> The "urge to push" experienced by most women at the end of labor is a sign that delivery is near, usually within 30–60 minutes.

> **CAUTION**
>
> Never try to deliver a baby with a breech presentation in the field. Initiate transport to the hospital as soon as a breech presentation is identified, even if delivery seems imminent.

Summary of Triage of Patient in Labor

The responses to the three previously asked questions (Table 12-1), along with visual assessment of the perineum, provide the essential information to triage a laboring woman in the field. Known breech births and patients diagnosed with placenta previa require immediate transport, regardless of whether or not delivery is imminent. Other findings obtained from the maternal history and physical examination influence the decision whether to initiate transport or prepare for delivery on scene.

Preparation for Delivery

Resuscitation-Oriented History

Many factors in the mother's medical history affect the outcome of the baby and help predict the need for resuscitation of the newborn. However, once the decision has been made to deliver on scene, only four questions are pertinent for the immediate safety of the newborn (**TABLE 12-4**):

1. Is there more than one **fetus** present? If twins or multiple newborns are expected, prepare for more than one delivery. This may mean finding extra equipment, preparing an additional warm environment, and planning the management of the first baby while delivering the second. This usually requires calling for a second ambulance. In tiered EMS systems, an ALS ambulance should be requested.

2. When are you due to deliver? A significant number of out-of-hospital deliveries are preterm (less than 37 weeks' **gestation**), and the further from the expected delivery date, the greater the chances of delivering a depressed newborn. Knowing the due date is important for preparing the right resuscitation equipment for airway management and breathing support. Make sure there are masks

sized for preterm newborns less than 30 weeks' gestation. Have ready a size 0 **laryngoscope** blade and endotracheal tubes in sizes to fit the expected size of the newborn (**FIGURE 12-5**).

3. What color is the **amniotic fluid**? Greenish color in the amniotic fluid is a sign of passage of **meconium**, which is fetal stool. Meconium is released by the fetus during periods of intrauterine stress, especially hypoxia. If meconium is observed, be prepared to deal with a depressed baby

TABLE 12-4 Resuscitation-Oriented History: Four Essential Questions
Do you have twins or multiple fetuses?
When are you due to deliver?
What color is the amniotic fluid?
Are there any risk factors?

FIGURE 12-5 Special equipment for premature infant resuscitation: bag-mask device with small mask, size 0 laryngoscope blade, and endotracheal tubes sizes 2.5 and 3.0.

TIP

A large number of out-of-hospital deliveries are preterm, and the need for resuscitative efforts rises with the number of weeks of prematurity.

CASE STUDY 2

You are called to a residence by a woman in labor who has no transportation to the hospital. On arrival you find the woman lying on the floor screaming, "It's time!" She tells you that this is her sixth baby and the last one came "real quick." Her water broke 30 minutes ago, and it was clear. Your examination shows the baby is crowning and the mother has an urge to push.

1. What four questions are most appropriate to ask at this time to best prepare for delivery?

2. What equipment should be prepared for delivery?

or airway obstruction. Suctioning of the baby's mouth, oropharynx, and nose to clear the airway of thick meconium may be necessary.

4. Are there any risk factors? This can include gestational hypertension (**preeclampsia**), maternal diabetes, or maternal drug use. If the mother has preeclampsia, this puts her at risk for seizures. If she is a diabetic, the infant of a diabetic mother tends to be large, especially if postdates. If the mother is drug addicted, the infant may be born depressed (nonvigorous) and require assisted ventilation.

Assembling Equipment

If the triage decision is to deliver on scene, get the appropriate equipment ready. **TABLE 12-5** lists the essential ambulance equipment, best organized in a portable **obstetric** pack (**FIGURE 12-6**).

Warming the Environment

Avoiding hypothermia is an important part of newborn care. Before delivery, make the room or ambulance as warm as possible. Turn up the heat until it is uncomfortable for an adult. Air blowing across the newborn can lead to heat loss, so turn off all fans. If the setting allows, consider having a family member warm towels in the dryer in anticipation of the delivery.

TABLE 12-5	Contents of a Portable Obstetric Pack for Vaginal Delivery
Number	**Item**
1	Sterile disposable scalpel or scissors
3	Disposable towels
1	Receiving blanket
1	Sterile disposable bulb syringe
2	Sterile umbilical clamps or ties
1	Large plastic bag with twist tie (to store the **placenta**)
2	Plastic-lined underpads
1	Disposable plastic apron, mask, and protective eyewear

Positioning the Mother

Although it is a medical emergency for the patient and the family, the delivery of a baby is also a highly personal and emotional event. Establish a plan for positioning for delivery with the mother, but let her stay in a comfortable position and covered before delivery.

A safe maternal position for the delivery is lying supine (on her back) on one side of a bed. Allow her to deliver the baby onto the bed with minimal handling (**FIGURE 12-7**). Suctioning the baby's mouth and nose, if

FIGURE 12-6 Obstetric pack.

FIGURE 12-7 A safe position for delivery is with the mother lying supine on one side of a bed, allowing her to deliver the baby onto the bed with minimal handling.

necessary, before delivery of the body is difficult with the mother in this position because most infants are born face down. Another technique involves raising the mother's buttocks with a stack of folded towels to allow oropharyngeal suctioning of the baby, if necessary, after the head has been delivered.

Another safe position is the Sims position, in which the mother lies on her side with her back toward the attendant and her knees drawn toward her chest (**FIGURE 12-8**). In this position, the infant's head is easy to reach for suctioning if necessary. Additionally, the mother's perineum is still over the bed, so delivery onto the bed with minimal handling is still possible.

A third position to consider is with the woman lying supine and positioned sideways on the bed, with each foot on a separate chair and her perineum at the edge of the bed (**FIGURE 12-9**). After the baby's head is delivered, this position provides enough space to suction the mouth and nose if necessary before delivering the body. The disadvantage of this position is the lack of a supportive surface under the perineum, so that the prehospital professional must actually "catch" the baby.

Selecting a Clean Delivery Surface

Select a surface that is as clean as possible to conduct the immediate care of the child. Make sure everyone involved in the child's care has washed their hands and has several pairs of gloves.

Performing the Delivery

Most babies deliver themselves without assistance, especially if the laboring mother is lying supine or in the Sims position in bed. Although the prehospital professional may attempt to control the delivery as described next, only minimal interference with this natural process is necessary in most cases.

Use the following sequence for all deliveries:

1. Allow the mother to push the head out of the vaginal opening. You may need to place gentle pressure on the infant's head as it comes out to prevent too rapid of a delivery.
2. Next, with one finger, feel the infant's neck for the umbilical cord (**FIGURE 12-10**). If it is there, gently lift it over the baby's head. Do not pull hard on the cord because it may lead to avulsion of the cord with severe hemorrhage.
3. If the woman is delivering in bed, let the delivery proceed without intervention. Place one hand

FIGURE 12-8 The Sims position has the mother on her side with her back toward the attendant and her knees drawn toward her chest.

FIGURE 12-9 Alternate delivery position. The woman is perpendicular to the bed with each foot on a separate chair and her perineum at the edge of the bed.

FIGURE 12-10 Ensure the umbilical cord is not wrapped around the baby's neck.

FIGURE 12-11 Place a hand around the neck posteriorly and one underneath the infant to help control the delivery.

© Eddie Lawrence/Science Source.

FIGURE 12-12 On occasion, the infant's anterior shoulder may need to be pulled posteriorly to clear the mother's symphysis pubis. This can be accomplished by placing a hand on either side of the infant's head and gently pulling downward.

around the infant's neck **posteriorly** and one hand underneath the infant to help support the delivery (**FIGURE 12-11**). On occasion, the infant's anterior shoulder needs to be gently moved posteriorly to clear the mother's **symphysis pubis**. Place a hand on either side of the infant's head and gently pull downward (**FIGURE 12-12**).

4. For an infant (term or preterm) who is vigorous, position the infant on the mother's abdomen and delay cord clamping for 30–60 seconds. If the infant is not vigorous, or if there is concern for placenta abruption, clamp the cord and begin resuscitation.

FIGURE 12-13 Tie or clamp the cord in two places (approximately 3–4 inches from its insertion into the baby). Cut the cord between the two ties or clamps.

5. Tie or clamp the cord in two places, approximately 3–4 inches from its connection to the baby. Cut the cord between the two ties (**FIGURE 12-13**).

6. Dry and warm the baby with clean, warm towels. Gently clear the airway (mouth then nose) with bulb suction, if necessary. This removes amniotic fluid, prevents heat loss, and stimulates the newborn to breathe. Remove damp towels or blankets from around the baby, and replace them with clean, dry ones. If there are no complications, place the baby skin to skin on the mother's chest.

7. The last step in the delivery process is the delivery of the placenta. This generally occurs spontaneously 10–15 minutes after birth. Delivery of the placenta is not an emergency procedure and must not delay the transport of the mother and infant. Do not pull on the umbilical cord to hurry the process.

TIP

Recent research has shown benefits from delayed cord clamping, especially in preterm infants. While recommended times vary, 30–60 seconds is now recommended for vigorous term and preterm infants.

Separation of the placenta from the uterus is often signaled by a "gush of blood" from the vagina. After the placenta has separated from the uterine wall, gentle pulling on the cord removes it from the vagina. Too much pulling before it has separated naturally may lead to avulsion of the cord and bleeding. Place the placenta in a plastic bag and transport it with the patient for pathologic evaluation.

Maternal and Newborn Complications During Vaginal Delivery

Umbilical Cord Prolapse

Disruption of the oxygen and nutrients supplied to the fetus through the umbilical cord can cause devastating injury to the fetus, including fetal death. On rare occasions, the umbilical cord may enter the vaginal cavity before or simultaneously with a delivering fetus. The umbilical cord becomes compressed, and the fetal blood supply is compromised. During assessment the umbilical cord will be visible at the vaginal opening. When recognized in the prehospital setting, only one treatment option is available. The patient is placed into a knee-chest position (**FIGURE 12-14**), and the EMS provider inserts two fingers from a gloved hand into the vaginal cavity to prevent the presenting fetal body part from compressing the umbilical cord. One finger should be placed on either side of the cord to release pressure and allow blood to continue to flow through the cord. Transportation should commence immediately to a facility capable of performing an emergency cesarean section. Umbilical cord prolapse is more common in patients with premature rupture of membranes, premature delivery, multiple gestation, multiparity, and fetal breech presentations.

Nuchal Umbilical Cord

During the delivery, EMS providers should assess for the presence of a nuchal cord, which is the umbilical cord wrapped around the neck of a newborn as it delivers. Although it is more common to have the umbilical cord wrapped around the newborn's neck only once, it is possible for the umbilical cord to wrap around the

FIGURE 12-14 The knee-chest position.

neck multiple times. To reduce a single-wrapped nuchal cord, simply slide the umbilical cord from around the newborn's neck. When the cord is wrapped too tightly or around the neck multiple times, EMS providers should apply two clamps across the cord then cut the umbilical cord between the clamps. Multiple gestation pregnancies create a noteworthy hazard regarding nuchal umbilical cords, as it is possible for the umbilical cord of one fetus to strangle another fetus. Use extreme caution when considering whether to clamp and cut a nuchal cord when multiple gestation has not been excluded.

Meconium

Meconium is fetal stool passed in the uterus. It can be thin and watery or thick and sticky. If the newborn is vigorous (normal respiratory effort, muscle tone, and a heart rate >100 beats/min), no intervention is needed. Evidence does not support routine intrapartum oropharyngeal or nasopharyngeal suctioning, as these interventions do not prevent or alter the course of meconium aspiration syndrome. *Immediate endotracheal intubation and deep tracheal suctioning are no longer recommended when meconium is present and the infant is not vigorous* (see the procedure in the Specific Newborn Complications section). This is a significant change from previous versions of this text and other longstanding recommendations for resuscitation of newborn infants. Instead, simply use a bulb syringe or large-bore suction catheter (12F or 14F catheter) to clear the secretions and any meconium from the mouth and nose and perform resuscitation as needed.

Shoulder Dystocia/Cephalopelvic Disproportion

Shoulder dystocia is the mechanical entrapment of a fetus in the birth canal after the fetal head has successfully emerged from the vaginal introitus (**FIGURE 12-15**). Maternal diabetes, fetal macrosomia, maternal obesity, and fetal postdates are high risk for this condition. A relatively large or disproportioned fetus may not deliver through the vaginal canal without assistance from EMS providers. One or both fetal shoulders may become stuck within the maternal pelvis, typically against the symphysis pubis. The initial treatment is the McRoberts maneuver (**FIGURE 12-16**), which has two assistants sharply hyperflex the maternal thighs onto the abdomen, straightening of the maternal sacrum relative to the lumbar spine by rotating the pelvis anteriorly. This position resolves many episodes of shoulder dystocia. Some clinicians recommend combining suprapubic pressure with the McRoberts maneuver.

FIGURE 12-15 Shoulder dystocia.

Adapted from http://emedicine.medscape.com/article/1602970-overview.

FIGURE 12-16 The McRoberts maneuver.

If this fails, an additional "rescue" technique is to attempt delivery of the infant's arm or shoulder that is closest to the maternal rectum. This technique is likely to relieve the dystocia of the anterior shoulder. Cephalopelvic disproportion is a similar condition, where the fetal head is too large to pass through the pelvic opening. In true cases of cephalopelvic disproportion, a cesarean section is the only method available for successful delivery.

Postpartum Hemorrhage

The most common **postpartum** maternal complication and leading cause of maternal death is excessive bleeding after delivery. Usually, pregnant women lose 500 mL of blood with a vaginal delivery. Symptoms such as tachycardia and orthostatic hypotension begin to appear in the mother with 1,200–1,500 mL of blood loss. Because estimating blood loss is difficult, one must monitor the postpartum mother's vital signs carefully.

If a postpartum mother has excessive vaginal blood loss, perform uterine massage (**FIGURE 12-17**). To massage the uterus, place one hand with fingers fully extended just above the mother's pubic bone and

FIGURE 12-17 To massage the uterus, place one hand with fingers fully extended just above the mother's pubic bone, and use your other hand to press down into the lower abdomen and gently massage the uterus until it becomes firm.

use the other hand to press down into the lower abdomen and gently massage the uterus until it becomes firm. This should take from 3 to 5 minutes. As the uterus firms up, it should feel about the size of a softball or large grapefruit. If the infant is stable, encourage breastfeeding to increase uterine tone and to slow uterine bleeding.

ALS

Treatment of Postpartum Hemorrhage. Begin volume resuscitation with crystalloid fluid in the mother who continues to bleed after the placenta is delivered and has dizziness, pallor, tachycardia, or low blood pressure. Administer IV lactated Ringer's or normal saline solution during transport while continuing to monitor vital signs and clinical presentation of the patient. Maternal stability determines the rate and amount of IV fluids needed. In severe situations, massive amounts of IV fluids and blood products may be required. Persistent hemorrhage requires uterine exploration, surgical intervention, or uterotonic medications not generally available to EMS providers.

Summary of Vaginal Delivery

Delivery is a natural process that usually does not require much intervention. The birth attendant must simply control the environment to avoid things happening too fast. A history of prematurity, multiple fetuses, or meconium-stained amniotic fluid suggests higher probability of a depressed newborn. Review the steps for performing a vaginal delivery while on the way to the scene. Have the proper equipment ready, control the temperature of the environment, and position the mother to facilitate childbirth and care of the newborn. Control postpartum bleeding with uterine massage and encouragement of breastfeeding.

> **TIP**
>
> Encourage the mother to breastfeed the active, vigorous infant.

Immediate Care of the Newborn

A well-organized plan guides prehospital providers through the optimal care of the newborn. **TABLE 12-6** lists the five essential steps to care for every newborn in every setting. EMS providers should keep every infant warm and dry, maintain a patent airway, and support newborn respiratory and circulatory function when indicated. Most term newborns do not require any ALS interventions.

Vigor is an immediate assessment of a newborn infant's appearance. This determination is based on the quality of respirations or crying, skin color, and

TABLE 12-6 Organized Approach to Assessment and Care of the Newborn
Dry and warm the baby
Clear the airway, if necessary
Assess breathing
Assess heart rate
Assess color

muscle tone. This rapid visual assessment gives providers an immediate indication of the clinical status of a newborn infant and guides the approach to resuscitation. The APGAR score (**TABLE 12-7**) is a numerical representation of vigor obtained at 1 minute and again at 5 minutes after delivery, after initiating supportive and resuscitation measures. While this score may be requested on hospital arrival, EMS providers must not interrupt critical resuscitation procedures to obtain or calculate an APGAR score on an unstable newborn.

> **TIP**
>
> Perform the initial steps of drying, warming, and positioning on all newborns, whether active or depressed.

Dry and Warm the Baby

At birth, the baby is covered in amniotic fluid and can lose a lot of heat through **evaporation** unless immediately dried. Heat loss drastically increases the metabolic demand and oxygen consumption. Remove wet towels or blankets from around the baby after drying, and replace them with clean, warm, dry towels. This should take no more than 5–10 seconds.

Clear the Airway

Most infants need no suctioning or require only gentle suctioning of the mouth, then nose, with a bulb syringe. When meconium is present, prehospital professionals should anticipate the need for additional resuscitation measures. Routine endotracheal intubation and deep suctioning are no longer routinely recommended, even in nonvigorous newborns.

A newborn's head is larger than an older child's or an adult's compared to its overall body size, which leads to flexion of the neck in a supine position. This may cause airway **occlusion**. Extend the head slightly,

CASE STUDY 3

On arriving at the home of a family who had called 9-1-1 for labor, you find a woman lying on the floor who has just delivered an apparently term female. The infant is being held by the father, still attached to the umbilical cord. She is not moving or crying, is cyanotic, and appears limp.

1. What are the steps in the resuscitation of this newborn?
2. What is the role of vascular access?

TABLE 12-7 APGAR Scoring

Sign	0	1	2
Appearance: Color	Blue or pale	Acrocyanotic	Completely pink
Pulse: Heart rate	Absent	<100 bpm	>100 bpm
Grimace: Reflex irritability	No response	Grimace	Cry or active withdrawal
Activity: Muscle tone	Limp	Some flexion	Active motion
Respiration	Absent	Weak cry; hypoventilation	Good, crying

AAP, The APGAR Score, *Pediatrics* Vol. 117 No. 4 April 1, 2006, pp. 1444-1447.

and place a towel under the infant's shoulders to place the airway in a neutral position.

Assess Breathing

Most babies will be crying, indicating adequate respiratory effort. Breathing effort may be slightly irregular in normal newborns. Gasping and grunting are signs of increased work of breathing and indicate the need for **assisted ventilation**.

An **apneic** baby, with no visible respiratory effort, requires immediate treatment. Most apneic newborns start breathing simply with tactile stimulation. If the baby is completely apneic or only has gasping respiration after drying and suctioning, further stimulation is not likely to improve respiratory effort. Begin **positive-pressure ventilation (PPV)** via bag-mask at a rate of 40–60 breaths/min. The American Academy of Pediatrics has updated their guidelines for the routine use of supplemental oxygen in neonatal resuscitation. Initial resuscitation should be started without supplemental oxygen (21%) attached to the bag-mask device for infants >35 weeks' gestation. For those <35 weeks, start with a low oxygen concentration (21%–30%) and titrate oxygen based on pulse oximetry reading. (See preductal SpO_2 target in Figure 10-20. Do not expect newborns' oxygen saturation to be greater than 85%–95% until 10 minutes after birth.) This represents a huge paradigm shift from decades of resuscitation procedures.

TIP

Do not expect a newborn's pulse oximetry to be 85%–95% until 10 minutes after birth.

ALS

Treatment of an Infant Born to a Mother on Opiates. A special situation occurs when the prehospital professional encounters a newborn with respiratory depression after delivery by a narcotic-addicted mother. Do not give naloxone (Narcan) to the baby if the mother is addicted to narcotics. Reversal of narcotics may precipitate acute withdrawal symptoms and seizure activity. Assist ventilation with a bag-mask device, and follow the guidelines for care of a depressed newborn. Consider endotracheal intubation, depending on local protocols, if the infant requires prolonged ventilation or continued resuscitation measures.

TIP

Place pulse oximeter on the right finger or wrist of the infant, as this is preductal blood and better represents what is being supplied to the brain and heart.

Assess Heart Rate

Bradycardia in a newborn is usually caused by hypoxia, not primary cardiac disease. The crying, active baby usually has an adequate heart rate. Assess heart rate carefully in a baby who is not active or who requires assisted ventilation. This is most easily accomplished by palpating a pulse at the base of the umbilical cord (**FIGURE 12-18**). Count the number of beats over 6 seconds, and multiply this number by 10. This rapid assessment of heart rate is needed to assist

FIGURE 12-18 Feel for a pulse at the base of the umbilical cord.

decision making. Sometimes the umbilical vessels are constricted so that the pulse is not palpable. If a pulse cannot be felt, listen for the heartbeat over the left side of the chest using a stethoscope.

TIP

You may encounter pregnant women who have not received prenatal care or who are addicted to drugs. If the pregnant woman is "high," so is her baby. With such patients, it can be difficult to determine how long the woman has been in labor and what complications she has in addition to her drug addiction. Be prepared for anything.

CAUTION

Do not give naloxone to the newborn if you suspect the mother is addicted to narcotics.

Treat heart rates of less than 100 beats/min with bag-mask ventilation, even if the respiratory effort seems normal. Bradycardia usually responds rapidly to bag-mask ventilation, in which case no further treatment is necessary. Tachycardia (heart rate >160 beats/min) may also be present in a newborn. Severe physiologic stress, such as maternal infection or newborn hypovolemia, may cause an increased fetal heart rate.

Assess Color

Skin color assessment in newborns has several unique features. **In utero**, the fetus depends on placental delivery of oxygen, and blood oxygen concentrations are very low compared to conditions after birth. Therefore,

before the initiation of respiration after delivery, the infant appears cyanotic.

If the cyanotic newborn is apneic, immediately begin bag-mask ventilation. If the baby is breathing, but appears blue, determine if the cyanosis is central (on the trunk and face) or peripheral (limited to the hands and feet). This difference helps with decision making and therapy. If **central cyanosis** is present, a pulse oximeter with an infant probe should be applied to confirm hypoxemia. When hypoxemia is present, and the heart rate is >100 beats/min, administer supplemental oxygen and titrate based on pulse oximetry readings. Oxygen can be provided by a mask held loosely over the baby's face while squeezing the self-inflating bag. You can use the open tail of the reservoir of a self-inflating bag to provide oxygen as well.

Peripheral cyanosis, bluish skin color present only in the extremities, is also termed **acrocyanosis**. This is a common finding in newborns through the first 24–48 hours of life and requires no therapy.

TIP

Assist ventilation in an infant with a heart rate less than 100 beats/min with bag-mask ventilation. Bradycardia usually reflects inadequate respiratory effort.

Infant color and pulse quality provide an indication of overall perfusion status. Hypovolemia, shock, and congenital cardiovascular defects may present with central cyanosis, poor overall skin color, delayed capillary refill, or absent peripheral pulses. Persistent infant bradycardia, tachycardia, or alterations in perfusion may represent a severe condition requiring ALS intervention and transport to a specialty care center.

General Principles of Newborn Resuscitation

Newborn resuscitation includes a series of interventions designed to treat a variety of airway, respiratory, or cardiovascular problems after delivery in the prehospital setting. Most do not require the complex interventions discussed next. The initial steps of resuscitation are completed on every newborn. They include the following:

1. Dry the infant, remove all wet items, and place the newborn in the supine position in a warm environment.

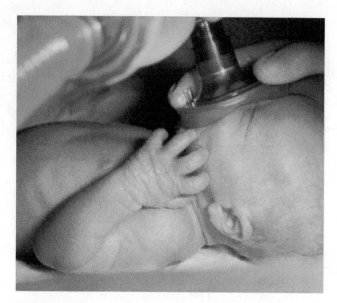

FIGURE 12-19 Using a bag-mask device on a newborn.

Courtesy of David J. Burchfield, MD.

2. Gently suction the mouth, then nose, if necessary.
3. Position the head in slight extension.
4. For infants who do not require resuscitation, place the newborn on mom for skin-to-skin contact.

When the baby remains depressed after initial drying, warming, and clearing of the airway, begin resuscitation. Use the following sequence:

1. Assess heart rate and breathing. If heart rate is >100 beats/min but the infant has labored breathing or persistent cyanosis, position and clear the airway, apply pulse oximeter, and provide supplemental oxygen as needed. If less than 100 beats/min, or if respiratory effort is absent or gasping, start bag-mask ventilation at 40–60 breaths/min (**FIGURE 12-19**).

2. Assess heart rate after 30 seconds of ventilation. If less than 100 beats/min but greater than 60 beats/min, then check that ventilation technique is resulting in adequate chest rise. If heart rate is less than 60 beats/min, begin chest compressions. Compressions should be delivered a depth of one-third the anteroposterior diameter of the chest. The "two thumb encircling hand" technique using two thumbs, positioned on the lower one-third of the sternum (just below the nipple line), with fingers encircling the chest and supporting the back is preferred because it generates superior coronary arterial perfusion pressure while also causing less fatigue in the provider. Deliver 90 compressions and 30 ventilations (120 events) per minute with a 3:1 compression to ventilation ratio (**FIGURE 12-20**). When compressions are begun, increase oxygen to 100%.

3. Reassess heart rate after 60 seconds. Continue compressions and positive-pressure ventilation until heart rate is more than 60 beats/min. Positive-pressure ventilations with 100% oxygen should be continued until the heart rate is more than 100 beats/min. If the heart rate remains below 60, consider intubation.

ALS

Endotracheal Intubation and Epinephrine Administration. Check the heart rate after 60 seconds of compressions. If less than 60 beats/min, prepare for endotracheal intubation as allowed by local protocol. IV or intraosseous (IO) access should be obtained as soon as possible. The recommended IV/IO dose of epinephrine is 0.01–0.03 mg/kg of a 0.1 mg/mL (or 1 mg/10 mL) concentration. The endotracheal route may be associated with lower blood levels of the drug, so a dose of 0.05–0.1 mg/kg of the 0.1 mg/mL (1 mg/10 mL) concentration may be required. Be sure to follow drug delivery by instilling 3–5 mL of saline down the endotracheal tube and aerosolizing it by providing ventilations.

Continue chest compressions, and give repeated doses of epinephrine every 3–5 minutes until heart rate is more than 60 beats/min.

Monitor blood glucose concentrations, especially if the infant has received prolonged or aggressive resuscitation measures. If a serum glucose of less than 40 mg/dL is documented in a depressed newborn, and an IV or IO line can be established during transport, give 10% **dextrose** in a 2-mL/kg bolus. Initiate prompt transport to a health care facility capable of neonatal stabilization.

The Inverted Pyramid. The inverted pyramid (**FIGURE 12-21**) illustrates the relative need for interventions in depressed newborns.

TIP

Good ventilation usually reverses bradycardia.

BLS is usually all that is required during deliveries and therefore comprises the largest area at the top of the inverted pyramid. In contrast, chest compressions and ALS interventions, such as intubation and medication administration, are rarely required and comprise the smallest area at the bottom of the inverted pyramid.

Antenatal counseling.
Team briefing.
Equipment check.

Birth

Term gestation?
Good tone?
Breathing or crying?

Yes → **Stay with mother for initial steps, routine care, ongoing evaluation.**

No

Warm, dry, stimulate, position airway, suction if needed.

Apnea or gasping?
HR <100 bpm?

No → **Labored breathing or persistent cyanosis?**

Yes ↓

Position airway, suction if needed.
Pulse oximeter.
Oxygen if needed.
Consider CPAP.

Yes ↓

PPV.
Pulse oximeter.
Consider cardiac monitor.

HR <100 bpm? — No → **Post-resuscitation care. Team debriefing.**

Yes ↓

Ensure adequate ventilation.
Consider ETT or laryngeal mask.
Cardiac monitor.

HR <60 bpm?

No

Yes ↓

ETT or laryngeal mask.
Chest compressions.
Coordinate with PPV-100% oxygen.
UVC.

HR <60 bpm?

No

Yes

IV epinephrine every 3-5 minutes.
If HR remains <60 bpm,
• Consider hypovolemia.
• Consider pneumothorax.

1 minute

Target Oxygen Saturation Table	
1 min	60%-65%
2 min	65%-70%
3 min	70%-75%
4 min	75%-80%
5 min	80%-85%
10 min	85%-95%
Initial oxygen concentration for PPV	
≥35 weeks' GA	21% oxygen
<35 weeks' GA	21%-30% oxygen

FIGURE 12-20 The Neonatal Resuscitation Program (NRP) Flow Diagram.

Weiner GM (Ed). *Textbook of Neonatal Resuscitation.* 8th ed. Itasca, IL: American Academy of Pediatrics; 2021.

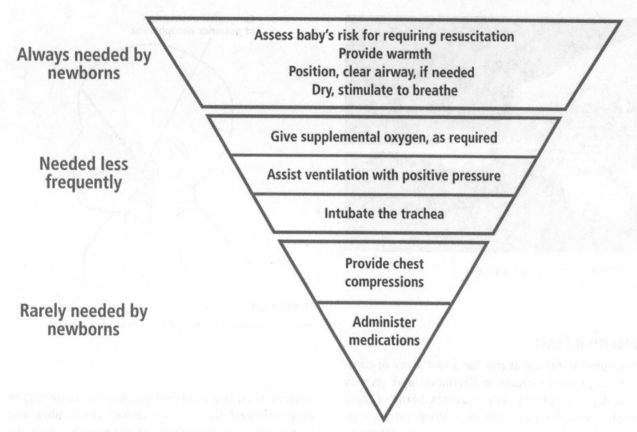

FIGURE 12-21 The relationship between resuscitation procedures and the number of newly born babies who need them.

Weiner GM, Zaichkin J ed. *Textbook of Neonatal Resuscitation*. 7th ed. Elk Grove, IL: American Academy of Pediatrics and American Heart Association; 2016.

Specific Newborn Complications

Meconium Aspiration

A child born with meconium-stained amniotic fluid who appears active and without respiratory distress needs no suctioning or only gentle oral then nasal suctioning as necessary, along with standard care of the newborn. Evidence does not support routine intrapartum oropharyngeal or nasopharyngeal suctioning, as these interventions do not prevent or alter the course of meconium aspiration syndrome. Provide adequate suctioning to remove meconium from the upper airway as necessary to clear the airway, but do not allow prolonged suctioning to delay assisted ventilation or other critical resuscitation measures. Overly aggressive suctioning may cause vagal stimulation and lead to bradycardia.

Treatment of Meconium Aspiration in a Nonvigorous Newborn. The presence of meconium in a nonvigorous newborn does not change the initial resuscitation steps. *This represents a significant change from previous newborn resuscitation guidelines and algorithms.* For newborns who have evidence of airway obstruction while receiving positive pressure ventilation (PPV), intubation and endotracheal suctioning can be beneficial, as allowed by local protocol. Intubate the infant's trachea with an appropriately sized endotracheal tube. Prehospital professionals can utilize either a 5F–8F suction catheter or a meconium aspirator device (**FIGURE 12-22**). Instead of a bag-mask device, a meconium aspirator is connected to the external end of the endotracheal tube. The other end of the meconium aspirator is connected to tubing from a wall or portable suction device. The port on the meconium aspirator is then occluded by a paramedic's gloved finger as the endotracheal tube is withdrawn from the trachea and mouth. If the infant's heart rate drops precipitously, terminate this procedure immediately and begin resuscitation measures. If no meconium is recovered, this procedure is stopped and initial resuscitation measures may begin. If no meconium aspirator is available, the suction catheter is inserted through the endotracheal tube and used in a similar manner, using sterile gloves (if available) and sterile technique.

FIGURE 12-22 A meconium aspirator.

Courtesy of Neotech Products.

Congenital obstruction
of posterior nasopharynx

FIGURE 12-23

Weiner, G.M., ed. Textbook of Neonatal Resuscitation. 7th ed. Elk Grove, IL: American Academy of Pediatrics; 2016.

Preterm Infants

Premature infants are at risk for a vast array of complications, which increase in likelihood and severity as the degree of prematurity increases. Many of these complications, such as acute respiratory distress syndrome, bronchopulmonary dysplasia, or intraventricular hemorrhage, cannot be adequately managed in the prehospital or transport setting because of the medications or procedures required. EMS providers need to provide the warmest environment possible during resuscitation and transport. Support ventilations as needed with bag-mask ventilation for those with apnea, labored breathing, cyanosis, or heart rate less than 100 beats/min.

Congenital Disorders

Choanal Atresia

Infants are occasionally born with a complete nasal obstruction. In severe, untreated cases, this condition may cause newborn death from hypoxia. Unless crying, newborn infants breathe exclusively through their nasal passages. Patients with choanal atresia may present with profound respiratory distress that resolves during crying episodes. If EMS providers suspect this condition, place an oral airway or endotracheal tube into the posterior pharynx (does not need to enter the trachea). The respiratory distress should improve. A more presumptive diagnosis may be made in EMS systems that carry small suction catheters, capable of being placed into the infant's nose. If the catheter cannot pass through either nasal passage into the posterior pharynx, **choanal atresia** is presumed (**FIGURE 12-23**). Do not use excessive force to try to pass a nasal suction catheter. A number of different

devices, such as a modified pacifier (tip removed) or oropharyngeal airways and endotracheal tubes, can be partially inserted into an infant's mouth to keep the airway open while the patient is being transported.

Pierre Robin Syndrome/Robin Sequence

Pierre Robin syndrome (also known as **Robin Sequence**) is another potential cause of airway obstruction in newborn infants (**FIGURE 12-24**). An underdeveloped mandible causes the tongue to obstruct the posterior pharynx. This can be treated in the prehospital setting by placing a suction catheter or endotracheal tube into the infant's nasal passage and placing the infant into a prone position, as long as resuscitation is not needed.

Congenital Diaphragmatic Hernia

It is possible for infants to be born without a completely intact diaphragm. The stomach or intestines may migrate into the chest cavity, collapsing lungs or inhibiting ventilation. EMS providers should suspect **congenital diaphragmatic hernia** when an infant presents with a flat (scaphoid) abdomen and respiratory distress (**FIGURE 12-25**). Prolonged bag-mask ventilations force additional air into the infant's stomach, worsening respiratory distress. Treatment in the prehospital setting requires prompt endotracheal intubation and decompression of the stomach with a gastric tube if available. Prompt transport and cautious bag-mask technique may be the only intervention available to BLS providers.

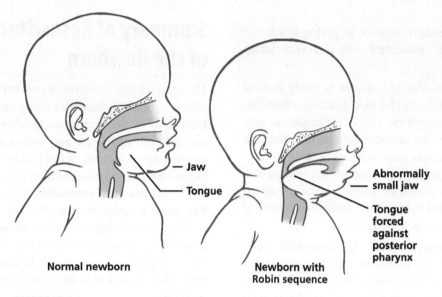

Jaw

Tongue

Normal newborn

Abnormally
small jaw

Tongue
forced
against
posterior
pharynx

**Newborn with
Robin sequence**

FIGURE 12-24

Weiner, G.M., ed. Textbook of Neonatal Resuscitation. 7th ed. Elk Grove, IL: American Academy of Pediatrics; 2016.

FIGURE 12-25

Weiner, G.M., ed. Textbook of Neonatal Resuscitation. 7th ed. Elk Grove, IL: American Academy of Pediatrics; 2016.

Congenital Cardiovascular Defects

Approximately 1% of infants are born with a congenital cardiovascular defect. Defects may involve several different parts of the heart and one or more of the great vessels in the chest. Diagnosis is often impossible without the assistance of a pediatric cardiologist or similar specialist, but certain cues may alert prehospital providers to newborns with these conditions. Cyanosis, shock, pulmonary edema, and altered peripheral pulses occur in infants with cardiovascular anomalies and may present across the full spectrum of severity. EMS providers should initiate immediate transport to a specialized facility capable of neonatal stabilization whenever a congenital cardiovascular

defect is suspected. Many types of defects present with persistent cyanosis that cannot be corrected in the prehospital setting, even with optimal resuscitation measures. Conversely, resuscitation with high concentrations of oxygen may actually worsen many of these conditions by altering the pulmonary circulation and vascular resistance. EMS providers are often limited to basic supportive care and prompt transport of newborns with suspected cardiovascular defects.

Shock

Shock at birth is most commonly caused by **asphyxia** (severe hypoxia in the uterus or during delivery) and **acidosis**. Blood loss during delivery caused by umbilical cord avulsion or fetal-placental transfusion is an uncommon cause of shock in the newborn. Signs and symptoms of shock, whatever the cause, include abnormal appearance (lethargy, hypotonia), abnormal skin color (pallor, mottling), tachycardia, and prolonged capillary refill time. Hypothermia may also mimic these findings.

ALS

Treatment of Shock. Because intrauterine or perinatal asphyxia is the most common cause of depression in the newborn, initial resuscitative efforts should ensure adequate oxygenation and ventilation. Volume resuscitation is rarely needed. In exceptional circumstances where hypovolemic shock is suspected, consider placing an IV or IO line. Isotonic crystalloid is recommended at a dose of 10 mL/kg. Fluid resuscitation should be cautious in premature infants, as giving fluids too rapidly has been associated with intraventricular hemorrhage.

Vascular Access. Vascular access is rarely needed in newborn infants in the field because resuscitation is largely focused on airway management and ventilation. In reality, establishing vascular access is challenging in infants, and its benefits must be carefully weighed against prolonged on-scene time and potential complications. IV access may be attempted in the antecubital fossa or the saphenous vein at the ankle. IO access is an alternative.

Newborn Hypoglycemia. The depressed newborn or prematurely delivered infant is at risk for hypoglycemia, but this complication is unlikely to develop in the first 30 minutes of life. If transport times are longer, measure a bedside glucose level at approximately 30 minutes after birth, or immediately in any newborn who has a drastic change in responsiveness or perfusion. If a serum glucose of less than 40 mg/dL is found in a depressed newborn, and an IV or IO line can be established in transport, give 10% dextrose in a 2 mL/kg bolus. Recheck serum glucose every 30 minutes during long transports. If the infant has documented hypoglycemia but is active, is in no respiratory distress, and has a suck reflex, allow the infant to breastfeed or offer the infant 20–30 mL of 5% dextrose by bottle.

When there is no IV or IO access, some resuscitation medications, such as epinephrine, can be given through the endotracheal tube. Do not give other solutions, such as dextrose, through the endotracheal tube.

CAUTION

Umbilical vein catheterization is a controversial field procedure. Although this route of vascular access is widely used in the neonatal intensive care unit, there are very few opportunities for the prehospital professional to practice and maintain this skill, and serious complications can occur.

TIP

IO infusion may be preferable if vascular access is clearly necessary for resuscitation delivery and a peripheral IV cannot be placed.

Summary of Resuscitation of the Newborn

Many newborn conditions present with airway, respiratory, or cardiovascular compromise. The primary treatment of the depressed newborn involves reversal of hypoventilation and hypoxia with immediate bag-mask ventilation. If the infant does not improve, begin chest compressions and provide oxygen. Consider endotracheal intubation per local guidelines if bag-mask ventilation is ineffective. Shock is rare and is most commonly the result of asphyxia. Hypovolemia is an uncommon cause of shock in the newborn. If hypovolemic shock is suspected, transport immediately and initiate volume resuscitation by IV or IO line.

Transport Considerations

Prehospital providers may need to transport healthy infants who have had an uncomplicated delivery or critical infants in continued cardiopulmonary arrest. The degree of monitoring and ongoing intervention depends entirely on the clinical status of the patient(s). All neonates require a warm environment. Every neonate needs to be secured during transport in a manner that will not cause devastating injuries if the transport vehicle is involved in a collision during the transport (see Chapter 16).

Healthy Infant

The active, term infant requires no intervention or electronic monitoring during transport. Be sure the infant is restrained as per local EMS system policy. Encourage the mother to breastfeed the active infant if possible. This may prevent hypoglycemia and promote maternal–infant bonding, uterine contractions, and decreased uterine bleeding.

Newborn With Complications
Oxygen Therapy

It is not appropriate to give supplemental oxygen to all newborn infants. Newborns with congenital cardiovascular defects and preterm neonates should receive only limited amounts of oxygen during transport. Most newborn conditions do not require any supplemental oxygen, provided that the infant's heart rate and oxygen saturation can be continuously monitored and remains stable. In the event that a newborn is having respiratory distress, carefully monitor the patient's condition and provide only the oxygen necessary, based on pulse oximetry.

Monitoring

After resuscitation, reassess the status of the infant throughout transport. Place cardiac leads in the same position as in an adult. A heart rate between 120 and 160 beats/min is normal in a newborn. If the heart rate decreases or increases unexpectedly, search for possible causes, which often include airway or respiratory compromise.

In newborn infants, the most accurate location for pulse oximetry sensor placement is the right hand or wrist due to alterations in blood flow related to the ductus arteriosus in the aorta. The pulse oximetry reading on the right upper extremity is termed the preductal pulse oximetry reading. Other sites are acceptable, but they may not be as reliable. Normal, healthy newborn infants have initial oxygen saturations between 60% and 65% immediately after birth, slowly increasing over the next 10 minutes. Oxygen saturations between 85% and 95% are normal after the first 10 minutes of life. Although there are negative effects of hyperoxia (high oxygen saturation) in the newborn infant, if the baby is distressed, the goal in the field should be to ensure adequate oxygenation through administration of supplemental oxygen and assisted ventilation when needed. Any supplemental oxygen should be titrated carefully to the infant's condition and targeted oxygen saturation based on pulse oximetry and the number of minutes since delivery.

Hypothermia

Hypothermia develops rapidly in newborn infants. Oxygen demand triples when skin temperature drops by 1 degree. Signs of hypothermia are similar to those of shock. Keep the newborn warm during transport. Have a small knit cap available to cover the infant's head. Turn the heat on in the ambulance, even at the risk of discomfort to the mother and crew. Prior to transport, place the baby on the mother's bare chest (skin-to-skin contact) and cover both of them to maintain the infant's temperature. Clear occlusive plastic bags, such as trash bags and food storage bags, are a very effective way to minimize hypothermia in preterm and low-birth-weight newborn infants, particularly in high-risk (cold) environments or when the infant cannot be held at the mother's chest during transport. The infant's torso and extremities, **not head**, are placed into the bag which is rolled loosely around the infant's neck. These bags also minimize the risk of dehydration from evaporative losses through the infant's skin. Use clear bags to allow continuous visual monitoring of the infant. Palpation of chest movement and auscultation can both be performed through the bag when needed.

Transport Destination

It is impossible to account for all potential variables when discussing transport destination. When choosing a receiving hospital, prehospital professionals should consider the condition of the mother and newborn, patient preference, transport times, and the obstetric and neonatal capabilities of the potential receiving hospitals. In many situations, it is appropriate to bypass a smaller community hospital to take the infant to a larger tertiary care center where specialty obstetric and neonatal services are immediately available. In other instances, prehospital professionals should transport to the closest facility available where the newborn can be stabilized for later transport. Contact online medical control when required by protocol or when the destination choice is not entirely clear.

Specialty Care Teams

Many regions of the country have specialty high-risk obstetric or neonatal transport teams, often comprising a physician, nurse, respiratory therapist, or specially trained paramedics. Consider activating these resources early when maternal, fetal, or newborn complications are present or expected. Prompt access to specialty care dramatically improves the outcome for many critical maternal or newborn patients.

Summary

EMS providers are in the unique position to provide assistance to women in labor outside the hospital setting, assist with delivery, and provide immediate lifesaving care to compromised mothers and newborns. Decisions and interventions performed by EMS providers have a potential to impact the health and lives of a pregnant mother and her child.

CASE STUDY ANSWERS

CASE STUDY 1

First, decide whether to transport the mother to the nearest hospital or to prepare for delivery of the newborn infant. Ask if this is a first pregnancy. If the mother has delivered before, ask her how long the labor was. Does the mother feel the urge to push? If the mother feels the urge to push, then examine for the presence of crowning. If crowning is not visible, wait and examine again during the next contraction.

If you decide to deliver at the scene, obtain a resuscitation-oriented history. Are twins present? What is the due date? What color was the amniotic fluid when the membranes ruptured? Are there any risk factors? These questions assist you in preparation.

If the child is crowning at the perineum, prepare the obstetric delivery pack, familiarize yourself with the contents, and make sure all necessary equipment is present. Warm the environment, and get clean towels to dry the baby. Find a clean delivery surface for the baby. Get or make a cap to place over the child's scalp to reduce heat loss from the head once delivered and dried.

CASE STUDY 2

If time allows, review the procedure for a vaginal delivery while on the way to the scene. On arrival, first plan for appropriate positioning of the mother. Discuss the position with the patient ahead of time so that she understands the plan for delivery. The woman should be lying supine with an object (e.g., stack of towels or a phone book) under her hips to allow for suctioning the mouth and nose if necessary. Alternatively, she can lie on her side facing away from you with her knees drawn toward the chest (Sims position).

Obtain resuscitation-oriented history. Are twins present? What is the due date? What color was the amniotic fluid when the membranes ruptured? Are there any risk factors?

Clear amniotic fluid implies there is no meconium. Meconium is fetal stool, which occurs in conditions of stress. Although the presence of clear fluid does not rule out the possibility of a depressed newborn, it is a reassuring sign and increases the chances of an active child who will need only the initial steps of standard newborn care.

Equipment prepared should include the obstetric delivery pack. Neonatal resuscitation equipment should be readily available.

CASE STUDY 3

The baby is in acute distress and needs immediate intervention. Thoroughly dry the baby, position her on her back, and suction the mouth, then nose, if needed. Tie or clamp the umbilical cord at 3 inches and 4 inches from the baby, and cut it in between the clamps. At this point, if the infant is still not breathing, begin bag-mask ventilation at 40–60 breaths/min and observe for chest rise. After 30 seconds of assisted ventilation, assess the heart rate. If the heart rate is less than 60 beats/min, begin chest compressions at 90 compressions and 30 breaths per minute with 100% oxygen. Administer three compressions followed by one bag-mask ventilation.

If the infant does not respond to these efforts with improvement in tone, color, and heart rate within 60 seconds, have one member of the team prepare for intubation and administration of epinephrine. Optimal cardiopulmonary resuscitation requires three individuals: one to assist ventilation, one to administer chest compressions, and one to prepare for intubation and possible administration of epinephrine. If only two prehospital professionals are present, as is frequently the case, get help from another adult to perform chest compressions if possible.

Epinephrine 0.1 mg/mL concentration (1 mg/10 mL) can be administered at a dose of 0.01–0.03 mg/kg (0.1–0.3 mL/kg) via IV or IO. The endotracheal dose is 0.05–0.1 mg/kg (0.5–1 mL/kg) Chest compressions and ventilations should be continued, with epinephrine given every 3–5 minutes, until the heart rate is more than 60 beats/min.

Although vascular access is not usually needed for newborn resuscitation, this baby is also at high risk for hypoglycemia and hypotension during transport and may benefit from IV access. Attempt an IV or IO line in transport. Check the serum glucose at 30 minutes of life, and treat for a level of less than 40 mg/dL. Because further resuscitation may be necessary, secure the infant to the stretcher and transport with continuous electrocardiogram and oxygen saturation monitoring. Consider transport to a facility with a neonatal intensive care unit, because this baby is likely to need ongoing critical care.

SUGGESTED REFERENCES

Textbooks

American Academy of Orthopaedic Surgeons. *Emergency Care and Transportation of the Sick and Injured.* 11th ed. Burlington, MA: Jones and Bartlett Learning; 2017.

Weiner GM, ed. *Textbook of Neonatal Resuscitation.* 7th ed. Elk Grove, IL: American Academy of Pediatrics; 2016.

Articles

Gherman RB, Chauhan S, Ouzounian JG, Lerner H, Gonik B, Goodwin TM. Shoulder dystocia: the unpreventable obstetric emergency with empiric management guidelines. *Am J Obstet Gynecol.* 2006;195(3):657–672.

Hamel MS, Anderson B. Rouse DJ. Oxygen for intrauterine resuscitation: of unproved benefit and potentially harmful. *Am J Obstet Gynecol.* 2014;211(2):124–127.

Leadford A E, Warren JB, Manasyan A, et al. Plastic bags for prevention of hypothermia in preterm and low birth weight infants. *Pediatrics.* 2013;132(1):e128–134.

Warland J. Back to basics: avoiding the supine position in pregnancy. *J Physiol.* 2017;595(4): 1017–1018.

Other Resources

American College of Obstetricians and Gynecologists. *Delayed Umbilical Cord Clamping After Birth. Committee opinion No 684.* Washington, DC: American College of Obstetricians and Gynecologists; 2017.

Declercq E, Stotland NE. Planned home birth. *Up to Date.* https://www.uptodate.com/contents/planned-home-birth. Accessed December 31, 2018.

Gray CJ, Shanahan MM. Breech presentation. In: StatPearls [Internet]. Treasure Island, FL: StatPearls Publishing; 2018. https://www.ncbi.nlm.nih.gov/books/NBK448063/. Updated October 27, 2018.

Isayama T, Dawson JA, Roehr CC, et al. Initial oxygen concentration for term neonatal resuscitation. Brussels: Belgium: International Liaison Committee on Resuscitation (ILCOR) Neonatal Life Support Task Force, November 12, 2018. https://costr.ilcpr.org/document/initial-oxygen-concentration-for-term-neonatal resuscitation.

Oyelese Y, Ananth CV. Placental abruption: Management. *Up to Date.* https://www.uptodate.com/contents/placental-abruption-management?topicRef=6826&source=see_link. Accessed January 11, 2019.

Rodis JF. Shoulder dystocia; Intrapartum diagnosis, management and outcome. *Up to Date.* https://www.uptodate.com/contents/shoulder-dystocia-intrapartum-diagnosis-management-and-outcome. Accessed January 11, 2018.

Roehr CC, Weiner GM, Isayama T, et al. Initial oxygen concentration for preterm neonatal resuscitation. Brussels: Belgium: International Liaison Committee on Resuscitation (ILCOR) Neonatal Life Support Task Force, November 16, 2018. https://costr.ilcpr.org/document/initial-oxygen-concentration-for-preterm-neonatal resuscitation.

United States Centers for Disease Control and Prevention (n.d.). Congenital Heart Defects (CHDs). https://www.cdc.gov/ncbddd/heartdefects/data.html. Accessed January 13, 2019.

United States Centers for Disease Control and Prevention (2014). Trends in Out-of-Hospital Births in the United States, 1990-2012. https://www.cdc.gov/nchs/products/databriefs/db144.htm. Accessed December 29, 2018.

© Mike Powell/Stone/Getty Images Plus/Getty Images.

CHAPTER 13

Sudden Unexpected Infant Death and Death of a Child

S. Heath Ackley, MD, MPH, FAAP

Keith Widmeier, BA, NRP, FP-C

LEARNING OBJECTIVES

1. Describe the common clinical presentations and risk factors for sudden unexpected infant death (SUID).
2. Understand the differences between SUID and a brief resolved unexplained event (BRUE).
3. Discuss the actions of the prehospital professional in the setting of suspected SUID.
4. Define a BRUE, and discuss assessment, management, and transport considerations.
5. Recognize responses of the family to the death of an infant or child.
6. Recognize emotional responses of prehospital professionals to the death of an infant or child.
7. List community resources for support after the unexpected death of an infant or child.

Introduction

Sudden unexpected infant death (SUID) and the death of a child are extremely difficult, emotional experiences for the prehospital professional. SUID was the second leading cause of infant death between 1 month and 1 year of age in 2017 in the United States.

The death of a child is an unparalleled family crisis and creates difficult emotional issues for the caregivers and the prehospital professional. The infant may be in the care of a parent, child care provider, or babysitter at the time of death and may not be at home. Absence of one or both parents may complicate field management and interactions at the scene.

Definition of SUID

SUID is the unexpected death of an infant younger than 1 year of age that occurs suddenly and unexpectedly and whose cause of death is not immediately obvious before investigation. The Centers for Disease Control and Prevention defines sudden infant death syndrome (SIDS) as "the sudden death of an infant <1 year that cannot be explained after a thorough investigation, including a complete autopsy, examination of the death scene, and review of the clinical history."

Therefore, SUID is considered a broader term, as it encompasses SIDS, unknown cause of death, and accidental suffocation and strangulation in bed. Hence, SUID cannot be diagnosed at the scene or in the emergency department.

SUID Epidemiology

Sometimes a sudden, unexpected infant death is not caused by SUID, and the medical examiner identifies a specific illness or injury as the cause. This group includes deaths caused by child maltreatment, as discussed in Chapter 11. On the scene, the prehospital professional cannot determine the true cause of death of an infant. Treat every caregiver as a grieving parent. *Never discuss child maltreatment as a possible cause of death while on scene.* Be sure, however, to note details of the death scene and record observations in the patient-care report. To help identify deaths that may not be from natural causes, document any observations related to the scene size-up, physical assessment, or focused history that seem atypical or inconsistent with SUID. For example, dangerous or unclean home conditions, bruises or burn marks on the child's body, or changing or implausible stories are possible red flags for child maltreatment that require explicit documentation, as discussed in Chapter 11.

SUID is the second leading cause of death in the postneonatal period (28 days to 11 months). A breakdown of SUID cases in 2017 demonstrated that 38% were SIDS, 36% unknown, and 26% accidental suffocation/strangulation in bed. Key information about mechanism for suffocation includes adults sharing a bed with the infant, soft bedding, and wedging and entrapment of the infant between two objects. Information provided by prehospital providers can assist in the later determination of the cause of death, so the scene survey is very important.

TIP

SUID is the second leading cause of infant death from age 1 month to 1 year.

CAUTION

Never discuss child maltreatment as a possible cause of death on the scene.

Important environmental factors include how the baby was positioned to sleep and what the baby was sleeping in. Many SUID cases were put down on their side or in the prone position, were covered with either an infant or an adult comforter, or were found with a blanket over their head. Risk factors for SIDS and SUID include low income and crowded houses.

Maternal risk factors include smoking and the use of drugs and alcohol.

Common Clinical Presentation of SUID

When evaluating an unresponsive infant, a thorough scene size-up is imperative. The scene may be potentially hostile because of the emotions present. Although emotional family members are rarely hostile toward prehospital providers, scene safety is a dynamic process, and the prehospital provider should constantly reevaluate the scene for hazards. A thorough scene evaluation can provide important clinical clues as to what may have caused the infant to become pulseless and apneic. Pay close attention to the environment. The provider should note any potential toxins that may have been within reach. Note any unusual conditions, such as high room temperature or odors. Look for street drugs and, if possible, bring all medications to the emergency department (ED). The provider should also pay attention to signs of abuse, as noted in Chapter 11.

The prehospital provider should note the time the infant was found, the position in which the infant was

---

CASE STUDY 1

You are dispatched for an infant not breathing. On your arrival you find a 4-month-old boy in his mother's arms, with dark purplish bruising on his face and chest. He has pink frothy sputum around his mouth and nose, and he is cold, pulseless, and apneic. His arms and jaw are stiff. His mother is weeping, "I think he is dead."

1. Is this a SUID death?
2. What can you do to assist the family with the death of their child?

TABLE 13-1 External Appearance of SUID Victims
Cold skin
Frothy or blood-tinged fluid in the mouth and nose
Lividity or dark, reddish-blue mottling on the dependent side of the body
Normal hydration and nutrition
Rigor mortis
Vomitus (uncommon)

TABLE 13-2 Key Questions in Focused History*
What happened?
Who found the infant and where?
What did the caregiver do?
Has the infant been moved?
What time was the infant last seen alive?
Had the infant been sick?
Was the infant receiving any medications?

*When asking these questions, use the infant's name rather than "the infant."

found, and the last time the infant was responsive. Pay close attention to the infant's position. Note if the infant is in a prone position. Evaluate how many pillows and plush toys are in the sleeping quarters. The provider should also note if the infant had a blanket over his or her head or if there was soft or loose bedding.

The infant will be unresponsive, pulseless, and apneic on arrival, and cardiopulmonary resuscitation (CPR) may be in progress. The provider should make it a point to evaluate central pulses. Pupils will be fixed and dilated. The advanced life support (ALS) provider will also notice asystole on the electrocardiogram (ECG) monitor. This should be confirmed in at least two leads, and additional strips may be required to hand over to the coroner/medical examiner. Along with the signs listed previously, the provider may also note lividity or rigor mortis. Lividity is reddish-blue mottling, caused by venous pooling, noted on the face and the dependent portion of the body. **TABLE 13-1** lists the signs of SUID. Some signs differ, depending on how long the infant has been dead. Some cases of SUID do not show any of these signs.

A thorough history is important for identifying potential causes of the infant's death. The provider should pay close attention to the patient history, which may include recent infections, potential birth defects, or a variety of other complications. The infant's prenatal history and the maternal gestational history should be noted in detail.

> **CAUTION**
>
> Refrain from asking judgmental or leading questions that suggest that the caregiver may be at fault for the infant's death.

Actions in Suspected SUID

The prehospital professional's first actions when SUID is suspected must always be to assess and treat the baby. Immediately begin resuscitation, using standard treatment protocols according to the current American Heart Association Guidelines and local protocols, unless the infant meets local emergency medical services (EMS) system criteria for death in the field. In many SUIDs cases, the baby has easily recognizable signs of death, and interventions or resuscitation are not indicated. If resuscitation is indicated, encourage the family to remain present during the resuscitative attempt, whenever possible.

After assessing the child's cardiopulmonary status, unless the patient meets local EMS system death in the field criteria, begin CPR if there is no detectable heart

> **TIP**
>
> The typical SUID scenario is an apparently healthy baby, usually younger than 1 year of age, who is found dead in his or her bed after having been seen alive a short time before.

Get a focused history at the scene if the child is not transported to the ED. *Refrain from asking judgmental or leading questions.* **TABLE 13-2** gives examples of key questions to ask. Always ask the baby's name at the beginning of the interview, and use his or her first name in all discussions with the caregiver.

rate or other signs of life. If resuscitation is started and the child responds, transport as soon as medically appropriate, as discussed in Chapter 16.

TIP

In all cases of cardiopulmonary arrest, immediately begin resuscitation using standard treatment protocol, unless the infant meets local EMS criteria for death in the field.

If resuscitation is considered to be futile on the prehospital professional's arrival at the scene or if the initial response to CPR is unsuccessful, it may be appropriate to leave the scene and allow the coroner or medical examiner to facilitate the death investigation. *The prehospital professional, however, should not leave the scene after a child has died until the appropriate authorities have arrived.* Notify medical oversight when there is uncertainty about treatment or transport. **TABLE 13-3** lists the pros and cons of transporting

TABLE 13-3 Pros and Cons of Transporting Suspected SUID Infants

Pros	Cons
ALS capability in ED	Caregiver concern about infant's body
Facilitation of autopsy	Disruption of scene investigation by medical examiner
More medical personnel to manage infant and caregivers	High costs in dollars, personnel, and equipment
Physician involvement in management	Possible violation of family's culture
Religious services	Removal of family from familiar setting
Social services for grief counseling	Transport liabilities, especially ambulance crashes and adverse bystander reactions

ALS, advanced life support; ED, emergency department.

suspected SUID infants. Because the prehospital professional cannot distinguish a child with SUID from any other child in cardiopulmonary arrest, use standard principles of treatment and transport for children in cardiopulmonary arrest, as discussed in Chapter 5.

ALS

Value of Transport After Failed ALS Treatment in Cardiopulmonary Arrest. The value of immediate or delayed hospital transport when a child does not respond to resuscitation is controversial. The chances of neurologic survival of a child in the ED, after failed ALS in the field, are almost zero, unless rare extenuating circumstances (e.g., profound hypothermia, barbiturate overdose) are present.

Sometimes, the child meets the EMS system's death in the field criteria or resuscitation is not successful, but grief counseling is not available at the scene. In this situation, consider transporting the baby to the hospital in a controlled transport mode (no lights or siren) with the caregiver, if possible. Transporting with lights and siren is the most dangerous transport that EMS providers perform and successful resuscitation on prompt transport for pulseless infants after failed ALS is extremely rare. The risks generally far outweigh the benefits of lights and siren transport. Allow the caregiver a chance to touch or hold the child before transport. This may be the last time the caregiver has to be with the child. This may not be possible if the scene is related to a crime, but is an important step in the grieving process.

TIP

Encourage family presence during the attempted resuscitation.

The prehospital professional's emotional support of the caregivers is extremely important. When possible, have one person stay with the caregiver to provide information and support. Let family or caregivers stay with the child and do not separate them, even during attempted resuscitation and transport. If family chooses to ride with the patient, ensure that they remain restrained with a seat belt according to manufacturer's recommendations and local protocols. *Be clear that the child is dead.* Do not use euphemisms, such as "Your child has left us" or "She has gone to a better place." Avoid well-intentioned but inappropriate remarks, such as, "You can always have other children," "I know how you feel," or "You will get over this in time." **TABLE 13-4** suggests specific ways to communicate with caregivers when there is an unexpected death of a child.

It is vital that providers create a clear picture of the events that occurred through their documentation, which should be objective in nature. Any statements that are pertinent to the documentation should be captured with quotation marks. This patient-care report should be extremely detailed and include dispatch information, a scene size-up, thorough head-to-toe assessment, interventions, response to interventions, transport decision and reasoning, and transfer of care. Also note any communication that occurs with the family, coroner, law enforcement, medical control, or any other entity involved. Failure to adequately document can cause a significant amount of stress on the provider and caregiver.

TABLE 13-4 Communicating About an Unexpected Death of a Child
Use the child's name.
Show **empathy** and express condolences.
Ask questions in a nonjudgmental manner. Never become hostile or angry.
Use a calm and directive voice.
Be clear with instructions and answers to questions.
Provide explanations to the caregivers about treatment and transport.
Repeat statements when necessary.
Reassure caregivers that there was nothing they could have done.
Allow the caregiver to accompany the baby if possible.

> **CAUTION**
>
> In discussion with the family, do not obscure the fact that the child is dead by using ambiguous language.

Summary of SUID

SUID is the most common cause of infant death. It is unpredictable and silent. The prehospital professional cannot "diagnose" SUID in the field, and the emergency physician cannot diagnose SUID in the ED. Determining the cause of death requires an autopsy. There are, however, common clinical signs and important risk factors that may be helpful in identifying probable SUID cases.

When faced with an infant in cardiopulmonary arrest, begin or continue CPR according to the local EMS system policies on death in the field. In some EMS systems, policy permits withholding or discontinuing resuscitation and focusing on the important tasks of talking to the family and helping them with their grief. **FIGURE 13-1** provides a typical sequence of events when there is a suspected SUID case. **TABLE 13-5** lists the responsibilities of the medical examiner and local health department in a case of suspected SUID.

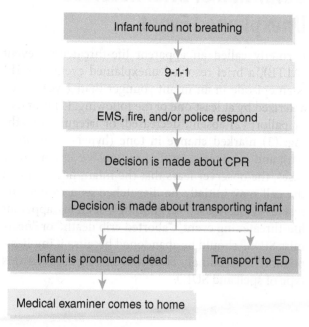

FIGURE 13-1 Flowchart of what to do in suspected SUID cases.

TABLE 13-5 Medical Examiner/Coroner and Local Health Department Responsibilities in Suspected SUID Cases

Medical Examiner/ Coroner Responsibilities	Local Health Department Responsibilities
Performs death scene investigation	Provides information and counseling
Performs autopsy	Provides referral information for peer support
Notifies local health department	Provides information to state program
Notifies state program	Performs periodic follow-up
Signs death certificate	Provides community education (with peer group)
Notifies parents of cause of death	

Definition of Brief Resolved Unexplained Event

Formerly called an apparent life-threatening event (ALTE), a brief resolved unexplained event (BRUE) is an episode in an infant younger than 1 year characterized by at least one of the following: (1) cyanosis or pallor; (2) absent, decreased, or irregular breathing; (3) marked change in tone (hyper- or hypotonia); and (4) altered level of responsiveness. In some cases, the observer fears that the infant has died and the call may initially be dispatched as a cardiac arrest. Previously used terminology, such as "apparent life-threatening event," "aborted crib death," or "near-miss SIDS," should be abandoned because it implies a possibly misleadingly close association between this type of spell and SUID.

CAUTION

ALTE is not an accurate or appropriate term for BRUE.

Common Clinical Presentation of BRUE

Similar to SUID, BRUE generally presents with a stressful scene. A thorough scene size-up should be used when evaluating scene safety, while ascertaining clinical clues that may have caused the event. Primary assessment should include evaluating the patient's appearance, the airway for patency, and circulation. The provider should evaluate the patient's breathing rate, depth, and quality. Breathing patterns may be slow, shallow, or have some other disruption in minute volume, causing breathing to be inadequate. The circulation should be assessed by palpating pulses for rate, regularity, and quality; assessing capillary refill; and assessing skin color temperature and condition. Pulses may be bradycardic and weak, capillary refills may be greater than 4 seconds, and skin may show signs of hypoperfusion or hypoxia.

A thorough history should be assessed using the SAMPLE mnemonic. Onset should be noted so a time line can be developed. The provider should note if anything makes the patient's symptoms better or worse. SAMPLE history can be obtained from the patient's family. Identify the patient's signs, and attempt to identify symptoms. If any allergies are known at this age, they should be noted. Any medications that the patient is taking should be evaluated for potential side effects and cross-referenced with any potential treatment plans. The patient's entire medical history is pertinent at this age. Ask if the infant is formula fed or breast fed. If the latter, ask if the mother is taking any medications, as some cross into the breast milk and can affect the infant. Identifying the patient's last oral intake and events leading up to it may help point toward a potential diagnosis.

Vital signs should be assessed on all BRUE patients. These should include pulse rate, respiratory rate, blood pressure, pulse oximetry, and blood glucose analysis. A thorough, hands-on, head-to-toe assessment should be performed, noting any abnormalities. Auscultation of lungs and bowel should occur. Reassessments should be done every 5–15 minutes, depending on severity and interventions.

Actions in Suspected BRUE

Clinical Interventions

Most BRUEs resolve before arrival of prehospital professionals, and it is common for the infant to appear normal on assessment (**FIGURE 13-2**). Do not be misled by the normal appearance of the patient. The caregiver

FIGURE 13-2 Most BRUEs resolve before arrival of prehospital professionals, and it is common for the infant to appear normal on assessment.

© Syda Productions/Shutterstock.

may imply that an evaluation is not needed because the child is fine. The prehospital provider should be clear that BRUE can be a precursor for an underlying issue and an evaluation at an ED is necessary to properly care for the patient. In this case, no immediate treatment is required, and the additional assessment can be completed on scene. If the child appears unstable or needs urgent treatment, complete the secondary assessment en route to the hospital. The prehospital professional must pay close attention to and protect the patient's airway as necessary. It is imperative that supplemental oxygen be placed on, or near if blow by is used, as early as possible if indicated. The ALS provider should be prepared to provide fluid resuscitation or cardiac medications as necessary and indicated. Always transport the baby, even if the complete assessment reveals no abnormalities. Serious illnesses in newborn and young infants are sometimes subtle and difficult to detect.

TIP

Consider every child with a reported BRUE to have a serious problem that requires evaluation in the ED.

Summary of BRUE

BRUE is a special clinical condition of young infants involving a sudden and transient change in appearance, respiratory effort, or perfusion. Examples of BRUE presentations include sudden loss of muscle tone, cyanosis, or cessation of breathing. Although

sometimes no cause is found despite hospital workup, a BRUE may be an indicator of serious **occult illness** or injury that may not be identified in the field. Perform a standard assessment and treat if there is a demonstrable physiologic or anatomic problem. In most cases, transport alone is the most important field intervention.

Responses to an Infant Death

Caregiver's Response

The prehospital professional is often the first responder on the scene following the discovery of the dead infant. Responses of the caregiver to the sudden and unexpected death of an infant are not predictable and may vary from numb silence to rage. Common reactions include denial, anger, hysteria, withdrawal, intense guilt, or no visible response. The caregiver may or may not accept that the infant is dead and that resuscitation is not possible. The caregiver may cling to the hope that the prehospital professional can do something to save the infant, even though the child is obviously dead.

The death of a child is likely the most stressful and tragic moment in the life of a parent or caregiver. It is not uncommon for caregivers in this situation to express strong preferences or make "demands" of the prehospital professional. Remember, this is that individual's last chance to fulfill his or her role of protecting and caring for the infant. Respond to the caregiver gently and professionally. The caregiver may do any of the following:

- Ask repeated questions
- Request that you not start care or that you stop resuscitation efforts
- Request to be alone with the infant
- Want to know the cause of death
- Physically interfere with care
- Insist on continuation of care or that resuscitation efforts begin

---

TIP

Responses of the caregiver to the sudden and unexpected death of an infant are not predictable and may vary from numb silence to rage.

When the caregiver or family expresses their preferences or asks difficult questions, use a calm and professional approach. Keep explanations simple. Be honest and direct with family members. Follow EMS system protocol for death in the field and maintain an empathetic and nonjudgmental attitude. Allow room for the family to grieve. Be respectful of the family's religious beliefs, customs, or traditions.

If there is no indication to attempt to resuscitate the infant, while awaiting the medical examiner or coroner at the scene, ask the family member or caregiver if someone can be called to give them support (**FIGURE 13-3**). This may involve calling friends, relatives, clergy, or public agencies to help care for other children at the home. If the scene is a child care setting, consider calling law enforcement to assist with other children and to contact the child's caregivers or the caregivers of other children present.

Prehospital Professional's Response

The prehospital professional has a difficult and sometimes agonizing role in the setting of unexpected infant or child death. After death is declared, comfort the parents. Never place blame on the parents or caregivers. Offering sensitive support to the family and gathering accurate information in a nonthreatening manner help surviving family members. This is often challenging, because the prehospital professional may be struggling with overwhelming personal emotional responses related to the loss of a patient.

Talking to the family or caregivers can be difficult. There are techniques that may improve the quality of these interactions:

- Use the child's name. This acknowledges the child as an individual rather than a "patient" and the unique, intensely personal nature of this child's death.
- Try to find a quiet area to talk to the caregivers. Often, the scene can become noisy with activity. Finding an area where the caregiver can concentrate on your conversation helps to keep your message clear.
- Use concrete terms. The use of euphemisms to soften the news can make it harder for the caregiver to understand what has happened. "Your child has died" has a finite meaning, whereas "Your child is in a better place" has infinite possibilities (the hospital is a better place).
- It is okay to show emotion. Parents whose child has died often comment on how meaningful it was to them that a health care provider clearly cared. Expressing your emotions is appropriate in such tragic circumstances, so long as the focus remains on the family and child and you are able to fulfill your professional duties at the scene.

FIGURE 13-3 Caregivers can react to the death of a child in many ways, but all need support. Attempt to contact identified individuals who might give comfort.

TIP

Ask the name of the child, and use it in any discussions with the caregiver.

CASE STUDY 2

You are called to an apartment complex that is home to a large number of immigrant families. On arrival, there is a large, agitated group congregated at the doorway to the apartment, speaking in a language that you do not understand. You enter the apartment to find a mother and father sitting on a couch, quietly weeping. They gesture toward a bassinet, where a stiff, cold 3-month-old infant with dependent lividity lies covered in a pile of blankets. Through a neighbor who speaks English, you explain that the baby is dead and ask if they would like to hold her. They decline and seem offended by the proposal.

1. How should you react?
2. What steps do you take from this point?

Sometimes there are cultural or language differences between the prehospital professional and the caregiver. There may be unfamiliar rituals and behaviors in how death is regarded or how grief is expressed. This presents another important challenge. *Respect cultural diversity. This is necessary to effectively communicate.* When cultural or language differences arise, attempt to find an interpreter to explain and translate.

Responses of the prehospital professional to the sudden and unexpected death of an infant may include one or more of the following:

- Anger or blame
- Identification with the caregiver
- Withdrawal
- Avoidance of the caregiver
- Self-doubt (if resuscitation is attempted and the child does not recover)
- Sadness and depression

The prehospital professional may have unrealistic expectations of how the caregiver should behave and respond or may believe that the caregiver was responsible for the baby's death. These feelings can become obstacles to communication, as outlined in **TABLE 13-6**.

TIP

The unexpected death of an infant or child is one of the most stressful experiences for the prehospital professional.

TABLE 13-6 Responses of Prehospital Professionals That Hinder Communication With Caregivers After an Unexpected Death

Having stereotyped expectations of how the caregiver should respond to the event

Judging a caregiver who did not initiate CPR

Distrusting a caregiver who has recognized the infant is dead and does not want resuscitation

Misunderstanding the mourning and grief behaviors of persons of different cultures or religious beliefs

CPR, cardiopulmonary resuscitation.

Critical Incident Stress

Stress is an unavoidable part of the prehospital professional's job. The death of a child may be the most stressful situation in the prehospital professional's career (**FIGURE 13-4**). Acknowledging emotions is a key element in successfully coping with stress and maintaining a healthy mental attitude. **TABLE 13-7** lists the frequent signs and symptoms of stress.

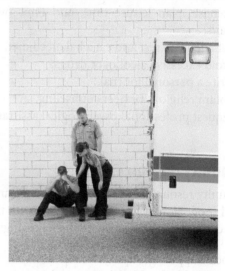

FIGURE 13-4 Stress is an unavoidable part of a prehospital professional's job. The death of a child can be agonizing.
© FangXiaNuo/E+/Getty Images.

TABLE 13-7 Signs and Symptoms of Critical Incident Stress

Anger and irritability

Changes in eating habits

Changes in sleeping patterns

Depression

Excessive alcohol consumption

Inability to concentrate

Mood changes and emotional instability

Physical illness

Recurring dreams or frightening images

Withdrawal

There are many ways to decrease the impact of stress related to the death of an infant or child. Critical incident stress management (CISM) may be an important technique for helping cope with the emotional toll of SUID and unexpected infant or child death. Other techniques to help decrease stress include the following:

- Talk to field supervisors and experienced prehospital professionals to share feelings.
- Maintain a well-balanced lifestyle outside of work. Exercise, plan leisure time, and limit overtime hours.
- Get adequate rest and eat a balanced diet.
- Avoid excessive alcohol or drugs.
- Write a personal journal.
- Obtain religious or peer counseling.
- Request professional psychological assistance.

Community Resources

Community resources available to caregivers and prehospital professionals to help them cope with the unexpected death of a child include the following:

- Local support groups
- Local public health departments
- First Candle/SIDS Alliance (1-800-221-SIDS)
- American SIDS Institute (https://sids.org)
- Professional counseling
- Emergency Services Chaplain

> **TIP**
>
> CISM may be an important technique for coping with the emotional toll of SUID and unexpected infant or child death.

> **CONTROVERSY**
>
> The value and appropriate timing of CISM are not known. Although the prehospital professional suffers predictable stress after the death of a child in his or her care, how and when such intervention should occur has not been studied.

> **CONTROVERSY**
>
> Risk reduction and risk counseling are important community prevention activities. Further research must help define the appropriate educational role of the prehospital professional at the scene of an injury or death.

> **TIP**
>
> Prehospital professionals can play a key role in educating parents in the community on ways to decrease the risk of SUID.

Risk Reduction Activities and Risk Counseling

In addition to community resource groups, prehospital professionals can also play a key role in educating parents in the community on ways to decrease the risk of SUID. This includes distribution of the American Academy of Pediatrics "Back to Sleep" brochures and active support of their recommendation to place babies on their backs to sleep. Although side-sleeping is several times safer than prone sleeping, the risk of SUID for the side-sleeping position is still double the risk of the supine position. Prehospital professionals can participate in community risk reduction by

---

CASE STUDY 3

You are dispatched to a coworker's home where a grandmother is weeping and largely incoherent. She leads you to a bedroom where a 3-month-old boy lies motionless in his crib, face down on a sheepskin. He is apneic and pulseless, has lividity on his chest and face, and is stiff. In between sobs, the grandmother tells you she put the baby to sleep 4 hours ago and found him this way when she checked on him 10 minutes ago. She asks you if he is dead.

1. What are your key medical actions?
2. How should you deal with the grandmother? The coworker?

advocating for firm, flat mattresses in safety-approved cribs and avoidance of soft or bulky blankets or comforters and overheating in the infant's sleeping area.

Recommendations for reducing the risk of SUID include the following:

- Place your baby to sleep on his or her back for every sleep.
- Place your baby to sleep on a firm sleep surface.
- Keep soft objects, loose bedding, or any objects that could increase the risk of entrapment, suffocation, or strangulation out of the crib. This includes pillows, blankets, and bumper pads.
- Place your baby to sleep in the same room where you sleep, but not the same bed.
- Breastfeed as much and for as long as you can.
- Schedule and go to all well-child visits.
- Keep your baby away from smokers and places where people smoke.
- Do not let your baby get too hot.

- Offer a pacifier at naptime and bedtime.
- Do not use home cardiorespiratory monitors to help reduce the risk of SUID.
- Do not use products that claim to reduce the risk of SUID, such as wedges and positioners.

Support of antismoking campaigns is also important. Recent research shows that the risk of SUID doubles among babies exposed to cigarette smoke after birth and triples for those exposed both during pregnancy and after birth. As for all infants, encouragement of breastfeeding is a useful action.

Prehospital professionals can also become involved in local or state child fatality review teams. These teams meet and discuss the community trends in infant and child deaths. They often review all sudden and unexpected deaths in children younger than 2 years of age to improve the accuracy of SUID as a diagnosis versus other natural and nonnatural causes, especially child maltreatment.

CASE STUDY ANSWERS

CASE STUDY 1

The infant has many findings commonly associated with a SUID death. Sleeping prone (indicated by the lividity on the chest and face), the pink frothy sputum, and the absence of traumatic injuries are the initial clues to a SUID death. However, remember that SUID is a diagnosis of exclusion made by a medical examiner or coroner at autopsy and cannot be made in the field.

In this setting, provide a direct and calm explanation to the parent that the child is dead. Find out the child's name and use it. Do not ask questions in a way that suggests blame. Use controlled and supportive dialogue with the parent. If the child is not transported, try to get grief counseling for the parent, contact the medical examiner or coroner from the scene, and consider CISM for yourself and your partner. Gather family support resources.

CASE STUDY 2

Different cultures have different beliefs about death, afterlife, and the proper handling of a dead body. There may be rituals or taboos with which you are unfamiliar and different ways of coping with loss. Because there is no medical intervention that will help this child, your focus must be on providing support to the survivors. Obtaining a professional interpreter, where available, is an important part of the scene management and the death investigation. Through an English-speaking neighbor, you can inquire about family needs, who they might want you to contact, and any way that you might assist them at the scene. Remember that even with an interpreter present, concepts may be difficult to translate and the family may have a very different belief system than do you with regard to illness, health care, and cause of death. If you cannot communicate the rationale for your treatment or nontreatment to the family, transport.

CASE STUDY 3

In most EMS systems, this child would meet death in the field criteria and would not require any resuscitation attempt. If you are uncertain about whether resuscitation is indicated, begin CPR and call medical oversight to clarify treatment options.

The grandmother may need to be medically evaluated if she cannot be calmed down. Provide a calm and controlled environment. Do not place blame.

Try to minimize radio communications if your coworker may be listening. If the employee is at work, have a supervisor contact the coworker and provide safe transportation to the scene. Contact other family, friends, or clergy if the situation warrants. Watch for symptoms consistent with that of critical incident stress and initiate CISM if indicated.

SUGGESTED REFERENCES

Articles

American Academy of Pediatrics. Taskforce on Sudden Infant Death Syndrome. SIDS and other sleep-related infant deaths: updated 2016 recommendations for a safe infant sleeping environment. *Pediatrics*. 2016;138(5):e20162938.

Goldstein RD, Trachtenberg FL, Sens MA, et al. Overall postneonatal mortality and rates of SIDS. *Pediatrics*. 2016;137(1).

Shapiro-Mendoza CK, Camperiengo L, Ludvigsen R, et al. Classification system for the sudden unexpected infant death case registry and its application. *Pediatrics*. 2014;134:e210–e219.

Tieder JS, Bonkowsky JL, Etzel RA, et al. Clinical Practice Guideline: brief resolved unexplained events (formerly apparent life-threatening events) and evaluation of lower-risk infants. *Pediatrics*. 2016:137(5):e20160590.

Other Resources

Centers for Disease Control and Prevention. About SIDS and SUID. https://www.cdc.gov/sids/index.htm. Accessed July 16, 2019.

Centers for Disease Control and Prevention. Sudden unexpected infant death and sudden infant death syndrome. http://www.cdc.gov/sids/index.htm. Accessed April 12, 2019.

Department of Health and Human Services, Center for Disease Control and Prevention. National Center for Health Statistics. Division of Vital Statistics. User Guide to the 2017 Period Linked Birth/Infant Death Public Use File. http://cdc.gov/nchs/linked.htm. Accessed April 12, 2019.

© Steve Jolicoeur/Shutterstock.

CHAPTER 14

Children in Disasters

S. Heath Ackley, MD, MPH, FAAP

Victoria Barnes, RN, BSN, EMT

LEARNING OBJECTIVES

1. Define disaster and mass-casualty incident, and list the phases of disaster response.
2. Discuss the modifications of the triage systems used by prehospital professionals to accommodate the special needs of children during disasters and mass-casualty incidents.
3. Recognize the anatomic, physiologic, and psychological features specific to children that increase their vulnerability and place them at special risk when disasters occur.
4. Differentiate the unique effects that chemical, biologic, radiologic, nuclear, and explosive (CBRNE) events may have on children.
5. Discuss pediatric issues related to the assessment and management of specific types of biologic agents.

Children in Disasters

Disasters have always been a dramatic part of human history, and community responses to disasters are a highly visible feature of modern emergency care systems. Indeed, catastrophic events have afforded a good deal of affirmation about the essential role of the emergency medical services (EMS) system, as well as highlighting its limitations. Disasters present unique difficulties to prehospital professionals, and children present additional complex challenges because of their special anatomic, physiologic, psychological, and transportation needs. There are limited data on the types and frequencies of children's injuries and illnesses during disasters, and additionally there are limited national guidelines on disaster triage, treatment, and transport of children. However, in such uncommon circumstances, chaos and an overwhelmed operating system are common, so planning and preparation are imperative. Hence, all prehospital professionals must have a basic understanding of the unique pediatric issues in disasters, and EMS agencies must possess a thorough, well-rehearsed disaster response plan that addresses children. Some disasters, such as school shootings, may primarily victimize children; the horrific idea of prehospital professionals responding to a scene that involves their own children, or children in the community whom they know, is also a distinct possibility. Postevent critical incident stress management (CISM) has become an integral part of long-term disaster response.

What Is a Disaster?

Disasters pose a significant local impact but may often also have a county-wide, state-wide, or regional impact. The definition of a disaster varies by the size and location of the event. For example, a bus crash in a large city will not have much of an impact on that EMS system, but the same incident in a small, rural town may exceed the community's response capabilities. Therefore, a **disaster** is an event or series of events that overwhelms the capabilities of the local emergency system and its mutual aid agreements.

Disasters are community emergencies that disrupt normal function and threaten the safety of citizens. Because the U.S. emergency care system is designed primarily around the care of adults, the infrastructure for the care of children in a disaster in most communities is likely to be inadequate, with fewer hospital beds, fewer specialists, and less experience with pediatric critical illness or injury.

A **mass-casualty incident (MCI)** is an event that generates more patients than available resources to care for them using routine procedures. An MCI may require multiple ambulances and additional help from another EMS provider agency. In some circumstances, an MCI may have an enormous impact on the EMS system.

A lower level MCI occurs when local medical resources are available and adequate, and regional backup resources may be put on alert. A moderate level MCI requires multi-jurisdictional medical mutual aid. Mutual aid agreements should be in place to provide backup for jurisdictions stripped of their local resources. The highest level MCI involves activation of the state disaster plan. Requests for federal assistance may be necessary.

There are two basic types of disasters: natural and man-made. **TABLE 14-1** lists common examples. Natural disasters are events caused by environmental perturbations, such as earthquakes, severe storms, flooding, wildfires, and natural epidemic disease outbreaks.

TABLE 14-1 Common Natural and Man-Made Disasters

Natural	Man-Made
Earthquake	Hazardous material spill
Hurricane	Structural fire
Tornado	Biologic exposure
Flood	Chemical exposure
Blizzard	Nuclear exposure
Wildland fire	Structural failure
Disease epidemic	School shooting/ Terrorism

Man-made disasters result from human errors, such as toxic spills; structural collapses; or malevolent intent, such as terrorism or mass shootings. Regardless of origin, disasters typically cause a significant increase in the incidence of pediatric injuries and illnesses.

Specific pediatric considerations in disasters and MCIs include the current lack of a universally accepted routine pediatric response and management plan, let alone a disaster response plan. States and territories have regional oversight of EMS activities, and there exists an overall diversity in the daily operating procedures for the coordination among first responders, recommendations for online or offline pediatric management protocols, and interfacility transfer guidelines and agreements. Additionally, there is often a lack of essential pediatric equipment on ambulances and first responder units and a lack of pediatric training requirements for emergency medical personnel.

CASE STUDY 1

Your community has been subjected to torrential wind and rain for 3 days. You are dispatched to an elementary school where wind gusts have blown out windows and, reportedly numerous children have been injured. While en route, you are notified that a nearby canal dam has just broken; the canal is one block away from the school, and water is pouring into the surrounding neighborhood. Your agency has a total of three ambulances, and one of those is already out of town on an emergent transfer.

1. What are your EMS and incident management priorities?
2. What are your specific concerns for the pediatric patients?

Roles of the Prehospital Professional in a Disaster

Predisaster Planning

EMS is a vital resource in predisaster preparedness and response. Prehospital professionals might be called on before a disaster to assist in evacuating hospitals, nursing homes, and other specific skilled care facilities and to provide medical staffing for evacuation shelters. After an MCI, EMS providers are responsible for performing search and rescue, providing medical care, and distributing information to the public.

Planning and preparation for such events are indispensable to the successful functioning of EMS before, during, and after a disaster. The most effective plans are often those that closely match an agency's daily activities. Unfortunately, because children are an infrequent part of an EMS provider's daily encounters, the child's needs are often only a small consideration in most EMS predisaster plans. Therefore, it is essential to include hospital-based pediatricians, nurses, and other personnel with expertise in pediatric illness and injury in the development process for EMS predisaster planning.

EMS can be of assistance in their communities by maintaining a presence in community disaster preparedness meetings and activities. Because 67 million children across the country are in school or child care centers during the weekday hours, considerations should be made for responding to disasters or hostile events at these locations. The following should be addressed prior to any disaster response:

- Know your community's Incident Command System (ICS), when and how it is activated, and what your role is at a disaster or hostile event
- Preplan responses to schools or buildings, and become familiar with the various rooms, sports fields, and layout of a school campus
- Know which agency takes the lead in evacuation, and if going in to an incident, when medical treatment is deemed safe
- Be aware of any children with special health care needs and any accommodations that may be needed
- Identify a process for transport tracking, with someone available on scene and at the receiving facility to assist in patient destination verification
- Maintaining adequate pediatric supplies and know who to call and where to get additional supplies and equipment in the event of a disaster
- Public information and outreach plans

The EMSC program is a federally funded program with the goal of ensuring that children receive state-of-the-art care in an emergency through the training of emergency medical personnel, both prehospital and in-hospital, and developing pediatric protocols, guidelines, policy statements, and educational resources for the triage and treatment of children. This includes resources in disaster preparedness involving children.

Phases of Disaster Response

Disaster response can be subdivided into three phases. The first phase is the **activation phase**. This occurs at the time of notification and initial response and includes initiation of the ICS and scene assessment. This is followed by the **implementation phase** during which there is search and rescue, victim triage, initial stabilization and transport of the injured, and definitive management of scene hazards and victims. Finally, the **recovery phase** occurs at the time of scene withdrawal, with return to normal operations and postincident debriefing.

Overall Response Strategy

Disasters often overwhelm prehospital professionals and the EMS system. Prehospital professionals must recognize that the incident will probably exceed their individual capabilities and should immediately activate an appropriate response plan with a preestablished unified command and management structure. The National Incident Management System (NIMS) provides a scalable framework for this collaborated response. With the activation of an ICS and an incident commander, a coordinated response can occur among various agencies and jurisdictions, with integration of facilities, personnel, and communication, all within a common organizational structure. This system provides structure and continuity for efficient management of the event. The goal in a disaster response is to do the most good for the most victims, and these actions allow optimal organization of the response.

Prehospital professionals must refrain from rushing into the scene and becoming victims themselves. This task is even more daunting when the victims are children and the impulse to help is powerful. *Remember that you cannot help if you become ill or injured.* Use appropriate safety gear and personal protective equipment (PPE) on every call when there is a potential that the rescuer may come in contact with contaminated patients. Chemical, biologic, and radiologic incidents require specific and specialized equipment. Therefore, before entering any scene, be sure it has been cleared by the appropriate authorities (e.g., law enforcement, fire, HazMat). Level C respiratory protection (a facemask with a canister filtration system) may be adequate for most conventional disasters; however, higher levels of protection may be required to meet the needs of the incident.

Prehospital professionals must also exercise the highest vigilance in securing communications between victims and families. This is especially important for children during disaster triage, treatment, and transport.

CAUTION

Prehospital professionals must refrain from rushing into the scene and becoming victims themselves. Injured and dead rescuers are not able to save anyone.

Pediatric Response Considerations

After initial recognition and general response to a disaster, the subsequent organization consists of four specific components: (1) staging, (2) triage, (3) treatment, and (4) transport, with attention to predisaster planning as an essential component to an organized response.

Planning

Before a disaster occurs, having the appropriate resources and training to treat pediatric patients is essential. Response vehicles should have pediatric supplies, including a range of pediatric airway equipment, pediatric-sized cervical collars, intraosseous needles, smaller gauge intravenous (IV) catheters, and methods to control hypothermia. In addition, having a system in place for patient tracking and reunification is essential, given the likelihood of family separation.

Staging

Staging occurs when ambulances and personnel arrive on the scene of a recognized disaster. Prehospital professionals should meet in an assigned location and await instructions from the staging officer. This ensures a quick and systematic deployment. Providers assigned to staging must remain close to their ambulances and equipment. For the ICS to function properly, all prehospital professionals need to coordinate their efforts to ensure appropriate and timely patient care. Pediatric specialty equipment should be identified by the staging officer.

Triage

Triage is the process of prioritizing patients based on the severity of their injuries and available resources. The goal of triage in the disaster setting is to make a daunting task manageable. The pediatric population can be challenging, because many patients are nonverbal, frightened, and separated from family members, and they may have injuries with which rescuers are unfamiliar (e.g., crush injuries, bomb blasts, chemical or radiologic exposures). Proper triaging of pediatric patients requires standardized triage algorithms.

The **Simple Triage and Rapid Treatment (START)** system is one recognized method for triage of adult disaster patients. The START triage system categorizes patients by color and allows the prehospital professional to quickly classify each patient according to physiologic status and urgency for treatment. It is difficult to apply the START concept to young children because this system uses adult vital sign measurements and requires that victims have the ability to verbally communicate and ambulate.

The JumpSTART triage system was devised as a modification of the START triage system for use in children younger than 8 years of age or less than 100 pounds. This triage system uses important assessment characteristics of infants and children to distinguish them from older patients. JumpSTART uses breathing as the cornerstone for triage decisions (**FIGURE 14-1**).

CASE STUDY 2

You are the first EMS provider to arrive on the scene of a reported shooting at a high school. The dispatch information conveyed that at least four people have been shot, and one perpetrator had been apprehended. It is not clear if there is still another perpetrator inside the school. When you arrive on the scene, law enforcement has not secured the area. Three students in the cafeteria and one adult on the second floor in the principal's office are seriously injured.

1. As you and your partner park and begin to pull your gear from the ambulance, what are your first considerations?
2. What pediatric issues are important to consider?

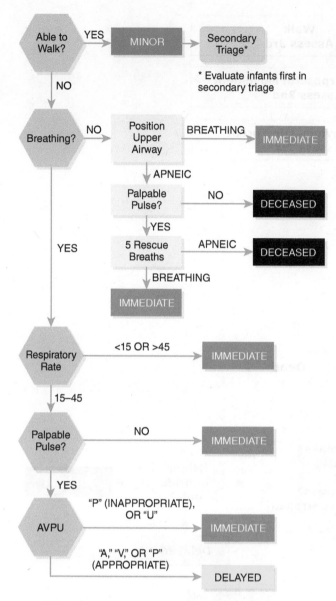

FIGURE 14-1 The JumpSTART triage system.

© 2002 Lou Romig, MD, FAAP, FACEP.

yellow category for "delayed" treatment. Children who have apnea responsive to positioning or rescue breathing, have respiratory failure, are breathing but do not have a palpable pulse, or have an inappropriate pain response should be assigned to the red category for "immediate" intervention. Children who are apneic and without a pulse, or apneic and unresponsive to rescue breathing, should be assigned to the black category and considered deceased or expectant deceased.

Another more recently developed triage system currently in use is the **Sort, Assess, Lifesaving interventions, and Treatment and/or Transport (SALT)** triage system (**FIGURE 14-2**). This guideline has the advantage of being applicable in adults and children. It describes four sequential activities that take place:

1. Global sorting of patients using voice commands often works for older children who can understand and follow a command to move to another location, but young children may not be able to respond.
2. Individual assessment and assignment of a priority category follow, starting with the individuals who were unable to respond first.
3. Lifesaving interventions that can be quickly applied may include rescue breaths for children who do not respond to positioning of the airway.
4. Finally, provision of treatment or transport completes the process.

There are a variety of triage algorithms available, and no current recommended pediatric standard. All prehospital professionals within an EMS system should be familiar with the method used by their EMS system and trained in its use. This system optimally should account for children in a disaster.

As in the START triage system, there are four triage categories in the JumpSTART system, designated by colors corresponding to different levels of urgency for treatment. Decision points include the following: ability to walk (except infants), presence of spontaneous breathing, respirations less than 15 or greater than 45 breaths/min, palpable peripheral pulse, and appropriate response to painful stimuli on the alert-verbal-painful-unresponsive (AVPU) scale.

Patients who are able to walk should be assigned to the green category for "minor" and are not in immediate need of treatment. Those breathing spontaneously, with a peripheral pulse and an appropriate response to painful stimuli, should be assigned to the

Treatment

Treatment of pediatric patients in disaster situations varies greatly depending on the specifics of the disaster, the exposure of the patient, and the availability of resources of the responding agencies. Treatment should always include removing the patient from the source of the threat or agent as immediately as possible, with due consideration to hot zone (contaminated area), warm zone (where full decontamination occurs), and cold zone (safe area); secondary threats; and the prehospital professional's safety.

After the patient is moved to safety, depending on the exposure, decontamination may be necessary. **Decontamination** is the physical process of removing or neutralizing potentially harmful substances from patients, personnel, equipment, and supplies.

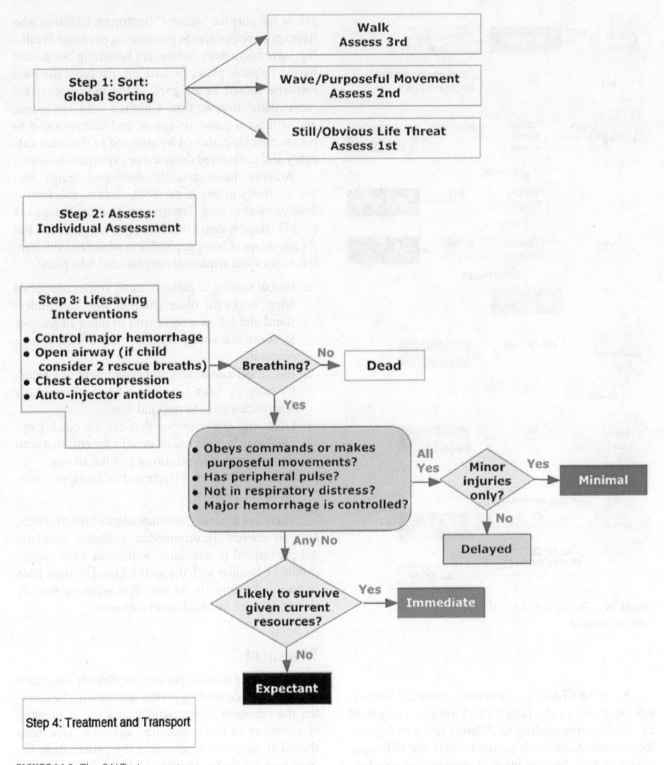

FIGURE 14-2 The SALT triage system.

Chemical Hazards Emergency Medical Management, U.S. Department of Health & Human Services, http://chemm.nlm.nih.gov/chemmimages/salt.png.

A person may become contaminated by contacting vapors, mists, solids, or liquids from a specific source or from others already contaminated. *Decontamination should be performed whenever an individual is actually or potentially contaminated with a hazardous substance.* Decontamination is designed to minimize the amount of a hazardous material that is available for absorption through a victim's skin and prevent contamination of the rescuers. Because of children's proportionally greater body surface area, and skin that is less keratinized and more permeable, they have an increased likelihood of systemic toxicity from agents that contact their skin; this underlies the importance of rapid decontamination in the pediatric population. Therefore, time is a critical consideration in effective decontamination of skin exposed to chemical agents. Even if large amounts of time have elapsed since the initial exposure, perform decontamination on the patient to eliminate any remaining agent and mitigate the risk of exposure to others.

Families are likely to be kept together during this process. However, lack of adequate protocols or preplanning may require that other adults or older children be recruited to assist in decontaminating younger children. Keeping families together reduces the risk of secondary contamination to responding health care providers and public safety personnel.

Because children lose body heat faster than adults, special care is indicated during decontamination because they are at an increased risk for hypothermia when exposed to the environment. Appropriate planning can ensure that there is warm water, warming equipment, and pediatric-sized clothing and blankets available after decontamination is complete.

When the number of patients exceeds the number of ambulances available for transport, designate and assign treatment areas and attempt to keep families together. After these patients have arrived at the treatment area, conduct a secondary triage to determine if the patient's initial triage status has changed. Essential medical equipment is vital to maintaining a functional treatment area. Each of the different triage divisions—red, yellow, green, and black—should have its own treatment area. The most experienced providers should treat the red- and yellow-designated patients.

Transport and Tracking

Early identification of patients by first responders in combination with patient tracking technology should be part of every disaster plan and drill. There are many patient tracking devices available. Coordination with regional resources (e.g., EMS agencies, hospitals, and emergency management personnel) is critical to ensuring compatibility and access.

The transport officer's duty is to get patients into ambulances and routed to appropriate hospitals. The transport officer must be flexible to ensure that the proper patients are transported to the proper facilities. Prehospital professionals must be cognizant of destination policies and guidelines so that children go to the hospitals best prepared for pediatric emergencies or for specific injuries, such as trauma and burns. Do not give pediatric patients priority for transport just because they are children. Assign transport priority based on the specific patient's condition.

Family Reunification

Although child and parent separation should be minimized during disaster response, one should anticipate and prepare for this situation. The parents and caregivers that children depend on may also be injured and incapacitated. For those pediatric victims and caregivers who require transport, it is necessary to track patients to ensure reunification.

Family reunification should not take place at the active disaster or hostile incident scene. A safe area well off site should be established; sometimes this is a location within the community or at the hospital. Children who are separated from their families are vulnerable and at great risk for physical and emotional trauma, as are parents who do not know the status of their child's well-being. In the case of a school disaster, much of the necessary information needed for safety and identification is addressed in the specific emergency planning. However, this can vary among locations, as there is no set national standard. Should a family reunification plan need to be activated, and EMS is involved, the following three separate areas should be set up:

- A reunification center, where children's information is gathered from family members or others charged with the children's care at the time. This helps avoid mass crowds showing up on the scene of a disaster or hostile incident and attempting to perform their own searches. Parents should wait here for further instruction.
- A pediatric safe area, where children who are medically clear but unable to be reunited with the parents or caregivers should be established. Activities and necessary supplies including games and snacks should be included in this section.
- A family reunification site, where actual reunification would take place. This should be separate from areas one and two to avoid further trauma to families and children still awaiting news.

All areas should include psychological first aid workers.

Natural Disasters
Earthquakes

North America is situated atop multiple seismically active fault lines. Faults are seams in the Earth's crust along which geologic plates slide. An earthquake is a sudden, rapid shaking of the ground caused by the breaking and shifting of rock beneath the surface along these fault lines. This shaking can cause buildings and bridges to collapse; disrupt gas, electric, and telephone service; and sometimes trigger landslides, avalanches, flash floods, fires, and huge destructive ocean waves (tsunamis). Ground movement during an earthquake is seldom the direct cause of death or injury. Most earthquake-related injuries result from collapsing walls, flying glass, and falling objects.

Damage from earthquakes can be extensive, and multiple types of injuries may occur. These injuries usually include blunt and multisystem trauma. *Seismic events have been known to also trigger illnesses, especially asthma.* The lack of appropriate shelter exposes children to environmental elements, such as stray animals, insects, hazardous chemicals, and exposed building materials. The additional psychological stress caused by earthquakes may also contribute to increases in domestic violence and child abuse.

TIP

A natural disaster or environmental disturbance, such as an earthquake, often causes a major increase in pediatric respiratory ailments, especially asthma.

Floods

Several environmental events can cause flooding, including heavy rains, rapid snow melt, and coastal storm surges (**FIGURE 14-3**). Unlike earthquakes, flooding is usually somewhat predictable and typically has a more gradual development. Therefore, family dislocation can be anticipated and plans can be implemented so that families are not separated unexpectedly. However, separation can occur during flash flooding. An additional public health consequence of flooding is contamination of drinking water and outbreaks of

disease. Because of their small size and relatively low fluid reserve, children are at a greater risk of dehydration from vomiting and diarrhea associated with drinking contaminated water.

Hurricanes, Tornados, and Severe Storms

Severe storms differ from one geographic region to another. Coastal areas are subject to hurricanes, whereas inland regions often experience more tornado activity (**FIGURE 14-4**). Much of the continent is at risk from blizzards, heavy rains, and high winds, and these often wreak havoc on communities. Prehospital professionals must be aware of the potential for pediatric patients to experience cold-related emergencies during severe snow storms or rainstorms, as infants and young children have a higher body surface area-to-weight ratio and lose heat more quickly than adults when their skin is wet or cold.

Hurricanes, tornados, and severe storms can lead to structural damage, loss of power, communication outages, and isolation. Floods may result. EMS providers must coordinate efforts with other local agencies, such as search and rescue, to help the victims. These events place children and the elderly at high risk of injury from environmental conditions and structural damage. There are also the added problems of asthma exacerbations, respiratory ailments, gastroenteritis, and emotional crises over family separation. Depending on the time of day the event occurs, there may be heavy concentrations of children in schools, child care facilities, and other locations. Younger children will have little understanding of the events, and they may be primarily focused on separation from loved ones. Being separated from their caregivers and not comprehending the current events make the management of their emotional needs difficult. *EMS systems must*

FIGURE 14-3 Flooding is a yearly concern in many areas of the country.
Courtesy of Dave Saville/FEMA.

FIGURE 14-4 Inland regions experience tornados.
© Clintspencer/E+/Getty Images.

anticipate these emotional crises and have a plan in place to establish communications and restore unity of families as quickly as possible.

> **TIP**
>
> EMS systems must anticipate emotional crises in children who are separated from their families during a disaster and have a plan in place to establish communications and restore unity of families as quickly as possible.

Disease Epidemics

Every year there are significant communicable disease outbreaks. Sometimes, the pediatric population is at the heart of these outbreaks. These outbreaks include infections, such as influenza, chickenpox, measles, and hepatitis. Sometimes viruses, especially influenza, may attack a community and greatly elevate requirements for prehospital and hospital services. Occasionally, the prehospital professional may be at risk for disease transmission from contact with an infected patient.

Man-Made Disasters

Man-made disasters include hazardous material incidents; structure failures; and criminal activities, such as school or mass shootings or other acts of terrorism. These events can have an extensive impact on children, including those not directly involved in the disaster, suffering from posttraumatic stress disorder (PTSD) or anxiety.

Hazardous Materials Exposures

In daily life, hazardous materials are everywhere (**TABLE 14-2**). Examples of these hazards include chemicals used in cleaning, refrigeration, and swimming pool maintenance; fuels; and agricultural products. Many of these materials are present in schools, other

TABLE 14-2 Examples of Common Hazardous Materials	
Diesel fuels	Insecticides
Gasoline	Fertilizers
Motor oil	Propane
Herbicides	Natural gas

public facilities, and in homes. Additionally, illegal activities, such as methamphetamine laboratories, use materials that are highly explosive and toxic, which may cause burns and serious injuries to bystanders, including children.

> **TIP**
>
> Children have a proportionally greater body surface area and thin skin, which make them more susceptible to injury from burns, chemicals, and absorbable toxins.

Structural Failures

Buildings, bridges, and platforms sometimes fail. These collapses typically cause multiple injuries. Victims may be hysterical and confused, and individuals may be buried under other victims. Children can be the primary victims, especially when structural failures involve schools or recreational facilities.

School and Mass shootings

A troubling trend is the targeting of children by their peers for criminal acts. These disasters may generate horrific mass casualties. School shootings are the most publicized of these types of disasters. School shootings pose many unique difficulties because of safety issues for prehospital professionals; communication requirements; emotional responses of victims, providers, and the community; and gross overextension of emergency resources. Even children uninjured in a school shooting incident will have emotional responses to the incident that could impact resource utilization.

Having a disaster plan for a school or mass shooting should focus on involvement of law enforcement, the safety of uninjured children, and reunification as mentioned earlier in this chapter.

Terrorism

Terrorism is an emerging threat in all regions of the world. Children are frequent targets, sometimes precisely because of the psychological impact of death and injury of vulnerable victims by the perpetrators (**FIGURE 14-5**).

> **TIP**
>
> A new and troubling trend is the targeting of children, sometimes by their peers, for school shootings and terrorism.

FIGURE 14-5 Evacuating children during a school terrorist attack.
© Mike Stocker/South Florida Sun-Sentinel/AP Images.

Vulnerable Pediatric Physiologic and Psychological Characteristics in Disasters

Because of their unique anatomy and physiology, children are especially vulnerable to the effects of disasters. In addition, their immature behavioral and psychological characteristics place them at higher risk for immediate injury and longer-term effects. **TABLE 14-3** summarizes vulnerable physiologic and psychological characteristics of children that place them at high risk during disasters.

Physiologic Considerations

Children have a higher respiratory rate compared to adults, which makes them more vulnerable to large quantities of inhaled chemical or biologic agents. Additionally, their shorter stature lowers their "breathing zone," potentially making them more susceptible to inhalation injuries from chemicals or fires where the materials are denser than air. Their increased respiratory rate also increases insensible fluid loss, further placing them at risk for dehydration. The characteristics of a pediatric patient's airway make them more susceptible to compromise. These features include a smaller-diameter airway that may easily become occluded with mucus, edema, or secretions.

Compared to adults, children have less fluid reserve and smaller circulating blood volumes, making them more prone to dehydration. Causes of dehydration include heat exposure, burns, vomiting, and diarrhea. An increased metabolism, compared to that of adults, often causes children to metabolize medications differently; this characteristic may require the

TABLE 14-3 Vulnerable Pediatric Characteristics

Pediatric Characteristic	Special Risk During Disaster
Respiratory	Higher minute volume increases risk from exposure to inhaled agents. Nuclear fallout and heavier gases settle lower to the ground and may affect children more severely.
Gastrointestinal	May be more at risk for dehydration from vomiting and diarrhea after exposure to contamination.
Skin	Higher body surface area increases risk of skin exposure. Skin is thinner and more susceptible to injury from burns, chemicals, and absorbable toxins. Evaporative loss is higher when skin is wet or cold, so hypothermia is more likely.
Endocrine	Increased risk of thyroid cancer from radiation exposure.
Thermoregulation	Less able to cope with temperature problems with higher risk of hypothermia.
Developmental	Less ability to escape environmental dangers or anticipate hazards.
Psychological	Prolonged stress from critical incidents. Susceptible to separation anxiety.

prehospital professional to adjust medications and dosages when administering antidotes.

Children with special health care needs (CSHCN) include children who may have chronic physical, developmental, behavioral, or emotional conditions that require health-related services beyond those required by children generally. In a disaster, these children may be at an increased risk for suboptimal outcomes. An emergency information form (EIF), which summarizes the child's critical medical information required for optimal care and support, may be available in these circumstances. See Chapter 10 for more information on CSHCN.

Emotional Responses of Children

Response to a disaster or MCI must include an assessment of the emotional state of a child and the child's caregivers. The mental health needs of children also must be recognized in the incident management system and when planning for disasters. *Appropriate mental health personnel with pediatric expertise have an important role in the aftermath of disasters to help ensure adequate stress management and counseling services.* Reuniting children with their caregivers is key to child and family–centered care. Children's and caregivers' emotional responses may range from fear and anxiety to depression, grief, and symptoms of posttraumatic stress. Children may be especially vulnerable to posttraumatic stress reactions. Pediatric aspects of shelter management need to be considered if children are separated from their caregivers. Each child will respond differently to a disaster, depending on his or her age, maturity, previous experience, and cultural background. However, children of all ages experience anxiety from disasters. Younger children may interpret the disaster as a personal danger to themselves and those about whom they care.

Effects of Chemical, Biologic, Radiation, Nuclear, and Explosive Disasters on Children

Chemicals

Millions of different chemicals in the world are potentially detrimental to human health (**TABLE 14-4**). Chemicals are transported throughout the country daily by trucks, trains, and planes, with a potential for unintentional or deliberate population exposure. Additionally, chemical weapons are an important consideration for the prehospital provider, causing injury, death, and disease.

When chemical spills are identified, officials trained to work with **hazardous materials (HazMat)** are a key resource for identification of the toxicity, relative risk, decontamination procedures, and specific treatments required.

Assessment and Treatment of Specific Chemical Agents

Nerve Agents

Nerve agents are extremely toxic and have very rapid effects. Common agents include tabun, sarin, soman,

TABLE 14-4 Common Chemicals Detrimental to Human Health

Alcohols, including antifreeze and windshield washer fluid	Hydrocarbons, including furniture polish, gasoline, lighter fluid, and paint thinner
Ammonia	Laundry pods
Asbestos	Pesticides
Bleach (laundry)	Rodenticides
Chlorine	Sulfuric acid
Drain and oven cleaners	Toilet bowl cleaner

VX, and organophosphates. The nerve agent, either as a gas, aerosol, or liquid, enters the body through inhalation or through the skin (transdermally). These two characteristics have a greater effect on children because of their faster respiratory rates and larger body skin surface-area-to-mass ratio. Poisoning may also occur through consumption of liquids or foods contaminated with nerve agents. All nerve agents produce toxic effects by preventing the proper operation of the chemical that acts as the body's "off switch" for glands and muscles. Without an "off switch," the glands and muscles are constantly being stimulated, causing the victim to tire and no longer be able to sustain breathing. Because of the extremely rapid onset of symptoms, it is likely that children exposed to these agents will develop symptoms before adults who are exposed to the same event.

The initial signs and symptoms of a nerve agent exposure include frontal headache, eye pain, miosis (pupil constriction), runny nose, anorexia (loss of appetite), nausea, excessive sweating, tightness in the chest, and heartburn. If the patient is exposed to large amounts of a nerve agent, abdominal cramps, vomiting, profuse sweating, dyspnea (shortness of breath), diarrhea, drooling and tearing, increased urinary frequency, involuntary urination or defecation, or excessive bronchial secretions with bronchospasm may occur. Children are more prone to dehydration because of gastrointestinal fluid losses, further complicating their management. Additionally, apnea, seizures, paralysis, and coma may ensue. Bradycardia is typical (although tachycardia may occur).

Treatment for nerve agents includes decontamination and use of **atropine, pralidoxime (2-PAM)**, and benzodiazepines. These can all be given intramuscularly (IM) with effective absorption. Use antidotes only for severe exposures exhibiting the signs and symptoms listed previously. Treat skin contact by undressing and decontaminating the patient with copious amounts of water. Atropine dosing is 0.05–0.1 mg/kg IV or IM (with maximum dose of 5 mg) repeated every 2–5 minutes as needed until there is marked drying of secretions and reversal of bronchospasm. Pralidoxime dosing is 25 mg/kg over 5–30 minutes, with a maximum dose of 1 g IV, or 2 g IM, repeated as needed in 30–60 minutes for persistent weakness. Midazolam 0.1 mg/kg IM or 0.2 mg/kg intranasal (maximum 10 mg) may be required for seizures. Personnel who are wearing PPE may find children challenging to care for because it is difficult for rescuers to perform procedures while simultaneously having to battle their own environmental conditions. In addition, prehospital personnel wearing PPE may frighten children and render the assessment more complicated.

Cyanide

Cyanide is a rapidly acting, potentially deadly chemical that can exist in various forms. Cyanide can be a colorless gas or may be found in a crystallized form. Cyanide sometimes is described as having a "bitter almond" smell, but it does not always give off an odor; if it does, it has been found that not everyone can detect this odor. Cyanide is released from natural substances in some foods and in certain plants. It is in cigarette smoke and the combustion products of synthetic materials, such as plastics (e.g., in house fires). Patients may be exposed to cyanide by breathing air, drinking water, eating food, or touching soil that contains cyanide. The extent of poisoning caused by cyanide depends on the amount of cyanide a patient is exposed to, the route of exposure, and the length of time that a patient is exposed.

Breathing cyanide gas causes the most harm, but ingesting cyanide can be toxic as well. Cyanide prevents the cells of the body from using oxygen. When this happens, the cells die. Cyanide is more harmful to the heart and brain than to other organs, because the heart and brain require more oxygen compared to other areas. Children exposed to a small amount of cyanide by breathing it, absorbing it through their skin, or eating foods that contain it may have some or all of the following symptoms within minutes: tachypnea, restlessness, dizziness, weakness, headache, nausea and vomiting, and tachycardia. Exposure to a large amount of cyanide by any route may cause convulsions, hypotension, bradycardia, loss of consciousness, lung injury, and respiratory failure leading to death.

Cyanide is highly volatile, and removing the patient from the environment is often all that is needed to decontaminate them. If the child is soaked from a spill, remove the clothing and wash the child with soap and warm water. Even though cyanide inhibits cellular oxygen usage, administration of 100% oxygen is still useful and should be employed. Most cases of cyanide poisoning respond to these simple steps.

The newer cyanide antidote, hydroxocobalamin, has a lower risk of toxicity than the old three-component kit. Hydroxocobalamin works by exchanging the hydroxyl group for cyanide, creating cyanocobalamin (vitamin B_{12}, a water-soluble vitamin excreted by the kidneys). The initial dose for adults is 5 g, and the pediatric dose is 70 mg/kg, IV over 15 minutes. A second dose may be given at the same initial dosage, or one-half the initial dosage (depending on patient's toxicity), with the second infusion rate ranging from 15 minutes to 2 hours after the first dose. Hypertension and reddening of the skin, mucosa, and urine are side effects of this antidote.

An important distinction by the prehospital provider is determining if the exposure in question was from a nerve agent or from cyanide, given the different immediate antidotes required in each scenario. One important distinction is that patients exposed to nerve agents are more likely to have cyanosis, altered vision with miosis, copious secretions, and bronchospasm.

TIP

Patients exposed to a small amount of cyanide by breathing it, absorbing it through their skin, or eating foods that contain it may have symptoms within minutes.

Pulmonary Intoxicants

Pulmonary intoxicants produce pulmonary edema. The most widely known agents are phosgene and chlorine. Patients typically exhibit eye and airway irritation, dyspnea, and chest tightness. In most cases, patients have shortness of breath caused by pulmonary edema hours after the exposure. Without supportive treatment, including decontamination and advanced airway management with intubation if necessary, patients may progress to respiratory failure.

Vesicants

Vesicants are chemicals that cause blistering of the skin, irritation and inflammation of the eyes and airways, and vomiting and diarrhea. Exposure to vesicants can be through inhalation, absorption, or ingestion. The most common vesicants are sulfur mustard (mustard gas) and lewisite. Blistering usually occurs hours after contact. Mustard gas has no immediate effects, while lewisite causes immediate irritation to the eyes, skin, and upper airways. Within seconds, lewisite liquid causes pain and burning on any surface with which it comes in contact.

Treatment for these chemicals includes decontamination with large volumes of warm, soapy water at low pressure; eye irrigation; airway control; and oxygen administration. Bandage wounds with dry dressings. Providers may consider administration of British anti-lewisite as an antidote for lewisite at a dose of 3 mg/kg IM; however, there is little experience with this antidote when used in children.

Biologic Agents

There are many different **biologic agents** that can pose a threat to humans (**TABLE 14-5**). They can be as common as influenza or as lethal as plague. Biologic weapons used by terrorists can cause widespread disease and death. Typical agents that may be weaponized include anthrax, smallpox, botulism, and plague. Terrorists could use these agents because they are fairly easy to purchase or formulate. An added incentive is that some of the agents are extremely contagious and can be spread to a large number of people, which very often includes children in schools and child care facilities.

TABLE 14-5 Biologic Agents That Pose a Threat to Humans

Anthrax	Plague
Botulism	Ricin
Cholera	Smallpox
Ebola	Tularemia
Influenza	

Assessment and Treatment of Specific Biologic Agents

Biologic Pathogens

Biologic pathogens, released intentionally or accidentally, or naturally occurring, can result in disease or death. Human exposure to these agents may occur through inhalation, cutaneous exposure, or ingestion of contaminated food or water. After exposure, physical symptoms may be delayed and are sometimes confused with naturally occurring illnesses. Biologic agents may persist in the environment and cause problems after their release.

Smallpox

Because of the global eradication of smallpox, with the last endemic case in 1977, and the subsequent discontinued use of the vaccine, a large segment of the population remains unvaccinated. This population at risk includes children and young adults. **Smallpox** is caused by the variola virus. The incubation period is about 12 days (range, 7–17 days) after exposure. Initial symptoms include high fever, fatigue, and head and back aches. A characteristic rash, most prominent on the face, arms, and legs, follows in 2–3 days (**FIGURE 14-6**). The rash starts with flat red lesions that evolve at the same rate. Lesions become filled with pus and begin to crust early in the second week. Scabs develop, then separate and fall off after about 3–4 weeks. The majority of patients with smallpox recover, but death occurs in up to 30% of cases. Smallpox is spread from one person to another by infected saliva droplets; this exposure is usually through a susceptible person having face-to-face contact with the ill person. Persons with smallpox are most infectious during the first week of illness, because that is when the largest amount of virus is present in the saliva. Airborne,

FIGURE 14-6 Smallpox.

Courtesy of CDC/Dr. John Noble, Jr.

droplet, and contact precautions are essential and should be initiated immediately, wearing gowns, gloves, N-95 respirators, and eye protection. Exposed lesions should be covered with a sheet, and the patient should wear a mask. For exposed individuals, vaccination with vaccinia within 4 days from exposure may prevent development of the disease. Those who have come in contact should be observed for 17 days after the last exposure, with fever being the criterion for isolation in a negative-pressure room.

Anthrax

Anthrax is an acute infectious disease caused by the spore-forming bacterium *Bacillus anthracis*. Anthrax most commonly occurs in hoofed mammals but can also infect humans. Symptoms of disease vary depending on how the disease was contracted, but usually occur within 7 days after exposure. The serious forms of human anthrax are inhalation anthrax, cutaneous anthrax, and intestinal anthrax. Initial symptoms of inhalation anthrax infection may resemble a common cold. After several days, the symptoms may progress to severe breathing problems and shock. Inhalation anthrax is often fatal. The intestinal disease form of anthrax may follow the consumption of contaminated food and is characterized by an acute inflammation of the intestinal tract. Initial signs of nausea, loss of appetite, vomiting, and fever are usually followed by abdominal pain, vomiting of blood, and severe diarrhea. For inhalational and gastrointestinal anthrax, direct person-to-person spread of anthrax is extremely unlikely; however, with cutaneous anthrax, contact precautions should be employed. The use of gloves when in contact with skin lesions, hand washing, and cleaning and sterilizing equipment are required. In situations where risk of exposure to spores exists, decontamination of patients is recommended with providers wearing gloves, gown, and mask when handling contaminated clothing or other fomites.

> **TIP**
>
> The serious forms of human anthrax are inhalation anthrax, cutaneous anthrax, and intestinal anthrax.

Plague

Plague is an infectious disease of animals and humans caused by the bacterium *Yersinia pestis*. *Y. pestis* is found in rodents and the fleas that feed on them in many areas around the world. Pneumonic plague occurs when *Y. pestis* infects the lungs. The first signs of illness in pneumonic plague are fever, headache, weakness, and a cough productive of bloody or watery sputum. The pneumonia progresses over 2–4 days and may cause septic shock and, without early treatment, death. Person-to-person transmission of pneumonic plague occurs through respiratory droplets, which can infect those who have face-to-face contact with the ill patient; therefore, droplet precautions must be used.

Ricin

Ricin is a potent protein synthesis inhibitor derived from the beans of the castor plant (*Ricinus communis*). The beans are available worldwide, and the toxin is fairly easily produced. When inhaled as a small-particle aerosol, this toxin may produce pathologic changes within 8 hours and have severe respiratory symptoms (chest tightness, shortness of breath, cough), fever, and myalgias. Within 36–72 hours, cyanosis with pulmonary edema and respiratory failure occurs. When ingested, ricin causes severe gastrointestinal symptoms with vomiting and bloody diarrhea. Ingested ricin exposure may eventually lead to hallucinations, seizures, and low blood pressure, followed by vascular collapse and death. Treatment is supportive depending on the symptoms, and early diagnosis may be difficult. Decontamination should occur in the warm zone at the site of release before transport, with a full chemical-resistant suit; gloves; surgical mask; and eye and face protection, such as a face shield and goggles. Clothing that has to be pulled over the head should be cut and double-bagged; there should be soap and water decontamination of the skin and irrigation to the eyes for 10–15 minutes, with disposal of contact lenses. Once decontaminated, ricin cannot be transmitted from person to person; therefore, standard precautions should be used.

TIP

Plague is an infectious disease carried by rodents and their fleas in many areas around the world.

Botulism

Botulinum toxins are created by *Clostridium botulinum*, an anaerobic bacterium found commonly in soil. Botulism is the result of exposure to these toxins and can occur naturally through the ingestion of contaminated food or through bioterrorism exposure. The toxins act primarily at the neuromuscular junction, preventing the release of acetylcholine and ultimately leading to flaccid paralysis. The toxin effects can take from 24 hours to several days to manifest, and patients exhibit eyelid droop, dilated pupils, blurry vision, slurred speech, difficulty swallowing, dry oral mucosa, flaccid paralysis, and respiratory failure. The distinguishing factors from nerve agent exposure are the lack of initial muscle fasciculations, the dilation of the pupils, dry mucous membranes, and the period from exposure to onset of symptoms.

Infants are particularly susceptible to botulism because of the potential for colonization of their gastrointestinal tract with the bacteria. This spore-forming bacterium can be introduced through environmental dust or by honey products. Therefore, it is recommended to avoid giving honey to children younger than 1 year of age. Treatment for this exposure is primarily supportive care with ventilator support. However, there may be benefit in using botulinum antitoxin, which is best given during the latent period after exposure. After the symptoms are recognized, this therapy may only reduce the further progression of symptoms. Botulism is not contagious, so standard precautions should be used for patient care.

Ebola

Ebola virus is in the family of filoviruses and can cause severe hemorrhagic fever in humans. Symptoms include fever, mucous membrane bleeding, unexplained hemorrhage, petechiae, muscle pain, weakness, diarrhea, and vomiting. The virus is spread by direct contact with blood or body fluids and objects (syringes, needles) contaminated with body fluids; it is highly contagious, but will not spread until the person develops symptoms. Symptoms occur from 2–21 days after exposure to the virus, so anyone with a fever who has travelled to a region within 21 days where there is an outbreak should be considered contagious. Treatment is supportive.

Specific Treatment of Biologic Disease

TABLE-14-6 summarizes the specific treatment of diseases caused by biologic agents, including pediatric doses.

Radiation

Radiation disasters, although rare, can occur wherever radioactive materials are used, stored, or transported. Nuclear power plants, hospitals, universities, research laboratories, industries, major highways, railroads, and shipping yards are all possible sites. Radioactive materials are dangerous because of the harmful effect certain types of radiation have on the cells of the body. The longer a person is exposed to radiation, the greater the risk. Children are more susceptible to radiation injury because of their rapidly reproducing cells. Radiation weapons include nuclear and "dirty" bombs. Radiation cannot be detected by sight, smell, or any other sense.

Nuclear

A **dirty bomb**, also known as a radiologic dispersal device, consists of a conventional explosive, such as dynamite, packaged with radioactive material that is meant to scatter when the bomb explodes. A dirty bomb can kill or injure by means of the initial blast of the conventional explosive or by airborne radiation and contamination (hence the term "dirty").

A **nuclear bomb** uses the power of nuclear fission or fusion to produce an intense pulse or wave of heat, light, air pressure, and radiation. In a nuclear blast, injury or death may occur as a result of the blast itself or as a result of debris thrown from the blast. Victims may experience moderate to severe skin burns, depending on their distance from the blast site. Those who look directly at the blast may experience eye damage, ranging from temporary blindness to severe burns on the retina. Individuals near the blast site may be exposed to high levels of radiation and develop symptoms of radiation sickness.

There are two types of exposure from radioactive materials from a nuclear blast: external exposure and internal exposure. External exposure occurs when patients are exposed to radiation outside of their body from the blast or its fallout. Internal exposure occurs when patients eat food or breathe air that is contaminated with radioactive fallout. Both internal and external exposure from fallout can occur miles away from the blast site.

Protection from radiation exposure can be attained by using a shield, minimizing exposure time, and maximizing the distance from the source.

TABLE 14-6 Medical Management of Bioterrorism Infections

Pre-exposure Vaccine and Dosing	Treatment Postexposure With Symptoms	Postexposure Without Symptoms
Anthrax, Inhalation Biothrax vaccine, 0.5 mL IM or SQ at weeks 0 and 4 and months 6, 12, and 18, then annual boosters This vaccine is NOT recommended for use in those younger than 18 years	Ciprofloxacin, 15 mg/kg IV twice daily (max 1 g/day) Or Doxycycline (if >8 years and >45 kg), load with 200 mg then 100 mg IV twice daily for 60 days If >8 years and <45 kg, 4.4 mg/kg load then 2.2 mg/kg/ twice a day for 60 days (If <8 years or <45 kg), 4.4 mg/kg load then 2.2 mg/kg/twice a day (max dose 200 mg daily) for 60 days	Ciprofloxacin, 15–20 mg/kg (max 1 g/day) orally twice a day for 60 days Or Doxycycline (if >8 years and >45 kg), 100 mg orally twice daily for 60 days If >8 years and <45 kg, 2.2 mg/kg/ twice a day orally for 60 days If <8 years or <45 kg, 2.2 mg/kg/ twice a day orally (max dose 200 mg daily) for 60 days
Smallpox ACAM 2000 vaccine No vaccine for infants younger than 12 months Not recommended for age 18 and younger for pre-event vaccination	No current treatment other than supportive care	Vaccination within 96 hours of exposure
Plague, Pneumonic Vaccine is not available	Gentamicin, 2.5 mg/kg IM or IV three times a day for 10 days Or Doxycycline (<45 kg), 2.2 mg/kg IV twice daily (max 200 mg daily) for 10 days Doxycycline (>45 kg), 200 mg once a day for 10–14 days Or Ciprofloxacin, 15 mg/kg IV twice daily for 10–14 days (maximum 1 g/day)	Doxycycline (<45 kg), 2.2 mg/kg orally twice daily (max 200 mg daily) for 7 days Doxycycline (>45 kg) 200 mg once a day for 7 days Or Ciprofloxacin, 20 mg/kg orally twice a day (max 1 g per day) for 10 days Or Chloramphenicol (>2 years), 15 mg/kg (maximum 1 g/day) orally four times daily for 10 days (not recommended for patients 0–2 years)

IM, intramuscular; IV, intravenous; SQ, subcutaneous.

Depending on the type of radiation emitted, different shielding may be required, with alpha particles being stopped by a sheet of paper, beta particles by a layer of clothing or less than an inch of most substances. Gamma rays require over 6 feet of concrete to be stopped. Because PPE cannot protect against high-energy, highly penetrating forms of radiation associated with most radiation emergencies, first responders should wear direct-reading personal radiation dosimeters to monitor radiation doses and stay within recommended dose limits for radiation workers. External decontamination of radioactive particulate can be accomplished by removal of all clothing, warm soap water irrigation, wound debridement with foreign body removal, oral rinsing, and eye and ear irrigation. A radiation survey meter should be used to monitor the decontamination progress, and there may be the need to cut hair if washing was insufficient to remove the radioactive particulates. The goal is to reduce the radiation level to no more than two times background radiation level. Care should be made to avoid the contamination of vehicles and equipment through onsite decontamination, and hospitals should not be used as decontamination centers. The management of internal radiation exposure varies by the radioactive element involved. Because radioactive fallout does enter the ecosystem and the foods that are consumed, radioactive iodine is a concern. In these cases, prophylactic treatment with potassium iodide prevents the radioactive form of the element from being absorbed into the thyroid gland, because children are vulnerable to late carcinogenic effects.

TIP

Perform decontamination whenever an individual is possibly contaminated with a hazardous substance.

CAUTION

Be sure children do not get hypothermic after decontamination. Immediately dry them and give them warm clothes.

Explosives

Explosive devices are frequently used for terrorism. Children are at risk for blast injury because of their size and susceptibility to head and abdominal injuries. Injuries from the blast wave, flying debris, and being thrown may have deadly results.

Critical Incident Stress Management

A **critical incident stress management (CISM)** team can provide support and counseling for prehospital professionals who have been exposed to stressful incidents in the course of providing EMS. The need for this may be especially acute after dealing with pediatric patients in disasters. A mental health professional is often part of the CISM team. The debriefing process is intended to be educational; CISM is not psychotherapy. The effectiveness of CISM after disasters for prehospital professionals and for children is not known.

Summary

Disasters are fortunately a rare occurrence, but when they happen they will likely involve children, either directly or indirectly. Preparation is the key to providing the best care possible. Using the National Incident Management System (NIMS) framework and the Incident Command System (ICS) will enable the responding team to acquire appropriate resources, personnel, and communication and to organize assistance from additional responding agencies. When children are triaged in a disaster scenario, there are several different triage methods used, which vary regionally. The JumpSTART triage system is one standardized method that takes into consideration the distinctive features of young children. Another recognized triage approach is the SALT triage system. However, these systems have not been validated; therefore, there is no nationally recognized recommendation for children.

Because of their physiologic, anatomic, and psychological differences, children present a unique challenge to the prehospital professional. Natural and man-made disasters necessitate that EMS preplan their response and rehearse their roles in an ever-changing world.

CASE STUDY 3

You are dispatched to a gymnasium, the scene of a high school dance on a hot evening. On arrival, you find 20 adolescents and 4 adult chaperones. They all have eye irritation, respiratory distress, chest tightness, and coughing. The pool is next door, and there is a cloud above the pool.

1. What is the likely agent?
2. How would you treat and transport these patients?

CASE STUDY ANSWERS

CASE STUDY 1

Your first action should be to confirm that your position is safe and to identify all other potential initial responders. Ask for an official determination about whether the school is in a flood zone, and consider the necessity of an evacuation order. Initiate the ICS, and identify a casualty collection point at the nearest safe location. Begin rescue and evacuation operations. Implement your disaster operations plan, and activate your mutual aid agreements as necessary. Have dispatch notify local medical facilities of the MCI/disaster, and ensure the necessary notifications are made to emergency relief agencies.

During your assessment of the children, determine the severity of injuries and triage them using an appropriate standardized technique, such as the JumpSTART triage system. Provide psychological support to the children by remaining calm, and attempt to reunite families when possible. Pediatric patients require additional care to maintain thermal balance during a weather-related emergency. Providing blankets and protection from the wind and rain is an important aspect of caring for these patients.

CASE STUDY 2

Scene safety must be your primary consideration. Law enforcement is in charge, and you will not be allowed inside the school until the scene is safe. Do not make yourself the next victim. While awaiting clearance, establish incident command if it has not already been established by the initial officers on scene, and determine staging and triage areas. Request appropriate response of other providers (basic and/or advanced life support) and ensure transportation or additional resources, such as an aeromedical team.

Determine the amount of pediatric equipment that is available and the level of care that may be needed, then request any additional resources you may need. Decide which hospitals in your area have pediatric trauma capability and how you will transport the patients. Do not forget to consider how best to plan for family reunification.

CASE STUDY 3

These students and chaperones have likely been exposed to a chlorine gas leak.

Begin by donning PPE including gowns, gloves, and masks. Treatment should begin by moving anyone who is able to walk outdoors. Call for a hazmat team to decontaminate the patients; request additional ambulances to provide oxygen, airway management, and hospital transport; and notify the local hospital and law enforcement.

SUGGESTED REFERENCES

Textbooks

Bledsoe B, Porter R, Cherry R. *Essentials of Paramedic Care*. Upper Saddle River, NJ: Prentice Hall; 2003.

Hogan D, Burstein J. *Disaster Medicine*. Philadelphia, PA: Lippincott Williams & Wilkins; 2002.

Shaw KN, Bachur RG, eds. *Fleisher & Ludwig's Textbook of Pediatric Emergency Medicine*. 7th ed. Philadelphia, PA: Wolters Kluwer; 2016.

Articles

American Academy of Pediatrics, Committee on Environmental Health and Committee on Infectious Diseases. Policy statement. Chemical-biological terrorism and its impact on children. *Pediatrics*. 2006;118(3):1267–1278.

American Academy of Pediatrics, Committee on Pediatric Emergency Medicine and Council on Clinical

Information Technology, American College of Emergency Physicians, Pediatric Emergency Medicine Committee. Policy statement. Emergency information forms and emergency preparedness for children with special health care needs. *Pediatrics*. 2010;125(4):829–837.

American Academy of Pediatrics Disaster Preparedness Advisory Council and Committee on Pediatric

Emergency Medicine. Ensuring the health of children in disasters. *Pediatrics*. 2015;136:e1407.

Ball J, Allen K. Consensus recommendations for responding to children's emergencies in disasters. *Natl Acad Pract Forum*. 2000;2:253–257.

Curtis T, Miller BC, Berry EH. Changes in reports and incidence of child abuse following natural disasters. *Child Abuse Negl*. 2000;24(9):1151–1162.

Freyberg C, Arquilla B, Fertel B, et al. Disaster preparedness: hospital decontamination and the pediatric patient: guidelines for hospitals and emergency planners. *Prehosp Disaster Med*. 2008;23(2):166–173.

Gausche-Hill M. Pediatric disaster preparedness: are we really prepared? *J Trauma*. 2009;67(suppl 2):S73–S76.

Ginter PM, Wingate MS, Rucks AC, et al. Creating a regional pediatric medical disaster preparedness network: imperative and issues. *Maternal Child Health J*. 2006;10(4):391–396.

Heffernan RW, Lerner EB, McKee CH, et al. Comparing the accuracy of mass casualty triage systems in a pediatric population. *Prehosp Emerg Care*. 2018;17:1–5.

Holbrook PR. Pediatric disaster medicine. *Crit Care Clin*. 1991;7:463–470.

Hoven CW, Duarte CS, Lucas CP, et al. Psychopathology among New York City public school children 6 months after September 11. *Arch Gen Psychiatry*. 2005;62(5):545–552.

Lerner EB, Cone DC, Weinstein ES, et al. Mass casualty triage: an evaluation of the science and refinement of a national guideline. *Disaster Med Public Health Prep*. 2011;5(2):129–137.

Lerner EB, Schwartz RB, Coule PL, et al. Use of SALT triage in a simulated mass-casualty incident. *Prehosp Emerg Care*. 2010;14(1):21–25.

Lerner EB, Schwartz RB, Coule PL, et al. Mass casualty triage: an evaluation of the data and development of a proposed national guideline. *Disaster Med Public Health Prep*. 2008;2(Suppl 1):S25–S34.

Lovejoy J. Disaster medicine: initial approach to patient management after large-scale disasters. *Clin Ped Emerg Med*. 2002;3(4):217–223.

Lozon MM, Bradin S. Pediatric disaster preparedness. *Pediatr Clin North Am*. 2018;65(6):1205–1220.

Markenson D, Redlener I. Executive summary. *Pediatric Preparedness for Disasters and Terrorism: National Consensus Conference*. 2006;12.

Waeckerle JF, Seamans S, Whiteside M, et al. Executive summary. Developing objectives, content, and competencies for the training of emergency medical technicians, emergency physicians, and emergency nurses to care for casualties resulting from nuclear, biological, or chemical (NBC) incidents. *Ann Emerg Med*. 2001;37:587–601.

Wallis LA, Carley S. Comparison of paediatric major incident primary triage tools. *Emerg Med J*. 2006;23(6):475–478.

Other Resources

American Academy of Pediatrics. Family Reunification following disasters: a planning tool for health care facilities. July 2018. https://www.aap.org/en-us /Documents/AAP-Reunification-Toolkit.pdf. Accessed July 15, 2019.

American Academy of Pediatrics. Children and disasters. https://www.aap.org/en-us/advocacy-and -policy/aap-health-initiatives/Children-and-Disasters /Pages/default.aspx. Accessed September 9, 2019.

Centers for Disease Control and Prevention. Anthrax. https://www.cdc.gov/anthrax/index.html. Accessed September 9, 2019.

Centers for Disease Control and Prevention. Bioterrorism. https://emergency.cdc.gov/bioterrorism/. Accessed September 9, 2019.

Centers for Disease Control and Prevention. Center for preparedness and response. https://www.cdc.gov /cpr/prepareyourhealth/index.html. Accessed September 9, 2019.

Centers for Disease Control and Prevention. Children in disasters. https://www.cdc.gov/childrenindisasters/. Accessed September 9, 2019.

Center for Disease Control and Prevention. Plague. https://www.cdc.gov/plague/healthcare/clinicians .html. Accessed October 31, 2019.

Centers for Disease Control and Prevention. Ricin. https://emergency.cdc.gov/agent/ricin/. Accessed September 9, 2019.

Centers for Disease Control and Prevention. Viral hemorrhagic fevers. https://www.cdc.gov/vhf/. Accessed September 9. 2019.

Emergency Medical Services for Children. Emergency Innovation and Improvement Center. Disaster planning. https://emscimprovement.center /education-and-resources/tooklits/pediatric -disaster-preparedness-toolbox/. Accessed September 9, 2019.

Federal Emergency Management Agency. Post disaster reunification of children: a nationwide approach. November 2013. https://www.fema.gov/media-library /assets/documents/85559. Accessed July 15, 2019.

Food and Drug Administration. Emergency preparedness, bioterrorism and drug preparedness. https://www.fda.gov/Drugs/EmergencyPreparedness. Accessed April 24, 2019.

Lindell M, Prater C, Perry R. Fundamentals of emergency management. 2006. http://em.fsu.edu/assets /outlines/Foundations_Online_Grad.pdf. Accessed September 9, 2019.

National Library of Medicine. JumpSTART pediatric MCI triage tools. Team Life Support. 2011. https:// chemm.nlm.nih.gov/startpediatric.htm. Accessed April 25, 2019.

START Adult Triage Algorithm. https://chemm.nlm .nih.gov/startadult.htm. Accessed April 25, 2019.

U.S. Department of Health and Human Services. Decontamination procedures. https://www.remm .nlm.gov/ext_contamination.htm. Accessed September 9, 2019.

U.S. Department of Health and Human Services. Emergency medical services and pediatric transport. https://archive.ahrq.gov/prep/nccdreport/nccdrpt4 .htm. Accessed August 7, 2012.

U.S. Department of Health and Human Services. Emergency worker exposure guidelines in the early phase. https://www.remm.nlm.gov/exposureonly.htm. Accessed April 25, 2019.

U.S. Department of Health and Human Services. Managing internal radiation. http://www.remm.nlm .gov/int_contamination.htm. Accessed April 25, 2019.

U.S. Department of Health and Human Services. Protective actions and protective action guides. https://www.remm.nlm.gov/pag.htm. Accessed September 9, 2019.

World Health Organization. *Psychosocial Consequences of Disasters—Prevention and Management.* Geneva: WHO, Division of Mental Health; 2002.

© Eddie M. Sperling.

CHAPTER 15

Medicolegal and Ethical Considerations

Andrew Bartkus, RN, MSN, JD, CEN, CCRN, CFRN, NREMT-P FP-C

Matthew R. Streger, Esq., MPA, NRP

Michael H. Stroud, MD, FAAP

LEARNING OBJECTIVES

1. Identify prehospital ethical and legal issues unique to pediatric emergency care.

2. Discuss the doctrine of implied consent in the prehospital treatment and transport of a minor.

3. Understand the different ethical and legal challenges in caring for older children and adolescents.

4. Outline the prehospital professional's responsibilities when a caregiver may refuse to grant consent to prehospital professionals to treat or transport a minor.

5. Review the legal and ethical considerations when faced with a child who has a "Do Not Resuscitate" status.

Introduction

The prehospital professional frequently encounters ethical and legal issues while caring for children. These may include the inability to obtain the legal guardian's permission to treat a child, refusal of consent by parents or older children, challenges of confidentiality, issues related to telling the truth, and the identification of possible child maltreatment. This chapter discusses these issues and emphasizes the importance of protocols and policies for prehospital professionals to address common pediatric ethical and legal concerns.

Consent

The requirement to obtain **informed consent** from a patient or legal guardian before delivering medical care is a central feature of American health care law and ethics. A legally competent individual may not be touched, treated, or transported without his or her consent. **Minors** (children younger than 18 years of age), however, present a special problem because, under most circumstances, they do not have the legal authority to give or refuse consent. Therefore, in most states, a parent or legal guardian must give permission before a minor can be medically treated or transported (**FIGURE 15-1**). Many states have provisions for minor children to consent to medical care for certain types of conditions. These provisions often involve access to reproductive health needs, treatment for sexually transmitted diseases, and access to behavioral health services. Prehospital professionals should consult local protocols or agency/department guidelines for requirements in a particular state or region.

State laws designate certain minors as "emancipated" and grants these **emancipated minors** the right to make decisions, including health care decisions. Adolescents who are legally emancipated may give consent for medical treatment and transport, they may refuse medical care or transport, and may give consent for the treatment and transport of their own minor children. Although emancipated minor laws vary from state to state, most states recognize minors to be emancipated if they are married, are pregnant, have a child, are economically self-supporting and not living at home or are on active-duty status in the armed services. In most jurisdictions, the actual determination of emancipation is established by court order.

In situations where a minor who is not emancipated, yet has a medical condition that represents a threat to life or health and a legal guardian is not readily available to provide consent, prehospital professionals can assess the child, provide necessary medical treatment, and transport the child. The legal basis for taking action in an emergency when consent is not available is known as the doctrine of **implied consent**. For minors, this means that the prehospital professional can presume consent and proceed with

appropriate treatment and transport if all of the following four conditions are met:

1. The child is suffering from an emergent condition that places his or her life or health in danger.
2. The child's legal guardian is unavailable or unable to provide consent for treatment or transport.
3. Treatment or transport cannot be safely delayed until consent can be obtained.
4. The prehospital professional administers only treatment for emergency conditions that pose an immediate threat to the child.

The doctrine of implied consent is based on the principle that all reasonable people want to live, and therefore would consent to the provision of essential emergency medical care if necessary to save an individual's life. Any time a minor is treated without consent, the burden of proof falls on the prehospital professional to justify that the emergency actions were necessary. The prehospital professional must fully and clearly document on the prehospital record the nature of the medical emergency, attempts to contact the legal guardian, and the reasons the minor required immediate treatment or transport.

If possible, contact online medical control for assistance when consent is unclear or unavailable. If the guardian is unavailable or cannot be notified, provide information about the destination emergency department (ED) to the most responsible person on scene (in writing whenever possible), with instructions to pass the information on to the minor's legal guardian. As a general rule, when the prehospital professional's authority to act is in doubt, always do what is in the best interest of the patient.

FIGURE 15-1 In most states, a parent or legal guardian must give permission before a minor can be transported.
© kali9/E+/Getty Images.

Refusal of Care or Transport
Guardian Refusal

A special situation occurs when the prehospital professional is faced with a legal guardian who refuses to give permission for medical treatment or transport of a child with an acute illness or injury. As long as a

CASE STUDY **1**

You are called to an apartment where you find a 3-year-old girl in mild respiratory distress. She is interactive and consolable, but has bilateral wheezes and a pulse oximeter reading of 94%. She is home alone with a 16-year-old babysitter who tells you that the child's parents will not return for several hours and did not leave information about their destination or contact information.

1. Can the babysitter give you legally valid consent to treat the child?
2. Can you legally provide care and transport this child?

child's legal guardian is of sound mind, he or she has the right to refuse medical care for his or her child. However, the guardian must act in the best interests of the child.

When a guardian refuses to allow provision of care or transport of a child whose life or health might be threatened, an important legal and ethical issue arises. In such circumstances, attempt to contact medical control for guidance. The medical control physician may speak directly to the legal guardian to convince the guardian to allow treatment and transport. If medical control agrees that the child's condition requires immediate treatment to prevent serious harm, yet the legal guardian continues to refuse consent for care, it may be necessary to enlist the assistance of law enforcement in placing the child in **emergency protective custody**. Likewise, when a legal guardian seems to be intoxicated, impaired, or has his or her decision-making capacity impacted by another circumstance, involvement of law enforcement officers may be necessary to place a minor in emergency protective custody. Local emergency medical services (EMS) pediatric guidelines and protocols should guide the prehospital professional's procedure in such situations.

CAUTION

When a legal guardian is not readily available to provide consent for a minor, the prehospital professional must provide only treatment and transport for emergency conditions that pose an immediate threat to the child.

TIP

When the prehospital professional's authority to act is in doubt, always do what is in the best interest of the patient.

Although emergency protective custody may allow the prehospital professional to transport a minor to a medical facility for purposes of medical evaluation, it does not give the prehospital professional the right to treat a minor for medical conditions that are not serious or life-threatening. *A prehospital professional can provide medical treatment without consent only when the child has a medical condition that poses a risk of death or serious harm, when immediate specific*

treatment is necessary to prevent that harm, and when only those specific treatments are provided. Discuss these situations with medical control before initiating treatment, whenever possible. Sometimes an intermediate solution is possible. Document everything fully and clearly about the medical condition of the child, the need for emergency care, and the basis for overriding the wishes of the legal guardian, including the involvement of medical control and/or law enforcement.

Every case of unclear consent or refusal requires careful scene management; notification of medical control, if available; and full and accurate documentation in the prehospital record.

Never confront the caregiver with accusations, moral judgments, or threats when difficult circumstances develop at the scene. This approach only aggravates the situation and does not help the patient. Try to establish whether the caregiver refuses all care and transport or only certain aspects of care. For example, some caregivers may prefer that prehospital professionals not initiate therapy, but permit the child to be transported to the hospital. If the child can be safely transported without initiating care, respect the caregiver's wishes concerning care. It may be appropriate for the caregiver of a child with a terminal illness or significant disabilities to restrict certain kinds of care for the child. Discuss these difficult situations with medical control.

TIP

Get police assistance when a guardian who is intoxicated, impaired, or has his or her decision-making capacity impacted by another circumstance refuses care or transport of an ill or injured child.

TIP

Never confront the caregiver with accusations, moral judgments, or threats.

Child Refusal

There are two instances in which a minor has the legal authority to refuse care and make decisions regarding his or her health care. The first situation is when the child is an emancipated minor, as previously discussed. A second situation in which a minor might have legal status to make decisions arises when a court has declared an individual a **mature minor**. This is different than an emancipated minor. In most states, mature minors are older than 14 years of age and have been formally declared adults by the court. **TABLE 15-1** lists the legal circumstances in which pediatric patients can provide or refuse consent for medical care and transport in most states. The mature minor doctrine most often applies to a child with a chronic medical condition who has demonstrated an active, informed role in managing his or her own care and may involve a life-threatening or terminal illness.

Because these laws vary, the prehospital professional should be familiar with the specifics of emancipated and mature minor laws in the state in which care is being provided.

If a child is not an emancipated or a mature minor, then he or she has no legal capacity either to give consent or to refuse medical care. Regardless of whether a child has the legal authority to provide or withhold consent, it is always prudent to get the child's agreement or assent to treat and transport, if possible. This approach respects the personal dignity and self-determination of the child-patient and minimizes

TABLE 15-1 Common Characteristics of Emancipated and Mature Minors

Emancipated Minor
Married
Pregnant
Has a child
Active-duty status in the armed services
15 years or older, economically self-supporting, and living apart from parents

Mature Minor
14 years or older and declared a mature minor by the state Superior Court
AND patient is not on a psychiatric hold
AND patient demonstrates competency to be involved in his or her own health care decision making

confrontation. A willingness to provide the child with some control and some choices may allow for a compromise that helps prehospital professionals to achieve a safe transfer. Avoid restraint use to transport a child except in those situations when the child is at risk of serious harm if he or she is not transported, and only after consultation with medical control.

TIP

A minor child cannot legally refuse care or transport when care is required.

Caregivers Who Disagree

One rare but confusing situation arises when the prehospital professional is confronted by caregivers who disagree about whether to consent to treatment and transport of a sick or injured child. In these cases, establish whether one or both caregivers are legal decision makers for the child. If both caregivers have legal authority, the prehospital professional may need to negotiate a plan that both find acceptable. Focus on the child's needs and the common desire to assist the child, while deflecting attention from the disagreement. Medical control may need to be involved to assist the prehospital professional in determining the proper course of action and to determine the need for law enforcement.

Custody Issues and Nontraditional Families

Parents who are legally divorced may disagree about the child's care or access to the child's medical records. One parent may accuse the other of harming the child or being a poor influence. There may be differing viewpoints between the biologic parent and the step parent. In another case, the biologic mother at the scene may refuse to allow the step mother, also at the scene, to participate in the child's care, give permission for any treatment, or have any access to knowledge about the child's condition. Perhaps one parent is the legal guardian, and the other parent's rights have been terminated. Another parent may refuse transport because he or she does not want to be billed, because that responsibility rests with the parent who is not available.

Many children live in nontraditional families in which they are cared for by grandparents, older siblings, same-sex parents, or foster parents. It may not be clear who has the responsibility of consenting for the minor child. In addition, these caregivers may be the only adults involved with the child on a regular basis despite the fact that they may not be legally accountable for that child. State statutes may have various mechanisms to allow nonparent caregivers to provide valid consent for minor children. These caregivers can stand **in loco parentis**, meaning "in place of the parent," with recognized rights to consent for medical care, make educational decisions, and perform other parental functions even though they have no other legal or biologic connection to the child. In general, health care providers can place reasonable reliance on statements made by individuals professing to be in a caregiver role for a child. Conversely, health care providers have a duty to investigate further if a purported caregiver's claims seem suspicious or questionable. Certain states may allow parents to convey certain parental rights to others through a power of attorney, guardianship, or a "Caregiver's Affidavit" without severing their parental ties to a child.

In these situations, determining legal guardianship for treatment and transport may be difficult. If the child is acutely ill or injured, there is not time to look at legal documents, even if they are available. Contact medical control for advice, and involve law enforcement if the situation becomes violent or may cause harm to the child.

CAUTION

Many children live in nontraditional families, and it may be unclear who has responsibility for consenting for the minor child.

Summary of Consent

Laws strictly protect the right of adult patients to accept or reject medical care. Interpreting these consent laws for children in a prehospital setting, however, can pose special challenges. The prehospital professional faces a difficult situation in cases where the caregiver refuses to consent or where consent to provide care and transport for a child cannot be readily obtained. Every case requires careful scene management; notification of medical control, if available; and accurate documentation in the prehospital record. EMS systems should provide clear

policies, procedures, and protocols based on state law to guide the prehospital professional or medical control. Local EMS policy on consent should clearly define the following:

- Who can refuse ambulance transport according to state law
- The process for field evaluation, consultation, and documentation
- The method for enlisting police and medical control when the patient's medical conditions and other scene factors warrant these resources

Confidentiality

Medical information is private. Carelessly or inadvertently revealing identifiable information is an ethical and legal risk that prehospital professionals face, because they frequently care for individuals in a public environment. *It is essential to remain aware of the potentially sensitive nature of identifiable information and to take every possible precaution to protect confidentiality.* Conduct all sensitive discussions, when possible, in a setting where bystanders cannot overhear. Avoid using last names, if at all possible, at the scene. Do not share private information with concerned bystanders (other than those legally responsible for the patient).

TIP

Prehospital professionals must be aware of the potentially sensitive nature of protected health information and take every possible precaution to protect confidentiality.

Respect for Cultural or Religious Differences

Cultural differences and religious beliefs may present exceptionally difficult situations. Although the care of the patient is always of primary concern, the prehospital professional must be sensitive to requests from the family or patient regarding preferences that may originate from their religious or cultural beliefs, especially when these do not interfere significantly with the provision of treatment to the child.

The prehospital professional must always remain nonjudgmental about requests that stem from cultural or religious beliefs, acknowledge the importance of these requests to the family, and attempt to accommodate them when possible. When the prehospital professional cannot accommodate requests that are based on cultural or religious beliefs because he or she would put a child at risk of serious harm, the reasons the requests cannot be accommodated must be respectfully explained and documented. Parents have great latitude to make medical decisions for themselves based on religious beliefs; however, this right does not extend to allow them to make martyrs of their children on the basis of religious beliefs. Medical control and police may need to be involved if parents refuse to consent to necessary care and the child is at risk of imminent harm.

TIP

The prehospital professional must always remain nonjudgmental about cultural or religious beliefs, acknowledge their importance to the family and the community, and attempt to accommodate them whenever possible.

Language barriers may also present a challenge as the prehospital professional attempts to communicate with a child's caregiver. The prehospital professional should be familiar with locally available resources to provide translation in a timely manner. Miscommunication can have a significant impact on patient care, especially if the prehospital professional is unable to obtain information about a child's underlying medical conditions, allergies, current medications, or other factors relevant to medical treatment. When available, professional translation services should be used instead of family members or bystanders. If translation

services are not available, a family member or neighbor may be asked to assist with translation, with the understanding that information may be inaccurate or incomplete. When using nonprofessional translation, care should be taken to avoid medical terminology when possible.

Patient Rights and Advocacy

For children, patient rights may be dependent on the wishes of the child's parents or legal guardians. However, emancipated minors have the ability to make decisions about their medical care and treatment, even though these decisions may not be accepted by other family members or the general public. The EMS system, the medical director, and the community's standard of care can compete with the wishes of patients. These competing interests can create an ethical conflict that needs to be resolved.

The decision to accept medical treatment may be a difficult one. Give the parents, guardians, or the emancipated minor time to consider what is most appropriate. In some instances, this emergency may be the first time the patient has had to face the reality of his or her medical condition. When in doubt, try to do what is in the best interest of the patient and rely on medical control for advice.

End-of-Life Issues

The caregivers of children who are terminally ill, usually in consultation with their primary physician, may decide on limitations to treatments and interventions. These decisions usually arise from the child's underlying condition and the desire to avoid futile or burdensome interventions if the child develops a life-threatening condition. Prehospital professionals,

---

CASE STUDY 2

You are called to care for a homeless 15-year-old boy whose friends called because he was not feeling well and was not acting normally. You find the young man lying on the sidewalk, complaining of a severe headache. When you attempt to assess him, he starts cussing, pushes you away aggressively, and demands to be left alone. He screams that he has rights and that he does not have to talk to you. He will not even answer questions that would allow you to assess his level of consciousness and orientation.

1. What rights does the teenager have to refuse care and transport?
2. What methods of persuasion can you use?

FIGURE 15-2 DNR order.

© Jones & Bartlett Learning. Courtesy of Glen Ellman.

in responding to a call about a sick child, may be confronted with a **Do Not Resuscitate (DNR)** order or **Physician Orders for Life-Sustaining Treatment (POLST)**. A DNR order must be signed by a physician to be valid (**FIGURE 15-2**). These orders inform health care providers that cardiopulmonary resuscitation (CPR) or additional resuscitation, such as defibrillation or advanced airway control, should not be initiated in the event of a cardiopulmonary arrest. Some local EMS regions do not recognize DNR orders for children. *Prehospital professionals must know the specifics of DNR and/or POLST guidance in their jurisdictions and develop protocols for dealing with them.*

A POLST form is a comprehensive document indicating goals of care, treatment that is permitted when the patient still has a pulse and is breathing, artificially administered nutrition, CPR and airway management permissions, as well as other directions to care (**FIGURE 15-3**). POLST form endorsement varies among states.

HIPAA PERMITS DISCLOSURE OF POLST TO OTHER HEALTHCARE PROFESSIONALS AS NECESSARY

NEW JERSEY PRACTITIONER ORDERS FOR LIFE-SUSTAINING TREATMENT (POLST)

Follow these orders, then contact physician/APN. This Medical Order Sheet is based on the current medical condition of the person referenced below and their wishes stated verbally or in a written advance directive. Any section not completed implies full treatment for that section. Everyone will be treated with dignity and respect.

PERSON NAME (LAST, FIRST, MIDDLE)   DATE OF BIRTH

A	**GOALS OF CARE** *(See reverse for instructions. This section does not constitute a medical order.)*	

B	**MEDICAL INTERVENTIONS:** *Person is breathing and/or has a pulse*
	 ❏ **Full Treatment.** Use all appropriate medical and surgical interventions as indicated to support life. If in a nursing facility, transfer to hospital if indicated. See section D for resuscitation status.
	 ❏ **Limited Treatment.** Use appropriate medical treatment such as antibiotics and IV fluids as indicated. May use non-invasive positive airway pressure. Generally avoid intensive care.
	   ❏ Transfer to hospital for medical interventions.
	   ❏ Transfer to hospital only if comfort needs cannot be met in current location.
	 ❏ **Symptom Treatment Only.** Use aggressive comfort treatment to relieve pain and suffering by using any medication by any route, positioning, wound care and other measures. Use oxygen, suctioning and manual treatment of airway obstruction as needed for comfort. Use Antibiotics only to promote comfort. Transfer only if comfort needs cannot be met in current location.
	 Additional Orders:_____	

C	**ARTIFICIALLY ADMINISTERED FLUIDS AND NUTRITION:** *Always offer food/fluids by mouth if feasible and desired.* ❏ No artificial nutrition.	❏ Defined trial period of artificial nutrition. ❏ Long-term artificial nutrition.
D	**CARDIOPULMONARY RESUSCITATION (CPR)** *Person has no pulse and/or is not breathing* ❏ Attempt resuscitation/CPR ❏ Do not attempt resuscitation/DNAR Allow <u>N</u>atural <u>D</u>eath	**AIRWAY MANAGEMENT** *Person is in respiratory distress with a pulse* ❏ Intubate/use artificial ventilation as needed ❏ Do not intubate - Use O2, manual treatment to relieve airway obstruction, medications for comfort. ❏ Additional Order (for example defined trial period of mechanical ventilation) _____
E	If I lose my decision-making capacity, I authorize my surrogate decision maker, listed below, to modify or revoke the NJ POLST orders in consultation with my treating physician/APN in keeping with my goals: ❏ Yes ❏ No ❏ Health care representative identified in an advance directive ❏ Other surrogate decision maker Print Name of Surrogate (address on reverse) Phone Number	
F	**SIGNATURES:** *I have discussed this information with my physician/APN.* Print Name_____ Signature_____ ❏ Person Named Above ❏ Health Care Representative/Legal Guardian ❏ Spouse/Civil Union Partner ❏ Parent of Minor ❏ Other Surrogate	Has the person named above made an anatomical gift: ❏ Yes ❏ No ❏ Unknown *These orders are consistent with the person's medical condition, known preferences and best known information.* PRINT - Physician/APN Name Phone Number Physician/APN Signature (Mandatory) Date/Time Professional License Number

4/12/17   SEND ORIGINAL FORM WITH PERSON WHENEVER TRANSFERRED

FIGURE 15-3 POLST form.

Regardless of the nature of the local law or prehospital policy, a legal guardian may always revoke a DNR or POLST order written on behalf of a child. When faced with a valid DNR or POLST order written for a child and a legal guardian requesting that the child be resuscitated, always follow the legal guardian's wishes. Even in the face of a valid DNR or POLST order, clarify with the legal guardian what kinds of interventions he or she does and does not consider acceptable. For example, oxygen delivery and transport may be acceptable and expected for some children with DNR orders.

Resuscitation

Sometimes resuscitation attempts are ineffective for children in cardiopulmonary arrest, and occasionally such attempts are unnecessary, as discussed in Chapter 5. Resuscitation policy should define circumstances when cardiopulmonary resuscitation must be initiated, when it may be withheld, and when it may be stopped. Personnel in rural and wilderness situations must also consider the time it takes for a patient to reach definitive care at the hospital. For pediatric patients, the policy should take a patient-focused approach, but allow appropriate withholding of resuscitation to focus on grief management and family interactions.

Local resuscitation policy may allow prehospital professionals to withhold or stop resuscitation when a child is clearly deceased, as defined by specific criteria (e.g., rigor mortis or injuries incompatible with life). This situation may be emotionally difficult for the prehospital provider, and all crew members must be in agreement with the decision to stop or to forego a resuscitation attempt. Likewise, it may be difficult emotionally for family members if prehospital professionals do not attempt resuscitation. *In cases where family members of the child are clearly distressed by the decision to forego resuscitation, consider providing resuscitative efforts as a gesture to the family that every effort has been made to save their child.* In such cases, the child can be treated with basic life support (BLS) measures only and transported to the ED, where physicians can formally pronounce the child dead and terminate resuscitation. Consider incorporating guidance on this topic into your local protocols.

EMS systems should have, as part of educational and training requirements for field personnel, a formal training program regarding sudden unexpected infant death syndrome (SUIDS; see Chapter 13). Local EMS policies should clearly establish the responsibility of the prehospital professional at death scenes regarding care of the body, notification of the coroner or medical examiner and law enforcement, and interaction with caregivers.

Organ Donation

A major issue in medical ethics involves the potential for patients with mortal injuries to donate organs. Donor organs are badly needed within the medical system, and many patients wait years or die while waiting for a match (**TABLE 15-2**).

Whether or not a child should be kept alive for the sole purpose of organ donation is an issue that prehospital professionals should discuss with medical control and the local hospital system. The parameters for viable organs should be clearly spelled out within the individual EMS system. Understanding state laws regarding organ donation helps the prehospital professional decide how to proceed.

Another helpful resource is the local organ transplant programs within the EMS service area. They may offer workshops or agree to come to the service to provide continuing education to increase awareness of the vital role of prehospital professionals, as well as help with protocol development.

Telling the Truth in Difficult Situations

Prehospital professionals should deal as honestly as possible with children and their caregivers. It is not

---

TABLE 15-2 Organ Donation Statistics

- As of December 2018, more than 113,000 were waiting for an organ transplant to survive. Of this number, almost 2,000 are pediatric patients.

- Another person needing a transplant is added to the waiting list every 10 minutes.

- Each day, approximately 20 people die waiting for a transplant.

- In 2018, there were 36,528 organ transplants performed.

- More than one-half of the adults in the United States are registered as organ donors, however only 0.3% of deaths allow for organ donation.

CASE STUDY 3

You respond to the scene of a motor vehicle crash where you find a 10-year-old child with facial bruising; a tense, tender abdomen; and an obviously deformed left thigh. The child is seat belted in the rear passenger seat of the car, which has been struck on the driver's door by a truck. The child seems scared and begins to cry as you begin your assessment. The adult woman who had been driving the car has obvious head injuries and lacks a pulse. Another team begins work on the adult while you tend to the child. As you stabilize the child for transport, she asks you if her mother is okay.

1. Would it be appropriate to tell the child her mother is okay to enable a safe and efficient transport?
2. How should you respond to this child's question?

unusual for caregivers to ask about the condition of a child or request information about a child's "chances of survival." In such situations, refrain from speculating, but respond instead with honest reassurance. For example, the statements "We'll take the best possible care of your child," or "He is in good hands; everything is being done to help him," provide an honest and reassuring response without speculating about uncertain outcomes.

The prehospital professional may also face situations in which multiple patients have sustained injuries and the parent or child requests information about others involved in the incident. It may be appropriate to deflect such questions, especially when the other party has suffered severe injuries or has died. The best tact may be to offer an honest statement of reassurance, such as "I need to focus on taking the best care of you right now. My partners are doing their best to take care of the others." Although there is an ethical obligation to be honest, it may be appropriate to delay sharing particularly distressing information until a patient has been transported safely and other sources of emotional support are available.

Physician on Scene

Prehospital care is under the authority of EMS medical control. Unless specifically authorized by medical control of the medical director of the EMS agency, prehospital professionals cannot carry out orders from other physicians, including the patient's private physician. These interactions are sometimes controversial. *Only medical control may allow the on-scene physician to assist prehospital professionals or transfer total authority to the on-scene physician.* If the on-scene physician takes responsibility for treatment, he or she must be available to accompany the child to the ED.

TIP

If the on-scene physician takes authority for care, he or she should be available to accompany the child to the ED.

CONTROVERSY

The role of the child's private physician in on-scene care is controversial. The prehospital provider must abide by local EMS system policy, but the precise limitations to an on-scene physician providing assistance are sometimes unclear. Always act in the best interests of the child when the policy is confusing.

Hospital Destination

The hospital destination policy for children must define the following components:

1. Field triage criteria (which patients with what conditions go where)
2. Designated receiving hospitals
3. Specialized pediatric centers

The appropriate ED for a sick or injured child may differ from the ED appropriate for an adult with a similar condition. Some EMS systems may identify specialized pediatric centers (e.g., general trauma centers with pediatric capability, pediatric critical care centers, or pediatric trauma centers) as primary receiving facilities for certain pediatric patients. In some cases, a child may meet multiple conflicting triage criteria (e.g., should a severely burned child be transported to a regional children's hospital or a nonpediatric hospital with a regional burn center?). The destination policy must either provide guidance on where such patients should be transported or specify that medical control makes all complex triage decisions. If disagreement persists, try to explain your reasoning for choosing the destination. If not successful, call medical control and have them speak to the guardian. The prehospital professional must transport the child to the ED preferred by the legal guardian unless hospital destination policy requires an alternate facility; always objectively document your observations and decision making.

Pediatric Policies and Procedures

EMS systems should provide clear guidelines for common problems related to ethical and legal issues involving children. In addition, when available, online medical control provides the prehospital professional with the ability to obtain real-time consultation regarding particularly difficult situations, such as the inability to obtain consent, refusal of consent by a child or guardian, presence of a physician on scene, resuscitation or other clinical decisions, and suspected child maltreatment or sexual assault.

Protocols, Policies, and Procedures

Operations are the administrative backbone of the EMS system. The goal of operations is to manage day-to-day field care with standards established by the EMS system. An important part of operations is the policies, procedures, and protocols that define the medical responsibility and legal authority of the prehospital professionals and medical director within the EMS system. These written directives assist the prehospital professional in knowing what to do in complicated prehospital situations. These written directives, along with education and training, also help set performance standards.

Because the needs of children differ from those of adults, pediatric-specific protocols, policies, and procedures are necessary tools for a comprehensive EMS system. Protocols define explicit field treatments or the order and type of medical interventions for specific illness and injury conditions. They give appropriate pharmacologic options, including drug doses, routes of delivery, and methods of administration. Most EMS systems have prehospital pediatric advanced life support (ALS), medical emergency, and trauma treatment protocols. Appropriate treatment protocols for prehospital BLS personnel and for first responders are also important. **TABLE 15-3** lists some common EMS pediatric treatment protocols.

Policies and procedures reflect the expectations of the community for prehospital care, quality management, and system accountability. These forms of regulation consist of clear, written directives to guide prehospital professionals. They are intended to help with decision making in difficult or legally sensitive pediatric field situations, such as those discussed previously in this chapter. Policies usually explain how the prehospital professional should handle certain situations and the reasoning behind them, rather than medical treatment. Procedures describe the sequence of actions for the prehospital professional in applying medical protocols or medicolegal policies. The field policies with the most

TABLE 15-3 Examples of Pediatric Treatment Protocols
Airway obstruction
Allergic reaction and anaphylaxis
Altered mental status
Bradycardia
Burns
Cardiopulmonary arrest
Hypoperfusion or shock
Neonatal resuscitation
Seizures
Respiratory distress
Tachycardia
Toxic exposures
Trauma

frequent application to pediatric care include the following:

- Consent for care or transport
- Refusal to consent for care or transport
- Death in the field
- Triage guidelines
- Hospital destination
- Child maltreatment

Each state has statutes to establish basic requirements for local EMS systems; provide guidelines for quality management, accountability, and enforcement; and establish provider scope of practice. Policies, procedures, and protocols may be very different from one EMS system to the next. Mutual aid agreements between bordering geographic areas are especially useful because resources, equipment, and personnel for specialized care of children are not evenly distributed. Specialized trauma care and critical care centers for children are usually only available at major hospitals in large urban areas. In some states, no specialized centers at all exist for children.

Child Maltreatment and Sexual Assault

Education of prehospital professionals in identifying possible maltreatment is an essential component of initial education and continuing medical education in pediatrics (see Chapter 11). A policy and procedure for reporting suspected cases of maltreatment and for appropriate patient transport to an ED are important components of every EMS system. The prehospital professional must ensure that victims of maltreatment or sexual assault are initially evaluated in a careful, compassionate, and respectful way. Transport these patients to an ED staffed by clinicians experienced in working with child victims of maltreatment and sexual assault and equipped with the appropriate ancillary and follow-up services. Never confront the caregiver or others with accusations, moral judgments, threats, or suspicions. Although these situations are emotionally difficult, the immediate goal must always be to provide necessary treatment and ensure the safe transport of the child.

Medical Control for Pediatrics

Medical control, medical direction, or medical oversight are the mechanisms by which physicians, nurses, and EMS officials supervise field practice. Medical control includes direct and indirect methods.

Online (Direct) Medical Control

Online or **direct medical control** refers to any communication between the prehospital professional and medical control by telephone or radio. This form of control is required by some local EMS systems for many or all cases involving children younger than 18 years of age (**FIGURE 15-4**) because decisions about pediatric ALS treatment (e.g., intravenous lines [IVs], drug routes, and doses), triage, scene control, and transport are often difficult. Online medical control can be very useful and should be employed in cases of high-risk pediatric refusals. Online medical control is usually a recorded line and any conversation with the parent while speaking with medical control can also be recorded. In the cases of high-risk refusals with a life threat, the medical control physician should speak directly with the parent or guardian via the recorded line. **TABLE 15-4** lists some examples of problems in pediatric field practice that often require online physician input or direct medical control.

Offline (Indirect) Medical Control

Offline or **indirect medical control** involves prospective and retrospective guidance. Prospective indirect control consists of planning for expected educational and operational requirements within the prehospital professional's scope of practice. Retrospective

FIGURE 15-4 Direct medical control can be extremely helpful when the prehospital professional confronts medical and legal problems with children.
© Jones and Bartlett Learning. Courtesy of MIEMSS.

TABLE 15-4 Possible Pediatric Issues Needing Direct Medical Control

Pediatric Issue	Possible Scenario
Type of field treatment	IV or rectal diazepam for status epilepticus
Hospital destination	Appropriate ED for infant trauma patient
Specialized scene control	Hazardous materials exposure in school
Transport	Requirement for ED care after minor poisoning

TABLE 15-5 Indirect Medical Control

Examples of Prospective Control
Pediatric BLS and ALS ambulance equipment and drugs
Pediatric prehospital treatment protocols
Skills training
Airway foreign body removal
Endotracheal intubation
IO needle insertion
Rectal diazepam
Pediatric-specific policies
Hospital destination
Triage
Transport
Refusal of care
Suspected SUIDS
Maltreatment
Examples of Retrospective Control
Review of compliance with treatment, triage, and transport policies
Review of success, failure, and complications of pediatric procedures and patient outcomes
Epidemiologic data on types of pediatric illness and injury
Review of ED or hospital capabilities for the care of children

indirect control involves review of individual and overall system performance against expectations or standards of care to provide accountability. **TABLE 15-5** lists common examples of how indirect control creates and monitors different types of policies, procedures, and protocols for children.

Summary of Rationale for Protocols, Policies, and Procedures

Pediatric-specific guidelines (as defined in protocols, policies, and procedures) help set standards of care for children. Medical control is especially important in the delivery of prehospital services to families and children because of the unusual circumstances that often arise medically and legally.

CASE STUDY ANSWERS

CASE STUDY 1

Although a babysitter (even an adult babysitter) cannot provide valid consent to treat, the doctrine of implied consent allows you to treat and transport this child who is in respiratory distress. She suffers from an emergent condition that places her at risk, her legal guardian is unavailable, and it would be unsafe to delay treatment. If the babysitter has a telephone number for the parents, call them, apprise them of the situation, and ask permission to provide necessary treatment and transport. If there is no way to reach the parents, you should provide treatment for the child's wheezing and respiratory distress with oxygen and a bronchodilator and transport her to an appropriate facility. Finally, make sure this 16-year-old babysitter is safe, and leave a note with her to give to the child's caregivers that explains what happened and where you have transported the child.

CASE STUDY 2

Unless you can persuade the child to allow you to deliver care, this will be a difficult situation. As a homeless adolescent, most states would consider this child to be a ward of the state, not an emancipated minor. However, despite the fact that he cannot legally refuse treatment and transport, every effort must be made to show respect, involve him in decisions, and avoid the use of force. If he persists in his refusal to be evaluated, contact medical control. If his combativeness seems to be the result of a medical condition that impairs judgment (e.g., meningitis, a head injury, intoxication), call law enforcement to provide assistance in restraining the adolescent sufficiently to allow a safe assessment and transport.

As a practical matter, respect the boy's dignity, but be firm that transport to an ED is necessary. Try to establish rapport and do not be judgmental. If a friend or counselor is available, try to get assistance in persuading the teenager to agree to care and transport.

CASE STUDY 3

Carefully consider your answer to this child's concerned question. On the one hand, avoid being dishonest. Because you do not know whether her mother will survive, you should not assure the child that her mother will be okay. On the other hand, it would be appropriate to withhold your concerns and suspicions about the mother's condition until the child has been transported safely, more is known about the mother's condition, and there are resources (e.g., a social worker) available to assist the child in receiving what may be terrible news. One honest answer might be, "I know you are worried about your mother. My partners are taking good care of her. I need to take good care of you, and I'm going to take you to the hospital. Once we get there, we'll try to find out more about your mother."

SUGGESTED REFERENCES

Textbooks

American Academy of Orthopaedic Surgeons. *Nancy Caroline's Emergency Care in the Streets*. 8th ed. Burlington, MA: Jones & Bartlett Learning; 2018.

McWay DC. *Today's Health Information Management: An Integrated Approach*. Clifton Park, NY: Delmar Cengage Learning; 2008.

Wertz Evans EM. Children and youth with special health care needs. In: Thomas D, Bernardo L, eds. *Core Curriculum for Pediatric Emergency Nursing*. 2nd ed. Chicago, IL: Emergency Nurses Association; 2009.

Articles

American Academy of Pediatrics, Committee of Pediatric Emergency Medicine & Committee on Bioethics. Consent for emergency medical services for children and adolescents. *Pediatrics*. 2011;128(2):427-433.

Larkin G. Essential ethics for EMS: cardinal virtues and core principles. *Emerg Med Clin North Am*. 2002;20:887–911.

Schears R, Marco C, Iserson K. "Do not attempt resuscitation" in the out-of-hospital setting. *Ann Emerg Med*. 2004;44:68–69.

Other Resources

American Medical Association. What you need to know about the new HIPAA Breach Notification Rule. https://www.ama-assn.org/practice-management/hipaa/hipaa-breach-notification-rule. Accessed October 8, 2019.

Center for Democracy and Technology. Stronger protections for, and encouraging the use of, de-identified (and "anonymized") health data. https://www.cdt.org/insight/stronger-protections-and-encouraging-use-of-de-identified-and-anonymous-health-data. Accessed Oct 8, 2019.

Centers for Medicare and Medicaid Services. HIPAA basics. https://www.cms.gov/Outreach -and-Education/Medicare-Learning-Network -MLN/MLNProducts/MLN-Publications-Items /ICN909001.html. Accessed October 8, 2019.

Centers for Medicare and Medicaid Services. HIPAA—General information, 2010. http://www .cms.gov/HIPAAGenInfo/ 01_Overview.asp. Accessed September 12, 2012.

Donate Life America. Organ donation. https://donate life.net/statistics. Accessed October 8, 2019.

Privileged Communication. *Encyclopedia Britannica*. https://www.britannica.com/topic/privileged -communication. Accessed October 7, 2019.

United States Department of Health and Human Services. Organ Donation Statistics. https://www .organdonor.gov/statistics-stories/statistics.html. Accessed October 8, 2019.

© Steve Jolicoeur/Shutterstock.

CHAPTER 16

Transportation Considerations

Michael J. Stoner, MD, FAAP

LEARNING OBJECTIVES

1. Discuss transport considerations for pediatric encounters in an ambulance.
2. List the considerations used to determine the mode of transport for children in an ambulance.
3. Discuss advantages and disadvantages of transporting caregivers in the ambulance.
4. Identify and discuss current guidelines for child restraint systems in ambulances.
5. Identify issues related to choice of destination when making pediatric transport decisions.
6. Outline issues involved in transporting multiple children.

Pediatric Transport

Although pediatric patients make up a small portion of EMS runs, every prehospital professional is faced with the decision of when and how to transport a child. Whether the child is a patient or accompanying an adult, the transport decision involves many facets. One must consider current and potential circumstances when making the decision on how, or even if, to transport the child. The prehospital professional must know the local emergency medical services (EMS) protocols for safe transport of children, the state motor vehicle

CASE STUDY 1

You arrive on scene to find a 27-year-old single mother who fell down the steps in her home. She had a brief loss of consciousness and sustained a head laceration. Her ankle is also swollen, and she cannot bear weight on it, so she requires transport. Her 6-month-old daughter is asleep in her crib. The patient agrees to be transported, but not without her child. No other family members or neighbors are available at this time.

1. Is it appropriate to transport the child with the mother?
2. What issues are involved when transporting children who are not patients?

laws addressing child occupants in vehicles, the local resources and equipment that may be available, and the EMS regulations that govern the treatment of children en route. Most importantly, the prehospital professional must be able to address the urgent and changing medical needs of the patient as well as the operational issues involved in transport.

The decision process about whether a child should be transported in the ambulance if he or she is accompanying an adult patient should be handled through policies and protocols, with forethought and resource guidelines before an on-scene decision. If that is not available in the system, it is important to understand that ambulances were not designed to transport pediatric occupants, and so ambulance design challenges even the most experienced personnel with regards to safe options for nonpatient pediatric occupants.

When the child is the patient and transport is necessary, the position in which the patient is secured usually depends on the stability of the child and whether or not interventions are needed en route. Rapid transport depends on multiple factors. In a basic life support system, early transport is appropriate if the scene is unsafe for the child, caregiver, or prehospital professional or if the child has any of the following:

- A serious mechanism of injury
- A history compatible with serious illness
- A physiologic abnormality noted during the primary assessment
- A potentially serious anatomic abnormality
- Significant pain

In an advanced life support (ALS) system with more extensive treatment options in the field, the transport decision is often complicated. Major factors to consider include the following:

- Type of clinical problem (injury versus illness)
- Expected benefits of ALS treatment in the field
- Local EMS system treatment and transport policies
- The ALS provider's comfort level

> **TIP**
>
> Many EMS systems have clear policies or protocols that define pediatric transport practices, whether at the local or state level, but not all do. While there is no regulation, there are national guidelines about safe transport of children in ambulances.

Another consideration is choice of destination; not all areas have pediatric centers and may rely on local hospitals for stabilization. This should be addressed within local EMS protocols. Many states have pediatric hospital designation agreements and other pediatric-specific programs accomplished through the Emergency Medical Services for Children program.

How to Begin Transport

Is the Child the Patient?

Why a child is being transported is the first factor in determining how to transport. Is the child the patient, or is the child with a caregiver who needs ambulance transport? *Children who are not patients and only need transport because they must accompany the patient are best transported properly restrained in a vehicle other than an ambulance whenever possible.* There are few safe options available to secure a child properly, and there may be risk of injury while transporting any patient in an ambulance. Ambulances are not designed for transporting children who are not patients.

Many communities have coalitions for pediatrics that may be able to act as resources to transport children who are not patients in alternate vehicles. Public safety disaster plans and school resources in the local area are good places to start when looking to develop partnerships. Agreements can be set up ahead of time to have alternate transport options when these situations arise. Working with partners, prehospital professionals may be able to provide a system that affords a variety of child restraints and safe vehicles. Providers should explain that the need for safe transport of additional family members may require separating the family temporarily.

> **CAUTION**
>
> Avoid transporting a child who is not a patient in an ambulance.

When a Sick Child Is the Patient

If the child requires airway, breathing, or circulatory support beyond simple oxygen delivery or nebulized bronchodilators, or if the child requires ALS monitoring or treatment, secure him or her to the stretcher in a supine or **semi-Fowler's position**. This is a position that best and most safely allows the prehospital professional to perform ongoing assessment and treatment en route.

TIP

Except in the case of mild illness or injury, transport a sick child appropriately secured on a stretcher in a supine or semi-Fowler's position. This provides the safest and most effective position for ongoing assessment, monitoring, and treatment.

When the Child Is the Patient but is Not Sick

Often, the primary assessment reveals that the child has only minimal or mild illness or is not seriously injured, but still requires transport to a medical facility. There are numerous options on how to transport that protect the child's safety, permit appropriate monitoring, and provide comfort. Many children who are strapped supine to a stretcher become distressed from the effects of restraint, stranger anxiety, fear, and pain. When possible, attempt to transport children who are only mildly ill or injured in an upright position, to minimize the emotional distress and discomfort from an uncomfortable stretcher. Integrated child restraints for the EMS provider and pediatric transport devices that attach to stretchers are becoming more readily available and can provide more options for safe transport.

When a child is the patient, consider carefully how to position him or her to maximize effectiveness of interventions, to allow appropriate monitoring, and to preserve safety and comfort. If the child has any immediate or anticipated requirements for interventions other than oxygen delivery or simple wound care, appropriately secure the child to a stretcher in a supine position. If the child only requires monitoring, attempt to transport the child appropriately restrained in an upright position that allows observation, enhances safety, and promotes comfort. **Do not secure the child in the parent's arms.**

CAUTION

It is never acceptable to secure the child in the parent's arms.

Taking Caregivers in the Ambulance

Taking parents or caregivers in an ambulance is usually regulated by local EMS protocols. Often, the caregiver can decrease the anxiety of the child during the transport, especially age groups that are more likely to experience emotional distress when transported without familiar caregivers. Dealing with emotional distress of children is an important principle in prehospital pediatric care and represents a key ingredient in quality care. The presence of family or a caregiver on the effectiveness and comfort level of the prehospital professional is not known but has been associated with higher satisfaction in pediatric care delivery in other settings and may reduce ongoing parental and child anxiety (**FIGURE 16-1**).

FIGURE 16-1 Allowing a parent to accompany a child may reduce the child's anxiety, but make sure all occupants are safe.

CASE STUDY 2

You arrive on the scene of an 18-month-old toddler who has altered mental status. She is limp in her mother's arms and does not respond to your arrival in the room. She is pale but does not seem to have increased work of breathing or noisy respirations. The patient has been sick for 24 hours with nausea and vomiting and could not be awakened from her afternoon nap. The child responds to painful stimuli and is wearing a dry diaper. Vital signs show heart rate of 160 beats/min, respiratory rate of 40 breaths/min, and blood pressure of 70 mm Hg/palp. She weighs 22 pounds (10 kg).

1. Should this child be transported in a car seat?
2. Should the mother be transported with the child?
3. Discuss the possible transport modes and destination for this patient.

Some prehospital professionals may feel less comfortable when a caregiver is present in an ambulance during a resuscitation or when an advanced procedure, such as endotracheal intubation, is being performed. One way for the prehospital professional to help address his or her own comfort level is to get involved with child advocacy and increase pediatric training and exposure.

If local EMS policy allows caregiver transport with the child, it should specify where the child and caregiver should be positioned during the transport. One common place for a caregiver during transport is in the front seat of the ambulance. As with any passenger, make sure the caregiver fastens his or her seat belt correctly and remains seated. Another possible place to seat a caregiver is in the rear of the ambulance when it is appropriately configured with secure seating options for both crew and the caregiver. This allows a child to visualize the caregiver and may provide

FIGURE 16-2 If caregivers are allowed to ride in the ambulance with the child, make sure all equipment and personnel are securely fastened.

some emotional consolation. Ensure that all occupants and equipment are secured; unsecured items and occupants have been shown to pose a great threat to the patient's safety in the event of vehicular events (**FIGURE 16-2**).

Child Restraint Systems in Ambulances

Dangers Facing Children During Transport

There are several factors that can decrease the possibility of additional injury to a child during ambulance transport. These factors include how the child is secured, the configuration of the ambulance, and whether the crew and the equipment are secured. The National Association of State EMS Officials (NASEMSO) considers safe transport as standard of care, along the lines of airway, breathing and circulation. Their recommendation is to have **child restraint systems (CRS)** that cover a minimum weight range from 5 to 99 pounds. This can range from a car seat to a harness attached to the cot, depending on the child's presentation.

The first step in deciding how to transport a child is to determine what assessment, monitoring, and treatment are necessary during transport. The Working Group Best-Practice Recommendations for the Safe Transportation of Children in Emergency Ground Ambulances gives recommendations for five scenarios (**TABLE 16-1**).

If the patient is stable and no interventions are anticipated, then transport the infant or child using a CRS that meets the injury criteria of the Federal Motor Vehicle Safety Standard No. 213. This consists of a car seat secured with appropriate restraining devices in

TABLE 16-1 Working Group Best-Practice Recommendations for the Safe Transportation of Children in Emergency Ground Ambulances Recommendations	
Scenario	**Description**
1	For a Child who is uninjured/not ill
2	For a Child who is ill and/or injured and whose condition *does not require* continuous and/or intensive medical monitoring and/or interventions
3	For a Child whose condition *requires* continuous and/or intensive medical monitoring and/or interventions
4	For a Child whose condition *requires* spinal immobilization and/or lying flat
5	For a Child or Children who *require* transport as part of a multiple patient transport (newborn with Mother, multiple children, etc.)

Working Group Best-Practice Recommendations for the Safe Transportation of Children in Emergency Ground Ambulances, DOT HS 811 677, September 2012.

the ambulance to the cot. *If the child requires continuous medical attention or spinal motion restriction, a car seat would be inappropriate, and appropriate CRS attached directly to the cot or backboard is necessary.* If there are concerns for spinal injury, then the child should be transported with spinal motion restriction (SMR). This can be in the form of an ambulance cot, vacuum splint, or similar device. SMR cannot be obtained with the head elevated more than 30 degrees or without securing the child in such a manner as to restrict movement of the neck and spine. Pediatric evidence supports using a cervical collar with any of the following presentations: neck pain, inability to move neck, neurologic deficit, altered mental status, high-risk mechanism (high-speed motor vehicle collision, diving accident), torso trauma, or predisposing condition. If using a backboard, such as in a situation where a child is critically injured or unresponsive, secure the child to the backboard, then secure the backboard to the cot with three horizontal restraints across the torso (at the chest, waist, and knees) and a vertical restraint over each shoulder. When possible, tether the foot end of the backboard to the cot to prevent forward movement during rapid decelerations. Due to skin breakdown, backboards should be used for the shortest time possible.

When using a CRS in the ambulance, decide where to position the device. Car seats are designed to restrain a child during a front-end or rear-end collision; they provide only moderate lateral stability. This means that these seats cannot be secured sideways to a bench seat. This limits the choices about where to position the CRS in the rear of an ambulance to the cot or the EMS provider's seat at the head of the stretcher.

TIP

Convertible child restraint devices are acceptable seats to use on the stretcher, or on a rear-facing or forward-facing EMS provider seat.

TIP

Transport stable children in a car safety seat properly secured in the ambulance.

CAUTION

Never secure car seats to a bench seat in the ambulance.

CAUTION

"Rear-facing-only" or "infant-only" child restraint seats cannot be secured properly to the ambulance cot or rear-facing EMS provider seat because they have only one belt pathway to secure the device and are not engineered to be restrained on a rear-facing seat.

Choosing a CRS

While there are many car safety seats and CRSs available for the ambulance, there are no federal regulations and very limited testing of these devices. Car safety seats designed for passenger vehicles are tested to meet Federal Motor Vehicle Safety Standard 213 (FMVSS 213); convertible car safety seats carrying weights specific to the individual car seat (usually up to 40–50 pounds) and a car bed using two belt paths have been tested and meet the injury criteria of FMVSS 213. There are a few integrated seats and restraints that are permanently mounted on the rear-facing captain's chair (**FIGURE 16-3**), and some restraint systems designed to be secured on a rear-facing stretcher. These options have variable recommendations for use, and some have been

FIGURE 16-3 An integrated child restraint system.
Courtesy of Serenity Safety Products.

tested to ensure they meet the injury criteria of FM-VSS 213, as no standards have been developed that are ambulance specific. *Rear-facing-only child safety seats (formerly called infant-only seats) are designed for infants who weigh from 4–5 pounds up to 22 or 30–35 pounds, depending on the model. Convertible car safety seats are for children of different ages and weighing up to 40–50 pounds. They are usually recognized by having two belt paths for both forward and rear facing.* Some recently manufactured seats have raised the limit to 80 pounds, but none has been tested for use on an ambulance stretcher in children over 40 pounds (**FIGURE 16-4**). In addition to securing the child in the car safety seat, the seat must be attached to the ambulance stretcher using two belt paths to prevent rearward and forward motion. Only convertible car safety seats have two belt paths and are the only seats that can safely be secured to a stretcher. The back of the stretcher is elevated to an upright position, and the seat is secured to the stretcher with belts through both the forward-facing and rear-facing belt paths.

Rear-facing-only seats are usually limited to those infants weighing less than 30–35 pounds and are designed only to be used in a rear-facing position. They cannot be secured to the stretcher safely, as they have only one belt path. However, there is one infant car bed that can be secured to the stretcher in a side-facing orientation.

If a booster seat is used, it should only be used on forward-facing captain's chairs with lap/shoulder belts available. *Other specialty restraints include vest and harness devices that may be available to specialty crews with additional training in how to install and secure a patient for transport. Detailed instruction for selection and installation of ambulance restraints is available from EMS providers who have taken the EMS training course on child transportation in ambulances.*

FIGURE 16-4 Convertible child safety seat for children 5–40 pounds.
Thinkstock/Getty Images.

> **TIP**
>
> Practice installing child seats to the stretcher as part of training, or bring in a certified child passenger safety technician with training in ambulance transport to help familiarize the service with the installation process.

A CRS should be cleaned and maintained. Pads that are removable and surfaces that can be wiped down are preferable. Check with the manufacturer to see what cleaning materials are acceptable for the seat. If there is a dedicated ambulance CRS, check with the EMS policy and the manufacturer to make sure there have been no safety recalls.

CASE STUDY 3

You are called to the scene of a vehicle crash involving two automobiles that collided at slow speed in a downtown intersection. There are three patients. One is the restrained driver of the vehicle that struck another vehicle broadside. The other patients are the restrained driver of the second vehicle and an 11-month-old boy, who was fully restrained in a rear-facing convertible car seat on the opposite side of the point of collision. The airbags did not deploy. The two drivers have minor wounds and no significant physiologic abnormalities. Assessment of the child reveals a crying infant with no signs of injury.

1. Should the child be transported?
2. Should the child be transported in his own car seat or an ambulance car seat?

Using Car Seats After a Collision

If the ambulance does not have a CRS and a stable child requires transport, an important dilemma arises when the child's own car seat is available. If local EMS policy permits using a personal car seat, be sure that it is fully intact. If the device shows any signs of damage, do not use it in the ambulance. The National Highway Traffic Safety Administration (NHTSA) recommends that child restraints should be replaced after a moderate or severe crash to ensure a continued high level of crash protection for child passengers; however, reuse of a child safety seat that has been involved in a minor crash is an option if the crash meets certain criteria (**TABLE 16-2**).

Securing a Car Seat to the Stretcher

Transport children weighing less than 40–50 pounds in a rear-facing convertible car seat unless medical attention is indicated. This is easily accomplished using the ambulance stretcher. Use a convertible car seat that meets the national standard, and place it flush with the raised back of the cot. Secure the car seat tightly to the cot using straps through both the forward-facing and the rear-facing belt paths of the seat (**FIGURE 16-5**). Adjust the car seat harness to be at or below the shoulders of the child, connect the harness, and pull it snug, then place the harness clip at the level of the child's armpit (**FIGURE 16-6**).

TABLE 16-2 Recommendations for the Use of a CRS After a Crash
It is safe to reuse a child safety seat that has been involved in a minor crash if:
■ The vehicle was able to be driven away from the crash site.
■ The vehicle door nearest the safety seat was undamaged.
■ There were no injuries to any of the vehicle occupants.
■ The airbags, if present, did not deploy.
■ There is no visible damage to the safety seat.

U.S. Department of Transportation. Car Seat Use After a Crash. Retrieved from https://www.nhtsa.gov/car-seats-and-booster-seats/car-seat-use-after-crash.

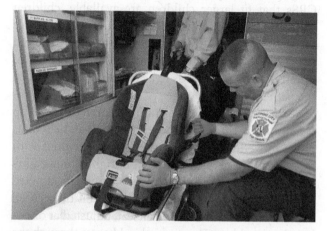

FIGURE 16-5 Place the car seat on the stretcher and use one belt through the rear-facing belt path and one through the forward-facing belt path of the car safety seat.

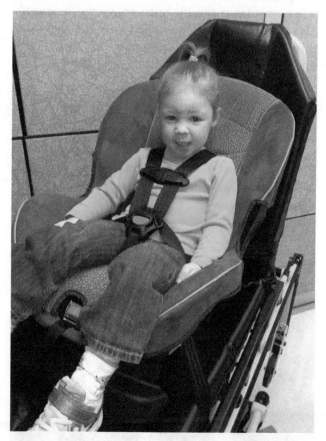

FIGURE 16-6 Child properly positioned in a convertible car seat with harness snug and chest clip at level of the armpits.

Securing Older Children to the Stretcher

Children weighing more than 40 pounds are too large for a car safety seat on a stretcher, but they are *not* yet large enough to fit into adult-sized restraint systems. As previously mentioned, NASEMSO's recommendation is to have CRSs that cover a minimum weight range from 5 to 99 pounds. When ambulance-specific CRSs that fit larger children are available, children should be transported in an appropriate device secured to the cot. If a CRS is unavailable, the child needs to be secured to the stretcher. The position of the stretcher straps needs to be adjusted for the size of the patient.

During an ambulance crash, children can slide up the stretcher. The use of shoulder straps can help minimize this effect, but there are some difficulties with these straps because they do not fit tightly on a child's shoulders or prevent the child from moving upward during a crash. Ideally, the straps should be secured similarly to those used in a car seat, adjusted at or below the shoulders. The straps should enter through the padding and be secured to the frame of the stretcher at the height of the shoulders. Unfortunately, this is not possible with most of today's stretchers. There are a few ambulance-specific restraint systems now available that make securing a child to the stretcher safer. These devices must be first secured to the stretcher, and then adjusted to fit the patient (**FIGURE 16-7** and

> ### TIP
>
> It is extremely important to secure all occupants and equipment during transport. Just applying the brakes hard can cause harm to the patient from unrestrained objects.

FIGURE 16-7 An ambulance-specific child restraint accommodating children 10–40 pounds.

FIGURE 16-8). The use of the pediatric restraint devices made for stretcher application helps to more properly secure most pediatric patients.

Other Dangers in Transporting Children

Placing the child in an appropriate transporting device is the first means of creating a safe mode of transport. It is important to recognize that crew members, parents/caregivers, and flying debris can create a significant hazard to the patient during a collision. When transporting a child, secure or store all loose equipment before leaving the scene. Monitors, portable oxygen containers, equipment bags, and all other loose pieces can create missile-like objects that have been shown to be potentially dangerous to crew members and patients. Keep crew members and parents/caregivers secured in a seat-belted position throughout the transport. Crash testing of ambulances has shown that unrestrained passengers in the patient compartment present a risk to the patient during a collision by being launched and landing on the patient.

FIGURE 16-8 An ambulance-specific child restraint accommodating children.

Courtesy of Quantum EMS LLC.

Summary of CRSs

Whenever possible, use a size-appropriate CRS to transport a stable child in an upright position. This is the preferred position for transport. There are important guidelines for proper use of car seats for children of different weights and how to secure the devices to the ambulance to maximize safety during transport. If local EMS policy allows use of the child's own car seat in the ambulance, be sure it is not damaged, meets all the NHTSA criteria for use of a car seat after a crash, and is properly secured to the ambulance. Also, if EMS policy allows and he or she can be properly restrained, encourage the presence of the caregiver in the ambulance to provide comfort and solace to the child and to improve ongoing assessment.

Transport Mode

Emotions can run high on pediatric calls, and prehospital professionals may feel a strong desire to transport quickly to the emergency department. However, lights and sirens transport, especially through crowded urban areas in the daytime, is fraught with risk to ambulance occupants and innocent bystanders. A way to minimize the dangers of transport to ambulance occupants and the public is to determine the best mode of transport before moving. Transport mode should be based on the type of call, the presenting illness or injury, and the degree of physiologic instability of the patient. The child with the highest priority for rapid transport is the critically injured child who needs blood products and/or operative interventions. This

child always requires a time-sensitive response, and a lights and sirens transport is often indicated. Children with severe illness or physiologic abnormality are also important candidates for lights and sirens mode.

Transport Destination

The decision of where to transport the pediatric patient depends on the physiologic condition of the patient, the cause of the illness or injury, and the stability of the patient, coupled with local EMS policy, weather, and resources. It is important to be aware of all the factors that affect the decision based on the situation. Air transport may be appropriate for some patients, but remember to add in the extra facet of potential separation from the caregiver, as not all air transport can accommodate caregivers. For further guidance on making transport destination decisions, consult local protocols.

Multiple Patients

If there are multiple pediatric patients, extra transportation units may be required to transport the children safely. There are limited locations to properly secure a car seat and limited ability to adjust the adult straps to fit the child in the patient compartment of the ambulance.

Summary of Transport Mode and Multiple Patients

Children are often the source of great provider stress. Transport mode is best determined before beginning transport. Although lights and sirens is the fastest method, this mode is more dangerous and is best reserved for unstable trauma cases and illness cases. When there is more than one child at the scene, activate additional units to avoid logistical problems with safely securing multiple child restraints in the ambulance.

CASE STUDY ANSWERS

CASE STUDY 1

This case demonstrates an important dilemma. Although family-centered care is highly desirable, this must take place without placing the patient, family member, accompanying child, or provider at increased risk. Whenever possible, arrange alternative safe care and/or transportation for the child so that the attention of the medical providers can be centered on the patient. This includes care by or transportation with a competent adult, ensuring that appropriate child restraints are available and in use. Additional potential options for transporting the child could include a supervisor's, auxiliary, or child service's transportation vehicle. Transporting the child in the front seat of the ambulance or in the rear seat of a police car or other emergency vehicle is dangerous. A vehicle where the CRS is to be used in the front seat must have an airbag deactivation switch.

Parent and child separation, however, may cause undue distress to the mildly injured parent. In that case, if the system allows the transport of the child in the ambulance, follow proper procedures to secure the child in the appropriate restraint system and in the correct position. This method of transportation must include enough participants to meet the child's and the patient's needs and to ensure that observation or immediate needs of either one does not detract from those of the other. This is an option that is often unavailable because of space or personnel resource limitations.

CASE STUDY 2

This is a case where the patient needs appropriate positioning, airway and vascular access, monitoring, and perhaps intervention during the transport process. "Stabilization" in a car seat affords none of those requirements and therefore should not be used. This is a child who should be restrained using an appropriate CRS on the ambulance stretcher, with attention to airway positioning, vascular access, and appropriate observation. Here, accompaniment of the parent can often be advantageous to parent and child. Although the medical team can attend to the physiologic needs of the child, they cannot meet the child's emotional needs. Be sensitive to the parent's need to offer support to his or her child and ability to keep the child calm. The parent may also be able to provide additional history and assist in reassessments. The parent cannot be allowed to carry the child during transport, either on his or her lap while seated or with the parent and child secured together to a stretcher.

Local protocol often dictates where and how this patient should be transported, as well as whether a parent can accompany his or her child and specific requirements for this process. These protocols should include preferred parental seating location and safety instructions for the parent before transport. Parents must be instructed that the primary role of the providers is to care for the sick child and that precious attention cannot be diverted from that task. Having the parent sit in the front is one way to include him or her in the environment, while allowing some separation for the providers.

Providers may express concern that parents will critique their techniques or skills during the transport or that the providers will be nervous when confronted with this environment. Parents, however, generally report very positively about the experience and comment mostly on the caring nature of the providers, not their technical capabilities.

CASE STUDY 3

Assessment of infants after a collision is very difficult in the best of environments. The significant mechanism of this incident necessitates assessment during the transport process and medical evaluation of the infant at the appropriate emergency department. The question then is how to best transport the child. If a careful inspection of the child yields no physiologic or anatomic abnormality requiring further stabilization or intervention, and the child is accessible to completely assess and reassess as needed when secured in the car seat, this method is appropriate. If a detailed inspection of the child's convertible car safety seat does not yield evidence of fracture or abnormality, it is an appropriate seat for the child's weight, it is not damaged and meets NHTSA criteria, and EMS policy allows, then use this seat and secure in the usual rear-facing position in the emergency vehicle, unless the ambulance has its own CRS or local EMS policy forbids this practice. If there is any question as to the appropriateness or the structural integrity of the child's car seat, then use another, more-appropriate car seat. Remember that a rear-facing-only or infant-only car seat cannot be safely secured to the ambulance cot and may only be secured to a forward-facing attendant seat.

SUGGESTED REFERENCES

Textbook

Bledsoe BE, Porter RS, Cherry RA. *Paramedic Care: Principles & Practice*. 5th ed. London, UK: Pearson, 2017.

Articles

Becker LR. Relative risk of injury and death in ambulances and other emergency vehicles. *Accid Anal Prev.* 2003;35(6):941–948.

Bledsoe BE. Emergency EMS Mythology, Part 4. Lights and sirens save a significant amount of travel time and save lives. *Emerg Med Serv.* 2003;32(6):72–73.

Bull MJ, Weber K, Talty J, Manary M. Crash protection for children in ambulances. *Annu Proc Assoc Adv Automot Med.* 2001;45:353–367.

Fischer PE, Perina DG, Delbridge TR, et al. Spinal motion restriction in the trauma patient – a joint position statement. *Prehosp Emerg Care.* 2018; 22(6):659–661. DOI: 10.1080/10903127.2018 .1481476

Kahn CA. Characteristics of fatal ambulance crashes in the United States: an 11 year retrospective analysis. *Prehosp Emerg Care.* 2001;5(3):261–269.

Leonard JC, Browne LR, Ahmad FA, et al. Cervical spine injury risk factors in children with blunt trauma. *Pediatrics.* 2019;144(1):e20183221.

Warren J. Guidelines for the inter- and intrahospital transport of critically ill patients. *Crit Care Med.* 2004;32(1):256–262.

Other Resources

Automotive Safety Program. http://www.preventinjury .pediatrics.iu.edu. Accessed June 21, 2019.

Health Resources and Services Administration and National Highway Traffic Safety Administration. The do's and don'ts of transporting children in an ambulance. https://one.nhtsa.gov/people/injury/ems /Archive/New%20Folder/childam.html. Accessed June 21, 2019.

National Association of State EMS Officials. Safe transport of children by EMS: Interim guidance. https://nasemso.org/wp-content/uploads/Safe -Transport-of-Children-by-EMS-InterimGuidance -08Mar2017-FINAL.pdf. Accessed June 21, 2019.

National Highway Traffic Safety Administration, Office of EMS. Working Group best practice recommendations for the safe transportation of children in emergency ground ambulances. https://www.ems .gov/pdf/811677.pdf. Accessed December 23, 2019.

© Eddie M. Sperling.

CHAPTER 17
Making a Difference

Joyce Foresman-Capuzzi, MSN, APRN, CCNS, CEN, CPEN, CTRN, TCRN, CPN, EMT-P, FAEN

William Krost, MD, MBA, NRP

LEARNING OBJECTIVES

1. Describe Emergency Medical Services for Children (EMSC) and the EMS-EMSC continuum.
2. Discuss how EMS can interface with public health and the EMS role in injury and illness prevention and promotion.
3. Identify primary and secondary prevention strategies involved in injury prevention.
4. Outline the three components and the three phases of an injury event.
5. Discuss EMSC partnerships with other injury-prevention agencies and programs.
6. Define the role of the child's "medical home," and identify its importance in the EMS-EMSC care continuum.
7. Identify unique quality and safety issues for children in prehospital care.
8. Discuss the importance of data collection and information management in EMSC.

Introduction

Emergency care for children involves the work of many health care professionals, inside and outside of the community's hospitals. To provide safe and effective emergency care, these professionals must work together as a team to develop and implement comprehensive clinical services and oversight mechanisms designed specifically for children suffering acute illness and injury. Professionals must also

CASE STUDY 1

You have been called to the scene of a motor vehicle crash between a compact car and a minivan. A 3-year-old girl, who was not properly restrained at the time of the crash, was thrown from the minivan and lies approximately 15 feet from the vehicle. She is unconscious; has no abnormal airway sounds, retractions, or nasal flaring; and is cyanotic. Respiratory rate is 6 breaths/min, heart rate is 40 beats/min, and blood pressure is difficult to palpate. You transport the child to the nearest emergency department (ED), but the child dies shortly after arrival.

1. How could this have been prevented?
2. What could you do to help others avoid this type of tragedy?

recognize the limitations of an emergency care system largely oriented toward treatment after an illness or injury occurs and embrace the essential role of prevention. Of all community activities that can improve children's overall health and well-being, prevention of acute injury and illness is by far the most cost-effective. Making a difference means practicing prevention as part of day-to-day work duties and stepping into a role as a community leader and health advocate. Making a difference entails professionals getting involved in injury and illness prevention in innovative ways. This includes understanding and supporting the prevention and safety programs conducted through Emergency Medical Services for Children (EMSC) and prevention programs within local emergency medical services (EMS) systems. EMS has the opportunity to make a substantial difference in a community through advocacy and involvement. Prehospital providers can act as the link between programs and intended recipients, bringing resources and education to those who are in need. Although one provider can make an incredible difference, together an EMS system can create a stable infrastructure for its community through advocacy.

Emergency Medical Services for Children

Children are a unique group of EMS patients. They have special needs and problems that are different from those of adults. They require equipment, tools, and medications designed for smaller bodies with different anatomy and physiology. Children also have different emotional and developmental needs that require a modified approach to assessment and treatment. Although children younger than 18 years of age account for only 10% of prehospital transports; evaluating, treating, triaging, and transporting this group can create significant stress and multiple challenges for prehospital professionals.

EMSC is a federal program initiated more than 30 years ago to ensure high-quality care of children within the EMS system. With federal grant funds and sustained EMSC program support, EMS communities across the country have developed pediatric-specific policies, procedures, and protocols to assist prehospital professionals in pediatric care at the local level. These pediatric considerations may be outlined in a state or local EMSC plan or in pediatric components within a general EMS plan. For example, most EMS systems now have pediatric treatment and transport policies. Most systems have pediatric-specific equipment and supplies and allow special pediatric procedures, such as **intraosseous** infusions and intranasal medication delivery administration. In addition, most EMS systems also have specialized operational policies that address unique pediatric legal considerations, such as a pediatric refusal policy that recognizes the legal issues surrounding consent and provision of care to unaccompanied minors.

The umbrella of EMSC is broad and includes prehospital and in-hospital care within general hospitals and specialized pediatric hospitals. Because there are relatively few specialized pediatric centers (**pediatric critical care centers** and **pediatric trauma centers**), most children receive emergency care in general hospitals. Hence, **universal standards for pediatric emergency care** in all EDs within an EMS system (urban and rural, general and specialized) are an important part of EMSC development.

The **EMS-EMSC continuum** (**FIGURE 17-1**) is the planned and organized interface among the clinical services of the EMS system itself, other prehospital emergency care resources, the community's primary child health services, and the in-hospital system. The five major phases in the overall continuum include (1) prevention, (2) primary care and the child's "medical home," (3) prehospital care, (4) hospital care, and (5) rehabilitation. These phases represent a cycle of care for a single event that should bring the child back to prevention and the child's medical home. The prehospital professional has the responsibility to support children's emergency care throughout all phases of the continuum. An active partnership with public health programs, collaboration with the community, and continued advocacy through prevention and training empower EMS to make a difference.

Summary of EMSC

EMSC began as a federal grant program to improve prehospital pediatric services within the community EMS system. Over the past three decades, the prolific work in the field has forged a broad concept of EMSC as a continuum of multiple clinical services in the community that are coordinated and child specific. The essential phases of the EMS-EMSC continuum include prevention, the medical home, prehospital care, in-hospital care, and rehabilitation.

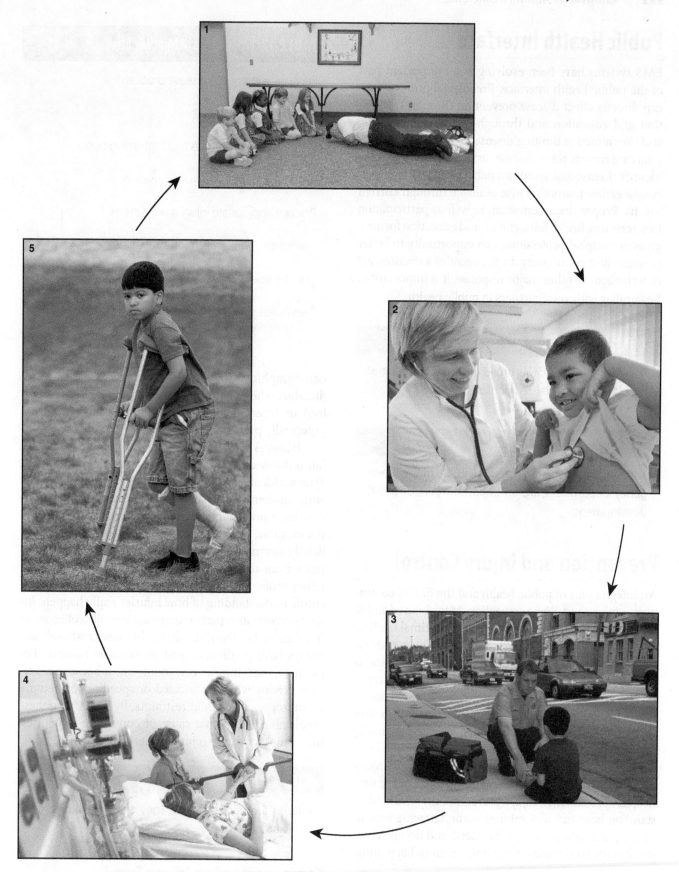

FIGURE 17-1 EMS-EMSC continuum: **1** prevention, **2** primary care and the medical home, **3** out-of-hospital care, **4** hospital care, and **5** rehabilitation.

Public Health Interface

EMS systems have been evolving as an important part of the public health interface. Prehospital professionals can directly affect disease prevention through vaccination and education and through continued screening and care aimed at limiting disease progression. Prehospital care reports act as disease surveillance in helping to identify disease and symptom patterns, identifying outbreaks earlier than otherwise available through current means. Proper documentation, as well as participation in screenings, health fairs, clinics, and education forums, gives prehospital professionals an opportunity to better prepare their community. In the event of a disaster, act of terrorism, or other major response, it is important to be familiar with your partners in public health.

> **TIP**
>
> The umbrella of EMSC is broad and includes general hospitals and specialized pediatric hospitals.

> **TIP**
>
> Standards for pediatric emergency care in the emergency department are an important part of EMSC development.

Prevention and Injury Control

An integral part of public health and the EMSC continuum is injury and illness prevention. Many injured and ill children die each year, despite receiving optimal medical care. To affect these numbers, injury and illness prevention must be increased. Injury and illness prevention is more effective at saving lives than optimal medical care.

Prevention is the first phase of the EMSC continuum. Although prevention does apply to illness and injury, prehospital services have concentrated primarily on injury control. **TABLE 17-1** lists the eight identified elements of injury prevention; these elements make injury prevention an objective and scientific effort. For the prehospital professional, injury prevention involves understanding how and why injuries occur, knowing how to identify the risks in the environment, and doing something in the community to stop injuries from happening.

Injuries Are Not Accidents

When injury patterns are carefully studied, it is clear that injuries, like illnesses, vary with the seasons, can occur in epidemics, and often have local trends and

TABLE 17-1 Elements of Injury Control

Recognize injury as a disease process.
Maintain a reliable database.
Identify problem injuries and high-risk groups.
Identify the factors in injury causation.
Practice appropriate injury **assessment**.
Formulate injury-prevention strategies.
Select efficient, practical injury-prevention strategies.
Reevaluate selected injury-prevention strategies for the desired effects.

demographic distributions. Injuries are largely predictable, whether they are unintentional (e.g., drowning) or intentional (e.g., handgun assaults) and are potentially preventable.

Webster's Dictionary defines the word accident as, "an unforeseen and unplanned event or circumstance." True accidents that cause injuries are rare. Even apparently random events, such as lightning strikes or tornados, have predictable features and can be anticipated. For example, weather forecasting can predict potentially deadly storms and alert the public to their path. "Injuries are not accidents" has become a common slogan by injury professionals. The slogan reflects the current scientific understanding of how injuries really happen. Injury prevention experts refer to automobile collisions as "crashes" rather than "accidents," because crashes almost always have predictable and preventable features. For example, crash injuries commonly occur because of persons driving while intoxicated or speeding, or because of improper use of child restraints. By identifying these predictable factors that cause or contribute to injuries, the "setup" for future injury events can be eliminated.

> **TIP**
>
> Injuries are not accidents. They are usually predictable and preventable.

Components of an Injury Event

Part of understanding how injuries occur involves looking at the three components of an injury event: (1) the host, (2) the agent, and (3) the environment (**FIGURE 17-2**).

FIGURE 17-2 Components of an injury event: the host, the agent, and the environment. The child is the host, the heat from the boiling water is the agent, and the dangerously placed handle is the environment for a burn injury.
© Libortom/E+/Getty Images.

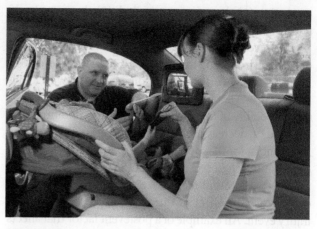

FIGURE 17-3 EMS professionals can become involved directly in injury prevention by attending a child safety seat technician training program and then by providing a child safety seat checkpoint program.
© Jones & Bartlett Learning. Courtesy of Glen Ellman.

The **host** is the person who is the recipient of the injury. An injury occurs when potentially destructive energy is too much for the host to tolerate. Human hosts have different levels of tolerance. Children, because of their unique **anatomic** and **physiologic** features, are particularly vulnerable to high-energy transfers. Their smaller body size means the energy that is transferred to the body during a collision transfers over a larger percentage of body surface, placing the child at higher risk for serious injuries from a multiple trauma event.

The **agent** is a form of energy. The major agents of injury are kinetic, thermal, chemical, electrical, and radiation energy. Most injuries are associated with these types of energy. Kinetic energy is the most common injury agent in circumstances that involve prehospital professionals. For example, falls, automobile-passenger injuries, and pedestrian-versus-automobile and bicyclist-versus-automobile events all involve a human as the host and kinetic energy as the agent. Burns, in contrast, involve thermal, chemical, or electrical energy.

The **environment** is the setting where the agent meets the host. The environment causes or influences the injury event. Some examples are an unfenced swimming pool, a poorly maintained road, or an open upper-story window without a protective barrier. Any of these factors may provide the environment for an injury event to occur that might involve a young child as a host and kinetic energy as the agent.

Looking at injury events, the prehospital professional should consider what components of an injury can be modified to prevent future occurrences (**FIGURE 17-3**). Modifying the host's behavior to prevent

FIGURE 17-4 When worn correctly, bicycle helmets significantly reduce the complications and incidence of death from closed-head injuries. Prehospital professionals have an important community role in teaching simple injury-control strategies.
© Monkey Business Images/Shutterstock.

drowning or head injury, for example, may involve education in swimming skills or driving techniques. Modifying the agent may include providing bicycle helmets (**FIGURE 17-4**) or installing soft stopping surfaces in playgrounds to reduce the effect of kinetic energy on vulnerable brain tissue. Modifying the environment may include fencing of swimming pools or setting up window bars.

Phases of Injury

Just as there are three components in every injury event, there are also three separate phases of every injury that need to be considered when devising control strategies: (1) the pre-event period, (2) the event itself, and (3) the postevent period (**FIGURE 17-5**).

Pre-event factors are conditions in the host, the agent, or the environment that make an injury more or less likely to occur. For example, riding a bicycle with a helmet is a pre-event factor that might significantly decrease the probability of injury. Event factors are conditions that increase or decrease the effect of the agent on the host. An event factor that decreases the risk of injury in a vehicle crash is seat belt use in the automobile at the time of the crash. Postevent factors are conditions that increase or decrease the effect of the agent on the host after the injury event. An example of a postevent factor that affects the outcome in a severely head-injured child is on-scene airway management by the prehospital professional.

Traditionally, prehospital care has focused almost exclusively on the postevent period, or medical care and transport after the injury has occurred. Prehospital professionals must now recognize their potential to influence the pre-event and event phases of injury by acting as community educators and advocates. Data collected from patient-care reports help identify patterns and incidences that can steer prevention programs. **TABLE 17-2** provides examples of injury control strategies aimed at modifiable factors in different phases of injury. The prehospital professional has an important role in all of these prevention strategies. Prevention is best achieved through partnerships accentuated through EMSC and other local health care systems and services.

TIP

Prevention is an essential feature of all EMS systems and represents an opportunity for prehospital professionals to profoundly affect the health and well-being of their own children and every child in their community.

CONTROVERSY

Until recently, prehospital professionals were not taught injury or illness prevention. Although adding prevention to the prehospital professional's scope of practice has exciting potential, the role of EMS in injury prevention has not yet been fully explored.

A **B**

FIGURE 17-5 The first two phases of an injury. **A.** The pre-event period. An unlocked medicine cabinet invites an adventurous toddler. **B.** The event itself. A toddler will put anything into his mouth, including dangerous medications.

TABLE 17-2 Modifiable Factors in Different Phases of an Injury

Phase	Examples of Modifiable Factors
Pre-event	Maintaining child restraint seats Installing proper fencing around pools Ensuring that smoke detectors work in homes Wearing bicycle helmets
Event	Properly using child restraint seats Cars with front and side air bags
Postevent	Performing pediatric airway management skills Proper spinal motion restriction Choice of an appropriate transport destination for an injured child

Summary of Prevention and Injury Control

Injury and illness prevention are key features of EMSC, and the first phase of the EMS-EMSC continuum. Injuries are not "accidents" and are almost always preventable. Prehospital professionals have a unique role in community injury control. They are at the scene and able to accurately assess the principal components in an injury or illness event. This includes assessing the child or host, the energy type or agent of injury, and the environment, as well as understanding the pre-event, event, and postevent phases of injury. National and state EMSC resources allow for collaboration with other programs to provide additional resources.

The Medical Home

The second vital link in the EMS-EMSC continuum is the child's primary care provider, or **medical home**. The American Academy of Pediatrics defines a medical home as the child's primary source of medical care. Creating an effective medical home requires that infants, children, and teenagers have accessible, continuous, comprehensive, family-centered, coordinated, compassionate, and culturally effective services in a geographically close location. The child and family need to know the primary care provider and develop a partnership of mutual responsibility and trust. This is especially important for children with special needs (see Chapter 10) who often require specialized medical care. Trained pediatricians and family physicians create the medical home. They should not only manage and facilitate ongoing pediatric primary care, but also have a linkage to the EMS system in case a child requires emergency services beyond what is offered by the office or clinic. In some offices, there are written protocols and procedures that define how to identify an emergency requiring EMS services, when to summon 9-1-1, and what care should be immediately provided in a medical emergency. The providers in the medical home should have an accurate understanding of the pediatric capabilities of the prehospital professional and EMS system; know the closest hospital for pediatric care; and know the local EMS system's policies and procedures regarding triage, transport, and treatment of children.

> **TIP**
>
> Communication and teamwork are essential features in the linkages between all components of the EMS-EMSC continuum.

CASE STUDY 2

You are dispatched to a local elementary school for a 7-year-old girl with a history of cerebral palsy and seizures. On arrival, the nurse states the patient has been seizing for 15 minutes and she has just administered clonazepam through the patient's G-tube. The patient is no longer seizing; is sleepy, but responds to voice; and has no increased work of breathing; her skin is pink. She has respirations of 20 breaths/min, a heart rate of 120 beats/min, a blood pressure of 92/64 mm Hg, and a blood glucose of 86 mg/dL. The child's father arrives and states the patient is demonstrating her usual presentation after a seizure. He requests transport to the children's hospital 45 minutes away and states he will take her if you cannot go that far, refusing ambulance transport to the local ED. The child is now awake, alert, at her normal developmental level, and deemed medically stable after discussion with medical command.

1. What are your options in the care and transport of this child?
2. How can you assist the parents with safe transportation for this child?

The Prehospital Professional and the Medical Home

Traditionally, prehospital professionals have had little contact with the primary care physicians who provide the medical home, although both are part of the community settings in the EMSC continuum. There are many opportunities for collaboration between the physicians and providers in the child's medical home and the prehospital professionals in the EMS system. Under some conditions, with the permission of a parent or guardian, the primary provider can offer valuable history and information to the prehospital professional. This may be especially important in evaluating and treating children with special health care needs. This information may be communicated in the form of a written care plan or by a telephone consultation on scene. This does not require the prehospital professional to delay care or transport of a critically ill or injured child, but can take place as part of an EMS system optional procedure for history gathering in stable patients. Sometimes the primary physician can deliver emergency care on scene with the prehospital professionals and accompany the child to the ED. *Effectively treating a child with the assistance of prehospital professionals requires that the primary physician understand the local scope of practice, drugs, equipment, and supplies available for children within the local EMS system.* The prehospital professionals should have a "physician on scene" policy that defines the relative roles and responsibilities of the parties in such circumstances.

Communication from the medical home is especially important when assisting children with special needs and should include the **emergency information form (EIF)**, as described in Chapter 10 (**FIGURE 17-6**). This form can provide invaluable information to the prehospital provider when called on to care for a patient. Communicating with the family before the emergency can also allow for familiarity with the child's "regular" status, thereby allowing for a higher comfort level during an emergency response for all involved. Communication and teamwork are essential features in the linkages among all components of the EMSC continuum.

Summary of the Medical Home

The medical home is the child's primary medical provider, usually a pediatrician or family physician, sometimes in concert with other medical practitioners. The medical home is the source of key information and decision making for the child. When appropriate, use the expertise of the primary provider in information gathering and in decision making about emergency care. Always ask caregivers of a child with special needs if they have an emergency information form. Primary care physicians should be aware of the pediatric capabilities and scope of practice of the prehospital professionals and local hospitals and about the services of the other components of the EMSC continuum.

Quality and Safety in EMSC

Quality improvement (QI) has long been recognized as methods of ensuring efficiency, decreasing waste, and increasing customer satisfaction in industrial settings. Over the past few decades, the concept of continuous QI has been adopted by the health care industry. The ingredients of health care quality now defined in health institutions include *patient-centered care, efficiency, effectiveness, timeliness, equity,* and *safety.* All of these domains are relevant to pediatric prehospital care:

- *Patient-centered care* is "respectful of and responsive to individual patient preferences, needs, and values."
- *Efficiency* avoids waste, including waste of equipment, supplies, ideas, and energy.
- *Effectiveness* entails treatment grounded in the best scientific evidence that links clinical practice to improved patient outcome. To date, there has been limited research on the effectiveness of prehospital interventions for children. A commitment to participating in clinical research studies is an important element of an EMS program.
- *Timeliness* has always been a primary goal of EMS systems, where treatment and transport delays have long been linked to adverse outcomes for cardiac and trauma patients.
- *Equity* implies providing the same level of care to all patients and families, regardless of socioeconomic status, race or ethnic background, disability, or language barriers.

Safety is a paramount concern for every health care professional, and certainly for the prehospital professional, who faces unique risks in the prehospital setting. Medical error and safety in the prehospital environment are issues now receiving increasing attention. Error rates—in terms of medication dosing and administration, performance of critical procedures, and misdiagnosis—are higher in children than in adults. This discrepancy is probably related to the limited number of pediatric calls and limited opportunities to reinforce pediatric knowledge and skills in the field. EMS efforts to improve pediatric patient safety might include competency-based pediatric training

Last name:

Emergency Information Form for Children With Special Needs

American College of Emergency Physicians®

American Academy of Pediatrics

| Date form completed | Revised | Initials |
| By Whom | Revised | Initials |

Name: Nickname:

Birth date:

Home Address: Home/Work Phone:

Parent/Guardian: Emergency Contact Names & Relationship:

Signature/Consent*:

Primary Language: Phone Number(s):

Physicians:

Primary care physician: Emergency Phone:
                                               Fax:

Current Specialty physician: Emergency Phone:
Specialty: Fax:

Current Specialty physician: Emergency Phone:
Specialty: Fax:

Anticipated Primary ED: Pharmacy:

Anticipated Tertiary Care Center:

Diagnoses/Past Procedures/Physical Exam:

1.   Baseline physical findings:

2.

3.   Baseline vital signs:

4.

Synopsis: Baseline neurological status:

*Consent for release of this form to health care providers

Last name:

Diagnoses/Past Procedures/Physical Exam continued:

Medications: Significant baseline ancillary findings (lab, x-ray, ECG):

1.

2.

3.   Prostheses/Appliances/Advanced Technology Devices:

4.

5.

6.

Management Data:

Allergies: Medications/Foods to be avoided   and why:

1.

2.

3.

Procedures to be avoided   and why:

1.

2.

3.

Immunizations (mm/yy)

Dates						Dates					
DPT						Hep B					
OPV						Varicella					
MMR						TB status					
HIB						Other					

Antibiotic prophylaxis: Indication: Medication and dose:

Common Presenting Problems/Findings With Specific Suggested Managements

Problem	Suggested Diagnostic Studies	Treatment Considerations

Comments on child, family, or other specific medical issues:

Physician/Provider Signature: Print Name:

© (Year) (Company name). Permission to reprint granted with acknowledgement.

FIGURE 17-6 Emergency information form. A computerized emergency information form created by the American College of Emergency Physicians is available at https://www.acep.org/globalassets/uploads/uploaded-files/acep/clinical-and-practice-management/resources/pediatrics/medical-forms/eifspecialneeds.pdf.

© American College of Emergency Physicians and American Academy of Pediatrics.

FIGURE 17-7 Pediatric medical decision support software systems will soon be available for prehospital professionals on vehicle computers and cell phones.

© Jones & Bartlett Learning. Courtesy of Glen Ellman.

modules, use of length-based tapes or medical software to assist in equipment sizing and medication dosing, the development and dissemination of guidelines of care for common or critical pediatric emergencies, and routine run reviews to identify factors that contribute to adverse outcomes related to field care. The emerging availability of computer-based decision support systems that prehospital professionals can access by mobile computers or cell phones (**FIGURE 17-7**) may help to reduce pediatric errors. EMSC has been instrumental in the development of regional prehospital pediatric protocols for offline medical control, pediatric hospital destination agreements, and pediatric care policies. These resources better prepare the prehospital professional for pediatric calls.

Data and Information Management

To improve systems of care, providers must have substantive knowledge of how the system currently works. This requires collection and analysis of data on system performance at baseline and after a process or procedure has been introduced or modified. Change for the sake of change does not necessarily represent improvement. Therefore, before any QI initiative is undertaken, the following three questions should be answered:

1. What are we trying to accomplish?
2. What changes can we make that will result in improvement?
3. How will we know that a change is an improvement?

A Prehospital QI Case Study

Consider the following hypothetical scenario: An ED physician contacts the manager of your EMS agency with concerns about two children who were transported over the past month after scene endotracheal intubations following apparent febrile seizures. Both had been treated in the field with intravenous (IV) diazepam, suffered brief respiratory depression, received endotracheal intubations, and were extubated shortly after arrival in the ED. A query of your agency's electronic database reveals a total of 10 children over the past year with a diagnosis of seizure who were intubated in the field after treatment with IV diazepam. Knowing that most febrile seizures are brief and self-limited, you are concerned that the potential complications of intubation likely outweigh the benefits of diazepam therapy. You bring this to the QI committee for review. They ask the following questions:

> *Question #1: What are we trying to accomplish?*
> Answer #1: We want to decrease the incidence of children experiencing respiratory depression and intubation caused by benzodiazepine treatment for seizures.
> *Question #2: What changes can we make that will result in improvement?*
> Answer #2: Possible changes might include education of advanced life support (ALS) personnel on indications for benzodiazepine administration in children with seizures, adding computer-based decision support software or length-based resuscitation tapes to each drug box to promote accurate dosing of benzodiazepines, switching from IV to rectal diazepam administration for prolonged seizures, and teaching the technique of nasal airway placement and bag-mask ventilation.
> *Question #3: How will we know if a change is an improvement?*
> Answer #3: Our intubation rate for children with seizures will drop, without an associated increase of children with low oxygen saturation on arrival to the ED.

Together with your medical control physician, you develop a new protocol for assessing and managing seizures in children, provide in-service training with your ALS personnel, and develop a data sheet to be filled out after every seizure call. After 6 months, you find that your intubation rate for children with febrile seizures has been cut by 75%. This data-driven approach is based on examining the status quo and looking for opportunities to improve prehospital practice.

Importance of Data Collection and Information Management in EMSC

Injury prevention begins with an understanding of the community's injury problems. Data, when correctly collected, integrated, and interpreted, become useful information. A properly maintained injury database can be analyzed to identify patterns of preventable injury in a community, which then can be used to generate financial and political support for focused prevention programs. These data also allow an evaluation of the effectiveness of targeted programs in reducing the frequency and severity of injuries.

Elements of an injury database that would be useful in EMS system management include the type, severity, and frequency of fatal and nonfatal injuries; persons at risk; geographic location; time of day and year; and contributing factors, such as alcohol, weather, and lack of (or improper use of) protective devices. Analysis of these data can help set the agenda for program planning and evaluation. For example, the data indicate that a community is experiencing a high rate of injury among unrestrained young children in car crashes. An injury prevention effort must then examine why the injured children are not restrained. The problem may be an issue of education or accessibility. Perhaps the problem is a community cultural belief that a baby is always safest in a mother's arms. Understanding the basis of the problem is critical in determining the best intervention strategy.

> **TIP**
>
> Data, when correctly collected, integrated, and interpreted, become useful information.

Summary of Quality, Safety, Data Collection, and Information Management

QI is now a key feature of EMSC. There are many opportunities to evaluate clinical practice with children and to implement system improvements to reduce error. Appropriate data collection is a key to improvement. There are many types of EMS data that pertain to children. Simply collecting data is not enough. For data to be useful, they need to be accurately collected and then reviewed with a problem orientation. When data are effectively managed, the essential information can be used for focused education and program development.

Prevention: The Prehospital Professional's Role

Prehospital professionals have a responsibility to affect their communities through illness and injury prevention. *They can have a greater impact on health by reducing illness and injury through prevention than they can through treatment alone.* However, to be effective in this new role, prehospital professionals need education and training. Recognizing how injuries can be avoided is the first step in developing prevention activities in the community.

> **TIP**
>
> Prehospital professionals can have a greater impact in reducing the incidence and impact of illness and injury through prevention than through treatment.

CASE STUDY 3

You are called to a recreational complex for an 8-year-old male student who was hit in the chest with a baseball and collapsed. Before your arrival, his coach and teammates started CPR and attached an automated external defibrillator (AED); the patient was subsequently defibrillated but is still in ventricular fibrillation. As you arrive on scene, you are told what happened and what care was administered prior to your arrival. As you continue resuscitation efforts, you calculate medications and equipment size with a length-based tool. The patient has return of spontaneous circulation prior to transport. He is awake on arrival to the ED and after hospitalization and implantation of an automated internal cardiac defibrillator, he is able to participate in sports again.

1. How did the community prepare for this event? How did EMS?
2. What resources are available in a community?

Before the Call

Prevention can be started before the call through preparedness. Working with your community on such programs as Community Emergency Response Team, the emergency information form, CPR and first aid training, babysitting classes, and car seat safety checks helps to strengthen the infrastructure needed to handle emergencies. Educational programs and skills training also serve to hone your response to pediatric calls. The better prepared your community is to recognize and respond to an event, the more likely prevention programs and response will be successful.

Role on Scene

Prevention actions of the prehospital professional begin during the scene size-up and include ensuring scene safety and performing an **environmental assessment**. Ensuring scene safety involves prevention of injury and illness to the prehospital professional and to other medical and law enforcement personnel. This includes identification of possible communicable diseases in the child that can be transmitted to unwary scene personnel unless proper body substance precautions are observed. Ensuring scene safety also may prevent an injury to the child or to the caregiver.

Performing an environmental assessment adds a crucial piece to the overall picture at the scene. ED providers cannot do an environmental assessment. Observation and documentation of the physical and interpersonal environment by the prehospital professional may provide the basis for important prevention actions. Such actions may include providing information directly to the caregiver on safety hazards in the home.

Another type of environmental assessment involves observing and noting any evidence of possible maltreatment by the caregiver and then communicating these concerns to the ED physician. This preventive action may be lifesaving to the child, as explained in Chapter 11.

Role in Safe Transport

Another important aspect of childhood injury prevention for the prehospital professional is safe vehicular transport. *Most serious and fatal vehicular injuries occur to occupants who are improperly restrained.* This pertains to ambulance transport and automobile transport. The key steps for safety of the prehospital professional AND the patient are the simplest: Wear a seat belt, secure all equipment, and secure the pediatric patient in a child restraint device for the entire transport.

For a child who requires spinal motion restriction, use a device secured to the ambulance stretcher to package the child safely, as described in Chapter 16. If the child is critically ill, treat and transport the child secured in a **supine** or **semi-Fowler's position** on a stretcher. This position allows rapid management and monitoring of the child's airway, breathing, and circulation. For a child with mild to moderate illness or injury not requiring spinal motion restriction or a supine position, transport in an upright position on the stretcher or use an age-appropriate and locally approved approach to restraint, as described in Chapter 16, if available. For some children with respiratory problems, an upright position of comfort is important, as explained in Chapter 3. The child with cardiopulmonary or neurologic disabilities may require a specialized child seat to breathe effectively, as described in Chapter 10.

In addition to passengers, unsecured items and equipment move like unsecured people in the back of an ambulance. If the transport requires additional equipment for special patient care, such as a drug box or medication pump, then secure the items before transport. There is always the potential for an ambulance crash, or even just a hard stop, and preparation and prevention avert damage and injury.

> **TIP**
>
> Wear your seat belt and secure all portable items in the ambulance.

Role in the Community

Detailed and accurate observations at the scene may serve to start or support community-wide strategies for injury and illness control. For example, in Europe and Australia, prehospital professionals played a key role in recognizing the relationship between sleep position and **sudden unexplained infant death (SUID)**. Scene observations were part of the scientific studies that confirmed the increased risk of SUID in babies who slept **prone** and assisted in the campaign that has decreased SUID **mortality**. Chapter 13 discusses SUID in more detail.

Prehospital professionals can help in the understanding of community injury and illness patterns by documenting the mechanism and scene circumstances of an acute event in the prehospital record and by assisting in other local data-collection efforts. **TABLE 17-3** lists some specific community injury prevention activities that prehospital professionals might consider in

TABLE 17-3 Examples of Common Injuries and Possible Prevention Strategies

Injury	Prevention
Vehicle trauma	Infant and child restraint seats
	Seat belts and air bags
	Pedestrian safety programs
	Motorcycle helmets
Cycling	Bicycle helmets
	Bicycle paths separate from vehicle traffic
Recreation	Appropriate safety padding and apparel
	Cyclist/skateboard/skater safety programs
	Soft, energy-absorbent playground surfaces
Drowning	Four-sided locked pool enclosures
	Pool alarms
	Immediate adult supervision
	Caretaker CPR training
	Swimming lessons
	Pool/beach safety instruction
	Personal flotation devices
Poisoning and household items	Proper storage of chemicals and medications
	Child safety packaging
Burns	Proper maintenance and monitoring of electrical appliances and cords
	Fire/smoke detectors
	Proper placement of cookware on stove top
Other	Discouragement of infant walker use
	Gated stairways
	Babysitter first aid training
	Child care worker first aid training

their expanded roles as community advocates, public educators, and teachers.

> **TIP**
>
> Scene observations were part of the scientific studies that confirmed the increased risk of SIDS in babies who slept prone.

Summary of Roles in Prevention

The prehospital professional has many opportunities to teach and practice prevention on the job and as a community member (**FIGURE 17-8**). Recognition of scene safety issues, documentation of suspicious home circumstances, and recording of injury mechanisms are fundamental information for EMS systems. Error reduction through careful equipment sizing and drug dosing prevents adverse outcomes as a result of medical care delivered in the field. Fulfilling the dual agendas of ensuring the child passenger's safety in the event of an ambulance crash and permitting ongoing monitoring and treatment continues to represent a challenge for EMS professionals. Last, there are many opportunities as a community member to advocate for injury control and illness prevention as a member of the EMSC continuum.

Call to Action: Advocacy for EMSC

Advocates can support EMSC on and off the ambulance. There are numerous roles for the prehospital professional in the clinical and operational aspects of

FIGURE 17-8 Prehospital professionals have the opportunity to teach prevention.
© Holly Parker/The Saginaw News/AP Images.

EMSC, and there are endless problems to undertake in every community. National and state EMSC programs offer many excellent models and templates for system improvement and often provide funding to support new programs for children. New pediatric-specific software is available to support bedside clinical care of children. In addition, many funding agencies, public and private, have resources to support children's services and enhancements in pediatric emergency care in the community. Advocacy for EMSC includes looking creatively for sources of support outside traditional EMS to help or strengthen pediatric services.

Possible roles to advance children's issues within EMS may involve participation on EMSC committees and advocating on a day-to-day basis for training, equipment, policies, procedures, and protocols that pertain exclusively to children. Other roles may include serving as a volunteer educator at school, developing school first aid services, becoming a CPR trainer, or joining community programs on injury control and children's health issues. National associations, such as the American Academy of Pediatrics, American College of Emergency Physicians, and the Emergency Nurses Association, and local fire departments and prehospital organizations sponsor programs for pediatric illness and injury prevention, but these visionary programs require advocacy and participation for success.

Partnerships created within your community can help empower tomorrow's generation through education today. A child who understands he or she is not helpless in times of emergency becomes a powerful ally on the scene, while allowing for less psychological trauma. Civil organizations have been successful with affecting lives through preparedness, and EMS has an opportunity to further those efforts exponentially. Through training and education, we can make a difference.

There is unprecedented potential for exciting improvements in saving lives, decreasing pain and suffering, preventing injury and illness, and facilitating the complex interface of prehospital pediatric care with community and in-hospital services through participation with public health. Preserving the health and safety of children demands constant advocacy and vigilance from all prehospital professionals to sustain quality pediatric services in EMS systems now and to continue the evolution of EMSC tomorrow.

CASE STUDY ANSWERS

CASE STUDY 1

Factors that may have helped prevent or modify the injuries include car safety education in schools and communities, especially use of seat belts and child restraint seats; reduced vehicle speed; and better traffic signs for drivers.

For the prehospital professional, the key prevention steps in this case are to do the scene size-up, document the important scene conditions, provide appropriate on-scene care, and rapidly transport the child to the appropriate facility. Documenting the mechanism and informing hospital professionals of the preventable aspects of the injury (unrestrained child) have many benefits. It is highly unlikely that any type of medical care would have changed this child's outcome. Hence, although the prehospital professional's interventions after an injury event are few and futile in such cases, there are many useful preventive interventions before the event.

Careful documentation of the circumstances of injury also contributes to vital data collection and helps define patterns of injury within the community. The prehospital professional can become a community advocate for injury prevention, helping to educate parents and policy makers about known risks and identifying and promoting solutions to the important public health problems of childhood injury. Consider use of a critical incident response team for a psychological first aid debriefing before going back into service and per protocol. The hospital staff also may initiate this and invite EMS to participate.

CASE STUDY 2

This child's primary care physician plays an active role in managing her chronic illness and is likely best qualified to make care decisions. Given the child's medically stable status after treatment, contact with medical control to discuss transport destination is reasonable. Effective prehospital care is a phase of the EMS-EMSC continuum and requires not only appropriate equipment and education of prehospital personnel, but also teamwork, knowledge of community resources, and expert communication. Transport of this child to her "medical home," if allowed by local EMS policies, may have advantages that must be weighed against potential risks of further physiologic compromise. When local protocols do not allow transport beyond local facilities, alternative safe transport should be sought. If the patient has an emergency information form, it also can act as a resource to the patient's regular status and response and provide information before the parent's arrival.

CASE STUDY 3

The rapid response, scene efficiency, and lifesaving skills provided by the community before EMS arrival serve the patient and the bystanders. Through education, training, equipment procurement, and emergency preparedness, the potential for a community to handle an emergency with the best outcomes is allowed. The ability to respond and react appropriately ensures the continuum of care is served. CPR training, AED placement, community response teams, pediatric training, and tools create a community empowered to make a difference. Access to a computer-based decision support software program or length-based tool can assist the prehospital professional in choosing the appropriately sized equipment and the correct dosages of medications. Having pediatric equipment well organized and accessible facilitates the search for the correct equipment size and safeguards the care of the child. Using computer software tools or length-based tapes may elevate critical thinking; reduce cognitive load; and allow the prehospital professional to focus on assessment, prioritization, medical interventions, and transport.

Training and education allow the community to take an important role in the patient's care and subsequent outcome. Prehospital professionals have the ability to help prepare and empower their communities through EMSC resources and community collaboration.

SUGGESTED REFERENCES

Textbooks

Aehlert B. *Paramedic Practice Today: Above and Beyond*. St. Louis: Elsevier-Mosby-JEMS; 2010.

Barss P, Smith G, Baker S, Mohan D. *Injury Prevention: An International Perspective*. New York: Oxford University Press; 1998.

Seidel J, Knapp J. *Childhood Emergencies in the Office, Hospital, and Community: Organizing Systems of Care*. 2nd ed. Chicago: American Academy of Pediatrics Committee on Pediatric Emergency Medicine; 2000.

Articles

American Academy of Pediatrics. Medical Home Initiatives for Children with Special Needs Project Advisory Committee: the medical home. *Pediatrics*. 2002;110(1):184–186.

American Academy of Pediatrics, Committee on Pediatric Emergency Medicine. The role of the pediatrician in rural emergency medical services for children. *Pediatrics*. 2012;130:978–982.

Gausche M. Out-of-hospital care of pediatric patients. *Pediatr Clin North Am.* 1999;46(6): 1305–1327.

Horowitz L. Mental health aspects of emergency medical services for children: summary of a consensus conference. *J Pediatr Psychol.* 2001;26(8): 491–502.

Other Resources

EMSC Improvement and Innovation Center. https://emscimprovement.center.

Emergency Information Form. https://www.pediatrics .aappublications.org/content/125/4/829 and https:// www.acep.org/globalassets/uploads/uploaded-files /acep/clinical-and-practice-management/resources /pediatrics/medical-forms/eifspecialneeds.pdf. Accessed January 10, 2020.

Sia C. The medical home: closing the circle of care. In: Seidel JS, Henderson DP, eds. *Emergency Medical Services for Children: A Report to the Nation.* Washington, DC: National Center for Education in Maternal and Child Health; 1991.

Procedures

Procedure 1: Field Reporting   336

Procedure 2: Length-Based
Resuscitation Tapes   340

Procedure 3: Oxygen Delivery   342

Procedure 4: Suctioning   347

Procedure 5: Airway Adjuncts   353

Procedure 6: Foreign Body
Obstruction   356

Procedure 7: Bronchodilator
Therapy   360

Procedure 8: Bag-Mask
Ventilation   363

Procedure 9: Pulse Oximetry   367

Procedure 10: Orogastric and
Nasogastric Tube Insertion   369

Procedure 11: Endotracheal
Intubation   373

Procedure 12: Confirmation of Endotracheal
Intubation and End-Tidal Capnography   383

Procedure 13: Advanced Airway
Techniques   389

Procedure 14: Intramuscular
Injections   398

Procedure 15: Intranasal Medication
Administration   402

Procedure 16: Intravenous
Access   405

Procedure 17: Intraosseous Needle
Insertion   409

Procedure 18: Cardiopulmonary
Resuscitation   415

Procedure 19: AED and
Defibrillation   420

Procedure 20: Endotracheal Tube Drug
Instillation   425

Procedure 21: Rectal Administration
of Benzodiazepines   427

Procedure 22: Spinal Motion
Restriction   430

Procedure 23: Needle
Thoracostomy   435

Procedure 24: Removing and Replacing
a Tracheostomy Tube   437

Procedure 25: Tourniquet
Application   441

Procedure 1: Field Reporting

S. Heath Ackley, MD, MPH, FAAP

Jennifer L. Stafford, BSN, CEN, CFRN

Introduction

Gathering and organizing pertinent information about pediatric patients to report to other prehospital professionals, medical oversight, and the receiving emergency department (ED) are important pieces of the continuum of care. Clear, concise communication is imperative when describing children and their clinical problems to medical oversight personnel, when informing a receiving ED about an incoming patient, and before transferring patient care. Field reporting should be clear, concise, organized, and pertinent and should be done in a manner that protects the privacy of the patient. The reporting is usually done via a secure radio transmission, a telephone, or another form of secure real-time communication. Different emergency medical service (EMS) regions may have unique requirements for field reporting to medical oversight and to receiving EDs.

In addition to the spoken presentation format for field reporting, pediatric-specific documentation is also essential for later review and analysis. EMS agencies typically have their own reporting form or template on which the prehospital professional must record clinical facts, as well as the necessary information for billing and for detailed incident or system analysis.

INDICATION

Utilize appropriate field reporting procedure in any radio, telephone, facsimile (fax), or personal communication with medical oversight, a receiving ED, or other prehospital providers regarding on-scene or inbound pediatric emergency patients. Utilize appropriate pediatric-specific documentation for written reports or records.

CONTRAINDICATION

The only relative contraindication to appropriate field reporting is the child with a physiologic abnormality requiring constant hands-on care. This situation may make it difficult for the prehospital professional to communicate fully with a receiving ED or medical oversight during transport. In most cases, a coworker, such as a partner, can assist with notifying pertinent parties that a distressed child is en route. However, complete reporting of patient assessment, treatment, and response to treatment may not be possible. There are no contraindications to accurate reporting through written documentation.

EQUIPMENT

Equipment requirements vary depending on the EMS system. Equipment may include telecommunications equipment, computerized real-time data transmission, or video. The patient care record is essential, as are other assessment worksheets in some EMS systems.

Rationale

A logical and descriptive format for presentation of key information about ill or injured children is essential for everyday field practice. It promotes the cost-efficient use of communications equipment and personnel time. Proper field reporting also integrates efforts from all emergency care professionals (prehospital professionals, nurses, and doctors) and helps ensure that vital data are transmitted completely and concisely. Pediatric-specific reporting techniques complement appropriate age-related modifications in assessment, treatment, triage, and transport.

Preparation

1. The prehospital professional should prepare for and practice field reporting on pediatric patients.
2. It is helpful to have a field reporting format that is agreed on by the EMS agency, medical oversight, and the transport providers. The desired format can be an actual document or checklist; this may help facilitate the gathering of patient information during situations when the prehospital professional has multiple tasks and when the environment or equipment makes communication difficult.

Possible Complications

Using incorrect, deceptive, or unclear terminology, or failing to distinguish the pediatric report from the more frequent adult-oriented report, may delay medical oversight and preparation by the receiving ED.

> **TIP**
>
> 1. Field reports should be approximately 30 seconds in length and give enough patient information for the ED and/or medical oversight to determine the appropriate level of care.
> 2. Utilize the Pediatric Assessment Triangle (PAT) for assessment reporting.

Components of a Prehospital Field Report

1. Unit's identification and level of service (advanced or basic life support)
2. Patient's age, gender, and approximate weight
3. Chief complaint
4. Brief, *pertinent* history of present illness or injury
5. *Pertinent* medical history, medications, and allergies
6. Pertinent physical exam findings (Pediatric Assessment Triangle)
7. Significant findings in airway, breathing, circulation, and level of consciousness (AVPU or pediatric Glasgow Coma Scale [GCS]).
8. Diagnostic findings (e.g., glucose)
9. Treatments and responses
10. Estimated time of arrival (ETA)
11. Request for orders from or further questions for medical oversight
12. Repeat medical oversight orders to confirm understanding if given

Procedure 1-1

Field Reporting

1. State the child's age, gender, and estimated body weight. For a step-by-step explanation, see **Length-Based Resuscitation Tapes, Procedure 2**.

2. Give the child's chief complaint.

3. Provide, in one sentence, the mechanism of injury or history of illness, and state pertinent past medical history, medications, and allergies (usually none or brief).

4. Summarize the assessment and establish the level of severity and urgency for treatment using the PAT. Address all three elements of the PAT, using appropriate descriptive words and terms, as listed in **TABLE P1-1**.

Appearance / Work of Breathing / Circulation to Skin

5. Report any abnormalities in airway, breathing, circulation, or level of consciousness. Avoid focusing on vital signs. Use AVPU or pediatric GCS for level of consciousness.

6. Report any diagnostic findings.

7. State treatment and response.

8. Estimate time of arrival.

9. Request agreement from medical oversight with interventions and request additional orders as per local EMS protocol.

10. Repeat medical oversight orders to confirm understanding. **TABLE P1-2** is a sample pediatric reporting template.

TABLE P1-1 Examples of Pediatric-Specific Terminology for PAT

Appearance (use TICLS mnemonic to recall individual features)	Work of Breathing	Circulation to Skin
Tone Active, vigorous, good muscle tone Limp, listless, motionless, will not sit or walk	Apneic	Pink, good color
Interactiveness Alert, interactive, attentive, playful Restless, agitated, screaming	Abnormal positioning (sniffing position, tripoding)	Mottled, dusky
Consolability Consolable or distractible by caregiver, comfortable Cannot be consoled	Abnormal airway sounds (snoring, stridor, wheezing, grunting)	Pale
Look/Gaze Fixes gaze, maintains good eye contact Will not engage or make eye contact	Retractions (supraclavicular, intercostal, subxiphoid)	Cyanotic
Speech/Cry Strong cry, normal speech Weak cry, cannot speak	Nasal flaring	

TABLE P1-2 Sample Pediatric Reporting Template

We are [on scene] or [en route to (name of ED)] with a [state age in days, weeks, months, or years as appropriate] [state male or female] patient weighing [state approximate body weight in kilograms].

CC	The patient's chief complaint is [state chief complaint in one or two words].
HPI	State brief history of present illness/injury.
PMH	State brief, pertinent, medical history, medications, and allergies (note: usually there is none).
PAT	Appearance: Describe the patient's appearance using descriptive terms.* Work of breathing: Describe the work of breathing using descriptive terms. Circulation to skin: Describe the circulation to skin using descriptive terms.
Initial ABCDEs assessment	Summarize key findings from the ABCDEs (see Chapter 1 for more information on the AVPU Scale and Chapter 7 for more information on the pediatric GCS).
Diagnostic findings	Summarize any diagnostic findings.
TX	Report the treatment and the patient's response. Use these elements as the basis for ongoing assessment: the PAT, the ABCDEs, repeating vital signs, and reassessing of positive anatomic findings in distressed children who have received the focused and detailed exams.
ETA	Our ETA to [state receiving ED] is _____ minutes. Do you have any advice or questions? [Request additional orders as per local protocol at this point.]

* See Table P1-1 for examples of pediatric-specific descriptive terminology.

Procedure 2: Length-Based Resuscitation Tapes

S. Heath Ackley, MD, MPH, FAAP

Jennifer L. Stafford, BSN, CEN, CFRN

Introduction

Selecting the appropriately sized equipment or calculating drug dosages is often challenging during pediatric resuscitations. Use of a length-based pediatric emergency resuscitation tape in the prehospital setting is associated with significantly fewer medication dosing errors. There are several different types of length-based systems that are useful for determining correct equipment sizes and drug doses. The pediatric length-based resuscitation tape is a simple and effective tool to measure body lengths and to determine approximate weights.

INDICATION

Pediatric patients weighing 3–36 kg requiring appropriate-sized equipment as well as accurate volume and medication dosing based on weight

EQUIPMENT

Length-based resuscitation tape
Pediatric drug doses based on length-based resuscitation tape on computer or cell phone

Rationale

Treatment of infants and children in the prehospital setting is difficult. Equipment size, volume resuscitation, and medication dosages are all weight based in the pediatric population. Mistakes are common when selecting appropriate equipment and medications in critically ill pediatric patients without the benefit of an accurate weight. Pediatric resuscitation equipment/methods for such calculations use weight or length as a valid marker of size-specific equipment and medication needs. These devices are portable, easy to use, and applicable to all prehospital equipment and medications. The use of a computer- or cell phone–based application to determine the correct drug dose in milliliters (versus milligrams) is beneficial, but it is important to verify the concentrations of the particular drug to ensure it is the same being used by your agency.

Possible Complications

- Incorrect measurement
- Incorrect drug concentration

TIP

Store the length-based resuscitation tape in a place that is easily accessible, such as the pediatric equipment kit.

TIP

Set up your pediatric medication bag thoughtfully to minimize the risk of error. For example, avoid putting "look-alike" drugs in close proximity.

Procedure 2-1

Length-Based Resuscitation Tape

1. Place the patient in a supine position.

2. Extend the patient's legs.

3. Measure the child's length from head to heel with the tape, with the red portion at the head ("red to head"). Note and verbalize the weight in kilograms that corresponds to the child's measured length at the heel. If the child is longer than the tape, use adult equipment and medication doses. From the tape, identify appropriate equipment sizes as well as appropriate medication doses and fluid volumes.

There are several different brands of length-based pediatric resuscitation tapes which are based on an average sized US child. Studies have shown these tapes underestimate the weight of obese children, especially toward the longer lengths. However, the equipment sizes are still accurate based on length.

CAUTION

Measuring to the child's toes (instead of heel) adds a number of kilograms to the estimated weight and may result in equipment sizes that are too large or excessive drug doses.

CONTROVERSY

Pediatric length-based resuscitation tapes are based on ideal body weight. With the epidemic of obesity in children, there is concern about the accuracy of length-based resuscitation tapes. However, most emergency medications are dosed on what a patient should ideally weigh—their ideal body weight. Thus, there is rarely a need to increase resuscitation medication doses in obese children.

Procedure 2-2

Pediatric Resuscitation Software

1. Pediatric drug dosage calculators based on length-based resuscitation tapes now exist for a computer or cell phone. It is crucial to use a length-based method to determine the weight of the child. Do not use software to determine the weight. You can then use software to help you determine a drug dose; it is usually in milliliters, rather in milligrams, but look carefully to determine the unit. In addition, it is crucial to verify the concentration of the particular drug to ensure it is the same being used by your agency (e.g., atropine and naloxone come in different concentrations).

2. Enter the child's weight into the software program, then select the clinical condition or type of resuscitation. The software calculates the drug dose for the child's weight.

Procedure 3: Oxygen Delivery

Michael H. Stroud, MD, FAAP

Sam Vance, MHA, LP

Introduction

Hypoxia in the infant or child causes cardiopulmonary distress and may lead to organ failure. Careful assessment of the child's cardiopulmonary status includes standard physical assessment techniques, pulse oximetry, and end-tidal CO_2 ($EtCO_2$). A normal room air pulse oximetry reading is equal to or greater than 94%. A pulse oximetry value of less than 94% on room air is an indication for supplemental oxygen; a value less than 90% with the child on 100% oxygen is also an indication for ventilatory support. Maintain the airway and administer oxygen as appropriate with a target of achieving >94% SpO_2. Some respiratory problems will improve with simple measures. Rapid intervention may slow or reverse cardiopulmonary distress or failure and avoid the need for additional ventilatory support. The goal is to stop progression from respiratory distress so that the child does not develop respiratory failure. This can happen quickly in infants and children. Although respiratory disease is usually the cause of hypoxia in children, other conditions, such as hypovolemic shock, severe poisonings, or seizures, may also result in hypoxia.

There are different procedures for giving oxygen to children that vary the amount of actual oxygen supplementation. Use an oxygen delivery technique that matches the child's clinical condition, age, and need for oxygen. When necessary, escalate support methods to maintain normal oxygenation. For example, give oxygen by nasal cannula or simple mask to the child in no or mild distress who has an open airway; give oxygen by a nonrebreathing mask or bag-mask device to the child with moderate to severe respiratory distress. For severe respiratory distress or impending respiratory failure, more advanced methods of oxygen delivery may be required, such as continuous positive airway pressure (CPAP), bilevel positive airway pressure, intermittent positive pressure breathing, humidified high-flow nasal cannula, and/or bilevel nasal CPAP. Use caution with use of positive-pressure delivery methods in children with bronchospasm; use of such methods can lead to air leaks such as pneumothoraxes and pneumomediastinum. Rarely, a critical child requires endotracheal intubation for positive-pressure ventilation and oxygen administration. When supplemental oxygen does not improve the child's condition, consider other possibilities, such as a cardiac disorder (e.g., cyanotic congenital heart disease); a circulatory disorder (e.g., hypovolemic shock); or, rarely, a toxicologic disorder (e.g., methemoglobinemia).

Under some circumstances, giving blow-by oxygen may avoid agitating the child and increasing his or her distress. In a newborn, be careful about oxygen delivery; it is unnecessary if the newborn is vigorous and pink, and a high concentration of supplemental oxygen may be harmful to the immature brain.

INDICATIONS

- Cardiac arrest
- Respiratory distress
- Pulse oximetry less than 94% on room air
- Respiratory failure
- Partial upper airway obstruction
- Partial lower airway obstruction
- Worsening of chronic lung disease
- Status epilepticus
- Overdose
- Shock from any cause
- Multiple trauma
- Any condition possibly causing decreased oxygen delivery to tissues
- Smoke inhalation
- Carbon monoxide poisoning

There are few absolute contraindications to oxygen delivery to a child who may be hypoxic. A relative contraindication is a child with known cyanotic heart disease. It is important to ask the parent or caregiver what the child's normal pulse oximeter reading should be. You can then provide oxygen to meet this oxygen saturation. Oxygen has proper doses and routes of administration for maximum benefit, minimum toxicity, optimal feasibility, and reasonable cost.

Rationale

A child's immature anatomy and physiology make respiratory distress and failure common pediatric emergencies. When apnea or hypoventilation occurs, hypoxia develops quickly. Therefore, give oxygen to any child with clinical signs of cardiopulmonary distress or failure, or with a history suggesting possible abnormalities in gas exchange. *Children seldom have a condition where excess oxygen suppresses their respiratory drive, so it is better to overtreat with oxygen than to undertreat.*

TIP

The appropriate oxygen delivery technique is based on the child's condition, age, and need for oxygen.

Preparation

1. Connect the pressure regulator and flow meter to the oxygen source. Turn on the tank.
2. Match the correct oxygen delivery device with the patient assessment (child's condition, age, and need for oxygen; **TABLE P3-1**).

Equipment

- Infant and pediatric nasal cannula
- Pediatric mask sizes
- Pediatric nonrebreathing mask
- Oxygen connecting tubing
- Oxygen source
- Pulse oximeter and probes

Possible Complications

Injury, if the pressurized tank is punctured or a valve breaks off.

Potential for fire, because oxygen supports combustion.

In preterm newborns, there is a risk of brain injury due to unnecessary high concentrations of supplemental oxygen.

CAUTION

Do not give oxygen to a newborn who is not hypoxic. It is also important to realize that the normal preductal SpO_2 is 85%–95% at 10 minutes after birth.

TIP

An oxygen mask may frighten a child.

CAUTION

Do not force the child to lie down, because it may increase the child's anxiety and agitation.

TIP

Add humidification to nasal cannula flow to avoid nasal irritation and bleeding, which helps to loosen secretions.

TIP

For nasal cannula: The percentage of oxygen delivered is affected by respiratory rate, tidal volume, and extent of mouth breathing. An infant may receive higher FiO_2 concentration than older patients (e.g., 30%–35% with 1 L/min oxygen, 26%–32% with 0.5 L/min oxygen).

TABLE P3-1 Oxygen Delivery Technique and Patient Assessment

Device	Flow Rate	Concentration Delivered	Considerations
Nasal cannula	1–6 L/min	21%–44%	<ul><li>Low-flow system</li><li>Least restrictive</li><li>Slowly start flow of oxygen after cannula is secured to avoid frightening child</li><li>May help to tape cannula to child's cheeks</li><li>Use in infants who are obligatory nose breathers or if there is difficulty in obtaining a correctly sized mask</li></ul>
Simple mask	6–10 L/min	35%–60%	<ul><li>Low-flow system</li><li>Infant-, pediatric-, and adult-sized masks are available</li><li>At least 6 L/min flow rate is needed to prevent re-breathing of exhaled CO_2</li></ul>
Nonrebreathing mask	10–15 L/min	60%–95%	<ul><li>High-flow system mask</li><li>Consists of face mask and reservoir bag with a valve on the exhalation mask port to prevent drawing in room air during inhalation, and a valve between the reservoir bag and mask to prevent exhalation of air into the reservoir bag</li><li>Use in spontaneously breathing patients who require highest concentration of oxygen available (children with respiratory distress and shock)</li><li>Make sure the flow rate keeps the reservoir bag inflated</li><li>With a snug fit, delivers highest oxygen concentration available by mask</li><li>Pediatric and adult masks are available</li><li>Partial rebreathing masks are indicated in neonates and infants who cannot overcome valve resistance</li></ul>
Blow-by	10 L/min	Approximately 30%–40%; dependent on proximity to face	<ul><li>Indicated for infant or young child requiring oxygen who will not tolerate mask on the face</li><li>Start oxygen flow through simple mask, corrugated tubing, or oxygen tubing threaded through the bottom of a cup</li><li>Hold the delivery device as close to the child's nose and mouth as tolerated</li></ul>

Modified from American Heart Association. *ACLS Provider Manual Supplementary Material*. 2016.

Procedure 3-1

Oxygen Delivery

1. Explain to the child and family why oxygen is needed and how the device works. Use developmentally appropriate language. **TABLE P3-2** suggests methods to ease anxiety in the child who does not want to cooperate with oxygen delivery. For blow-by oxygen using a paper cup, punch a hole in the bottom of the cup and insert the tubing through the hole. Placing stickers on the cup or drawing smiley faces may decrease the child's anxiety. Also consider attaching the oxygen tubing to a favorite toy and encourage the child to hold the toy near their face.

2. Allow the child to remain in a position of comfort, which may be sitting on the caregiver's lap. In the ambulance, the child must be safely restrained.

3a. To apply a mask, select the correct size. The mask should extend from the bridge of the nose to the cleft of the chin. Avoid placing pressure on the eyes.

3b. Place the mask over the child's head, starting from the nose downward. Squeeze the nose clip and adjust the head strap.

4. To apply a nasal cannula, curve the plastic prongs back into the nostrils. Loop the tubing around the ears.

5. For blow-by oxygen, instruct the caregiver to hold the tubing, paper cup, or favorite toy close to the child's face to maximize oxygen delivery.

TABLE P3-2 Methods to Gain Child's Cooperation for Oxygen Delivery

Allow the child to hold the mask before placing it on his or her face.

Allow the child to feel the flow of oxygen before placing the mask on his or her face.

Describe the mask in appealing terms, such as a space mask or superhero mask.

If the child struggles, consider using the blow-by technique to avoid agitation and increasing the oxygen demands. Placing stickers or drawing smiley faces on the cup may decrease the child's anxiety. Also consider attaching the oxygen tubing to a favorite toy and encourage the child to hold the toy near their face.

CONTROVERSY

The amount of oxygen to give to children with chronic lung disease is unknown and probably differs for each individual. In some children, oxygen delivery may have the unexpected effect of worsening hypoxia. That said, administration of oxygen to patients with chronic lung disease who retain carbon dioxide at baseline rarely results in hypoventilation in pediatric patients. If the child has a history and assessment suggesting acute hypoxia and increased work of breathing, give oxygen but be ready to assist ventilation with a bag-mask device.

SUGGESTED REFERENCES

American Heart Association. *Web-based Integrated Guidelines for Cardiopulmonary Resuscitation and Emergency Cardiovascular Care – Part 12: Pediatric Advanced Life Support.* Dallas, TX: American Heart Association, Inc; 2015.

National Association of State EMS Officials. *National Model EMS Clinical Guidelines Version 2.0.* Falls Church, VA: NASEMSO; 2017.

Procedure 4: Suctioning

S. Heath Ackley, MD, MPH, FAAP

Victoria Barnes, RN, BSN, EMT

Introduction

Children of all ages are prone to airway obstruction from secretions, vomitus, pus, blood, edema, and foreign bodies. In newborns, airway obstruction from amniotic fluid, meconium, and blood is a common and potentially critical problem that is usually treatable with suction alone. In infancy and childhood, conditions such as closed-head injury or status epilepticus may cause the loss of airway protective reflexes and put the child at risk for loss of airway patency from aspiration or airway obstruction. Children needing endotracheal intubation often have diseases or trauma associated with fluid in the endotracheal tube and airway sacs; this fluid must be removed to ensure adequate oxygenation and ventilation. Children with tracheostomy tubes may get secretions or mucus in the tubes, which must be evacuated.

INDICATIONS

- Some newborns
- Infants or children with fluids or foreign bodies in the nasopharynx or oropharynx
- Intubated patients with fluids or secretions in the endotracheal tubes
- Patients with tracheostomy tubes with secretions or mucus in the tubes

CONTRAINDICATIONS

- Children with severe airway obstruction and suspected airway foreign body, prior to seeing the airway with laryngoscopy
- Minimize suctioning in intubated children with increased intracranial pressure and herniation.

EQUIPMENT

- Bulb syringes, one- and two-piece types
- Endotracheal tube suction catheters, sizes 8 to 14 French
- Feeding tubes, size 5 or 7 for small infants
- Large-bore rigid suction catheter

Rationale

Suctioning is a basic technique to maintain an open airway. Children have small airways that are easily obstructed. The type of suction device and suctioning procedure depend on the child's age and clinical problem (**TABLE P4-1**). Bulb syringes remove thin secretions from newborns or infants, but do not permit deep suctioning. When suctioning newborns, avoid suctioning vigorously or deeply. Deep suctioning can cause vagal stimulation, bradycardia, and laryngospasm in the newborn, particularly in the first hours during initial transition to extrauterine life. Brief, gentle suctioning with a bulb syringe (mouth, then nose) is usually adequate to remove secretions. Suction catheters remove thin secretions from the mouth, nose, or throat and are useful in all age groups. Suction catheters are also necessary for endotracheal tube suctioning. Large-bore rigid suction catheters are useful in infants and children (not newborns) to remove thick secretions, vomitus, pus, blood, or particulate matter from the mouth.

TABLE P4-1 Suction Technique Based on Age and Type of Obstructing Material

Newborns	Bulb syringe or suction catheter
Infants and children with thin secretions	Bulb syringe or suction catheter
Newborns, infants, and children with endotracheal tube	Suction catheter
Infants and children with thick secretions or particulate matter	Large-bore suction catheter

Preparation

1. Use personal protective equipment.
2. Select an appropriate suction device based on clinical condition or type of obstruction and age. If there is no functioning negative-pressure or

suction source (vacuum outlet, battery-powered or electric portable suction, or hand-powered portable suction), use a bulb syringe for thin secretions.
3. Make sure the suction device is operational.
4. Determine correct catheter size with the pediatric length-based resuscitation tape. The suction catheter should be smaller than the nostril.
5. Open catheter package.
6. Connect suction tubing or rigid suction catheter to connecting tubing and suction source.
7. Set suction vacuum (maximum, 120 mm Hg), being careful to avoid injuring sensitive tissues.

Possible Complications

- Injury to the mouth, nose, airway, or lung
- Gagging, vomiting
- Aspiration of stomach contents
- Hypoxia from prolonged suctioning
- Pushing foreign body into trachea with suction device
- Increased intracranial pressure

Procedure 4-1

Oropharyngeal/Nasopharyngeal Suctioning With Bulb Syringe

1. Squeeze the bulb away from the infant to remove air. Suction the mouth, then the nose.

2. Open the mouth and insert the syringe tip at the side of the mouth, and then advance the syringe to remove thin secretions. Avoid inserting the syringe tip into the deeper soft tissues at the back of the mouth. Do not use a two-piece bulb syringe in the mouth because it may come apart.

3. Lift the nostril slightly and suction the nose. Insert the syringe tip straight back into the nostril or at a right angle to the face.

Procedure 4-2

Oropharyngeal/Nasopharyngeal Suctioning With Suction Catheter

1. Suction the mouth, then the nose. Open the mouth, and advance until the tip touches secretions.

2. Block the side port and begin suctioning. Do not do deep suctioning beyond what is in direct vision. Remove catheter with twisting motion.

3. Insert the catheter into the nostril.

4. Block the side port to begin suctioning when the tip touches secretions. Remove the catheter with a twisting motion. Never suction longer than 5 seconds.

> **TIP**
>
> In suspected foreign body aspiration, look at the airway prior to suctioning.

> **TIP**
>
> Suction for less than 5 seconds, but use enough time to remove secretions.

Procedure 4-3

Tracheal Tube Suctioning With Suction Catheter

1. Ask your partner to preoxygenate the patient with five to six breaths from a bag-mask device using 100% oxygen.

2. With thumb off the side port, insert suction catheter through endotracheal tube and down the trachea until resistance is met.

3. Apply suction off and on by placing thumb over the side port while withdrawing and twisting the catheter (maximum, 5 seconds).

4. Irrigate catheter with normal saline.

5. Ask your partner to oxygenate five to six times. Repeat, as necessary.

Procedure 4-4

Oropharyngeal Suctioning with Large-Bore Rigid Suction Catheter

1. Open the mouth and advance catheter until it touches secretions.

2. Close the side port or turn on suction to begin suctioning. Remove the catheter with a twisting motion. Do not suction more than 5 seconds.

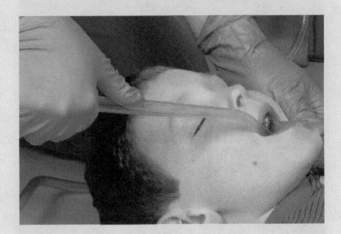

SUGGESTED REFERENCE

American Academy of Pediatrics, American Heart Association. *Textbook of Neonatal Resuscitation.* 7th ed. Elk Grove, IL: AAP; 2016.

Procedure 5: Airway Adjuncts

Victoria Barnes, RN, BSN, EMT

Toni M. Petrillo, MD, FAAP

Introduction

An oropharyngeal (OP) or nasopharyngeal (NP) airway adjunct is often helpful to maintain an open airway for optimal ventilation. Sizing is important, because improperly sized OP or NP airways may cause further obstruction. The prehospital professional must know when to use an OP or NP airway adjunct, how to determine the proper size, and how to insert the adjunct safely and effectively.

INDICATIONS

- Respiratory insufficiency
- NP or OP airway obstruction
- Seizures, including postictal state (NP airway)

CONTRAINDICATIONS

OP airway:
- Intact gag reflex
- Ingestion of a caustic or petroleum product

NP airway:
- Complete nasal obstruction
- Possible basilar skull fracture
- Major nasofacial trauma

EQUIPMENT

- NP airways
- OP airways

Rationale

Opening the airway of a small infant or child by positioning alone, with the head-tilt/chin-lift maneuvers or jaw thrust, may not keep the tongue from obstructing the airway. Adequate ventilation often requires placement of airway adjuncts. They are easy to insert and may markedly improve airway patency. Adjuncts may immediately improve the efficacy of the child's spontaneous ventilation. In addition, they may allow more effective bag-mask ventilation, reduce gastric inflation, and avert the need for endotracheal intubation.

Preparation

1. Position patient's airway:
   Medical patient
   - Perform the head-tilt/chin-lift maneuver to open the airway. Avoid hyperextension of the neck because it may cause airway obstruction.
   - Use a towel under the shoulders of an infant or small child to get neutral airway position.
   Trauma patient
   - Use the modified jaw thrust maneuver with in-line spinal stabilization to open the airway.
2. Select the properly sized adjunct:
   OP airway
   - Use resuscitation tape (see Procedure 2) OR
   - Measure the device on the patient:
     - Place OP airway next to face with the flange at the level of the central incisors (front teeth) and the bite block segment parallel to the hard palate.
     - The tip of the appropriately sized OP airway should reach the angle of the jaw.
   NP airway
   - Use resuscitation tape (see Procedure 2) OR

- Measure the device on the patient:
  - The outside diameter of the NP airway should be less than the diameter of the nostril.
  - Place the NP airway next to the face and measure from the tip of the nose to the tragus of the ear.
  - Adjust movable flange (if present) up or down to get appropriate length.

Procedure 5-1

OP Airway Insertion

1. Depress tongue with a tongue blade (if available). Next, insert oral airway with the tip down, to avoid injury to the palate, until the flange rests against lips.

2. If a tongue blade is not available, insert the airway sideways, with the tip to the side. Then, rotate down over the base of the tongue.

3. Insert OP airway until the flange is resting against the lips.

Procedure 5-2

NP Airway Insertion

1. Lubricate NP airway.

2. Insert with bevel toward septum (center of nose).

3. Advance tip along floor of nasal cavity.

4. If using the right nostril, advance until flange is seated against outside of nostril. The tip should be in the nasopharynx.

5. If using the left nostril, begin inserting the airway with the curvature upward until resistance is felt (about 2 cm), and then rotate the device 180 degrees and advance until flange is against outside of nostril.

Possible Complications

OP Airway

- If OP airway is too small, the tongue may get pushed back into the pharynx, obstructing the airway
- If OP airway is too large, it may obstruct the larynx
- Pharyngeal bleeding
- Laryngospasm
- Vomiting

NP Airway

- Adenoidal tissue laceration
- Pharyngeal bleeding
- Obstruction of tube with fluids or soft tissues, causing airway obstruction
- If an NP airway is too long, vagal stimulation or esophageal entry with gastric distention may occur
- Laryngospasm
- Vomiting

CONTROVERSY

The use of airway adjuncts in facial trauma is controversial. If the child has an open fracture of the craniofacial bones, the device could penetrate into the brain and cause further brain injury or hemorrhage. The devices should not be used in the setting of major facial bone injury.

CAUTION

Never attempt to insert an OP airway in a conscious child.

CAUTION

Do not insert an OP airway that is too small, or it will push the tongue back and obstruct the airway.

Procedure 6: Foreign Body Obstruction

Michael J. Stoner, MD, FAAP

Introduction

Foreign body obstruction of the airway is common in toddlers and preschool children, who place objects in their mouths as part of the exploratory behavior normal for patients in these age groups. Fortunately, hypoxic brain injury and death are uncommon outcomes. Liquids are the most common cause of choking in infants, whereas balloons, small objects, and food (e.g., hot dogs, round candies, nuts, and grapes) are the most common causes of foreign body airway obstruction (FBAO) in children. The infant or child with a completely obstructed airway poses the ultimate medical challenge because a moment's delay can result in permanent disability or be fatal. When treating a patient with foreign body obstruction, it is important to begin with basic maneuvers to clear the airway, but sometimes more advanced techniques are necessary.

INDICATIONS

Severe airway obstruction

Severe partial airway obstruction and respiratory failure

CONTRAINDICATION

Partial airway obstruction with maintenance of the airway

EQUIPMENT

Laryngoscope and straight blades (Miller sizes 1 and 2)

Pediatric Magill forceps
Bag-mask devices (infant and pediatric)

Rationale

In the setting of severe airway obstruction, prehospital professionals can make the difference between life and death. Immediate removal of an airway foreign body can often be achieved using basic life support (BLS) procedures, yet every year many children suffer grave injury and death because of failure to use basic clearance maneuvers. Sometimes, the foreign body is deeper in the airway or embedded in tissue, so that basic maneuvers are unsuccessful. In such cases, using Magill forceps and direct laryngoscopy may be the best option for removal.

CAUTION

Do not perform blind finger sweeps, which may push the foreign body further into the airway.

Preparation

1. Attempt BLS maneuvers first (see **Procedure 6-1**).
2. Move to advanced life support (ALS) maneuvers if BLS maneuvers fail.
3. Attach appropriately sized straight blade to laryngoscope handle.
4. Ensure light is working on laryngoscope blade.

Possible Complications

- Hypoxia
- Foreign body is pushed farther into airway
- Laryngeal and tracheal injury
- Teeth and mouth injury

Procedure 6-1

BLS Maneuvers

1. If FBAO is mild, do not interfere. Allow the victim to clear the airway by coughing while you observe for signs of severe FBAO.

2. If the FBAO is severe (i.e., the victim is unable to make a sound), you must act to relieve the obstruction.

3. For a child, perform subdiaphragmatic abdominal thrusts (Heimlich maneuver) until the object is expelled or the victim becomes unresponsive. One study suggests abdominal thrusts administered with the child in a prone position may increase the chances of successfully clearing an FBAO.

4. For an infant, deliver repeated cycles of five back blows (slaps) followed by five chest compressions until the object is expelled or the victim becomes unresponsive. Abdominal thrusts are not recommended for infants because they may damage the infant's relatively large and unprotected liver.

5. If the victim becomes unresponsive, start cardiopulmonary resuscitation (CPR) with chest compressions (do not perform a pulse check).

6. If alone after 30 chest compressions, open the airway. If you see a foreign body, remove it; however, do not perform blind finger sweeps, because they may push the obstructed object farther into the pharynx and may damage the oropharynx. Attempt to give two breaths and continue with cycles of chest compressions and ventilations until the object is expelled.

Procedure 6-2

Laryngoscopy and Magill Forceps (ALS Procedure)

1. Grasp laryngoscope handle in the left hand. Use trigger-finger technique.

2. Open mouth by using thumb pressure on chin. Insert pediatric straight laryngoscope blade into mouth.

3. Lift tongue with blade. Exert gentle traction upward along the axis of the laryngoscope handle at a 45-degree angle. Do not use teeth or gums for leverage. Advance blade. Watch the tip until foreign body is visible. Do not go past vocal cords. Use suction to improve visibility and maintain airway.

CAUTION

Suctioning may push the foreign body farther into the airway, so look at the airway before suctioning.

4. Grasp closed Magill forceps in right hand, palm down. Insert Magill forceps into mouth, tips closed. Open forceps and move tips around foreign body. Grasp foreign body and remove while looking directly at it. Look at the airway and make sure it is clear of foreign bodies or debris. Remove laryngoscope blade. After removal of foreign body, reassess respiratory status. Use suction if needed. Attempt to ventilate if the child does not breathe spontaneously. Return to BLS maneuvers if no foreign body is seen by direct laryngoscopy.

TIP

Repeat BLS procedures if no foreign body is seen by direct laryngoscopy.

TIP

Attempt BLS maneuvers before using Magill forceps.

SUGGESTED REFERENCES

Berg MD, Schexnayder SM, Chameides L, et al. Part 13: Pediatric basic life support: 2010 American Heart Association Guidelines for Cardiopulmonary Resuscitation and Emergency Cardiovascular Care. *Circulation*. 2010;122(suppl 3):S862–S875.

Ichikawa M, Oishi S, Mochizuki K, Nitta K, Okamoto K, Imamura H. Influence of body position during Heimlich maneuver to relieve supralaryngeal obstruction: a manikin study. *Acute Med Surg*. 2017;4:418–425.

Procedure 7: Bronchodilator Therapy

S. Heath Ackley, MD, MPH, FAAP

Thomas Herron Jr., AAS, NRP

Introduction

Wheezing from bronchospasm is one of the most common prehospital pediatric problems. Children who are wheezing are usually in acute respiratory distress and are often anxious, agitated, and uncooperative. The prehospital professional must use a developmentally appropriate approach with the child and the caregiver when giving general noninvasive respiratory care and using beta agonists with or without anticholinergic medications. The caregiver can help by holding, soothing, and supporting a scared child. One way to give aerosolized beta agonist and anticholinergic medication is with an oxygen-powered nebulizer. Another way is the metered-dose inhaler (MDI) with a spacer, although this inhalation technique has not been studied adequately in the prehospital setting. If the child is uncooperative or unable to use inhaled beta agonist therapy, intramuscular (IM) drug delivery is another possibility.

INDICATION

Wheezing

CONTRAINDICATION

Known sensitivity to bronchodilator drugs

EQUIPMENT

Inhalation therapy (nebulizer)
>An oxygen-powered nebulizer that aerosolizes the liquid bronchodilator to small particle size that can reach the bronchioles

Oxygen source set to 6 L/min minimum

Mask or mouthpiece with liquid reservoir

Beta agonist
>**Albuterol** solution (1.25 mg/3 mL, 2.5 mg/3 mL, prediluted solutions for nebulization; 5 mg/mL solution for nebulization [dilution required])

Anticholinergic
>**Ipratropium** solution 0.02% (500 mcg/2.5 mL)

Inhalation therapy (MDI)
>MDI, mask, and spacer

Beta agonist drugs
>Albuterol MDI (90 mcg/puff)

Anticholinergic
>Ipratropium (MDI) (17 mcg/puff)

IM therapy
>Tuberculin (TB) or 3-mL syringe

22- to 27-gauge needle

Bronchodilator
>**Epinephrine** 1 mg/mL concentration

Rationale

For asthma, early bronchodilator therapy, on scene and en route to the emergency department (ED), helps immediately open airways, relieve respiratory distress, and improve oxygen delivery. Early bronchodilator therapy may reduce the need for more aggressive hospital therapy, shorten ED and hospital times, and decrease chances of complications or death. The addition of anticholinergic medication may also be beneficial. *Inhalation treatment with a nebulized beta agonist is the best initial approach with severe wheezing and respiratory distress.*

Preparation

Inhalation Therapy

1. Have the caregiver hold the child on his or her lap. An older child can sit alone.
2. Have the child in an upright position of comfort.
3. Explain what is happening. Most children need only inhalation bronchodilator therapy by oxygen-powered nebulizer or with an MDI and spacer.

Intramuscular Therapy (Epinephrine)

1. Position the child on the caregiver's lap or straddling the caregiver's leg.
2. Expose the thigh or deltoid area for injection (see **Procedure 14, Intramuscular Injections**).

Possible Complications of Albuterol and/or Ipratropium

Anxiety	Nausea
Chest pain	Nasal stuffiness
Cough	Palpitations
Dizziness	Restlessness
Dry mouth	Tachycardia
Dysrhythmias	Tremors
Headache	Vomiting
Hypertension	

Procedure 7-1

Inhalation Therapy

1. If the child can cooperate, deliver nebulized beta agonist with or without anticholinergic medication through a mouthpiece or mask. The caregiver can hold the mask to the child's face, if necessary.

2. If an MDI is used, attach spacer and mask when the child is too young or unable to trigger aerosol effectively.

3. Monitor respiratory rate, heart rate, and pulse oximetry during therapy.

© Jones & Bartlett Learning.

© Jones & Bartlett Learning.

The role of the MDI in prehospital beta agonist therapy is not known. Although ED studies have shown that the MDI is as effective as inhaled drugs for most children, it has not been studied adequately in the prehospital setting. MDI with mask and spacer, however, can probably deliver an adequate beta agonist dose to most children older than 2 years of age.

Use beta agonists for children who are wheezing from asthma.

In children unable to cooperate with a nebulized treatment and/or patients who are unable to properly utilize an MDI, the EMS provider can remove the bag from a nonrebreathing mask and insert the medication reservoir into the opening. This allows passive administration of the nebulized medication via mask. Oxygen settings remain the same as if utilizing a nebulizer in the normal manner.

The nebulizer may also be placed in-line on a bag-mask device when ventilating a patient with wheezing who needs assistance with ventilation.

Procedure 7-2

Intramuscular Therapy

1. If the child is in significant respiratory distress or if the child cannot cooperate with inhalation therapy, give epinephrine by IM injection. Use one of two anatomic locations: lateral aspect of deltoid in upper arms (older child) or anterolateral thigh.

2. Inject the medication intramuscularly.

Avoid injectable drugs in cooperative, wheezing patients. The procedure is painful and no more effective than an inhaled beta agonist.

Procedure 8: Bag-Mask Ventilation

J. Joelle Donofrio-Odmann, DO, FAAP, FACEP, FAEMS
John A. Erbayri, MS, NRP, CHSE

Introduction

Bag-mask ventilation is a highly effective way to deliver assisted ventilation to a child in respiratory failure. Oxygen at 60%–95% concentration can be given safely by choosing a well-fitted mask, connecting the oxygen reservoir to a supplemental oxygen source at 15+ L/min, disabling the pop-off valve, and ventilating at an age-appropriate rate.

INDICATIONS

Apnea or respiratory arrest
Respiratory failure
Cyanosis despite supplemental oxygen*

Consider when oxygen saturation (SaO$_2$) less than 90% despite administration of 100% oxygen by nonrebreathing mask

EQUIPMENT

Transparent masks with soft rim, sizes neonate through adult

Self-inflating resuscitator (bag), at least 450 mL in volume

*N.B. Children with uncorrected cyanotic heart disease may have low oxygen saturations at baseline.

Rationale

Assisted ventilation is a way to oxygenate and ventilate a child who is unable to breathe adequately on his or her own. Although the technique does not provide the definitive airway control that endotracheal intubation does, in many cases bag-mask ventilation will be the best technique for assisting ventilation during resuscitation and transport. Effective bag-mask ventilation is one of the prehospital professional's most useful skills in pediatric prehospital care.

Preparation

1. Measure the mask on the patient. The mask should extend from the bridge of the nose to the cleft of the chin, avoiding compression of the eyes. The right-sized mask will have a small volume to minimize dead space and to prevent rebreathing of expired carbon dioxide. Transparency allows the rescuer to observe the child for cyanosis of the lips and for emesis.

2. Select an appropriate resuscitator bag. Although a small child can be safely and effectively ventilated using an adult bag, a pediatric bag will not work for a large child, adolescent, or adult. Pediatric tidal volume is approximately 8 mL/kg, so the pediatric bag should have a volume of 450–750 mL. An adult bag (1,200 mL) is acceptable for larger children or adolescents.

3. If a pop-off valve is present, it may need to be disabled to permit higher inspiratory pressures and achieve chest rise.

4. Connect one end of oxygen tubing to the resuscitator bag and the other end to the flow meter, set to 15 L/min.

Possible Complications

- Hypoxia
- Barotrauma
- Gastric distention
- Emesis and aspiration

Procedure 8-1

Bag-Mask Ventilation

1. Open airway. *Medical patient*: Use head-tilt/chin-lift maneuver. *Trauma patient*: Use jaw thrust with in-line manual cervical spine stabilization.

2. Ensure neutral positioning (sniffing position). Because infants and toddlers have large heads, place a small roll under the shoulders to achieve the sniffing position. Avoid hyperextension of the neck because this may cause airway obstruction or spinal injury.

3. Insert appropriate airway adjunct if airway patency cannot be maintained with the head-tilt/chin-lift or jaw thrust maneuvers (see **Procedure 5, Airway Adjuncts**). Use an oropharyngeal (OP) airway if the patient does not have a gag reflex, or use a nasopharyngeal (NP) airway if the patient has an active gag reflex.

4. Begin ventilation. Ensure no air leak around the mask. Common problem areas include near the eyes and chin.

CAUTION

Avoid hyperextension of the neck, which may cause airway obstruction or spinal injury.

TIP

In children with pending respiratory failure due to an obstructive process (i.e., status asthmaticus), listening for the end of expiration may minimize risk of barotrauma.

TIP

Use an OP or NP airway with the bag-mask device if airway patency cannot be maintained with the head-tilt/chin-lift or jaw thrust maneuvers.

Procedure 8-2

Bag-Mask Ventilation Using One-Rescuer Technique

1. Apply the mask to the face and get an airtight seal by placing the thumb and index finger on the mask, and place the third, fourth, and fifth fingers on the bony portion of the jaw (mandible). This is called the E-C clamp technique.

2. Pull the child's jaw into the mask, instead of pushing the mask into the face, to establish a seal. Failure to provide a tight seal may result in delivery of lower oxygen concentrations or an inadequate volume of air. Avoid placing pressure on soft tissues under the chin because this may compress the airway. Squeeze the bag with the dominant hand, watching for chest rise. Squeeze the bag only until the chest rise is visible, then release. Say, "squeeze, release, release" during ventilation to achieve the correct inspiratory volume and to allow for expiration. Child and infant: 12–20 squeezes/minute. Adult: 12–16 squeezes/minute.

3. Assess effectiveness of ventilation. Look for adequate bilateral rise and fall of chest. Auscultate for lung sounds at the midaxillary line bilaterally. Monitor oxygen saturation. Consider monitoring end-tidal CO_2.

TIP

Pull the jaw into the mask, instead of pushing the mask into the face.

TIP

Seeing the chest rise is the best indicator of adequate tidal volume.

CONTROVERSY

The relative value of bag-mask ventilation versus endotracheal intubation in respiratory failure is not known. Bag-mask ventilation may be as good as endotracheal tube ventilation in the prehospital setting in children with acute illness or injury.

Procedure 8-3

Bag-Mask Ventilation Using Two-Rescuer Technique

The two-rescuer technique is preferable in trauma patients or if the one-rescuer technique does not create an effective seal.

1. Rescuer applies the mask to the face and maintains a seal. *Medical patient*: Hold the mask to the face with the thumb and index fingers of both hands; use the other fingers to perform a chin lift (bilateral E-C clamp technique). *Trauma patient*: Perform a jaw thrust maneuver, lifting the jaw into the mask with both hands, while maintaining in-line cervical spine manual stabilization.

2. Pull the child's jaw into the mask, instead of pushing the mask into the face, to establish a seal. Avoid placing pressure on soft tissues under the chin because this may compress the airway.

3. Second rescuer ventilates. Avoid gastric distention. Watch the abdomen for signs of enlargement during

ventilation. If this happens, reposition the airway and observe the chest rise carefully, squeezing the bag only until the chest starts to rise. If bag-mask ventilation is to be considered during transport, consider placement of an orogastric or nasogastric tube for gastric decompression.

TIP

The two-rescuer technique is preferable in a trauma patient or if the one-rescuer technique does not get a good seal.

CAUTION

A bag less than 450 mL will not generate enough inspiratory pressure to ventilate a large child, adolescent, or adult.

Procedure 9: Pulse Oximetry

S. Heath Ackley, MD, MPH, FAAP

Thomas Herron Jr., AAS, NRP

Introduction

Pulse oximetry, which measures oxygenation and pulse rate, can be a useful adjunct in the management of the ill or injured child. Use of the pulse oximeter does not replace clinical assessment of the child. Monitoring changes in pulse oximetry readings may help the prehospital professional to determine the patient's response to interventions and guide additional interventions.

However, there are caveats. If the child is in shock, inadequate circulating red blood cells may have such low flow states that the pulse oximeter probe will be unable to sense flow, resulting in an inability to obtain a reading or waveform. Where there is suspected carbon monoxide (CO) poisoning, do not rely on conventional pulse oximetry. Oximetry detects gaseous saturation of the hemoglobin molecule and cannot discriminate between oxygen and CO unless the oximeter is specially designed to also measure CO being carried in the blood, which may be carried by some agencies. A child with CO poisoning may have a pulse oximetry reading of 100% and still be hypoxic.

INDICATIONS

Hypoxia
Need for oxygen therapy
Respiratory distress

Major trauma or other clinical conditions with the potential for hypoxia

EQUIPMENT

Pulse oximeter probes in sizes for newborns, infants, and children

Monitoring cable and pulse oximetry monitoring device

Preparation

1. Prepare the child for application of the pulse oximeter probe. This may be explained as being similar to putting on a band-aid.

CAUTION

Do not rely on pulse oximetry in carbon monoxide poisoning.

Possible Complications

Using incorrect probe placement
Poor perfusion with poor tracing or waveform
Inability to obtain a SpO_2 reading

Causes of Inability to Obtain a Reading or Waveform

Using incorrect probe placement
Poor perfusion with poor tracing or waveform

Procedure 9-1

1. Obtain equipment in the appropriate size. Place probe on a fingertip, toe, earlobe, or wrist, as indicated in the manufacturer's instructions.

2. Connect the probe to the monitoring cable. Some portable monitoring devices have a reusable probe that has a spring-loaded clip for use only on a fingertip or toe. Note oxygen saturation (SpO_2) and document. If the monitoring device being used shows a waveform, observe for correlation with heart rate.

TIP

Use pulse oximetry in the primary assessment of every acutely ill or injured child.

CAUTION

Even when the pulse oximetry is normal, if there is increased work of breathing or significantly increased respiratory rate, the child may need additional therapy.

CAUTION

Pulse oximetry is a very useful tool for measuring oxygen saturation; however, it should not replace a thorough assessment including respiratory rate, auscultation of lung sounds, and palpation of a pulse.

Procedure 10: Orogastric and Nasogastric Tube Insertion

S. Heath Ackley, MD, MPH, FAAP

Keith Widmeier, BA, NRP, FP-C

Introduction

Gastric tube insertion has many purposes, such as emptying the stomach, evaluation and treatment of gastrointestinal hemorrhage, and gastric decompression in cases of bowel obstruction or distention from assisted ventilation or severe respiratory distress. In the prehospital setting, gastric tube insertion is indicated for decompression of the stomach during assisted ventilation or decompression of the stomach when distention impedes adequate ventilation in an infant or child with severe respiratory distress. The tube may be placed into the stomach through the nose (nasogastric [NG] insertion) or through the mouth (orogastric [OG] insertion).

INDICATIONS

Gastric distention that impeded ventilation

Abdominal distention resulting from severe respiratory distress

CONTRAINDICATIONS

NG and OG insertion

Unconscious child with poor or no gag reflex and unsecured airway: In this case, perform endotracheal intubation first to decrease risk of vomiting and aspiration. Alternatively, an extraglottic airway should be placed with a gastric tube inserted in accordance with the manufacturer's recommendation.

Caustic ingestions: In a child who has ingested a caustic substance, there is a risk of esophageal damage with passage of the tube.

NG insertion

Perform OG insertion to avoid intracranial passage of the NG tube when the child has any of the following findings: severe head or facial trauma, especially with midfacial injuries, nasal bleeding, or clear nasal secretions.

Infants with nostrils too small to accommodate the tube: OG insertion is preferred for infants younger than 6 months of age.

EQUIPMENT

Gastric tube

30- to 60-mL syringe with funnel-tipped adaptor for manual removal of stomach contents through tube

Mechanical suction

Adhesive tape

Nonpetroleum lubricant

Rationale

During assisted ventilation or in a child with significant respiratory distress, it is common to inflate the stomach as well as the lungs with air. Gastric inflation with air slows downward movement of the diaphragm and decreases tidal volume, making ventilation more difficult and necessitating higher inspiratory pressures. In the spontaneously breathing child, gastric inflation decreases tidal volume and significantly increases the work of breathing. In addition, inflation of the stomach with air increases the risk that the patient will vomit and aspirate. Gastric tube insertion with an NG or OG tube decompresses the stomach and makes assisted ventilation or spontaneous breathing easier.

Preparation

1. Select the proper size tube. Sizing techniques are outlined in **TABLE P10-1**.
2. Measure the tube on the patient. The length of the tube should be the same as the distance from the lips or tip of the nose (depending on if the route OG or NG is used) to the left ear PLUS the distance from the left ear to the left upper quadrant of the abdomen, just below the costal margin (**FIGURE P10-1**).
3. Mark this length on the tube with a piece of tape. When the tip of the tube is in the stomach, the tape should be at the lips or nostrils.
4. Place the patient in a supine position.
5. Assess the gag reflex. If the patient is unconscious and has a poor or no gag reflex, perform endotracheal intubation before gastric tube insertion.
6. In a trauma patient:
   - Maintain in-line stabilization of the cervical spine if a neck injury is suspected.
   - Choose the orotracheal route if the patient has severe head or facial trauma or has serious midfacial injuries.
7. Lubricate the end of the tube.

Possible Complications

- Placement of the tube into the trachea with hypoxia
- Vomiting and aspiration of stomach contents
- Airway bleeding or obstruction
- Passage of tube into brain when head/facial trauma is present

FIGURE P10-1 Technique for measuring the distance to insert an NG or OG tube.

CONTROVERSY

The value of NG and OG insertion is unproven. Although these procedures are routine in emergency departments, no studies have tested the benefit of easier ventilation against the potential complications of hypoxia from endotracheal intubation or aspiration of stomach contents.

CAUTION

Never use force to pass an NG tube. If the tube is having difficulty passing, consider attempting the other nostril.

CAUTION

Do not perform OG tube insertion on a conscious patient because he or she is at risk for aspiration.

TABLE P10-1 Methods for Determining NG/OG Tube Size

1. Refer to a length-based resuscitation tape or resuscitation software (see Procedure 2).

2. Select a tube size that is the same as the size of the patient's nostril, through which it should pass with minimal resistance.

3. Use a tube size twice the endotracheal (ET) tube size (a child who needs a 5.0-mm ET tube needs a 10.0 French NG or OG tube).

Procedure 10-1

NG Insertion

1. Pass the tube gently through the nostril, directing the tube straight back. Do not angle the tube superiorly.

2. If the tube does not pass easily, try the opposite nostril, or a smaller tube. Never force the tube. If NG passage is unsuccessful, use the OG approach.

Procedure 10-2

OG Insertion

1. Insert the tube over the tongue, using a tongue blade if necessary to help insertion.

2. Advance the tube into the hypopharynx, then insert rapidly into the stomach. If coughing, choking, or change in voice occurs, immediately remove the tube. It may be in the trachea.

Procedure 10-3

Check Placement of NG or OG Tube

1. Check tube placement by aspirating stomach contents. An additional method of checking tube placement is to use a syringe with appropriate adaptor to quickly instill 10–20 mL of air through the tube while auscultating over the left upper quadrant. If there is a rush of air over the stomach region, the placement is correct. If correct placement cannot be verified, remove the tube.

2. Secure the tube to the bridge of the nose or to the cheek, using adhesive tape. Aspirate air from stomach, using a 30- to 60-mL catheter-tipped syringe, or connect to mechanical suction at low, continuous, or intermittent setting.

TIP

Perform OG insertion in infants younger than 6 months of age.

TIP

Talking or crying during the procedure is a good indication that the gastric tube is not in the trachea.

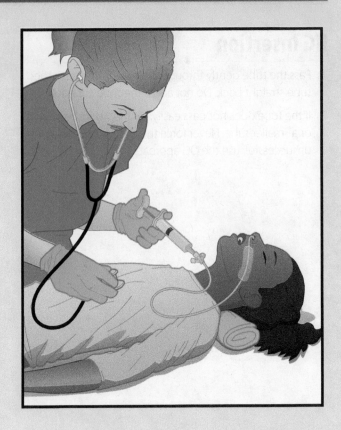

Procedure 11: Endotracheal Intubation

Sylvia Owusu-Ansah, MD, MPH, FAAP

Sam Vance, MHA, LP

Introduction

The airway of a neonate, infant, or child should be managed in the least invasive way possible. Supraglottic devices and endotracheal intubation should only be utilized if bag-mask ventilation fails. Performing the procedure quickly and safely in the field can be difficult. Malposition of the ET tube (ETT) or aspiration can be nearly three times as common in children as compared to adults. Inappropriate or unsuccessful intubation attempts may result in hypoxia, aspiration, oral trauma or injury to the child's airway, worsening of cervical spine injury, or malposition of the ETT (right mainstem intubation, esophageal intubation). This is especially important in children because endotracheal intubation is an infrequently performed skill in this age group and has not been shown to improve outcomes.

There are several anatomic considerations that make the pediatric airway different from the adult airway:

- The child's vocal cords are more anterior and superior.
- The tongue is proportionally larger.
- The mandible and oral cavity are smaller.
- The diameter and length of the trachea are less.
- The soft tissues are more fragile.
- The narrowest area of the airway for children 5 years of age and younger is the cricoid cartilage.
- Airway is more pliable and hyperextension or hyperflexion could cause complete occlusion of the airway
- Epiglottis is larger and omega shaped (U-shaped) and can be more difficult to position upon intubation.
- Anatomy: Larger head and shorter neck are important for positioning of the airway to avoid hyperflexion/extension of neck and to align airway axes.
  - Placement of towel roll under head in patients ≥8 years
  - Placement of towel roll under shoulders in patient <8 years

EQUIPMENT

Length-based resuscitation tape OR a reference material that provides appropriate guidance for equipment sizing based on length/age

Pediatric laryngoscope handle with extra batteries and bulbs

Pediatric laryngoscope blades, curved (sizes 2–4) and straight (sizes 0–4)

Video laryngoscopy (if available)

Endotracheal tubes sizes 2.5–5.5 mm cuffed and/or uncuffed and 6.0–8.0 mm cuffed

10-mL non-Luer Lock syringes

Stylets for endotracheal tubes, pediatric and adult

Bougie for endotracheal tubes, pediatric and adult

Magill forceps, pediatric and adult

End-tidal CO_2 ($EtCO_2$) detection capability, pediatric and adult

Waveform capnography (preferred)

Pulse oximeter with pediatric and adult probes

Rescue airway device such as a supraglottic airway or laryngeal mask airway

Portable and fixed suction apparatus with a regulator, per federal specifications

Wide-bore tubing, rigid pharyngeal curved suction tip; tonsil and flexible suction catheters, 6F–16F

Water-soluble lubricant

Oropharyngeal airways sizes 0–5; infant, child, and adult

Bag-mask device; hand-operated, self-expanding bag; adult (>1,000 mL) and child (450–750 mL) with oxygen reservoir/accumulator; valve; and adult-, child-, infant-, and neonate-size masks

Adhesive tape

Commercial ETT securing devices

Skin adhesive

Oxygen source, capable of metered flow with adequate tubing

Drug-Assisted Intubation (DAI)/ Rapid Sequence Intubation (RSI)

Drug-assisted intubation (formerly known as rapid sequence intubation) is a technique for relaxing a child's muscles and central nervous system in preparation for intubation. The medications available can be divided into neuromuscular blockers (succinylcholine, rocuronium) and analgesics/sedatives/anxiolytics (midazolam, diazepam, fentanyl, ketamine). See **TABLE P11-1.** Local protocols define the medications used. It is important to realize that each drug or combination of drugs have important benefits and risks. Atropine as a premedication to prevent bradycardia can be used in infants (use only if heart rate is <100). The induced muscular paralysis allows the prehospital professional to insert an ETT with no resistance and, hence, improve success and decrease complications. However, it is not appropriate to induce paralysis without the addition of a medication (awake intubation) that provides some degree of sedation and even unconsciousness. One must also realize that the induction of muscular paralysis renders the patient apneic. *Therefore, if DAI/RSI fails, bag-mask ventilation is essential for the child to survive. Medication doses vary with the changing weight of the child. Medication doses are important causes of error.*

Indications

- Failed endotracheal intubation (ETI)
- Severe head trauma requiring hyperventilation

Contraindications

- Abnormal airway anatomy
- Upper airway obstruction
- Laryngeal fracture

Equipment

- ETI equipment
- RSI medications

Preparation

1. Prepare the child for ETI.
2. Double-check suction, oxygen source, oxygen tubing, endotracheal confirmation device, and monitor.
3. Ensure stable IV or IO line (if available).
4. Double-check doses per kilogram on length-based resuscitation tapes (Procedure 2).

TABLE P11-1 Drug-Assisted Intubation Medications

Drug	Type	Dose
Midazolam	Anxiolysis/sedative	0.1 mg/kg IV/IO/IM 0.2 mg/kg Intranasal
Diazepam	Anxiolysis/sedative	0.1 mg/kg IV/IO
Lorazepam	Anxiolysis/sedative	0.1 mg/kg IV/IO/IM
Fentanyl	Analgesia	1 mcg/kg IV/IO 1–2 mcg/kg Intranasal
Ketamine	Analgesic/anesthetic	1–2 mg/kg IV/IO 3–4 mg/kg IM
Succinylcholine	Paralytic/neuromuscular blockade	1–2 mg/kg IV/IO/IM
Rocuronium	Paralytic/neuromuscular blockade	1 mg/kg IV/IO
Atropine (infants)	Anticholinergic	0.02 mg/kg IV/IO Use only if HR <100

IM, intramuscular; IO, intraosseous; IV, intravenous.

Procedure 11-1

RSI/DAI Steps

1. Prepare equipment and medications.
2. Preoxygenate.
3. Premedicate with atropine (as needed).
4. Administer sedation/analgesia/anxiolysis.
5. Administer a neuromuscular blockade.
6. Intubate (can apply cricoid pressure as needed for visualization).
7. Confirm ETT placement (chest rise, breath sounds, end-tidal CO_2).
8. Tape ETT in place (or use commercial device if available).

TIP

The induced muscular paralysis from RSI allows the prehospital professional to insert an ETT with no resistance and, hence, improves success and decreases complications from forced insertion attempts.

CAUTION

If RSI fails, bag-mask ventilation is essential for the child to survive.

TIP

Preferred resuscitation medication delivery is by intraosseous (IO) or intravenous route (IV). Only LEAN (lidocaine, epinephrine, atropine, and naloxone) medications can be given through the ETT route (doses must be increased two to three times for lidocaine, atropine, and naloxone and increased 10 times for epinephrine).

Rationale

Successful ETT placement allows optimal oxygenation and ventilation, provides a tube for medication delivery, and decreases the risk of aspiration and loss of airway control. A properly placed and secured ETT is a good tool for managing critical patients, but the procedure can take a long time, there are frequent and serious complications, and it has not been shown to improve outcomes in children.

Preparation

1. Make sure oxygen delivery equipment is connected to an oxygen source.
2. Select an appropriately sized ETT (**TABLES P11-2** and **P11-3**) for oral endotracheal intubation.
3. For a properly selected uncuffed ETT:
   - Allow a minimal air leak. The absence of an air leak may indicate excessive pressure at the cricoid cartilage.

TABLE P11-2 Suggested Endotracheal Tube and Suction Catheter Sizes

Age	ETT Size (mm) Uncuffed	ETT Size (mm) Cuffed	Suction Catheter Size (French)
Premature newborn	2.0–2.5		5
Newborn to 3 months	3.0		6–8
6 months	3.5	3.0	8
12–18 months	4.0	3.0	8
3 years	4.5	4.0	8
5 years	5.0	4.5	10
6 years	5.5	5.0	10
8 years	6.0	10	10
12 years	6.5	12	12
16 years		7.0–8.0	14

- Tracheal perfusion pressure is between 35 and 40 cm H_2O, such that the cuff pressure should be less than 25 cm H_2O.
4. For a properly selected cuffed ETT: Check cuff for leaks, maintaining aseptic technique, as follows:
   - Inflate cuff with appropriate volume of air.
   - Remove syringe.
   - Feel cuff for integrity.
   - Deflate cuff before insertion.
5. Attach blade to laryngoscope handle, and make sure the bulb is secure and works.
6. Test the large-bore rigid suction catheter.
7. Insert stylet into the ETT, stopping the stylet at least 1 cm from the end of the ETT.
8. Bend the ETT into a gentle upward curve. In some cases, bend the tube into the shape of a hockey stick.
9. Lubricate tube with a water-soluble lubricant (optional).
10. Prepare device for confirmation of ETT placement.
11. To predict correct ETT tube position at gum line, either:
    - Check resuscitation tape, or refer to computer software
    - Calculate ETT position with formula: gum line position (in cm) = ~3 × tube size
12. Have partner prepare for:
    - Ongoing patient assessment
    - Providing time counts for ventilation rates
    - Watching monitors (heart rate, pulse oximetry)
    - Handling suction devices
    - Handling ETT
    - Applying gentle cricoid pressure, as necessary.
    - Stabilizing neck, if child has possible spinal trauma
13. Position patient (avoid hyperextension or hyperflexion of neck).
    - Medical patient: Place the child in the "sniffing" position.
    - If spinal trauma is a possibility, place the child in neutral position with in-line manual cervical spine stabilization.

TIP

Make sure proper equipment is available and functioning before intubation attempt.

CONTROVERSY

The value of performing endotracheal intubation in children in the prehospital setting is controversial. The airway of a neonate, infant, or child should be managed in the least-invasive way possible. Supraglottic devices and endotracheal intubation should only be utilized if bag-mask ventilation fails. Performing the procedure quickly and safely in the field can be difficult. Malposition of the ETT or aspiration can be nearly three times as common in children as compared to adults. Inappropriate or unsuccessful intubation attempts may result in hypoxia, aspiration, oral trauma or injury to the child's airway, worsening of cervical spine injury, malposition of the ETT (right mainstem intubation, esophageal intubation). This is especially important in children because endotracheal intubation is an infrequently performed skill in this age group and has not been shown to improve outcomes.

TABLE P11-3 Selecting Endotracheal Tube Size

Uncuffed	Cuffed

Length-based resuscitation tapes are more accurate than age-based formula estimates of ETT size for children up to 35 kg.
Newborns and infants
    Preterm infants: 2.0- or 2.5-mm tube
Term newborns or small infants: 3.0- or 3.5-mm tube
Infants 6–12 months: 3.5-mm tube
Infants 12–18 months: 4.0-mm tube
Children >1 year:
OR
The diameter of the tracheal tube is approximately the same size as the width of the child's fingernail on the fifth finger.
For a child ≥2 years old: size = (age in years/4) + 4
	Length-based resuscitation tapes are more accurate than age-based formula estimates of ETT size for children up to 35 kg.
	It is appropriate to approximate:
	    3.0 or 3.5 ETT for a child younger than 1 year old
	    3.5 or 4.0 ETT for a child 1–2 years old
	    For a child 2–10 years old (age in years/4) + 3.5
	Or calculate uncuffed tube size and use a tube 0.5 mm smaller

Procedure 11-2

Insert Endotracheal Tube

1. Oxygenate and ventilate patient for 1 to 2 minutes with bag-mask device and 100% oxygen, at a rate of one ventilation every 3-5 seconds. Say "squeeze, release, release" to reinforce proper rate.

2. Grasp laryngoscope in left hand. Stop ventilating and begin timing, giving 20- to 30-second counts.

3. Open mouth by applying thumb pressure on chin; check mouth for foreign bodies or loose teeth; remove oropharyngeal airway if present.

4. There is insufficient evidence to recommend routine cricoid pressure application to prevent aspiration during endotracheal intubation in children.

5. Hold laryngoscope in trigger finger position.

6. Insert laryngoscope blade into the right side of the mouth.

7. Lift tongue with blade and sweep to the left.

8. Exert gentle traction upward along the axis of laryngoscope handle at a 45-degree angle. Do not use teeth or gums to gain leverage.

9. Advance blade straight along tongue. Continue looking at blade tip, until tip is just beyond epiglottis. Do not take your eyes off of the vocal cords once visualized. Your partner should be handing the ETT to you while you are maintaining visualization.

10. If there is difficulty seeing the vocal cords, have partner apply cricoid pressure. If there is difficulty seeing the vocal cords, consider the following: (1) advance or retract laryngoscope blade; (2) remove vomitus, blood, other fluids, or particulate matter with rigid, large-bore suction device; (3) have assistant apply backward-upward-rightward pressure (BURP) to the larynx; or (4) reposition the head or degree of extension.

11. Continue to look at vocal cords and suction.

12. Remove large solid matter with pediatric Magill forceps, if necessary.

13. Insert ETT. Hold tube in dart-like fashion with right hand and insert tip of tube from right corner of mouth down between vocal cords. Do not insert tube in channel of laryngoscope blade because this blocks the view of the vocal cords. Watch the ETT go through the vocal cords. Advance tube until vocal cord marker on ETT is situated beyond the vocal cords with an un-cuffed tube. Advance a cuffed tube until the balloon passes through the vocal cords. Look for centimeter marking on ETT in relation to the gum line.

14. Remove laryngoscope blade, holding ETT in place.
15. Remove stylet from ETT.

16. If using an ETT with a cuffed end, inflate cuff with pilot balloon. Maintain tube position by holding ETT against upper lip. If large amount of fluid is evident in ETT, use a suction catheter to clear the airway. Have partner maintain ETT position and ventilate patient with bag-mask device.

17. Confirm ETT correct placement using waveform capnography, bilataral breath sounds, and absent gastric sounds.

18. Assess correct position in trachea. Do general patient evaluation (appearance, heart rate, pulse oximetry). Look for bilateral chest rise. Make sure there are no bubbling or gurgling sounds in epigastric area indicating air-water interface (check for two breaths). Auscultate for bilateral lung sounds at the midaxillary line, third intercostal space (check for two breaths on right and then two breaths on left). Use device to confirm endotracheal positioning. If breath sounds are heard only on one side (usually the right), pull back ETT slightly until breath sounds are heard on both sides.

19. Record tube position on permanent record. Use centimeter mark at teeth or gum line or mark on ETT with indelible pen and monitor frequently for tube movement/displacement.

20. Secure tube with tape or commercially available ETT securing device. Reassess proper location of tube, and make sure the patient is stable.

21. Cervical collar and/or cervical immobilization device may help reduce neck movement and risk of tube displacement.

22. Ventilate with minimal volume to see chest rise, approximately 6–7 mL/kg ideal body weight. Overinflation may be detrimental.

23. Adult: 10–12 breaths/minute; older children: 20 breaths/minute; infants and young children: 30 breaths/minute.

24. Continuously monitor $EtCO_2$ to maintain $EtCO_2$ of 35–40 mm Hg.

25. Consider sedation with sedative or opioid medications if agitated.

26. Gastric decompression may improve oxygenation and ventilation, so it should be considered when there is obvious gastric distention.

27. Transport to the closest appropriate hospital for airway stabilization when respiratory failure cannot be successfully managed.

Indications for Tube Removal

Immediate Tube Removal

- No chest rise with ventilation
- Presence of epigastric gurgling sounds
- Failure to confirm endotracheal placement with detection device

CAUTION

Beware of inadequate spinal stabilization during intubation attempts in trauma patients.

CAUTION

Never assume the ETT is in the trachea unless you see the tube passing through the vocal cords.

CAUTION

Providers who do not routinely use medications for RSI should not use RSI on children and should be reserved for providers with a comprehensive program with ongoing training and quality assurance measures.

CAUTION

Use continuous waveform capnography to detect $EtCO_2$, as this is the standard to confirm supraglottic airway and endotracheal tube placement.

CAUTION

In addition to preoxygenation, apneic oxygenation (high-flow O_2 by nasal cannula) may prolong the period before hypoxia during an intubation attempt.

CAUTION

Misting in the tube is not a reliable method of tube placement confirmation.

CAUTION

Video laryngoscopy may enhance intubation success rates and should be used when available.

CAUTION

Because pediatric intubation is an infrequently used skill for many prehospital providers, ongoing education and hands-on practice are essential.

CAUTION

Acute worsening of respiratory status or evidence of hypoxemia can be secondary to displacement or obstruction of the airway device, pneumothorax, or equipment failure.

Procedure 11-3

Secure Endotracheal Tube

1. Continuously secure tube manually until secured with tape, twill, or a commercial tube holder.

Always reassess tube location after patient movement or when there is a change in patient status.

Procedure 11-4

Reconfirm Endotracheal Tube Placement

1. Recheck to make sure there is no bubbling or gurgling noise in epigastric area (air-water interface) for two breaths.

2. Reassess breath sounds bilaterally at the midaxillary line, third intercostal space (two breaths on right and then two breaths on left). Take extra care handling an ETT in a pediatric patient because it can be easily dislodged. Reassess after patient is in ambulance (and after change of position or change in patient status). Report and record findings.

CAUTION

Ongoing assessment is critical when an airway device is in place.

Possible Complications

- Aspiration of stomach contents
- Dislodgment of ETT from trachea
- Esophageal intubation
- Tracheal tube malposition
- Hypoxemia
- Tube obstruction
- Barotrauma
- Adverse events from medications
- Hypoxia
- Increased intracranial pressure
- Laryngeal, tracheal, pharyngeal, or esophageal injury
- Teeth and mouth injury
- Vocal cord injury

Procedure 11-5

Extubation

1. Postresuscitation extubation is rarely indicated in the field. All three situations must be present: (1) spontaneous breathing with adequate rate and tidal volume, (2) conscious patient, and (3) coughing and gagging causing inability to maintain oxygenation and ventilation. Ensure rigid large-bore suction device is functioning.

2. Suction oropharynx.

3. Turn patient on left side.

4. Deflate cuff completely (if cuff is inflated).

5. Remove ETT quickly at end-inspiratory phase, while suctioning.

SUGGESTED REFERENCES

Articles

American Academy of Pediatrics, American College of Emergency Physicians, American College of Surgeons Committee on Trauma, Emergency Medical Services for Children, Emergency Nurses Association, National Association of EMS Physicians,

National Association of State EMS Officials. Joint policy statement – equipment for ground ambulances. *Prehosp Emerg Care.* 2014;18(1):92–97. doi:10.3109/10903127.2013.851312.

Other Resources

DeCaen, AR, Macononochie IK, Aickin R, et al. *Pediatric Advanced Life Support.* Part 12 American Heart Association Guidelines Update for Cardiopulmonary Resuscitation and Emergency Cardiovascular Care. *Circulation.* 2015;(18Suppl2) 3 November 2015, pp. S521–S542.

National Association of State EMS Officials. *National Model EMS Clinical Guidelines Version 2.2.* NASEMSO; 2019. https://nasemso.org/projects/model-ems-clinical-guidelines/. Accessed September 18, 2019.

Procedure 12: Confirmation of Endotracheal Intubation and End-Tidal Capnography

S. Heath Ackley, MD, MPH, FAAP

Keith Widmeier, BA, NRP, FP-C

Introduction

Performing pediatric endotracheal intubation in the prehospital setting may be difficult or impossible even for experienced prehospital professionals. Confirming position of the endotracheal tube (ETT) in the trachea is a major challenge because esophageal intubation is a common and potentially lethal complication of endotracheal intubation. Intubation is often not necessary in the field if there is effective bag-mask ventilation with appropriate chest rise. Furthermore, portable quantitative capnography, as well as continuous waveform capnography, do not require intubation and may be used in line with bag-mask ventilation as long as there is a good mask seal on the patient's face. Currently there are several methods to confirm placement of the ETT:

1. Waveform capnography (gold standard)
2. Use of exhaled carbon dioxide detection device
3. Use of digital capnometry (quantitative end-tidal CO_2)
4. Clinical assessment

INDICATIONS

Endotracheal intubation
Insertion of a supraglottic device

Ventilations with a bag-mask device

CONTRAINDICATION

An adult carbon dioxide detector cannot be left in place in a child weighing less than 15 kg.

EQUIPMENT

Stethoscope
Colorimetric end-tidal carbon dioxide detector device, or quantitative end-tidal CO_2 capnometry

End-tidal CO_2 ($EtCO_2$) waveform capnography

Rationale

Properly positioned ETTs and supraglottic devices make it possible to effectively oxygenate and ventilate children with critical illnesses or injuries. Esophageal placement of an ETT, however, is usually harmful or lethal. Moreover, if the child is moved, a correctly placed ETT may easily dislodge from the trachea to the oropharynx or esophagus. Delayed detection may result in hypoxia. Clinical assessment of placement of the ETT can be inaccurate, especially in infants and small children. Often, there is a lot of noise in the surrounding area (family members or traffic) that may make it difficult to hear breath sounds. Also, breath sounds may be transmitted from the esophagus or stomach throughout the chest of a child and mislead the listener. Fortunately, several mechanical adjuncts are available to supplement clinical assessment, help confirm correct ETT placement in the trachea, and help the emergency medical services (EMS) provider continuously monitor correct airway placement.

Preparation

1. Determine the weight of the patient.
2. Intubate the infant or child with a correctly sized ETT (see Procedure 11, Endotracheal Intubation) or insert the correctly sized supraglottic device (see Procedure 13, Advanced Airway Techniques).
3. Suction any fluid from the ETT.

End-Tidal CO_2 (EtCO$_2$) Waveform Capnography

1. Connect device to end of endotracheal tube.
2. Observe for a waveform and a numerical value.
3. A flat waveform or value of 0 means the ETT is in the esophagus.

Colorimetric Exhaled Carbon Dioxide Detector

1. Determine correct size of the carbon dioxide detector.
   - Use a pediatric device if the child weighs less than 15 kg.

- Use an adult device if the child weighs 15 kg or more.
- If an adult device is used on a small child, remove after six breaths (initial confirmation of placement).

2. Check the expiration date on the carbon dioxide detector package.
3. Remove the carbon dioxide detector from its packaging.
4. Inspect the carbon dioxide detector before use for bright purple color and dryness.

Digital Capnometry

1. Place sensor as indicated by manufacturer.
2. Attach sensor probe to monitoring cable.
3. Observe for the presence of a numerical value that indicates correct ETT placement.
4. Absence of a numerical value indicates improperly placed ETT.

Procedure 12-1

Clinical Assessment

1. Look for bilateral rise and fall of the chest. Listen for breath sounds over the stomach. If gurgling is present (like a straw in milk), the ETT is in the esophagus. If there is an absence of an EtCO$_2$ waveform or numerical value, desaturations, or bradycardia, remove the ETT. However, if you do not hear breath sounds and the patient is hemodynamically stable (blood pressure, heart rate, and oxygen saturation are adequate), then provide six breaths and monitor for color change.

2. Listen for breath sounds in the right midaxillary line, then in the left midaxillary line. If breath sounds are equal, secure the tube. If breath sounds are greater on the right side than on the left side, then the tube may be in the right mainstem bronchus. Slowly pull back the ETT until breath sounds are equal.

CAUTION

Do not remove the ETT just because breath sounds are heard in the stomach. They may be transmitted sounds from the lungs. If the patient has continued desaturations or bradycardia, perform a direct laryngoscopy to ensure the ETT is through the vocal cords. If it is not, or you are unsure, and the patient has continued desaturations despite giving effective breaths with positive end-expiratory pressure (PEEP), then remove the ETT and deliver oxygen with bag-mask ventilation.

Procedure 12-2

End-Tidal CO$_2$ (EtCO$_2$) Waveform Capnography

Waveform capnography is the best diagnostic study to determine EtCO$_2$, as it gives both a waveform and number. This may be used as a standalone device or it may be built into a cardiac monitor used by EMS. The capnograph is the waveform that shows how much CO$_2$ is present at each phase of the respiratory cycle, and it normally has a rectangular shape. Capnography also measures and displays respiratory rate. In patients who require assisted ventilation, another adapter can be attached to a bag-mask device and used with an advanced airway device or a mask.

The number is capnometry, which is the partial pressure of CO$_2$ detected at the end of exhalation. This is EtCO$_2$, which is normally 35–45 mm Hg.

Capnography, the shape (amplitude and width) of the waveform, can provide clues about respiratory effort and causes of respiratory distress and gives real time feedback on how management is working (**FIGURE P12-1**). For example, a shark fin waveform can indicate constriction (**FIGURE P12-2**). Capnography can also detect shock and

FIGURE P12-1 Capnography monitor.

- A-B (Phase I) Respiratory baseline
- B-C (Phase II) Expiratory upstroke
- C-D (Phase III) Expiratory alveolar plateau
- D-E (Phase IV) Inspiration down stroke

A

B

FIGURE P12-2 A. A normal waveform. **B.** A shark fin waveform can indicate constriction.

assist with determining the effectiveness of cardiopulmonary resuscitation (CPR) **(FIGURE P12-3)**.

Once the waveform capnography is connected, it is important that a waveform and number are observed on the monitor. A flat wave indicates that the ETT is not in the airway and is likely in the esophagus. If there is an initial waveform that then flattens, this is an indication that the ETT has become misplaced.

FIGURE P12-3 Capnography can also with determining the effectiveness of CPR.

the lungs. If the format has continued as this is an initial through the vocal cords. If it is not or vocal tissue, are the patient has initially easily positive and expiratory pressure (PEEP) then delivers the ETT and deliver oxygen with bag-mask ventilation.

TIP

Continuous $EtCO_2$ monitoring will show real-time changes within seconds.

Procedure 12-3

Colorimetric Carbon Dioxide Detector Device

1. Attach the device to the end of the ETT, and attach the other end to the bag-mask device.

2. Begin ventilation.

3. Observe the carbon dioxide detector for color change during exhalation. Read only after a total of six breaths. Check the color and act accordingly **(TABLE P12-1)**. Regardless of whether the ETT is in the trachea, the carbon dioxide detector will change to a purple color when 100% oxygen is squeezed through the bag device and ETT into the lungs. The color on exhalation is the one to pay attention to because a yellow color in the expiratory phase of breathing reflects carbon dioxide production. However, do not leave an adult carbon dioxide detector in place after initial confirmation of tube position on a patient weighing less than 15 kg, because the adult device has too much dead space and an infant can rebreathe carbon dioxide if it is left in line. Document observations and interventions.

TABLE P12-1 Use of Colorimetric Exhaled Carbon Dioxide Detector in ETT Placement

Color	Patient With Pulse	Patient Without Pulse
Yellow	Yes—tube correctly placed Leave tube in place and secure it	Yes—tube correctly placed Leave tube in place and secure it
Tan	Think about it Ventilate six more times (while reassessing tube placement)	Think about it Ventilate six more times (while reassessing tube placement)
	Reassess detector for color change. If still tan, leave tube in place and secure it	Reassess detector for color change. If still tan, leave tube in place and secure it
	Attempt to correct any possible cause of low perfusion or low carbon dioxide	Attempt to correct cause of low perfusion or low carbon dioxide
Purple	Problem—tube incorrectly placed or the child is in cardiac arrest and is not producing measurable amounts of carbon dioxide or delivering it to the lungs. Extubate Ventilate with bag-mask device Reintubate	Problem—tube may be incorrectly placed, or the child is dead and not producing measurable amounts of carbon dioxide

		Look at vocal cords with laryngoscope
		If tube is incorrectly placed:
		    Extubate
		    Ventilate with bag-mask device
		    Reintubate
		
		If tube is between vocal cords, and vocal cord marker is below vocal cords:
		    Leave tube in place
		    Check adequacy of CPR
		    Proceed with ALS protocol

ALS, advanced life support; CPR, cardiopulmonary resuscitation.

TIP

Remove the carbon dioxide detector from the ETT if endotracheal drugs are given, because a wet detector may not show a correct color change from purple to yellow.

TIP

If the child is in cardiac arrest and not receiving chest compressions, no color change will occur, even if placement is correct, because there is no carbon dioxide being delivered to the lungs.

TIP

If the child weighs less than 15 kg, use a pediatric colorimetric exhaled carbon dioxide detector.

Procedure 12-4

Quantitative End-Tidal CO₂ (EtCO₂) Capnometry

1. If quantitative EtCO₂ capnometry is used, a number should register quickly. Accuracy of the EtCO₂ number relies on a good mask seal if the patient is not intubated OR minimal leak if an ETT or supraglottic device is in correct airway position.

2. Remember that the number will be low in cardiac arrest and will hopefully improve with high-quality CPR and return of spontaneous circulation (ROSC).

3. Use waveform capnography tracing for quantitative assessment.

A

B

TIP

If there is a lot of pulmonary edema or pulmonary hemorrhage, an EtCO₂ value may not register.

TIP

Pulse oximetry requires a pulse and will not register with a cardiac arrest and may be difficult to pick up with delayed capillary refill as may be seen with shock.

TIP

If the child is pulseless and no chest compressions are being performed, there will be a very low (or zero) number on quantitative assessment. Assess quality of CPR (depth, rate, recoil).

Procedure 13: Advanced Airway Techniques

J. Joelle Donofrio-Odmann, DO, FAAP, FACEP, FAEMS

Introduction

Rarely, standard bag-mask ventilation fails, and endotracheal intubation (ETI) is difficult or impossible. Examples of such patients are children with massive head trauma and airway edema or hematomas of the mouth or upper airway, children with multisystem injuries and long transport times, or infants with significant congenital or acquired airway abnormalities that cannot be ventilated. In such dire circumstances, some emergency medical services (EMS) systems allow prehospital professionals to perform advanced airway techniques. These include use of the supraglottic airways (e.g., laryngeal mask airway [LMA], i-gel) or laryngeal tubes (e.g., King Airway, Combitube), the gum elastic bougie, and drug-assisted intubation (DAI). Needle cricothyrotomy is another option and is explained in detail in this procedure. None of these techniques has been well evaluated in children in the prehospital setting, and each procedure has important benefits, limitations, and contraindications.

Characteristics of children that are red flags for possible problems managing the airway include the following history or physical findings:

History:

1. Past history of difficult intubation or problems with ventilation
2. Children with congenital anomalies affecting facial bones and oropharyngeal structures including the tongue, such as Down syndrome and Pierre Robin sequence
3. History of recurrent stridor or upper airway obstruction

Physical Findings:

1. Unable to open the mouth widely
2. Difficulty in fully extending the neck
3. Presence of a large tongue or dysmorphic facial features
4. Inability to visualize the entire uvula when depressing the tongue with a tongue blade
5. Trauma to the face, mouth, tongue, or neck

A good mnemonic for predicting a difficult airway is LEMON.

- L: LOOK externally for signs of difficult airway, such as trauma and large tongue.
- E: EVALUATE the 3-3-2 rule using the size of the patient's finger. The mouth should open at least 3 fingerbreadths, the hyoid/mental distance should be at least 3 fingerbreadths, and the thyroid to mouth at least 2 fingerbreadths.
- M: MALLAMPATI. The Mallampati score should be at least 3 (**FIGURE P13-1**).
- O: OBSTRUCTION. Look for conditions that may cause an obstructed airway such as tumors, hemangiomas, and/or trauma.
- N: NECK MOBILITY. Ability to position the head and neck.

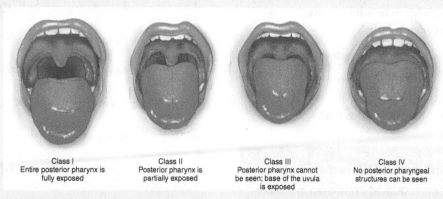

Class I	Class II	Class III	Class IV
Entire posterior pharynx is fully exposed	Posterior pharynx is partially exposed	Posterior pharynx cannot be seen; base of the uvula is exposed	No posterior pharyngeal structures can be seen

FIGURE P13-1 The Mallampati classifications.

Supraglottic Airway Device

Laryngeal Mask Airway (LMA)

The LMA is a device used frequently in emergency departments (EDs) and hospitals to ventilate children. It consists of a tube with a distal inflatable mask that is inserted into the mouth. When the mask is inflated, air goes into the trachea. A self-inflating bag can then be connected to the tube to provide rescue breathing. There are multiple types of LMAs available in the pediatric population, some with the option to deflate gastric secretions and/or intubate through the LMA. The LMA has classically been the alternative airway of choice for in-hospital pediatric difficult airway algorithms. There is little prehospital experience with LMAs, and the few reported trials are in adults. Hence, the safety and efficacy of this procedure in children in the prehospital setting are unknown. However, the procedure is simple and fast, the success rates in hospitals are excellent, and the risks are small. Some EMS systems have introduced the LMA for pediatric rescue breathing, and it may be an easier rescue technique than ETI in children who cannot be effectively ventilated by a bag-mask device. This technique requires special equipment and special training. Also, the epiglottis may flip over and interfere with good positioning of the LMA device.

INDICATIONS

A child who requires ventilation
Difficult or failed bag-mask ventilation

Failed ETI attempt

CONTRAINDICATIONS

Severe upper airway obstruction
An awake patient with intact airway reflexes
Patients requiring very high pressures to ventilate (asthma, bronchiolitis)

A relative contraindication is a full stomach, because the LMA does not fully protect against aspiration

EQUIPMENT

LMAs have eight sizes: 1, 1.5, 2, 2.5, 3, 4, 5, and 6
Water-soluble lubricant
Syringe
Oxygen source

Suction
Ventilation bag
Monitors (pulse oximeter, capnography)

Preparation

1. Select the LMA size for the patient (see **TABLE P13-1** for sizing).
2. Select an appropriate resuscitator bag; although a small child can be safely and effectively ventilated using an adult bag, a pediatric bag will not work for a large child. Pediatric tidal volume is approximately 6–8 mL/kg. The bag should have a volume of 450–750 mL. An adult bag (1,200 mL) is acceptable for larger children or adolescents.
3. Connect the oxygen tubing.

TIP

The LMA is a fast and simple device and is widely used for children in the ED and hospital.

CONTROVERSY

The LMA has not been studied in children in the prehospital setting, and risks and benefits are unknown.

4. Once inserted, connect the bag device to the end of the LMA.

TABLE P13-1 LMA Size/Cuff Volume by Weight

LMA Size	Cuff Volume	Weight of Patient
1	4 mL	<5 kg
1.5	7 mL	5–10 kg
2	10 mL	10–20 kg
2.5	14 mL	20–30 kg
3	20 mL	30–50 kg
4	30 mL	50–70 kg
5	40 mL	>70 kg
6	50 mL	>100 kg

Procedure 13-1

LMA Insertion Methods—Classic

1. Deflate the cuff of the mask.

2. Hold the LMA like a pen, with the index finger of the dominant hand at the junction of the mask and the tube.

3. Slide the LMA along the hard palate, pushing it back against the palate as it is advanced toward the hypopharynx. This prevents the tip from folding over on itself and reduces interference from the tongue.

4. Advance with gentle pressure until resistance is met.

5. If necessary, continue pressure on the tube with the nondominant hand to fully advance the LMA to its proper position.

6. Once in place, loosen grip. Then, inflate the cuff, allowing it to acquire its natural position.

7. Attach to bag device.

Procedure 13-2

LMA Insertion Methods—180-Degree Rotation

1. Invert the deflated mask "inside-out."

2. Insert the LMA into the mouth in a 180-degree rotated position, with the mask's orifice facing the palate.

3. Push the LMA toward the hypopharynx until it enters the pharynx (detected by a sudden loss of resistance). In contrast to the classic method, do not use the index finger as a guide.

4. Turn the LMA 180 degrees back to its normal position.

5. Inflate the cuff. Apply a water-soluble lubricant to the posterior surface. Rub the lubricant over the anterior hard palate.

6. Attach to bag device.

i-gel Supraglottic Airway

The i-gel is a supraglottic airway device with a soft, gel-like, noninflatable cuff that is designed to fit over the laryngeal inlet. This device is unique, as no cuff inflation is required. As with other supraglottic airways, it can be used with positive-pressure ventilation and spontaneously breathing patients. Also, as with all supraglottic airways, the i-gel may not fully protect from regurgitation and aspiration.

The i-gel was designed for ease and speed of insertion, reduced trauma, gastric access, bite block, superior seal pressure, and noninflatable cuff.

CAUTION

Do not allow peak airway pressures during ventilation to exceed 40 cm H_2O.

INDICATIONS

- Failed ETI attempt
- Failed bag-mask ventilation

CONTRAINDICATIONS

- Responsive patients with an intact gag reflex
- Patients with known esophageal disease
- Patients who have ingested caustic substances
- Trismus; limited mouth opening; pharyngoperilaryngeal abscess, trauma, or mass

PREPARATION

1. Choose correct size based on patient's height (see **TABLE P13-2** for sizing).
2. Inspect packaging to ensure no damage.
3. Apply water-soluble lubricant to integral bite block, back, sides, and front of device.
4. Inspect the device to ensure airway is patent and there are no foreign bodies or lubricant obstructing the opening of the airway or gastric port.
5. Check that the 15-mm connector fits the patient connection.
6. Place the patient in the sniffing position.

TABLE P13-2 i-gel Sizing and Information

i-gel	Neonate	Infant	Small Pediatric	Large Pediatric	Small Adult	Regular Adult	Large Adult
Size	1	1.5	2	2.5	3	4	5
Connector color	Pink	Blue	Gray	Clear	Yellow	Green	Orange
Recommended patient weight	2–5 kg	5–12 kg	10–25 kg	25–35 kg	30–60 kg	60–90 kg	90+ kg

Source: https://www.intersurgical.com/info/igel

Procedure 13-3

i-gel Insertion

1. Grasp the lubricated i-gel firmly at the integral bite block, and position the device so the i-gel cuff outlet is facing toward the chin (soft gel toward the tongue with hard tip toward roof of mouth).

2. With patient in sniffing position and with head extended, open mouth by pressing chin down.

3. Introduce leading top into the mouth toward the hard palate.

4. Glide the device down and back along the hard palate with gentle continuous push until resistance is felt.

Sometimes a feel of "give-way" is felt before the end resistance is met due to the passage of the bowl of the i-gel through the faucial pillars (pharyngo-epiglottic folds).

5. Hold the i-gel in correct position while device is being secured.

Instead of the chin-lift method, a laryngoscope or tongue depressor can be used to lift the tongue anteriorly to allow easy advancement of the tube.

Laryngeal Tubes

King Airway

This device can be used with positive-pressure ventilations as well as in spontaneously breathing patients. It is designed for esophageal intubation. It differs from an LMA in that it has two areas that inflate: the proximal cuff inflates near the base of the tongue and separates the laryngopharynx from the oropharynx and nasopharynx, and the distal cuff inflates in the esophagus, which prevents insufflation of the stomach. A single valve inflates both the proximal and distal cuffs. There are two main ventilation outlets on the anterior

A King Airway may not fully protect from regurgitation and aspiration.

surface and three small bilateral "eyes" for additional ventilation on the sides of the tube.

Failed ETI attempt
Difficult or failed bag-mask ventilation

Responsive patients with an intact gag reflex
Patients with known esophageal disease
Patients who have ingested caustic substances

Preparation

1. Choose correct size based on patient's height (see **TABLE P13-3** for sizing).
2. Test cuff inflation system for air leak.
3. Apply water-soluble lubricant to distal tip.

TABLE P13-3 King LT-D Sizing and Information

King LT-D Size	0	1	2	2.5	3	4	5
Connector color	Transparent	White	Green	Orange	Yellow	Red	Purple
Recommended patient height (weight)	(< 5 kg)	(5–12 kg)	35–45 inches (12–25 kg)	41–51 inches (25–35 kg)	4–5 feet	5–6 feet	>6 feet
Cuff volume	10 mL	20 mL	25–35 mL	30–45 mL	40–60 mL	50–70 mL	60–90 mL

Source: http://www.scdhec.gov/health/ems/ResourcesKingLT.pdf

Procedure 13-4

King Airway Insertion

1. Deflate the cuffs, and apply water-soluble lubricant to distal tip.

2. Hold the King Airway with your dominant hand. With the nondominant hand, hold the mouth open and apply chin lift.

3. Using lateral approach, insert the King Airway into the mouth, at a 45–90-degree angle.

4. Advance the tube behind the base of the tongue while rotating the tube back to midline so that the blue orientation line faces the chin of the patient.

5. Without excessive force, advance the tube so that the base of the connector is aligned with the teeth or gums.

9. If necessary, adjust cuff inflation to obtain a seal for the airway at the peak ventilation pressure used.

6. Inflate cuffs with appropriate volumes (see Table P13-3).

7. Attach the bag to the connector.

8. While bagging the patient, gently withdraw the tube until ventilation becomes easy.

TIP

Instead of the chin-lift method, a laryngoscope or tongue depressor can be used to lift the tongue anteriorly to allow easy advancement of the tube.

TIP

Insertion can also be accomplished midline by applying a chin lift and sliding the distal tip along the palate and into position in the proximal esophagus. Head extension may also be helpful. .

CONTROVERSY

Initially placing the tube deeper, inflating the cuffs, and then retracting until ventilation becomes easy and free flowing is preferred, because a shallow insertion requires deflation of the cuffs to insert the tube deeper.

Gum Elastic Bougie

Sometimes it is difficult to visualize the vocal cords for ETI. There are many reasons for failure to see the anatomy, especially if the child has increased muscle tone. The gum elastic bougie or endotracheal tube (ETT) introducer is a long, flexible stylet that facilitates insertion of an ETT. There are several versions of this device that are available and may prove useful in facilitating intubation. The classic bougie has a 5-mm diameter and is for use with endotracheal tubes larger than 5.0. If the child is old enough, usually >8 years, the trachea will have formed cartilaginous rings that allows the operator to feel the gum elastic bougie in the correct location. The semi-rigid tube or rod can be angled to pass into the trachea and, as the device brushes against the tracheal rings, the rod can be palpated to be in position. Once in place, the device serves as a guide for placement of the ETT. For endotracheal tubes 5.0 and smaller, there is a 10 French (3.3-mm) version that allows use down to a 3.5 tube. The pediatric version does not have the 38-degree distal bend. Airway injury is a risk. Recent literature has shown improved first-pass success with intubation in the ED with bougies.

An adjunct for the difficult airway when direct visualization of the vocal cords is impossible because of secretions or blood obstructing the view

Major facial trauma
Laryngeal fracture
Severe upper airway obstruction
Endotracheal tube is too small to pass over the bougie

Gum elastic bougie device in pediatric and adult sizes
All equipment described under ETI

Preparation

1. Prepare the child for ETI (see Procedure 11).
2. Ensure the gum elastic bougie points upward in a J-shape configuration.

A gum elastic bougie is particularly helpful when a very anteriorly placed larynx makes visualization of the cords difficult.

Procedure 13-5

Gum Elastic Bougie Device

1. Place the lubricated ETT over the straight end of the gum elastic bougie.

2. Visualize the cords with laryngoscopy.

3. Insert the J-shaped end of the gum elastic bougie through the cords, advancing the device until clicks are palpated indicating the presence of tracheal rings (if the child is >8 years old).

4. Slide the ETT over the gum elastic bougie into the trachea.

5. Remove the laryngoscope, then the gum elastic bougie.

6. Ensure the ETT is in the trachea by end-tidal CO_2 detection or an esophageal detector device and that the tube has a correct position at the lips.

7. Attach to the bag-mask device.

8. Secure the ETT.

Procedure 14: Intramuscular Injections

Claudia L. Phillips, MSN-Ed, RN, CEN, CPEN

Michael H. Stroud, MD, FAAP

Introduction

The intramuscular (IM) route is acceptable for giving several important medications to children. These medications include epinephrine and morphine sulfate. The IM route has limitations, but when inhalation, intravenous (IV), or intraosseous (IO) delivery of medication is not possible, IM administration may be lifesaving.

INDICATION

Administration of medications when vascular access or other routes are not possible or practical

CONTRAINDICATIONS

Poor perfusion

Availability and practicality of alternative effective routes: oral, inhalation, IV, intranasal, or IO

EQUIPMENT

Tuberculin or 3-mL syringe, 22- or 25-gauge needle (⅝- to 1½-inch for IM injection)

Rationale

IM administration allows the medication to absorb slowly but steadily. The effects of IM medications may take 10–20 minutes. The advantages of the IM technique are easy delivery and high safety. The disadvantages are poor patient acceptance and delayed effect. Avoid IM medications in patients with low perfusion because absorption is unpredictable. Sometimes, in situations involving a child with low venous pressures, such as in anaphylaxis, IM is an excellent first choice for delivery while vascular access is attempted.

The IM route may result in nerve damage, particularly if the injection is in the buttocks of an infant or small child.

Preparation

1. Prepare the child to help decrease stress and anxiety. Explain the procedure using developmentally appropriate terminology. Avoid using the word "shot" or "stick" because the child may associate this with being shot by a gun or being hurt with a stick. Be honest and tell the child it will hurt but be over as quickly as possible. Describe the needle stick as a pinch or a bee sting.
2. Select the medication. Confirm any medication allergies the child may have.
3. Select the appropriate syringe and needle. Keep needles out of the child's sight.
   Needle Length for IM Injection
   - For the ventrogluteal or dorsogluteal sites, use a needle slightly longer than one-half of the distance between the thumb and finger when the skin at the injection site is grasped.
   - For the deltoid and vastus lateralis sites, use a 1-inch needle if the skin is grasped. If the muscle is stretched, use a 5/8-inch needle.
4. Cleanse the top of the medication vial with an alcohol wipe or open the ampule.
5. Withdraw the appropriate volume of medication, based on the child's milligram per kilogram dose. Calculate the dose or obtain from length-based

resuscitation tape or resuscitation software (see Procedure 2).

- The maximum volume IM per age is as follows:
  - ○ 2 mL in older children
  - ○ 1 mL in small children and older infants
  - ○ 0.5 mL in small infants
6. Select the appropriate injection site (**TABLE P14-1**). Consider the following factors:
   - The volume of medication
   - The condition of the muscle
   - Level of muscle development
   - The type of medication
   - The child's ability to be properly positioned
7. Position and secure the child. Consider letting the caregiver hold the child in one of the following ways:
   - Have the child sit on the caregiver's lap, facing to the side. Put one of the child's arms around the caregiver's waist and have the caregiver hold the child close to his or her chest. The caregiver can hold the child's arms or legs.
   - Position the child straddling the caregiver's lap, sitting chest to chest. Tell the caregiver to hug the child. The caregiver can help to hold an arm or leg.

Possible Complications

- Abscess
- Cellulitis
- Damage to blood vessel, nerve, or tendon
- Redness or swelling at the site
- Adverse reaction to the medication
- Pain at site
- Injection into the joint space

TABLE P14-1 Appropriate Sites for IM Injections

Site	Indications	Landmarks	Considerations	Disadvantages
Vastus lateralis muscle: largest muscle group in children under 3 years of age (thigh)	Use in infants and small children Preferred site for all ages	Palpate the greater trochanter and the knee joint; divide the distance into thirds Use middle third for injection site	Can be used for IM injections in young children	Possible thrombosis of the femoral artery More painful than deltoid or gluteal sites
Ventrogluteal muscle: large muscle with few nerves and blood vessels (lateral upper thigh/buttocks)	Use in children older than 3 years of age	Have the child lie on his or her side and bend the upper leg forward in front of the lower leg Palpate greater trochanter and anterior and posterior iliac crests Place palm over greater trochanter with fingers open in a V shape pointing toward iliac crests Inject into center of the V shape	Well-defined landmarks to identify the site	None

(Continues)

Site	Indications	Landmarks	Considerations	Disadvantages
Dorsogluteal site (buttocks)	Use in children older than 3 years of age	Have the child lie on his or her stomach and rotate the legs and toes inward Palpate greater trochanter and posterior iliac spine; draw an imaginary line between these two points Inject lateral and above the imaginary line	In an older child, larger volumes of medication (2 mL) can be injected because the muscle mass is larger	Contraindicated in children younger than 3 years of age and those who have not been walking for at least 1 year Medication may inadvertently be given into fat in older child with a large fat mass May damage the sciatic nerve, which tracks out from the lower lumbar spine and goes underneath the gluteal muscles
Deltoid (upper arm)	Use for small volumes of medication. Do not exceed volume of 1 mL This is the preferred site for children ages 3–18	Palpate the acromion process and go two fingerbreadths (3–5 cm) below Give the injection in the upper third of the muscle	Faster absorption rate than gluteal site Fewer side effects from the injection and less painful site	May damage the radial nerve in young children Because of the limited muscle mass, only small volumes of medication can be injected

IM, intramuscular.

Procedure 14-1

IM Injection

1. The vastus lateralis site is preferable. Use the ventro-gluteal or dorsogluteal sites if the thigh muscle is not accessible in children older than 3 years.

2. Stretch the skin, and insert the needle at a 90-degree angle.

3. If the patient's muscle mass is small, grasp the body of the muscle between the thumb and forefingers.

4. Apply gentle pressure to the site with a gauze pad. Do not massage the site.

TIP

Select the injection site based on age, anatomic considerations, muscle development, and volume of medication to be given.

CAUTION

Avoid injecting close to a major nerve because it may cause nerve damage.

Procedure 14-2

After the Injection

1. Activate safety over the needle, if applicable.

2. Dispose of the syringe and needle in a sharps container.

3. Praise the child. Apply an adhesive bandage to the site.

4. Write down the name of the medication, dosage, route, time, location of the injection, and any effects.

TIP

Some experts believe that the dorsogluteal site should not be used until the child has been walking for at least 1 year.

SUGGESTED REFERENCE

Rishovd A. Pediatric intramuscular injections. *Am J Maternal/Child Nurs.* 2014;39(2):107–112.

Procedure 15: Intranasal Medication Administration

David LaCovey, BS, EMT-P

Michael J. Stoner, MD, FAAP

Introduction

Intranasal medication administration has become a popular route for delivering certain medications in the prehospital setting. It is particularly important when there is no IV access established and urgent medication administration is necessary. Such instances include medications that are needed for pain control, anxiolysis, seizures, and opioid reversal. The highly vascular nasal mucosa allows certain medications to rapidly achieve therapeutic drug concentrations. Delivery of intranasal medication is also relatively painless and easy and can be administered via the droplet or atomized method.

INDICATIONS

Pain control
Anxiolysis
Sedation

Seizure control
Opioid reversal

CONTRAINDICATIONS

Secure intravenous (IV)/intraosseous access (relative)
Cardiac arrest
Head trauma with altered level of consciousness

Facial trauma
Nasal deformity, obstruction, or recent surgery
Epistaxis

EQUIPMENT

1-mL Luer Lock syringe
Blunt filtered needle (if drawing from a glass ampule)

Mucosal Atomization Device (MAD)
Gloves

Rationale

The rich vascular plexus of the nasal cavity provides a direct route into the bloodstream for small, simple, lipophilic molecule medications to easily cross mucous membranes. The direct absorption into the bloodstream of many intranasal medications bypasses the first-pass metabolism of enteric medications and allows for plasma concentrations to be comparable to IV medications and typically better than subcutaneous or intramuscular routes. Intranasal drug administration is essentially painless and is often an easier route to administer certain medications than intravenously when an IV line has not already been established.

Limitations

Only a limited number of medications have data to support their administration via the intranasal route. The following are some common examples: midazolam, fentanyl, ketamine, hydromorphone, haloperidol, naloxone, and glucagon.

Studies suggest the ideal volume per nostril is 0.2–0.3 mL. In practice, the maximum volume for single administration into one nostril is 0.5 mL in pediatric patients and 0.1 mL in neonates. Larger volumes should be divided equally between both nostrils (i.e., half the dose in each nostril). Given this, the concentration of the medication can act as a limitation.

The molecular size and composition of the medication also play a role. Medications that are lipophilic and have a small molecule size have the best absorption. The physiologic pH of the nasal mucosa is 5.0–7.0. Medications outside of this pH range may cause irritation and affect absorption.

This delivery route will be less effective if there is something interfering with absorption. This can include nasal foreign body or significant congestion, such as seen with allergies or an upper respiratory infection.

Preparation

1. Perform hand hygiene, and don gloves.
2. Ensure the medication can be administered via the intranasal route.

3. Determine the volume of medication to be administered. If the volume of medication is greater than 0.5 mL, then divide the volume equally between each nostril. If the volume per nostril exceeds 0.5 mL, the dose should be administered in two separate applications 5–10 minutes apart. Spacing between doses allows the previous dose to be absorbed.
4. Draw the prescribed amount of medication into a 1-mL Luer Lock syringe. If using a MAD, draw an additional 0.1 mL of medication to account for dead space in the syringe and MAD.
5. Remove the needle from tip of syringe, and dispose of properly.
6. Administer medication into the nostril.

Procedure 15-1

Intranasal Administration Utilizing a MAD

1. Connect the MAD to the syringe by twisting in place.

2. Inspect the nostril for anything that might impair the absorption of the medication.

3. With the patient supine, use your free hand to hold the crown of the head stable.

4. Place tip of the MAD into the nostril, aiming it up and slightly outward (toward the top of the ear).

5. Briskly compress the syringe plunger to deliver medication.

6. Remove the syringe from the patient's nostril.

TIP

Ensure the atomizer is firmly attached to the tip of the syringe.

TIP

In neonates or small children, removal of the foam tip may provide a better fit.

Procedure 15-2

Intranasal Administration Utilizing the Drip Method

1. Inspect the nostril for anything that might impair the absorption of the medication.

2. With the patient supine, use your free hand to hold the crown of the head stable and place the patient's head into a sniffing position.

3. Slowly depress the syringe plunger to drip the medication into the patient's nostril, and give a few drops at a time.

SUGGESTED REFERENCE

Wolfe T. Therapeutic intranasal drug delivery. http://www.intranasal.net. Accessed September 18, 2019.

Procedure 16: Intravenous Access

J. Hudson Garrett Jr., PhD, MSN, MPH, MBA, FNP-BC, PLNC, IP-BC, AS-BC, NREMT, VA-BC, FACDONA, FAAPM, FNAP

Mary Otting, RN, BSN, CEN

Introduction

Establishing intravenous (IV) access is a time-honored method of fluid and drug administration. However, unlike the situation with an adult, securing IV access in a pediatric patient is often difficult or impossible in the prehospital setting. Fortunately, the majority of pediatric patients do not require IV access before emergency department (ED) arrival, and many prehospital medications do not require an IV route for administration.

INDICATIONS

Cardiopulmonary arrest
Shock
Trauma
Cardiac dysrhythmia

Illness or injury possibly requiring immediate IV drug or fluid administration
Consider vascular access on the way to the ED in the following situations:
Multisystem injury

CONTRAINDICATIONS

Availability of another reliable administration route
Brief transport time

Limited available vasculature (available vessels of substantial quality to access)

EQUIPMENT

IV catheters, 14- to 24-gauge
IV tubing (macrodrip or microdrip)
Extension connector
IV solution
Rubber band or elastic band tourniquet

Adhesive tape or adhesive transparent securement dressing
Gauze pad
Pediatric arm board

Rationale

IV access makes it easier to give medications and provides a route for fluid therapy in illness or injuries where there is possible blood or fluid loss. IV delivery is the gold standard for delivering medications because it permits predictable delivery and more rapid onset of action for most important drugs. The indications for IV access must be carefully weighed against common complications and possible risks associated with the procedure. These include distraction from airway and breathing management, possible delays to ED care, and excessive pain to the child. Also, there is a risk to the prehospital professional from exposure to bloodborne pathogens. However, in certain children, such as the critically ill child with shock, IV therapy in the field can be lifesaving.

Preparation

1. Assemble the equipment. Select the appropriate IV solution and tubing.
   - Inspect the solution for cloudiness, expiration date, leakage, or contamination. Verify the solution name.
   - Use microdrip IV tubing or saline lock for giving medications; for fluid administration, use a macrodrip.
   - For medication administration, consider a saline lock: male Luer lock device with injection port and sterile normal saline flush.
   - Spike the fluid bag with the tubing, clamp the tubing, squeeze the drip chamber until it is half full, open the clamp, and flush the tubing.
   - Select the appropriate catheter, depending on need for fluid volume. Use a smaller catheter when only medications are indicated.
2. Prepare the child and family for the procedure. Use developmentally appropriate language to explain the procedure.
3. Select the site.
   - The scalp is a potential site in newborns.
   - The best sites in the infant are the hands, antecubital fossa, and saphenous vein at the ankle or feet. The dorsum (back) of the hand is a good site in chubby infants. To access that site, grasp the child's hand with the fingers closed, and flex the wrist downward.
   - In toddlers and older children, potential sites are the hands and antecubital areas. Use the child's nondominant extremity if possible.
   - Ideally, avoid inserting the catheter over a joint.
   - Consider the antecubital fossa when fluid boluses are required because veins that are more distal in the forearm or hand are usually smaller.
   - Hand veins are often mobile under the skin and may move with contact with the catheter.

4. Position the patient supine, or in the caregiver's lap if the child is younger than school age. Secure the child's legs to avoid kicking. The caregiver can help hold the child and immobilize the insertion site.
5. Apply the rubber band or tourniquet proximal to the entry site. Do not make it too tight. The tourniquet should not block arterial flow. If it is necessary to make the vein more visible, do the following:
   - Place the extremity in a dependent position.
   - Tap or massage the site.
   - Ask the older child to clench and unclench his or her fist.
   Consider using a local anesthetic spray if permitted by local medical protocols to decrease patient pain.
6. Cleanse the site with antiseptic solution such as chlorhexidine gluconate with alcohol, isopropyl alcohol, or povidone iodine.

TIP

If IV access is for giving medication only, use microdrip tubing or a saline lock. For giving fluid, use macrodrip tubing.

CAUTION

Never delay transport in any critically injured infant or child; consider IV attempts while en route to the hospital.

TIP

Reward and comfort the child after the procedure.

Procedure 16-1

Intravenous Access

1. Insert the needle. Stabilize the vein by pulling the skin taut distally from the insertion site. Insert the catheter through the skin with the bevel up, at a 30-degree angle. Insert the catheter slowly; blood return may be delayed for a few seconds. When there is a flashback of blood, advance the needle and catheter into the vein and then remove the needle. Never pull the catheter back over the needle because this may cause shearing of the catheter tip. Release the tourniquet. Compress the vein proximal to the site to prevent blood loss through the catheter while connecting the tubing. It is also helpful to position a gauze pad under the catheter at this time. Connect the tubing or male Luer lock to the catheter. If a saline lock (male Luer lock with injection port) is used, a 2- to 5-mL saline flush should be used to maintain patency.

2. Stabilize the catheter with tape or adhesive transparent securement dressing. Avoid placing an excess amount of tape or gauze over the site because it obstructs the view of the site. Use a clear medicine cup or other device to protect the site while allowing access and visualization.

3. Immobilize the extremity. Be careful not to apply the tape too tightly, because this blocks the flow of blood through the vein.

4. Monitor the solution drip rate to avoid giving too much or too little fluid.

5. Dispose of the needle.

Troubleshooting

1. If the fluid is not infusing properly, assess the following:
   - Make sure the tourniquet has been released.
   - Make sure the child's arm is not bent.
   - Make sure the tape is not too tight.
   - Make sure the tubing is not kinked.
   - Make sure the clamp is open.
   - Lower the fluid bag below the extremity and assess for a backflow of blood into the tubing.
   - Raise the fluid bag higher, if possible.
2. If none of the above measures is effective, discontinue the IV and restart in another site.

Possible Complications

Pain

Infiltration (look for pain or edema at the site, inability to infuse fluids, or lack of blood return; discontinue IV, and insert at another site)

Hypothermia from giving too much room-temperature fluid to an infant

Skin or bloodstream infection

Extravasation (leaking of vesicant drugs into surrounding tissue)

Thrombophlebitis

Inadvertent fluid overload

Catheter shear

Inadvertent arterial puncture

CONTROVERSY

Few children require IV access in the field or on the way to the ED. The majority of injured children should be transported before attempting IV access. For ill children, especially if there is a short transport time, it is controversial which ones need IV access and whether IV access is beneficial to the patient or causes undue anxiety or stress to the child. It is important to carefully weigh the benefits versus risks prior to inserting a prehospital IV in a child.

CAUTION

Do not use words like "stick" or "needle" when describing the procedure to the child. Instead, consider an explanation such as, "I will be putting a soft tube into your arm to give your veins a drink."

CAUTION

Be careful not to secure the tape too tightly to immobilize the extremity, because this blocks blood flow in the vein.

TIP

Position the child and secure the site before beginning the procedure.

Procedure 17: Intraosseous Needle Insertion

Michael S. Riley, NRP, EMS-I

Michael J. Stoner, MD, FAAP

Introduction

Establishing vascular access is often difficult or impossible during life-threatening emergencies in infants and young children. The intraosseous (IO) route for the delivery of resuscitation fluids and medications has been used since the early to mid-1900s, and many studies have confirmed that the IO space is an excellent route for medications and fluids in children and adults. The primary technical problem is successfully piercing the bony cortex (outer layer of the bone) in older children. The bones of neonates and infants are usually soft and the intramedullary space is relatively large, so needle insertion is easier in children of these younger age groups. Good equipment, preparation, and effective technique are especially important for success.

INDICATION

Severe illness or injury requiring immediate drugs or fluids, when intravenous (IV) access is unsuccessful or unlikely to be possible

CONTRAINDICATIONS

Available secure IV line

Fracture or deformity in same bone as insertion site

Previous attempt in same bone

Skin or soft tissue infection over insertion site

Osteogenesis imperfecta

EQUIPMENT

IO needle/insertion device

Skin cleansing solution

Normal saline and IV tubing

10-mL syringe

Extension connector and three-way stopcock (optional)

Rationale

Using an IO needle to give drugs or fluids is an excellent alternative to cannulating peripheral veins in critically ill or injured children. The IO space is highly vascular and functions as a temporary, noncollapsible access. Needle insertion into this space is quick, simple, effective, and usually quite safe. There are several possible sites, but the easiest location is the proximal tibia. The IO space is suitable for infusion of all parenteral medications, crystalloid fluids, or blood products—which are quickly absorbed from small veins of the bone into the central circulation. Complications are usually minor and infrequent.

Preparation

Tibia and Femur Sites

1. Place the patient in the supine position.
2. Put a small towel roll under the knee.
3. Prepare the skin over the insertion site.

Possible Complications

- Compartment syndrome
- Failed infusion
- Growth plate injury
- Bone infection
- Skin infection
- Bone fracture

Procedure 17-1

Traditional IO Insertion

1. Pierce the bony cortex with a firm, twisting motion. Use a back-and-forth twisting motion to enter the marrow space. Do not push hard on the needle. A "pop" may be felt as the needle passes through the bony cortex and into the marrow cavity.

2. Remove the stylet, and aspirate marrow contents. Keep any bone marrow aspirate for glucose check or for other tests in the emergency department. Sometimes, marrow cannot be aspirated. Confirm correct placement by infusing 10 mL of normal saline without resistance.

3. Attach IV line to the hub, or to an extension connector and stopcock, and infuse fluids or drugs directly into IO space.

4. Secure the needle to the overlying skin with tape. Monitor the surrounding soft tissue to ensure that there is no swelling to indicate leakage of fluid.

5. Continuously infuse fluids to maintain patency of IO line.

6. Do not use an infusion pump to deliver fluids; use "push-pull" method by using a three-way stopcock, or use a pressure bag.

Procedure 17-2

EZ-IO Insertion

An alternate to the traditional manual IO is the EZ-IO (**FIGURE P17-1**). This device is cleared for IO access in the proximal humerus, distal femur, proximal tibia, and distal tibia in children.

FIGURE P17-1 EZ-IO.

Image courtesy of Teleflex Incorporated. © 2019 Teleflex Incorporated. All rights reserved.

1. After palpating the insertion site, select the appropriate needle for the patient based on the patient's weight, anatomy, and the clinical judgment. EZ-IO 45-mm Needle Set (yellow hub) should be considered for proximal humerus insertion in patients 40 kg and greater, and for patients with excessive tissue over any insertion site. EZ-IO 25-mm Needle Set (blue hub) should be considered for patients 3 kg and greater.

2. Attach the needle to the EZ-IO drill.

3. Position the needle and EZ-IO drill at 90 degrees to the bone for all sites except the proximal humerus, which should be at a 45-degree angle to the anterior plan and posteromedial. With the tip of the needle set touching bone, the 5-mm marker must be visible above the skin for confirmation of adequate length prior to drilling. Press the trigger on the drill handle and apply gentle pressure, while letting the drill do the work for you. When you feel the "pop," you're in; immediately release

the trigger, avoiding recoil. Do NOT pull back on the driver when releasing the trigger. As with traditional IO insertion, refrain from placing your other hand behind the insertion site to prevent possible palm penetration from excessive force.

4. Disconnect the EZ-IO drill while stabilizing the needle set to avoid dislodgement from the medullary space.

5. Withdraw the needle stylet and confirm placement by aspiration of blood with the syringe; however, the inability to aspirate blood does not necessarily indicate improper placement. Confirm correct placement by infusing 2–5 mL of normal saline without resistance.

CAUTION

If the drill stops, you are pushing too hard.

Procedure 17-3

Proximal Tibia Site

1. Use the flat surface of the proximal medial tibia, just below and medial to the tibial tuberosity on the flat side of the bone.

2. Introduce the traditional IO needle in the skin directed away from the growth plate or pointing toward the foot until the tip touches the bone. The EZ-IO is inserted at a 90-degree angle, but avoid the growth plate, and follow the prior steps for insertion into the intramedullary space.

Procedure 17-4

Distal Tibia Site

1. Use the flat surface of the medial distal tibia above the medial malleolus.

2. Introduce the traditional IO needle in the skin directed away from the growth plate or toward the knee until the tip touches the bone. The EZ-IO is inserted at a 90-degree angle, but avoid the growth plate. Follow the prior steps for insertion into the intramedullary space.

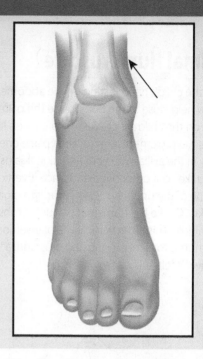

Procedure 17-5

Distal Femur Site

1. Use the distal third of the femur, estimate the distance through soft tissue to reach the bony surface of the femur, and ensure that the correct length needle is chosen or that the needle has been adjusted to a length that allows bony penetration.

2. Introduce the traditional IO needle in the skin, directed away from the growth plate or pointing toward the trunk until the tip touches the bone. The EZ-IO is inserted at a 90-degree angle, but avoid the growth plate. Follow the prior steps for insertion into the intramedullary space.

Proximal Humerus Site

1. With the child's hand resting on the abdomen and elbow held close to the body, place the palm of your hand on the child's shoulder. This area feels like a "ball" and is the proximal humerus. Then place one hand vertically in the axilla, with your fifth digit against the skin. Then take your other hand and place it vertically in the midline of the upper arm, with your fifth digit against the skin. Cradle the humerus so your thumbs meet in the middle. This is the vertical line of insertion. Then use one thumb to climb up the humerus until a "notch" or "groove" is felt, this is the surgical neck.

2. The insertion point for the IO needle is located approximately 1 cm above the surgical neck until the tip touches the bone, follow steps below for insertion into the intramedullary space.

3. Secure the arm in place to prevent accidental dislodgement of the IO catheter.

Elbow should remain adducted and posteriorly located

Place the hand over the umbilicus for humeral positioning and safety

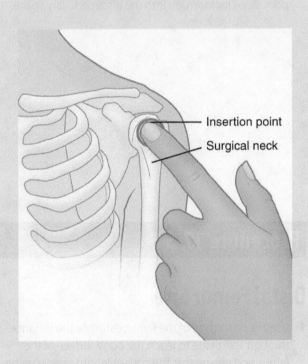

Insertion point

Surgical neck

CAUTION

The proximal humerus should only be utilized in children whose appropriate anatomic landmarks can be identified.

Procedure 18: Cardiopulmonary Resuscitation

John A. Erbayri, MS, NRP, CHSE

Michael H. Stroud, MD, FAAP

Introduction

Cardiopulmonary arrest (CPA) occurs when a patient's heart and lungs stop functioning. In children, CPA usually begins as a primary respiratory arrest. This is in contrast to adults, in whom CPA or "sudden death" is almost always a primary cardiac event that occurs with onset of ventricular fibrillation (VF) and an abrupt change in the heart's electrical activity. Because cessation of effective breathing is often the precipitating factor in pediatric CPA, airway management and ventilation are to children in CPA what defibrillation is to adults. Cardiopulmonary resuscitation (CPR) refers to chest compressions, airway management, and breathing via ventilations (CAB) to provide oxygen and circulation to core organs: the heart, brain, and lungs. In children, CPR has been shown to improve survival from drowning, and it may also benefit patients in CPA from other causes. Asphyxial cardiac arrest is more common than VF cardiac arrest in infants and children; thus, ventilation is extremely important in pediatric resuscitation.

INDICATIONS

Newborn, neonate, infant, or child of any age who is apneic and pulseless

Newborn, infant, or child with a heart rate less than 60 beats/min and not improving after positive-pressure ventilation

Neonates, infants, and children with a heart rate less than 60 beats/min and poor perfusion

CONTRAINDICATION

Newborn, infant, or child with effective perfusion (palpable central or peripheral pulse)

EQUIPMENT

Mouth-to-mask device
Bag-mask device, infant or child size

Airway adjuncts
Appropriate mask sizes

Rationale

CPR encompasses the basic procedures for sustaining critical oxygenation, ventilation, and perfusion recommended by the American Heart Association. The pediatric techniques are slightly modified from the adult techniques to reflect the known differences in CPA between age groups. Furthermore, there are specific differences between infants and children, including number of rescuers, placement of hands and fingers, rates of ventilation, and rates and depth of chest compressions.

Preparation

1. Position a child on a hard surface.

Pediatric Assessment

1. ABC assessment if patient is awake and moving.
2. If patient is unresponsive and not breathing (gasps do not count as breathing), perform the CAB assessment—begin with pulse
3. If no pulse detected in 10 seconds, or if the heart rate is less than 60 per minute, start chest compressions (see ratios in **TABLE P18-1**).

TABLE P18-1 Chest Compressions to Ventilation Ratios

Age	Compressions (min)/Ratios	Depth (inches)	Hand Placement
Newborn	3:1 ratio of compressions to ventilations (90 compressions to 30 breaths every minute)	Compress approximately one-third of AP chest diameter	Two thumbs encircling the chest and supporting back (may prefer higher coronary perfusion pressure than two-finger technique)
Infant	100–120/min; 30:2 ratio of compressions to breaths for lone rescuer; 15:2 if two rescuers	Compress at least one-third the depth of the chest or about 4 cm (1.5 inches)	One rescuer (whether lay rescuers or health care providers) should compress the sternum with two fingers placed just below the intermammary line; do not compress over the xiphoid or ribs
Child	100–120/min; 30:2 ratio of compressions to breaths for lone rescuer; 15:2 if two rescuers	Compress at least one-third of the AP dimension of the chest or approximately 5 cm (2 inches)	One rescuer (whether lay rescuers or health care providers) should compress the lower half of sternum with heel of one or two hands
Adolescent	100–120/min; 30:2 ratio of compressions to breaths	Compress at least one-third of the AP dimension of the chest or approximately 5 cm (2 inches)	Place the heel of one hand on the center of the chest (lower half of the sternum). Place the heel of your other hand over the first hand.

AP, anteroposterior.

4. If definite pulse is greater than 60 per minute, begin rescue breathing at a rate of one breath every 3 to 5 seconds.
   - Infant basic life support (BLS) guidelines apply to infants younger than 1 year of age.
   - Child BLS guidelines apply to children 1 year of age until puberty. For teaching purposes, puberty is defined as breast development in girls and the presence of axillary hair in boys.
   - Adult BLS guidelines apply at and beyond puberty.

High-Quality CPR

High-quality CPR is defined by the following:

1. Chest compressions of appropriate rate and depth
2. Push fast: Push at a rate of 100–120 compressions per minute.
3. Push hard: Push with sufficient force to depress at least one-third the anteroposterior (AP) diameter of the chest, or approximately 1.5 inches (4 cm) in infants and 2 inches (5 cm) in children.
4. Allow complete chest recoil after each compression to allow the heart to refill with blood. Incomplete recoil during CPR is associated with higher intrathoracic pressures and significantly decreased

TIP

Manipulation of the head to keep the airway in a neutral position is essential for effective ventilation. A towel roll under the shoulders of the infant or small child may help maintain neutral head position.

venous return, coronary perfusion, blood flow, and cerebral perfusion.
5. Minimize interruptions of chest compressions.
6. Avoid excessive ventilation.
7. See ratios in Table P18-1 for ratio of chest compressions to ventilation.
8. Rescuers should rotate the compressor role every 2 minutes to avoid fatigue.
9. Ratios do not apply if patient is intubated. Deliver breaths at a rate of 10 per minute (one breath approximately every 6 seconds), and provide continuous chest compressions.
10. If the patient has return of spontaneous circulation (ROSC) with a perfusing rhythm and pulse, then breaths can be delivered at a rate of approximately 20–30 per minute (one breath every 2–3 seconds).

Procedure 18-1

Performing CPR on an Infant

1. Position the infant on a firm surface. Place two fingers in the middle of the sternum just below a line between the nipples. Use two fingers to compress the chest at least one-third the AP diameter of the chest or about 4 cm (1.5 inches) at a rate of 100–120 per minute. Allow the sternum to return to its normal position between compressions.

3. If two rescuers are present, compressions can also be performed at a ratio of 15 compressions to two breaths using the two thumb-encircling-hands technique.

2. Coordinate compressions with ventilations in a 30:2 ratio (one rescuer) or 15:2 (two rescuers), pausing for two ventilations at the end of each cycle. Continue cycles of compressions and ventilations until an automated external defibrillator (AED) becomes available or the infant shows signs of spontaneous breathing.

Procedure 18-2

Performing CPR on a Child

1. Place the child on a firm surface. Prepare to place the heel of one or both hands in the center of the chest, in between the nipples, avoiding the xiphoid process.

2. Compress the chest at least one-third the AP diameter of the chest or approximately 5 cm (2 inches) at a rate of 100–120 per minute.

3. Coordinate compressions with ventilations in a 30:2 ratio (one rescuer) or 15:2 (two rescuers). At the end of each cycle, pause for two ventilations. Perform mouth-to-mask ventilation with 100% oxygen. Give two breaths of 1 second each.

4. Continue cycles of compressions and ventilations until an AED becomes available or the patient shows signs of spontaneous breathing. If the child resumes effective breathing, place him or her in a position that allows for frequent reassessment of the airway and vital signs during transport.

Possible Complications

- Coronary vessel injury
- Diaphragm injury
- Hemopericardium
- Hemothorax
- Interference with ventilation
- Liver injury
- Myocardial injury
- Pneumothorax
- Rib fractures
- Spleen injury

Use of End-Tidal Carbon Dioxide (EtCO$_2$) for Quality of Compressions

1. Exhaled CO$_2$ is reflective of cardiac output during a cardiac arrest, because pulmonary blood flow must exist for EtCO$_2$ to register, and is recommended for CPR in intubated patients.

2. Quantitative EtCO$_2$ may be used to monitor quality of CPR. Normal EtCO$_2$ with a good mask seal or if the patient is intubated is approximately

35–45 mm Hg. During a cardiac arrest, the $EtCO_2$ value will be much lower and can theoretically reach 0 if the patient has no pulse and is not receiving chest compressions.

3. $EtCO_2$ levels <10 mm Hg indicate chest compressions need improvement. $EtCO_2$ levels above 20 mm Hg indicate high-quality chest compressions.

4. If ROSC is achieved, the $EtCO_2$ will rise rapidly, reflecting increasing blood flow for cardiac output.

5. After circulation (ROSC) is restored, monitor systemic oxygen saturation. It may be reasonable, when appropriate equipment is available, to titrate oxygen administration to maintain the oxyhemoglobin saturation 94%–97%. Hyperoxia should be avoided after cardiac arrest, as it has been shown to induce free radical formation and worsen outcomes.

Procedure 19: AED and Defibrillation

John A. Erbayri, MS, NRP, CHSE

Michael H. Stroud, MD, FAAP

Introduction

Synchronized cardioversion for tachydysrhythmias has long been part of adult emergency care. However, ventricular dysrhythmias are rare in children, especially in infants, and pediatric supraventricular tachycardia (SVT) is usually treatable with medical therapy. All providers should be prepared to provide synchronized cardioversion or defibrillation in appropriate situations. Ventricular fibrillation (VF) is observed in 5%–15% of pediatric and adolescent arrests. However, when a child develops VF or pulseless ventricular tachycardia, defibrillation (unsynchronized cardioversion) may be lifesaving. Synchronized cardioversion may resuscitate a child in shock with SVT. Synchronized cardioversion provides a shock that is timed (synchronized) with the QRS complex, avoiding delivery during the refractory period of the cardiac cycle, when a shock could produce VF. Use the synchronized mode for selected cases of SVT or ventricular tachycardia with a pulse, and the unsynchronized (defibrillation) mode for VF or ventricular tachycardia without a pulse.

INDICATIONS

Ventricular fibrillation
Pulseless ventricular tachycardia
SVT with shock and no vascular access rapidly available (synchronized)

Ventricular tachycardia with shock and unresponsiveness with pulse
Atrial fibrillation or atrial flutter with shock

CONTRAINDICATION

Conscious patient with good perfusion

EQUIPMENT

Automatic external defibrillator with pads appropriate for age

Standard defibrillator with paddles or pads appropriate for age

Rationale

When a child's heart rhythm deteriorates into ventricular tachycardia or fibrillation, there is usually a severe systemic insult, such as profound hypoxia, ischemia, electrolyte abnormalities, electrocution, or myocarditis. Death may result if treatment is delayed. SVT, in contrast, is usually a more stable cardiac rhythm. When the child is pulseless and has VF or ventricular tachycardia, perform defibrillation as quickly as possible with the appropriate technique. If a child has ventricular tachycardia with a pulse or SVT with poor perfusion, use synchronized cardioversion. Do not attempt to perform synchronized cardioversion on a child with SVT who is well perfused.

Preparation

1. Open airway, and ventilate with bag-mask device with 100% oxygen if indicated, while assembling equipment for cardioversion or defibrillation.
2. If child is pulseless, begin chest compressions, until an automated external defibrillator (AED) or conventional defibrillator is available.

CAUTION

Do not deliver synchronized cardioversion to a conscious child with SVT or ventricular tachycardia unless the child is in shock and has no intravenous or intraosseous access rapidly available for medical treatment.

TIP

For a child with ventricular fibrillation or pulseless ventricular tachycardia, use the unsynchronized (defibrillation) mode.

Preparation

Conventional Defibrillator Use

1. Select the proper paddle or pad size. Use the 8-cm adult paddles if these will fit on the chest wall; otherwise, use the 4.5-cm pediatric paddles (**TABLE P19-1**).
2. Prepare paddles or skin electrodes with electrode jelly, paste, or saline-soaked gauze pads, or use self-adhesive defibrillator pads. Do not let jelly or paste from one site touch the other and form an "electrical bridge" between sites, which could result in ineffective defibrillation or skin burns.

3. Establish appropriate electrical charge (**TABLE P19-2**).
4. Select synchronized or unsynchronized mode.

TIP

Maintain high-quality chest compressions until defibrillator is charged when you are analyzing rhythm OR as long as possible when using AED mode. Immediately resume compressions once rhythm is analyzed and does not suggest a shock OR immediately after a shock is delivered.

CAUTION

Failure to firmly apply paddles to the chest wall decreases effective delivery of charge.

TABLE P19-1 Paddle Size

- 8-cm adult paddles (use in children older than 12 months of age or weighing more than 10 kg) on anterior chest wall OR anterior-posterior

- 4.5-cm pediatric paddles (use in infants up to 12 months of age or weighing less than 10 kg) on the anterior chest wall

TABLE P19-2 Appropriate Electrical Charge for Countershock

Dysrhythmia	Mode	Charge
Ventricular fibrillation Ventricular tachycardia without a pulse	Defibrillation (unsynchronized)	2 J/kg, then 4 J/kg Subsequent shocks >4 J/kg after CPR and each dose of medication Do not deliver more than 10 J/kg or adult dose.
Ventricular tachycardia with pulse, SVT	Synchronized cardioversion	0.5–1.0 J/kg Can increase to 2 J/kg if needed
Atrial fibrillation and atrial flutter with shock	Synchronized cardioversion	If no result with 0.5–1.0 J/kg, may use up to 2 J/kg

Procedure 19-1

Conventional Defibrillator Use

1. Apply the paddles or pads directly to the skin. Place one paddle or pad on the anterior chest wall on the right side of the sternum inferior to the clavicle and the other paddle or pad on the left midclavicular line at the level of the xiphoid process. The pads should not touch. If this occurs, use the anterior-posterior position.

2. Press charge button and clear the nearby area to avoid shocking someone. Announce, "I am going to shock on three. One, I am clear. Two, you are clear. Three, everybody is clear."

3. Begin recording rhythm. Deliver the electrical countershock with firm pressure if paddles are used.

4. If CPR was being performed prior to shock, resume CPR for 2 minutes. Then, check monitor for a change in rhythm and check pulse.

5. If the first electrical shock is unsuccessful, resume CPR, then reanalyze the rhythm after another 2 minutes (five cycles) of CPR. Give specific dysrhythmia treatment with epinephrine or other drugs, as per protocol. Treat bradycardia or other dysrhythmias.

CONTROVERSY

The preferred paddle location in children is controversial and no study in humans has compared the two techniques. Anterior chest wall placement has the advantage of a supine child and easier airway management. Anterior-posterior placement may allow larger paddles and more effective delivery of electricity.

TIP

Consider giving a benzodiazepine before cardioversion if patient is awake.

Procedure 19-2

One Rescuer With an AED

For children younger than 8 years of age, use a child-pad cable system if available.

1. Verify unresponsiveness.

2. Look for no breathing or only gasping and check pulse.

3. If not breathing but with a pulse, begin bag-mask ventilations.

4. If no pulse, begin CPR with 30 compressions and 2 breaths.

5. Apply AED as soon as it is available.

6. POWER ON the AED and follow voice prompts. Some devices will turn on when the AED lid or carrying case is opened.

7. ATTACH the AED. Select the correct pads for patient's size and age (adult versus child). Peel the backing from the pads. Attach the adhesive pads to the victim as shown on the pads. (If only adult pads are available, and they overlap when placed on the chest, use an anterior [chest] and posterior [back] placement.) Attach the electrode cable to the AED (if not preconnected).

8. Allow the AED to ANALYZE the victim's rhythm ("clear" patient during analysis). Deliver a SHOCK if needed ("clear" patient before shock). Reasonable variations in this sequence are acceptable.

9. Resume CPR.

Possible Complications

- Ineffective delivery of cardioversion because of failure to charge, improper positioning on the chest, incorrect paddle size, or improper conduction medium
- Burns on the chest wall

- Failure to "clear" before voltage discharge, leading to electrical shock of a team member or bystander
- Tachydysrhythmia
- Bradycardia
- Myocardial damage or necrosis
- Cardiogenic shock
- Embolic phenomena

Procedure 19-3

Two-Rescuer AED Sequence of Action

1. Verify unresponsiveness. Have your partner get the AED.

2. Look for no breathing or only gasping, and check pulse.

3. If no pulse, start CPR. If not breathing but with a pulse, begin bag-mask ventilation.

4. Apply AED as soon as it is available.

5. Attempt defibrillation with the AED if no signs of circulation are present. Place the AED near the rescuer who will be operating it. The AED is usually placed on the side of the patient opposite the rescuer who is performing CPR. The rescuer begins performing CPR while the rescuer who was performing CPR prepares to operate the AED. (It is acceptable to reverse these roles.)

6. The AED operator takes the following actions. POWER ON the AED first (some devices will turn on automatically when the AED lid or carrying case is opened).

7. ATTACH the AED to the patient. Select correct pads for the patient's size and age. Peel the backing from the pads. Ask the rescuer performing CPR to stop chest compressions. Attach the adhesive pads to the patient as shown on the pads. (If only adult pads are available,

and they overlap when placed on the chest, use an anterior [chest] and posterior [back] placement.) Attach the AED connecting cables to the AED (if not preconnected). ANALYZE rhythm. Clear the patient before and during analysis. Check that no one is touching the patient. Press the ANALYZE button to start rhythm analysis (some brands of AEDs do not require this step).

"Shock Indicated" message: Resume CPR until AED is charged and ready to deliver shock. Clear the patient once more before pushing the SHOCK button ("I'm clear, you're clear, everybody's clear"). Check that no one is touching the patient. Press the SHOCK button (patient may display muscle contractions).

"No Shock Indicated" message: Resume CPR immediately.

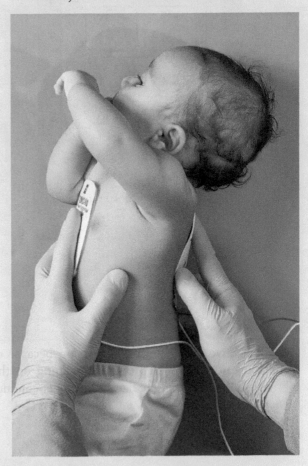

8. After two minutes of CPR (or when prompted by the AED), analyze rhythm, then follow the "shock indicated" or "no shock indicated" steps as appropriate.

Procedure 20: Endotracheal Tube Drug Instillation

Michael R. Aguilar, AA, EMT-P

Introduction

The ability of the airways of the lungs to absorb medicines has been recognized for more than a century. Giving medication through an endotracheal (ET) tube is an alternative to intravenous (IV) or intraosseous (IO) drug delivery in a cardiopulmonary resuscitation, when necessary. The airways are well vascularized and can absorb certain emergency medications. Drug dosages and dilutions in ET delivery are different from IV or IO administration. ET drug delivery has been deemphasized; while this route of administration is better than no drug delivery, it is less effective than IV or IO. Once vascular access has been achieved, consideration should be given to repeating drugs if there has been no response to the ET drug delivery.

INDICATIONS

Cardiopulmonary resuscitation

Lack of IV or IO access

CONTRAINDICATION

Functioning IV or IO access

EQUIPMENT

ET tube
Long catheter (feeding tube, suction catheter, nasogastric tube, or umbilical catheter)
Catheter size (in French units): approximately two times ET tube size (in mm) (TABLE P20-1)

Desired drug/diluent mixture
Normal saline
Self-inflating ventilation device
Use 1–3 mL of diluent in infants and 5–10 mL maximum in older children.

TABLE P20-1 Suggested Catheter Size per Tracheal Tube

Endotracheal Tube Size (mm)	Catheter Size (Fr)
2.5	5
3.0	6
3.5–4.5	8
5.0–6.5	10
7.0	12

Rationale

If neither IV nor IO access is available for giving drugs during cardiopulmonary resuscitation, the ET route is a good alternative for pediatric drugs (lidocaine, epinephrine, atropine, and naloxone [LEAN]). The absorption, blood levels, onset, and duration of action are different with each drug. ET doses are unique for each agent and are higher than IV or IO doses because absorption is not as good. While ET drugs are probably not as effective as IV or IO drugs, they can help improve the chances of successful resuscitation while IV or IO access is established.

Preparation

1. Intubate the patient.
2. Stabilize and secure the ET tube.
3. Preoxygenate and ventilate.

> **TIP**
>
> ET drug administration is a potential route for medications during early phases of resuscitation.

> **TIP**
>
> IV and IO are better routes of drug administration than the ET route.

Possible Complications

- Hypoxia
- Hypercarbia
- Pneumonitis
- Tracheal injury
- Adverse side effects of drug itself

Procedure 20-1

Endotracheal Drug Delivery

1. Draw the calculated drug dose into a syringe (doses must be increased two to three times for lidocaine, atropine, and naloxone, and increased 10 times for epinephrine).
2. Dilute the medication with normal saline.
3. Insert tip of small feeding tube or catheter past distal tip of ET tube.
4. Instill solution directly into the trachea.
5. Follow with positive-pressure breaths.
6. Ventilate three times with self-inflating ventilation device to disperse the solution into the entire lung. Repeat medications if indicated.

> **CAUTION**
>
> Never give sodium bicarbonate by the ET tube.

> **TIP**
>
> Doses via the ET route must be increased two to three times for lidocaine, atropine, and naloxone, and increased ten times for epinephrine.

> **TIP**
>
> Drugs approved for ET installation: lidocaine, epinephrine, atropine, and naloxone.

Procedure 21: Rectal Administration of Benzodiazepines

Wm. Travis Engel, DO, MSc

Claudia L. Phillips, MSN-Ed, RN, CEN, CPEN

Introduction

Rectal drug administration is a well-known delivery technique in children and is useful for many medications, including antipyretics and anticonvulsants. The only rectal medication approved in most emergency medical services (EMS) systems is diazepam for pediatric status epilepticus. Status epilepticus is a major pediatric medical emergency that may benefit from quick treatment. Although the first priority is airway and breathing, additional therapy may include medication to terminate the seizure. There remains significant controversy regarding the administration of rectal drugs from a safety and effectiveness stance. Rectal diazepam is an effective route with few added complications when other routes of administration are not immediately available. It is important to ask if the caregivers have administered a rectal gel form of diazepam prior to EMS arrival.

TIP

Many patients with a known seizure disorder will have diazepam prescribed to them for rectal administration in emergency situations. It is important to ask caregivers if any medication was administered prior to EMS arrival on scene.

INDICATION

Status epilepticus

CONTRAINDICATIONS

Newborn age (a month or less) (relative)

Recent rectal surgery (e.g., for Hirschsprung disease, imperforate anus) (relative)

EQUIPMENT

Lubricant
Tuberculin syringe, or 14- to 20-gauge over-the-needle catheter with 3- to 5-mL syringe

Intravenous (IV) solution of diazepam
Tape (optional)

Rationale

Establishing IV or intraosseous access is often time consuming and may delay delivery of essential advanced life support (ALS) drugs, especially in infants and toddlers. The rectum is an effective alternative route for emergency drug administration. The rectum is highly vascularized, and certain drugs are quickly absorbed through the lining or mucosa. Diazepam is a lipid-soluble benzodiazepine that is reliably absorbed through the rectum and terminates most seizures without further treatment. It takes a few minutes longer to stop the seizure after rectal administration of diazepam as compared to IV diazepam. Occasionally, as with the IV diazepam preparation, more than one dose of rectal diazepam is necessary. One reason is because of the drug's short duration of action and recurrence of seizure activity.

Rectal lorazepam also has been used in the treatment of status epilepticus. This is less frequently encountered in the prehospital setting because of the manufacturer's recommendations to keep this drug refrigerated. Lorazepam may be stored for up to 30 days unrefrigerated at room temperature.

Preparation

1. Use a pediatric resuscitation tape or resuscitation software to determine the weight of the child (see Procedure 2) or establish the patient's weight from information provided by the caregiver. Note: You may have to convert the given weight in pounds to kilograms (divide pounds by 2.2 to get kilograms).
2. Draw up the calculated dose of IV medication into a disposable tuberculin syringe or 3- to 5-mL syringe.
3. Lubricate the syringe or catheter:
   - If using the tuberculin syringe as the administration device, remove needle and apply lubricant to the tip of the syringe.
   - If using a 3- to 5-mL syringe (or tuberculin syringe, to draw up medication only), remove needle, attach over-the-needle catheter (plastic portion only), and lubricate catheter.

Possible Complications

- Respiratory depression
- Rectal trauma

Procedure 21-1

Rectal Administration of Benzodiazepines

1. Position the patient in the decubitus position, knee-chest position, or supine position with a second prehospital professional or the caregiver holding the legs apart.

2. Carefully introduce the lubricated syringe or over-the-needle catheter approximately 5 cm (2 in) into the rectum. Inject the solution into the rectum. Remove the syringe. Hold buttocks closed for 10 seconds. Tape buttocks closed (optional).

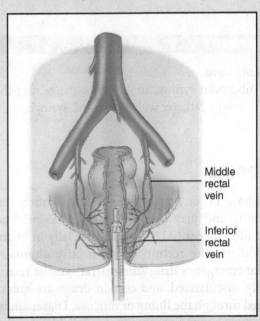

Middle rectal vein

Inferior rectal vein

TIP

The rectal dose of diazepam for infants, children, and adolescents is 0.5 mg/kg, to a maximum dose of 20 mg. Onset of action for rectal diazepam is slower than IV dose.

CAUTION

Administration of diazepam too high into the rectum may decrease its anticonvulsant effect, because the drug may be absorbed differently and broken down more quickly in the liver.

Procedure 22: Spinal Motion Restriction

Jennifer L. Stafford, BSN, CEN, CFRN

INTRODUCTION

Spinal injuries may be subtle or difficult to recognize because of altered mental status; distracting injuries; lack of obvious signs; or in infants and young children, the lack of verbal complaints about neck or back pain. Failure to recognize potential spinal injury can lead to death or permanent disability. Spinal motion restriction should be employed whenever there is a clinical suspicion of cervical spine injury, including high-risk mechanism of injury (where the head, neck, or spine may be involved), pain or tenderness of the spine, or signs or symptoms of weakness or loss of sensation.

INDICATIONS

Any significant mechanism of injury above the clavicles, including the head, neck, face, or axial spine

Acute weakness or loss of sensation after an injury

Pain or tenderness to the neck or spine

Deformity to the neck or spine

Altered mental status after an injury

CONTRAINDICATIONS

Presence of fixed neck deformity

Massive cervical swelling for which collar placement may impinge upon the airway

Need to perform cricothyrotomy

Attempts at applying cervical collar worsen neurologic symptoms or neck pain

The combative child is a relative contraindication because forceful restraint of a combative child with spinal or head injury can worsen the injury.

If the risks of agitation and increased spinal movement from spinal motion restriction are greater than the benefits, consider more acceptable but less definitive stabilization options, and document the circumstances clearly.

EQUIPMENT

Long spine board, scoop stretcher, vacuum splint, or approved EMS stretcher.

Padding materials (blankets, towels)

Rigid cervical collars in pediatric sizes

Straps with fastening device

Wide tape (2 or 3 in)

Optional equipment:

Head cushions from a cervical spine stabilization device (CID)

Rationale

The spinal column is made of 33 articulating bones, and its structure changes significantly during childhood growth. The age of the child and the physical state of spinal growth are important factors in the incidence and types of pediatric spinal injuries. Compared with adults, children younger than 8 years have relatively large heads, weak cervical muscles, and short necks, which make them particularly prone to axial cervical spine injury. The cervical spine matures, with adult patterns of injury, typically at 16 years of age. Whenever the mechanism of injury, signs, or symptoms suggests possible spinal injury, the entire spine must be stabilized. The neck is placed in a cervical collar, and the body is placed in the supine position and in a neutral, in-line position. In field situations where this stabilization technique is not possible, maintain the anatomic stability of the entire spinal column as carefully as possible, and use age-specific considerations in approaching the child to minimize spinal movement.

Procedure 22-1

Spinal Motion Restriction

1. Prepare the child and caregiver for the procedure by explaining actions.

2. Gently align the head and neck into a neutral position similar to the "sniffing position." Do not force neutral position if there is resistance to movement, crepitus, or increased spinal pain.

3. Have an additional rescuer(s) restrain other body parts as needed to reduce motion.

4. Have a second rescuer apply an appropriate-size rigid cervical collar. Evaluate the neck area that will be covered by the cervical collar. Determine the appropriate size with the manufacturer's recommendations. If a correctly sized cervical collar is unavailable, move on to the next step.

5. Logroll the patient while manual cervical spine motion is being restricted to facilitate supine placement onto the spinal restriction device, minimizing flexion, extension, or rotation of the possibly injured spine. Perform the clinical assessment of the patient's back and buttocks during the logroll process and be prepared to treat injuries. In young children, additional padding under the shoulders is often necessary to avoid excessive cervical spine flexion.

Possible Complications

Airway obstruction
Impairment of ventilation
Obscuring hemorrhage or other injuries
Spinal injury from improper technique
Back pain

Procedure 22-2

Securing a Patient to a Spinal Motion Restriction Device

1. Secure the patient's body to the device while manually maintaining the neutral alignment of the head and neck. To secure against lateral movement, pad along the patient's sides to the edge of the device, especially along the pelvis and legs.

2. Stabilize the cervical spine by using blanket rolls, or blocks from the CID, to restrict lateral head motion and rotation and to prevent upward motion of the shoulders. Secure against axial shifts if the board needs to be tilted (going down stairs, fitting into a small elevator, or for elevating the head in cases of head injury).

3. Place straps across the patient at the level of the **axilla**, pelvis, and legs. Do not place straps over the abdomen or use straps to impair movement of the diaphragm.

4. Further secure the head with tape directly above the patient's eyebrows. Avoid chin straps that may complicate airway maintenance.

CAUTION

Do not use sandbags or weighted material because of the risk of injury in the event of movement.

CAUTION

There is no role for spinal motion restriction in penetrating chest or abdominal trauma.

TIP

When using tape, use the longest strips possible to maximize adhesive surface and security.

Procedure 22-3

Releasing and Monitoring Spinal Stabilization

1. Do not release manual head and neck stabilization until the entire spine is properly stabilized.

2. Reassess airway, breathing, and circulation for possible compromise caused by spinal stabilization technique.

3. Assess the patient's distal neurologic status before and after spinal stabilization.

Never release manual neck stabilization until the entire spine is properly stabilized.

The time spent on rigid backboards should be minimized due to the risk of pain and pressure ulcers. Hospitals should be prepared to quickly and carefully remove patients from rigid backboards.

Procedure 23: Needle Thoracostomy

Toni M. Petrillo, MD, FAAP

Possible Complications

Introduction

A pneumothorax occurs when air gets between the two pleural membranes of the lung, a potential space that is virtually empty under normal breathing conditions. Tension pneumothorax develops when the air in the pleural space has enough pressure to shift the internal contents of the chest and impair the function of the lungs, heart, and great vessels. Reduction in blood return to the heart and diminished cardiopulmonary function results in shock and cardiopulmonary arrest if the tension pneumothorax is untreated. The child with tension pneumothorax has usually had positive-pressure ventilation in the field and has physiologic abnormalities on assessment, with evidence of increased work of breathing and hypoxia. While pneumothoraces can occur spontaneously in diseases such as asthma or cystic fibrosis, they rarely result in a tension pneumothorax. Classical adult physical findings, such as a shifted trachea or diminished breath sounds on the affected side, may not be detectable in an infant or child. If cardiac output is severely impaired by the tension pneumothorax, the child also exhibits shock.

INDICATIONS

Penetrating chest wall injury in a child with poor perfusion accompanied by respiratory distress and hypoxia

Blunt chest wall injury in a child with respiratory distress and hypoxia that worsens with assisted ventilation

CONTRAINDICATION

History of a severe bleeding disorder, such as hemophilia (relative)

EQUIPMENT

14- or 16-gauge over-the-needle catheter
30-mL syringe

Skin cleansing solution

Rationale

When the mechanism of injury, signs, and symptoms suggest tension pneumothorax in a child, create an opening between the pleural space and the atmosphere to immediately reduce elevated intrapleural pressure. This helps reexpand the lung, improve venous return, and restore cardiopulmonary function. The easiest method for creating a communication between the pleural space and the outside atmosphere is by producing an open pneumothorax. The technique requires inserting a large-bore needle into the pleural space and leaving it open to the air.

Preparation

1. Position the child supine.
2. Raise the arm above the head on the affected side, and have the caregiver or second rescuer hold it.
3. Select the site:
   - Second intercostal space at the midclavicular line OR
   - Fourth intercostal space at the anterior axillary line
4. Before preparing the site, count the ribs twice to ensure proper site location. The nipple is usually at the fourth intercostal space.
5. Prepare the site with skin cleansing solution.

Possible Complications

- Open pneumothorax
- Hemothorax
- Diaphragm penetration
- Bowel penetration
- Hemopericardium
- Intercostal nerve or vessel or other intrathoracic vessel injury

Procedure 23-1

Needle Thoracostomy

1. Attach the needle, with catheter in place, to the syringe.

2. Insert the needle through the skin at 90 degrees, and advance until the tip hits a rib.

Second intercostal space

90°

3. Advance the needle over the top of the rib margin.

4. Push the needle tip into the pleural space. A slight "pop" is usually felt when the needle pierces the outside pleural membrane or parietal pleura.

5. Pull back the plunger of the needle to aspirate air.

6. Remove the syringe and needle, and leave the catheter in the pleural space, anchored in the chest wall.

7. Monitor work of breathing, circulation to skin, heart rate, respiratory rate, and blood pressure. Consider doing contralateral needle thoracostomy if the child does not improve.

CONTROVERSY

The frequency of tension pneumothorax after blunt chest wall injury is not known, and the indications for needle thoracostomy in this prehospital situation are controversial.

CAUTION

A shifted trachea or diminished breath sounds may not be detectable in an infant or young child with a tension pneumothorax.

TIP

Suspect a tension pneumothorax when a child with chest injury worsens with assisted ventilation.

Procedure 24: Removing and Replacing a Tracheostomy Tube

Wm. Travis Engel, DO, MSc

Mary Otting, RN, BSN, CEN

Introduction

Children with tracheostomy tubes are increasingly common in the prehospital setting. Most of these children live at home and have trained caregivers.

Rarely, a tracheostomy tube problem occurs with a technology-assisted child and 9-1-1 is activated.

INDICATIONS

Decannulation

Obstruction

CONTRAINDICATIONS

Too small size tract or stoma for insertion of a new tracheostomy tube (in this case, insert an endotracheal tube)

Lack of a replacement tracheostomy tube or appropriately sized endotracheal tube

New tract and breathing adequately

EQUIPMENT

Suction device

Sterile suction catheters

Oxygen

Bag-mask device with a mask that is appropriately sized for the patient

Tracheostomy cannulas, appropriately sized for patient and one size smaller, if available

Endotracheal tubes, standard pediatric and adult sizes

Laryngoscope handle with blades

Tape or tracheostomy ties

Gauze pads

5- or 10-mL syringe

Water-soluble lubricant

Scissors

Sterile saline

Stethoscope

TIP

When a tracheostomy tube comes out, the stoma can decrease in size rapidly. Do not hesitate to consider a smaller-sized device if difficulty is encountered attempting to re-insert the tracheostomy tube.

Rationale

The tracheostomy complications most likely to be encountered by EMS personnel include obstruction (from mucus plugging) and displacement. While obstruction often responds to suctioning, in severe cases the mucus may be so thick that suctioning is ineffective. When a tracheostomy tube is displaced, the stoma will begin to close and significant respiratory distress can develop. Both of these scenarios require placement of a new tracheostomy tube or alternative airway management by prehospital personnel in order to save the child's life.

Preparation

1. Ask the caregiver if there are any special problems with the child's trachea or special requirements involving the child's tracheostomy.
2. Ask the caregiver if a replacement tracheostomy tube is available.

3. Speak directly to the child about what to expect, and attempt to enlist his or her cooperation.

4. Place child on pulse oximeter.

Possible Complications

- Creation of a false lumen
- Subcutaneous air
- Pneumomediastinum
- Pneumothorax
- Bleeding at insertion site
- Bleeding through tube
- Mainstem intubation with endotracheal tube (usually right mainstem)

Procedure 24-1

Removing an Old Tracheostomy Tube

1. Position the child with the head and neck hyperextended to expose the tracheostomy site.

2. Apply oxygen over the mouth and nose.

3. If the existing tube has a cuff, deflate it. Connect a 5- to 10-mL syringe to the valve on the pilot balloon. Draw air out until the balloon collapses. Cutting the balloon will not deflate the cuff.

4. Cut or untie the ties that hold the tracheostomy tube in place.

5. Withdraw the tracheostomy tube using a slow, steady, outward and downward motion.

6. Assess airway for patency and adequate ventilation.

7. Provide oxygen and ventilation as needed (through the stoma if necessary).

Procedure 24-2

Replacing the Tracheostomy Tube

1. Insert a tracheostomy tube of the same size and model whenever possible. If this is not available, use a smaller tube or an endotracheal tube of the same inner diameter as the tracheostomy tube.

2. If the tube uses an insertion obturator, place this in the tube. If the tube has an inner and outer cannula, use the outer cannula and obturator for insertion.

3. Moisten or lubricate the tip of the tube (and obturator) with water, sterile saline, or a water-soluble lubricant.

4. Hold the device by the flange (wings), or hold the actual tube like a pencil.

5. Position the head in a neutral or slightly extended position.

6. Gently insert the tube with an arching motion (follow the curvature of the tube) posteriorly and then

downward. Slight traction on the skin above or below the stoma may help.

7. Once the tube is in place, remove the obturator, attach the bag-mask device, and attempt to ventilate. If the tube uses an inner cannula, insert to allow mechanical ventilation with a bag-mask device.

8. Check for proper placement by watching for bilateral chest rise, listening for equal breath sounds, increase in pulse oximeter reading, and observing the patient. Signs of improper placement include lack of chest rise, unusual resistance to assisted ventilation, air in the surrounding tissues, no increase in pulse oximeter reading, and lack of patient improvement.

9. If the tube cannot be inserted, withdraw the tube, administer oxygen, and ventilate as needed.

10. Use a smaller-size tracheostomy tube for the second attempt. If still unsuccessful with a smaller tracheostomy tube, insert an uncuffed endotracheal tube through the stoma. Check the length of the original tracheostomy tube, note the markings on the endotracheal tube, and advance it to the same depth as the original tube. The inserted portion of the endotracheal tube will be approximately one-half the distance needed for oral insertion. Do not advance the tube too far, or it may go into a mainstem bronchus (usually the right).

11. If still unsuccessful, use a suction catheter as a guide. Insert a small, sterile suction catheter through the tracheostomy tube. Without applying suction, insert the suction catheter into the stoma. Slide the tracheostomy tube along the suction catheter and into the stoma until it is in the proper position. Remove the suction catheter. Assess ventilation through the tracheostomy tube.

12. If still unsuccessful, consider orotracheal intubation or transport the patient with ventilation through the stoma using a stoma mask or neonatal mask, or by placing a bag-mask device over the nose and mouth while covering the stoma with a sterile gauze.

13. After proper placement, cut the ends of the tracheostomy ties or tape diagonally (allows for easy insertion), pass through eyelets (openings) on the flanges, and tie around the patient's neck so that only a little finger can pass between the ties and the neck.

TIP

Talk to the caregiver about the size and type of tracheostomy tube and about known problems with the stoma or tube.

TIP

If the patient is in respiratory distress, it may be possible to assist his or her ventilations using a standard bag mask technique over the mouth and nose, so long as the stoma is occluded.

Procedure 54 Removing and Replacing the Tra...

TIP

If unable to reinsert a tracheostomy tube, use a similarly sized or smaller endotracheal tube.

TIP

Keep the suction catheter close at hand.

CAUTION

Do not force a tracheostomy tube, especially through a new stoma site. Consider inserting a smaller-size tracheostomy or endotracheal tube.

CAUTION

Do not advance an endotracheal tube too far through the stoma.

Procedure 25: Tourniquet Application

Wm. Travis Engel, DO, MSc

Mary Otting, RN, BSN, CEN

Introduction

Trauma and unintentional injury have long been the leading causes of mortality and morbidity for children living in the United States. Hypovolemia secondary to uncontrolled hemorrhage is the leading cause of shock in pediatric trauma victims, and the chances of death or disability rise rapidly once shock sets in. Advances in trauma care have demonstrated that hemorrhage control in the prehospital setting is achievable, and the use of tourniquets to meet this goal is both safe and effective. The probability of modern day EMS professionals encountering pediatric victims with uncontrolled bleeding is increasing, and the importance of hemorrhage control as an essential skill for the prehospital provider cannot be overstated.

Hypovolemia from uncontrolled hemorrhage is the leading cause of shock in pediatric trauma victims. Establishing hemorrhage control as quickly as possible to prevent blood loss and subsequent shock remains the highest priority when caring for a victim of trauma. Rapid placement of a tourniquet when direct pressure fails to control bleeding is often the single most important intervention prehospital providers can take to increase a victim's likelihood of survival.

INDICATION

Uncontrolled hemorrhage refractory to the application of direct pressure

CONTRAINDICATIONS

Embedded or impaled object at the site of intended application

Fracture at the site of intended application

EQUIPMENT

Tourniquet (commercial device or improvised)

Rationale

There are very few absolute contraindications to tourniquet application, and often they can be overcome. If there is an embedded object or fracture at the site of intended application, the prehospital provider should attempt to place the tourniquet at a more proximal location if possible. When it is not possible to position the tourniquet more proximally, then the provider should consider taking the necessary steps to control hemorrhage with pressure.

Junctional hemorrhage is bleeding due to an injury at or around the site where an extremity joins the torso. This includes the base of the neck, areas high in the groin region (proximal to the inguinal ligament), the gluteal region, the perineum, and the axillary region. Junctional hemorrhage is not amenable to tourniquet application due to anatomic location. While tourniquet application is not reasonable at these sites, junctional hemorrhage is compressible and will generally respond when the deep vessels proximal to the injury are compressed with significant force.

TIP

There are many styles of commercially available tourniquet devices. The type and style used by prehospital personnel are based on what device a particular agency chooses to use for their service. With this in mind, emergency medical services (EMS) professionals must practice often with whatever style device they will use in an emergency in order to maintain proficiency with that device.

TIP

When a commercially available tourniquet is unavailable, or if the patient is too small to properly use a commercial device, an improvised tourniquet is an acceptable alternative. Improvised tourniquets may be fashioned from common items including an item of clothing at least 2 inches wide with a windlass style device to apply sufficient pressure. A tightly inflated blood pressure cuff can serve as an improvised tourniquet if EMS personnel are equipped with the appropriate size. The cuff should be checked periodically to ensure there is no leak and it remains inflated.

TIP

Commercially available tourniquets are designed to tighten using one of two methods: a windlass-style device or a ratcheting mechanism. A windlass is a stiff rod that is inserted between the skin and the tourniquet or installed as part of a commercially available device. It is twisted to take up any slack and apply compression to the affected extremity. A windlass-type mechanism can be used with an improvised tourniquet.

A ratcheting device uses a lever-style mechanism to advance a ridged belt incrementally, locking it into position with each advancement. Each time it is advanced, it takes up the slack in the tourniquet and applies greater pressure. This style of mechanism cannot be improvised and is only available on commercial devices.

CONTROVERSY

There was a period of time where the use of tourniquets fell out of favor over concern that they cause ischemic injury and may lead to a higher incidence of limb loss when applied in the prehospital setting. There is now a mounting level of evidence that refutes these claims. Multiple studies have concluded that tourniquet use does not increase ischemic injury or limb loss when used to control massive hemorrhage. It has also been established that the benefit of hemorrhage control and increased chances of survival outweigh any negligible risk of limb ischemia and loss that may be present. The overwhelming consensus is that prehospital use of tourniquets for hemorrhage control saves lives and tourniquet application should happen as soon as possible for patients with uncontrolled hemorrhage.

Preparation

1. Place the patient in a position that protects the airway when possible (generally supine or recumbent).
2. If possible, expose the wounded area (do not delay treatment for this).
3. Select and prepare an appropriate commercial tourniquet device, or fashion an improvised tourniquet if a suitable commercial device is unavailable.

TIP

At the time of publication, the only commercially available device specifically designed for pediatric patients is the Child/Pediatric Ratcheting Medical Tourniquet®. The pediatric specification is designed for patients less than 55 kg or 120 lb. It is effective for limb circumferences as small as 2.5 inches (approximately 4 months and under). The combat application tourniquet (CAT windlass-style) can be tightened to a limb circumference of 5 inches, and could be used on an infant greater than 4 months. While other devices are not contraindicated in pediatric patients, they may be too large in some cases. If an appropriately sized commercially available tourniquet is unavailable, fashion an alternative device for use.

Possible Complication

- Limb ischemia (remote)

Procedure 25-1

Tourniquet Application

1. Have a partner or the victim apply direct pressure to the site of bleeding if possible.

2. Place the tourniquet on the affected limb, and position it 2–3 inches above the site of bleeding. Do not place the tourniquet on a joint; go above the joint. Wrap and secure the tourniquet device around the limb per the manufacturer's directions.

3. Pull the strap through the buckle device to draw the tourniquet down as tightly as possible before using the ratchet or windlass to apply compression. If more than two or three fingers can be inserted between into the

tourniquet and the limb, it should be tightened further before applying compression.

4. Turn the windlass rod or advance the ratcheting device until bleeding has stopped.

5. Secure the windlass rod or ratcheting device in place. Check again that bleeding has been stopped.

6. Secure any remaining tourniquet band or material so that it does not catch or snag when moving the patient.

7. Always indicate the time that the tourniquet was applied by writing it directly on the device once it is secured.

TIP

Generally, once a tourniquet is applied, it should not be loosened or removed unless directed to do so by medical control. In situations where transport may be significantly delayed, a physician may request that you either re-position the tourniquet to a location that is 2–3 inches proximal to the wound, or apply a second tourniquet 2–3 inches proximal to the wound and then release the original tourniquet. This will allow for blood flow to as much of the injured extremity as possible, without sacrificing hemorrhage control.

TIP

The tourniquet should be rapidly placed as proximally on the wounded extremity as possible to facilitate rapid application and eliminate unnecessary delay in hemorrhage control.

TIP

The use of hemostatic agents in conjunction with tourniquets or in situations where tourniquets are unavailable or impractical is becoming more common civilian EMS. When available, the use of hemostatic gauze and wound packing may be appropriate when a tourniquet is unavailable or ineffective. Follow local protocols and the advice of medical direction when performing these skills.

TIP

Continue to check periodically that bleeding remains controlled. Routinely assess distal pulses in the affected extremity to ensure they are absent and judge that the tourniquet has been tightened sufficiently.

TIP

If available, packing a wound and direct pressure remain the best options to control and stop pediatric hemorrhage.

SUGGESTED REFERENCE

Ross EM, Bolleter S, Simon E, et al. Pediatric extremity hemorrhage and tourniquet use. *J Emerg Med.* 2018. https://www.jems.com/2018/11/01 /pediatric-extremity-hemorrhage-and-tournquet-use. Accessed October 15, 2019.

Medication Formulary

Ali Paplaskas, PharmD, BCCCP

Michael J. Stoner, MD, FAAP

Note: The following drugs may be used for pediatric prehospital care. Certain drugs may not be available in some EMS systems per local policy. The drugs in tables designated by a green bar are core drugs commonly used in EMS systems. The drugs designated by a yellow bar are optional drugs that are sometimes used for children in EMS systems.

Acetaminophen, APAP

Use: Analgesic, antipyretic	**Recommended Dose**	**Precaution:** Ensure proper concentration. Use with caution in patients with liver disease.
	15 mg/kg (oral/G-tube)	
	15–20 mg/kg (rectal)	**Adverse Reactions:** Nausea, vomiting
	Maximum Dose	
	1 g	

Activated Charcoal

Use: Gastric decontamination	**Recommended Dose**	**Precaution:** Based on local EMS policy, the prehospital professional should consult either medical oversight or poison control (1-800-222-1222). Iron, lithium, alcohols, ethylene glycol, alkalis, fluoride, mineral acids, and potassium do not bind to activated charcoal.
	Initial dose:	
	<12 years: 1 g/kg (oral)	
	Maximum Dose	Administer as soon as possible after ingestion. Avoid aspiration. If airway reflexes are impaired, the risk of administering activated charcoal may outweigh the benefits. Commercially available preparations include charcoal with sorbitol (used to produce catharsis) and charcoal in water. Fatal hypernatremic dehydration has been reported after repeated doses of charcoal with sorbitol. Potentially fatal toxicities seen in neonates, such as seizures, lactic acidosis, and respiratory depression, have been seen with preparations containing propylene glycol.
	100 g	
		Adverse Reactions: Vomiting, constipation, obstruction, intestinal bezoar, diarrhea, dehydration, pulmonary aspiration, mouth discoloration

Adenosine

Use: Supraventricular tachycardia (SVT), regular monomorphic wide-complex tachycardia

Recommended Dose

0.1 mg/kg rapid IV or IO bolus over 1–2 seconds

Repeat at 0.2 mg/kg

Maximum Dose

First dose: 6 mg

Second dose: 12 mg

Precaution: Use continuous cardiac monitoring.

Avoid use in second- or third-degree AV block, sick sinus syndrome.

Administer at IV site closest to patient's heart, follow with a rapid saline flush (5–10 mL).

Adverse Reactions: Nausea, hypotension, dyspnea, bronchospasm, chest pain/pressure, tingling, heart block, dysrhythmias, facial flushing, metallic taste

Bronchoconstriction may occur in asthmatics.

Albuterol

Use: Prevention and acute relief of bronchospasm, prophylaxis for exercise-induced bronchospasm

Recommended Dose

Nebulizer solution (1.25 mg/3 mL, 2.5 mg/3 mL, 5 mg/mL)

Dose: 2.5 mg every 15–20 minutes for 3 doses. Repeat up to 10 mg every 1–4 hours as needed. Dilute in minimum of 2–3 mL of saline if needed for adequate nebulization. May use continuously for status asthmaticus.

MDI: 4–8 puffs (90 mcg/puff) every 15–20 minutes for 3 doses. Repeat every 1–4 hours as needed.

Maximum Dose

Not established for status asthmaticus

Precaution: Tremors and tachycardia are common.

Adverse Reactions: Nausea, palpitations, headache, dizziness, tremor, tachycardia

Amiodarone

Use: Life-threatening ventricular arrhythmias: ventricular fibrillation or tachycardia

Recommended Dose

5 mg/kg IV or IO push for ventricular fibrillation or pulseless ventricular tachycardia

5 mg/kg IV or IO infusion over 20–60 minutes for wide complex tachycardia

May repeat initial loading dose twice for acute treatment

Maximum Dose

300 mg/dose

15 mg/kg/day

Precaution: Must dilute with 20 mL of 5% dextrose prior to administration to avoid thrombophlebitis and hypotension.

May be given undiluted in pulseless VT of VF.

May cause hypotension and prolonged Q-T interval; slow rate of infusion if hypotension or bradycardia develop. Should not use in combination with procainamide.

Contraindicated in severe sinus node dysfunction, marked sinus bradycardia, second- and third-degree AV block.

Adverse Reactions: Hypotension, bradycardia, dysrhythmias, vomiting

Aspirin

Use: Analgesic, antipyretic

Recommended Dose

10–15 mg/kg

Maximum Dose

1 g

Precaution: Avoid use in children <18 years with chickenpox or influenza illness due to association with Reye's syndrome. Not routinely used in pediatrics.

Adverse Reactions: Nausea, vomiting, abdominal pain, ulcers, rash, urticaria, bronchospasm

Atropine

Use: Sinus bradycardia, chemical nerve gas and organophosphate pesticide poisoning

Recommended Dose

0.02 mg/kg IV or IO

0.04–0.06 mg/kg/dose if given via ET tube

May repeat dose every 5 minutes to maximum total dose of 1 mg for a child and 2 mg for an adolescent

Organophosphate/carbamate/nerve agent poisoning: 0.05–0.1 mg/kg IM, IV, or IO; repeat every 5–10 minutes as needed with doubling doses titrated to pulmonary status

Maximum Dose

Single dose: 0.5 mg for a child, 1 mg for an adolescent

Precaution: Atropine sulfate comes in different concentrations; calculate dosage accordingly. Avoid in tachydysrhythmias. Caution in children with brain damage or spastic paralysis.

Anticholinesterase poisonings may require large doses, so maximum dose above does not apply (will also need pralidoxime).

Slow IV injection may result in paradoxical bradycardia.

Adverse Reactions: Dry mouth, blurred vision, tachycardia, constipation, urinary retention

Calcium Chloride

Use: Ionized hypocalcemia, hyperkalemia, hypermagnesemia, calcium channel blocker toxicity

Recommended for cardiac resuscitation only in cases of documented hyperkalemia, hypocalcemia, or calcium channel blocker toxicity

Recommended Dose

20 mg/kg IV or IO slowly (if using 10% CaCl, dose is 0.2 mL/kg)

Inject slowly while monitoring heart rate.

Repeat dose in 10 minutes as necessary for desired clinical effects.

Maximum Dose

2,000 mg in cardiac arrest when hyperkalemia, hypocalcemia, or calcium channel blocker toxicity are present/suspected, 1,000 mg for all other indications

Precaution: Stop injection if symptomatic bradycardia occurs. Calcium chloride administration results in a more rapid increase in ionized calcium concentrations than calcium gluconate and is preferred for the critically ill child.

Infuse at a maximum rate of 50–100 mg/minute. During cardiac arrest, may administer over 20 seconds.

Extravascular administration can result in severe skin injury. Highly irritating to tissues. Avoid scalp vein, small hand or foot veins for IV administration.

Adverse Reactions: Tissue extravasation and necrosis; may exacerbate metabolic acidosis; hypotension, bradycardia, arrhythmias, ventricular fibrillation

Calcium Gluconate (preferred in neonates)

Use: Ionized hypocalcemia, hyperkalemia, hypermagnesemia, calcium channel blocker toxicity

Recommended for cardiac resuscitation only in cases of documented hyperkalemia, hypocalcemia, or calcium channel blocker toxicity

Recommended Dose

60 mg/kg IV or IO slowly (if using 10% calcium gluconate, dose is 0.6 mL/kg). Inject slowly while monitoring heart rate.

Repeat dose in 10 minutes as necessary for desired clinical effects.

Maximum Dose

3,000 mg in cardiac arrest

Precaution: Stop injection if symptomatic bradycardia occurs. Calcium chloride administration results in a more rapid increase in ionized calcium concentrations than calcium gluconate and is preferred for the critically ill child.

Infuse at maximum rate of 100 mg/minute.

Extravascular administration can result in severe skin injury. Highly irritating to tissues. Avoid scalp vein and small hand or foot veins for IV administration.

Adverse Reactions: Tissue extravasation and necrosis, hypotension, bradycardia, arrhythmias, ventricular fibrillation

Dexamethasone

Use: Croup, asthma

Recommended Dose

Croup:

0.15–0.6 mg/kg IV, IM, or PO

Asthma:

0.6–1.0 mg/kg IV, IM, or PO

Maximum Dose

16 mg/day

Precaution: Long-acting glucocorticoid

Parenteral dexamethasone may be mixed with an oral flavored solution and given orally.

Rapid IV administration is associated with perineal burning and tingling; infuse over 1–4 minutes to decrease perineal discomfort.

Oral liquid products may contain alcohol.

Adverse Reactions: Sodium and fluid retention, hyperglycemia

Diazepam

Use: Seizures, agitation

Recommended Dose

IV: 0.1 mg/kg every 5–10 minutes. Administer over approximately 2 minutes to avoid pain at intravenous site.

PR: 0.5 mg/kg up to 20 mg

Maximum Dose

IV: 10 mg/dose

PR: 20 mg

Precaution: There is an increased incidence of apnea when combined with other sedative agents or when given rapidly. Be prepared to provide respiratory support. Monitor oxygen saturation. Avoid extravasation to prevent venous thrombosis or phlebitis. Avoid prolonged use of parenteral diazepam because it contains 40% propylene glycol as a diluent.

Do not exceed 1–2 mg/minute administration time to prevent hypotension or respiratory arrest.

Adverse Reactions: Respiratory depression, drowsiness, bradycardia, hypotension, apnea, pain at injection site

Diphenhydramine

Use: Anaphylaxis, antihistamine

Recommended Dose

1 mg/kg IV or IO slow push, or PO

Maximum Dose

IV: 50 mg

Precaution: May cause sedation and respiratory suppression, especially if using other sedative agents. May cause hypotension. Overdose may cause hallucinations and seizures.

Rapid IV administration may precipitate seizures. Administer undiluted at a rate of ≤25 mg/minute.

All doses may cause paradoxical excitement or agitation.

Adverse Reactions: Drowsiness, dry mouth, constipation, urinary retention

Dopamine

Use: Hypotension, shock

Recommended Dose

Neonate: 2–20 mcg/kg/ minute IV or IO infusion

Children: 2–20 mcg/kg/minute IV or IO infusion

Titrate up to desired effect by 5–10 mcg/kg/minute increments:

  5 mcg/kg/minute = low dose (renal blood flow and urine output)

  10 mcg/kg/minute = moderate dose (beta activity—increases HR, contractility, and blood pressure)

  20 mcg/kg/minute = high dose (alpha activity— vasoconstriction and increasing blood pressure)

Maximum Dose

20 mcg/kg/minute

Precaution: Infusion rates greater than 20 mcg/ kg/minute may produce extreme peripheral vasoconstriction and ischemia. Mix with great caution. Extravascular administration can result in severe skin injury. Avoid small veins, central line preferred. Dopamine is inactivated in an alkaline solution. Correct hypovolemia prior to use.

Adverse Reactions: Ectopic beats, tachycardia, palpitations, vasoconstriction, dyspnea, vomiting

Epinephrine

Use: Croup, anaphylaxis, acute asthma, cardiac arrest, shock

Recommended Dose

Anaphylaxis: IM, 0.01 mg/kg/dose = 0.01 mL/kg/dose of 1 mg/mL concentration (maximum 0.3 mg = 0.3 mL). Repeat dose every 5–15 minutes.

Anaphylactic shock: IV 0.01 mg/kg of 0.1 mg/mL concentration (maximum 0.5 mg)

Cardiac arrest:

Newborn: IV/IO/ET 0.01-0.03 mg/kg of 0.1 mg/mL concentration

Infants and children: IV/IO 0.01 mg/kg of 0.1 mg/mL concentration

ET 0.1mg/kg of 1mg/mL concentration

Croup: 0.25–0.5 mg/kg of 1 mg/mL concentration in 3 mL of NS by inhalation (maximum 5 mL/dose)

Shock: 0.1–1 mcg/kg/minute 0.1 mg/mL concentration

Racemic epinephrine (2.25%) for croup: 0.1 mL/kg by inhalation (maximum 0.5 mL) in 3 mL of NS, may repeat every 20 minutes

Precaution: Use length-based resuscitation tape or computerized software to verify correct dose. Read concentration on label carefully. Incompatible with alkaline solutions. Extravascular administration can result in severe skin injury.

Anaphylaxis: Preferred location is IM anterolateral aspect of middle third thigh. Some anaphylactic reactions require large doses of epinephrine that may be administered IV.

Cardiac arrest: If administered through an endotracheal tube, follow with saline flush or dilute in isotonic saline flush (1 to 5 mL) based on patient length/weight.

Adverse Reactions: Tachycardia, palpitations, cardiac dysrhythmias, diaphoresis, vomiting, headache, dizziness

Fentanyl

Use: Analgesic, anesthetic for intubation and maintenance

Recommended Dose

IV: 1 mcg/kg/dose every 30–60 minutes

Intranasal: 1–2 mcg/kg

Maximum Dose

100 mcg

Titrate to effect

Precaution: There is an increased incidence of apnea when combined with other sedative agents, particularly benzodiazepines. Avoid rapid IV infusion; inject slowly over 3–5 minutes. If given rapidly IV, may cause chest wall or glottic rigidity, which may be reversed with a muscle relaxant.

Intranasal administration: Give one-half in each nostril using atomizer device or drip into nostril with syringe. Maximum dose is 1 mL/nare

Adverse Reactions: Apnea, bradycardia, nausea, vomiting

Flumazenil

Use: Reverse sedative effects of benzodiazepines, EXCEPT those receiving benzodiazepines for seizures

Recommended Dose

IV: 0.01–0.02 mg/kg over 15 seconds; repeat every 1 minute as needed. When IV access is unavailable, may be given IM.

Maximum Dose

0.2 mg/dose and to cumulative total dose of 0.05 mg/kg or 1 mg

Precaution: May precipitate acute withdrawal in dependent patients. May precipitate seizures in high-risk patients on chronic benzodiazepines, sedative/hypnotics, or other co-ingestants in an overdose. Observe for re-sedation. Avoid single bolus injection.

Adverse Reactions: Rebound sedation or respiratory depression due to its short duration of action; rebound sedation especially common in pediatrics age 1–5 years; flushing, nausea, blurred vision, agitation, thrombophlebitis, seizures

Do not give to patients receiving benzodiazepines for seizures.

Fosphenytoin

Use: Seizures, status epilepticus

Recommended Dose

Status epilepticus:

15–20 mg phenytoin equivalents (PE)/kg IV, IM, or IO. Do not administer faster than 2 mg PE/kg/minute or a total of 150 mg PE/minute.

Maximum Dose

1,500 mg PE

Precaution: Rate of infusion should not exceed 150 mg PE/minute or 2 mg PE/kg/minute. Reduce rate of infusion if heart rate decreases by 10 beats/minute or hypotension occurs. Dosages and concentrations are expressed as phenytoin sodium equivalents. Rapid IV administration may produce hypotension, may dilute in NS or D_5W.

IM administration not preferred, but may use quadricep area if needed.

Adverse Reactions: Hypotension, bradycardia, central nervous system depression, ataxia, dizziness, headache, paresthesia, pruritus; itching is common and is controlled by reducing flow rate

Furosemide

Use: Fluid overload, congestive heart failure, diuresis, edema, pulmonary edema, hypertension

Recommended Dose

Children: 1–2 mg/kg IV, IO, or IM

Maximum Dose

40 mg

Precaution: Do not give to child with hypovolemia. Contraindicated in anuria.

Adverse Reactions: Hypotension, electrolyte depletion, alkalosis, tinnitus, ototoxic

Glucagon

Use: Beta-blocker or calcium channel blocker overdose, hypoglycemia

Recommended Dose

Hypoglycemia due to insulin excess:

Children: 0.02–0.03 mg/kg for those <20 kg; for those >20 kg, 1 mg IV, IO, or IM; repeat every 20 minutes if needed for clinical effect. Total 3 doses.

Beta-blocker or calcium channel blocker overdose: IV: 0.05–0.15 mg/kg followed by 0.07 mg/kg/hour (maximum of 5 mg/hour) infusion.

Maximum Dose

Pediatric: 1 mg

Precaution: Use immediately after reconstitution. Caution in patients with pheochromocytoma. Supplemental carbohydrates (IV dextrose) should be given as soon as possible.

Adverse Reactions: Nausea, vomiting, hypotension, tachycardia. Nausea/vomiting incidence higher with rapid administration and higher doses.

Glucose (Dextrose)

Use: Hypoglycemia

Recommended Dose

Newborn: 2 mL/kg 10% dextrose IV or IO

Neonate: 5 mL/kg 10% dextrose IV or IO

<2 years: 5 mL/kg 10% dextrose IV or IO

>2 years: 1 mL/kg 50% dextrose IV or IO push or 2 mL/kg 25% dextrose IV or IO or 5 mL/kg of 10% dextrose IV or IO

Maximum Dose

Doses guided by repeated serum glucose level determinations

Precaution: Depending on situation, hypoglycemia may re-occur. Caution in multiple concentrations.

In emergency situations, 25% dextrose may be used peripherally in infants and 50% in adolescents.

Adverse Reactions: Hyperglycemia, thrombophlebitis, extravasation, hyponatremia

Hydrocortisone

Use: Acute adrenal insufficiency/adrenal crisis, septic shock

Recommended Dose

1–2 mg/kg IV, IO, or IM

Maximum Dose

100 mg

Precaution: Do not use for head injury. Use with caution in patients with hypertension, heart failure, renal or hepatic impairment.

If given IM, avoid deltoid muscle due to higher incidence of soft tissue atrophy.

Adverse Reactions: Arrhythmias, hypertension, adrenal suppression

Ibuprofen

Use: Analgesic, antipyretic

Recommended Dose

10 mg/kg/dose PO

Maximum Dose

400 mg in children <12 years of age

Precaution: Cross-reacts with aspirin allergy, gastrointestinal bleeding. Liquid products may contain alcohol. Do not use in patients with kidney disease.

Do not use in infants <6 months.

Verify concentration of liquid products.

Adverse Reactions: Vomiting, gastritis, ulcer formation, rash

Ipratropium

Use: Asthma

Recommended Dose

Nebulized solution (0.5 mg/2.5 mL):

Children <12 years: 0.25 mg nebulized every 20 minutes for three doses

Children >12 years: 0.5 mg nebulized every 20 minutes for three doses

Maximum Dose

0.5 mg

Precaution: Use with albuterol every 20 minutes x 3. May be administered with or without further dilution.

Adverse Reactions: Tachycardia, dry mouth, headache, cough, hoarseness, blurred vision

Ketamine

Use: Anesthesia for intubation, pain control, and agitation

Recommended Dose

IV: 1–2 mg/kg for intubation and pain control

IM: 4–5 mg/kg for intubation and pain, 4 mg/kg for agitation

Intranasal: 5 mg/kg

Maximum Dose

100 mg

Precaution: Administer slowly over 1 minute. Emergence reactions may occur up to 24 hours postoperatively: delirium, hallucinations, vivid dreams. Avoid use in patients with increased intraocular pressure or bowel obstruction.

Hypersalivation/lacrimation common in pediatrics, may be used in combination with anticholinergic to decrease incidence.

American College of Emergency Physicians considers the use of ketamine in those <3 months of age an absolute contraindication due to high risk of airway complications.

Several concentrations of products available. If giving Intranasal, use 50 mg/mL or 100 mg/mL, dilute to concentration of 20 mg/mL and administer half in each nostril using atomizer device or needleless syringe.

Adverse Reactions: Hallucinations, tonic-clonic movements, nausea, vomiting, decreased cough reflex, nystagmus, tachycardia, bronchospasm, hypertension, bradycardia, hypotension, apnea. May cause purposeless movements.

Lidocaine

Use: Ventricular tachycardia, ventricular fibrillation, wide-complex SVT

Recommended Dose

Shock-refractory VF or pulseless VT: IV/IO loading dose = 1 mg/kg; repeat in 10–15 minutes for two doses if needed; IV continuous infusion after loading dose: 20–50 mcg/kg/minute

ET: 2–2.5 times the IV dose

Maximum Dose

IV: 3 mg/kg

Precaution: Contraindicated in complete heart block and wide complex tachycardia due to accessory conduction pathways. Excessive dosage may result in myocardial depression, hypotension, agitation, or seizures. Hypersensitivity to amide anesthetics. If administered through an ET tube, follow the dose with saline flush or dilute in isotonic saline flush (1 to 5 mL) based on patient size.

Adverse Reactions: Arrhythmias, seizures, respiratory depression or arrest

Lorazepam

Use: Anticonvulsant, anxiety, sedation

Recommended Dose

Status epilepticus:

    0.05–0.1 mg/kg IV or IO over 2–5 minutes; repeat 0.05 mg/kg second dose in 5–15 minutes if needed

Sedation/anxiety:

    0.05 mg/kg IV or IO over 2–5 minutes; repeat 0.05 mg/kg second dose in 5–15 minutes if needed

Maximum Dose

4 mg/dose

Precaution: Beware of respiratory depression. There is an increased incidence of apnea when combined with other sedative agents. Monitor oxygen saturation, and be prepared to provide respiratory support. Do not reverse in patient with seizures.

Dilute with equal volume of D_5W or NS.

IV preparations contain alcohol.

Adverse Reactions: Bradycardia, hypotension, apnea, confusion, hallucinations, myoclonic jerking in preterm infants

Mannitol

Use: Diuresis, reduces intracranial pressure

Recommended Dose

IV: 0.25–1 g/kg

Maximum Dose

2 g/kg body weight

Precaution: Inspect vials for crystals; if present, re-dissolve by warming. Use 5-micron filter for 20% solutions or greater. Avoid excessive fluid loss with diuresis to prevent dehydration and electrolyte imbalance.

Administer over 20–60 minutes.

Adverse Reactions: Dehydration, fluid and electrolyte imbalance, headache, hypovolemia, seizures, water intoxication

Methylprednisolone

Use: Asthma, croup

Recommended Dose

1–2 mg/kg/dose IV or IO

Maximum Dose

60 mg/day

Precaution: Rapid IV push of high doses (>250 mg) in <20 minutes may cause hypotension, arrhythmias, and sudden death.

Caution multiple dosage forms, use methylprednisolone sodium succinate IV.

May contain alcohol.

Adverse Reactions: Edema, pituitary-adrenal suppression, hypokalemia, peptic ulcer, nausea, vomiting

Midazolam

Use: Anxiety, seizures

Recommended Dose

Status epilepticus:

IV or IO: 0.1 mg/kg; IM or intranasal: 0.2 mg/kg

May repeat in 5–15 minutes as needed

Sedation:

IV, IO, or IM: 0.05–0.1 mg/kg
Intranasal: 0.2 mg/kg

Maximum Dose

6 months to 5 years: 6 mg

>6 years: 10 mg

Precaution: Avoid rapid IV administration, which may produce respiratory arrest and seizures. There is an increased incidence of apnea when combined with other sedative agents, particularly benzodiazepines. Be prepared to provide respiratory support, regardless of route of administration. Monitor oxygen saturation. May be reversed with flumazenil. Myoclonus may occur in premature infants. Paradoxical excitation may occur in children. May be reversed with flumazenil.

Multiple concentration parenteral products available.

Use 5 mg/mL for intranasal administration, administer one-half dose in each nare using atomizer or needleless syringe (maximum 1 mL in each nostril).

Administer IM injection undiluted into large muscle, preferably anterior-lateral aspect of thigh in pediatric patients.

Adverse Reactions: Bradycardia, hypotension, cardiac arrest, apnea, respiratory depression

Morphine

Use: Severe acute and chronic pain

Recommended Dose

Neonates: 0.05 mg/kg IM, IV, IO

Infants and children: 0.05–0.1 mg/kg IM, IV, IO

Adolescents: 3–4 mg IV or IO, repeat in 5 minutes as needed

Maximum Dose

Neonates: 0.1 mg/kg

Infants, children, and adolescents: 10 mg

Precaution: Pediatric patients are more sensitive to the effects of opiates. Hypersensitivity to similar opiates. Some products may contain sulfites. There is an increased incidence of apnea when combined with other sedative agents, particularly benzodiazepines. Be prepared to provide respiratory support, regardless of route of administration. Monitor oxygen saturation. May be reversed with naloxone.

IM not preferred route of administration due to local tissue irritation, pain, variable absorption and lag time to peak effect.

Adverse Reactions: Respiratory depression, hypotension, rash, constipation

Naloxone

Use: Opiate intoxication

Recommended Dose

Pediatric: 0.1 mg/kg/dose IV, IO, IM, ET, intranasal

Repeat dose every 2–3 minutes if needed

If given via ET tube, administer 2–3 times IV dose

Maximum dose was 2 mg, but overdose with synthetic opioids need more

Precaution: Dilute to 1–2 mL with normal saline for ET use.

May induce acute withdrawal in opioid dependency. Patients who receive naloxone should be continuously observed for re-narcotization for at least 2 hours after last dose of naloxone. Doses may be repeated as needed to maintain opiate reversal. IM absorption may be erratic. Do not administer naloxone to a newborn whose mother is suspected of recently abusing drugs due to risk of acute withdrawal in the infant.

If administered intranasally, alternate nostrils for repeated doses.

Nitrous Oxide, Dinitrogen Oxide, N₂O, Laughing Gas

Use: Analgesia, sedation

Recommended Dose

25%–50% with oxygen 50:50

Maximum Dose

70%

Precaution: Asphyxiation may occur

Adverse Reactions: Malignant hyperthermia, cardiac dysrhythmias, nausea, vomiting, delirium

Norepinephrine

Use: Distributive shock

Recommended Dose

0.05–0.1 mcg/kg/minute IV, titrate to desired response

Maximum Dose

2 mcg/kg/minute

Precaution: Double check concentration and infusion rate. Avoid scalp veins.

Ensure adequate volume replacement prior to initiation.

Central line preferred, extravasation may cause severe tissue necrosis.

Adverse Reactions: Bradycardia, hypertension, arrhythmias, palpitations, pallor, ischemic necrosis, organ ischemia

Phenobarbital

Use: Status epilepticus, sedation

Recommended Dose

20 mg/kg IV or IO over 20 minutes (1 mg/kg/minute); not to exceed 30 mg/minute

May repeat once after 15 minutes if needed to maximum total dose of 40 mg/kg

Maximum Dose

1,000 mg

Precaution: There is an increased incidence of apnea when combined with other sedative agents. Be prepared to provide respiratory support. Monitor oxygen saturation. Avoid extravasation because parenteral solutions are very alkaline.

Parenteral formulations may contain alcohol.

Adverse Reactions: Drowsiness, hypotension, apnea, paradoxical excitation, respiratory depression, thrombophlebitis

Phenytoin

Use: Status epilepticus

Recommended Dose

Neonate: 10 mg/kg

Children: 20 mg/kg IV or IO over 20 minutes (1 mg/kg/minute); not to exceed 50 mg/minute

Maximum Dose

1,000 mg

Precaution: Incompatible with glucose solutions. Monitor heart rate and reduce infusion if rate decreases by 10 beats/minute. Rapid IV administration may trigger ventricular fibrillation and cardiac arrest. Avoid extravasation.

Injections may contain propylene glycol and benzyl alcohol.

0.22- to 0.55-micron in-line filter preferred for IV piggyback solutions.

Adverse Reactions: Bradycardia, hypotension, arrhythmias, cardiovascular collapse, nystagmus, drowsiness, purple glove syndrome

Pralidoxime Chloride, 2-PAM, 2-Pyridine Aldoxime Methochloride

Use: Organophosphate poisoning, carbamate insecticide poisoning with nicotinic symptoms, anticholinesterase poisoning

Recommended Dose

25–50 mg/kg IV over 5–30 minutes, then 10 mg/kg/hour or repeat load after 1 hour

IM: 15 mg/kg (up to 600 mg), repeat as needed every 15 minutes to a maximum of 45 mg/kg

Maximum Dose

2 g/dose

Large total amounts may be required in a severe poisoning.

Precaution: Rapid IV administration may cause tachycardia, laryngospasm, muscle rigidity, and transient neuromuscular blockade. Infuse IV loading dose over 15–30 minutes, not to exceed 200 mg/minute.

IV route preferred, but may be given IM when IV route is not immediately accessible.

May be used in conjunction with atropine.

Adverse Reactions: Nausea, headache, dizziness, diplopia, hyperventilation

Rocuronium Bromide

Use: Adjunct to general anesthesia to facilitate tracheal intubation and provide skeletal muscle relaxation during mechanical ventilation

Recommended Dose

IV: 1 mg/kg

Maximum Dose

1.2 mg/kg

Precaution: Ventilatory support is necessary. Prepare to respond with airway management. Do not mix with alkaline solutions. May interact with certain antibiotics that have neuromuscular blocking actions (e.g., aminoglycosides) and enhance neuromuscular blockade. Toxicity may be increased in patients with pulmonary disease.

Adverse Reactions: Muscle weakness, hypotension or hypertension, arrhythmias, tachycardia, bronchospasm, hiccoughs

Sodium Bicarbonate

Use: Cyclic antidepressant overdose, hyperkalemia

Recommended Dose

Pediatric: 1 mEq/kg IV or IO slowly

Maximum Dose

50 mEq/dose

Precaution: Do not mix with calcium, dopamine, or epinephrine. May cause tissue necrosis from IV extravasation. Caution with renal impairment. No more than 0.5 mEq/mL for neonatal use.

Adverse Reactions: Cerebral hemorrhage, edema, hypernatremia, hypokalemia, hypocalcemia, metabolic alkalosis

Succinylcholine, Suxamethonium

Use: Adjunct to general anesthesia, endotracheal intubation, mechanical ventilation

Recommended Dose

IV, IO, or IM: 1–2 mg/kg/dose

Precaution: Contraindicated in conditions associated with increased ICP, severe burns, spinal cord injury, neuromuscular disease, myopathy, or malignant hyperthermia. When these contraindications exist, use a nondepolarizing muscle relaxant such as rocuronium. Ventilatory support is necessary. If cardiac arrest occurs immediately after administration of succinylcholine, hyperkalemia must be suspected (particularly in males younger than 9 years of age). Toxicity is increased in patients with muscle injury, muscle myopathies, rhabdomyolysis, or low pseudocholinesterase levels. Children are more susceptible to developing bradycardia, cardiac arrest, and myoglobinemia. Atropine is recommended prior to the administration of succinylcholine in children.

Adverse Reactions: Bradycardia, hypotension, arrhythmias, apnea, cardiac arrest, hyperkalemia, malignant hyperthermia

Abbreviations: AV, atrioventricular; bpm, beats per minute; ET, endotracheal; HR, heart rate; ICP, intracranial pressure; IM, intramuscular; IO, intraosseous; IV, intravenous; MDI, metered-dose inhaler; NS, normal saline; PO, per os; PR, per rectum; SQ, subcutaneous; VF, ventricular fibrillation; VT, ventricular tachycardia.

Glossary

A

"alert, verbal, painful, unresponsive" (AVPU) scale A standardized method of assessing the level of consciousness in all patients; categorizes motor response based on responses to stimuli.

abdomen The anatomic portion of the anterior trunk below the ribs and above the pelvis; it contains the stomach, lower part of the esophagus, small and large intestines, liver, gall bladder, spleen, pancreas, and bladder.

abdominal excursions The work of abdominal muscles in infants during the breathing cycle.

abrasions A portion of skin or of a mucous membrane scraped away as a result of injury.

absorbed To take in or suck up.

abusive head trauma Seen in abused infants and children. The patient has been subjected to violent, whiplash-type shaking injuries inflicted by the abusing individual. This may cause coma, convulsions, and increased intracranial pressure due to tearing of the cerebral veins with consequent bleeding into the brain. (Old term: shaken baby/infant syndrome.)

acceleration-deceleration event A type of injury caused when a moving body part, such as the head, stops its forward motion suddenly.

acid A corrosive substance with low pH.

acidosis Excessive acidity of body fluids due to an accumulation of acids (as in diabetic acidosis or renal disease) or an excessive loss of bicarbonate (as in renal disease).

acrocyanosis Cyanosis of the extremities; acrocyanosis of the hands and feet may be normal in the infant within the first hour after birth.

activation phase First of three phases in disaster response. This is the notification and initial response phase which includes establishment of the Incident Command System organization and scene assessment.

acute Characterized by sharpness or severity, or having a sudden onset, sharp rise, and short course.

adenoidal Lymphoid tissue in the back of the mouth and oropharynx.

adrenaline Synonym for epinephrine. A hormone produced by the body that increases pulse rate and blood pressure; mediates the "fight-or-flight" response of the sympathetic nervous system when the body is under stress.

adrenergic agents Drugs that mimic the effects of epinephrine (adrenaline) and norepinephrine.

adsorb To take up and hold by adsorption.

afebrile seizure A seizure not accompanied by a fever.

agent Something that causes an effect; thus, bacteria that cause a disease are said to be agents of the specific disease. An injury agent is the energy causing the damage, such as thermal energy from a burn. A drug is a pharmacologic agent.

agonist A substance that stimulates or activates a specialized receptor on a cell and causes a response.

airway adjunct An artificial device to maintain an open airway.

aldosterone A steroid hormone produced by the zona glomerulosa of the adrenal cortex in the adrenal gland.

alkali A strong base with a high pH, usually corrosive to tissues.

alveoli The air sacs of the lungs in which the exchange of oxygen and carbon dioxide takes place.

amniotic fluid The liquid contained in the amnion, inside the uterus. This fluid is sterile, transparent, and almost colorless. The liquid surrounds and protects the fetus from injury and helps maintain an even temperature.

analgesia, analgesic A drug that relieves pain.

anaphylactic reaction An extreme, life-threatening systemic allergic reaction that may include shock and respiratory failure.

anaphylaxis A severe form of hypersensitivity reaction that produces dangerous physiologic changes, such as bronchospasm, shock, and airway edema.

anatomic Relating to the anatomy or structure of an organism.

androgens A group of hormones that play a role in male traits and reproductive activity.

antecubital fossa The triangular area lying anterior to and below the elbow, bounded medially by the pronator teres muscle and laterally by the brachioradialis muscles.

anthrax A deadly bacteria (*Bacillus anthracis*) that lies dormant in a spore (protective shell); the germ is released from the spore when exposed to the optimal temperature and moisture. The route of entry is inhalation, cutaneous, or gastrointestinal (from consuming food that contains spores).

antibiotics Any of a variety of natural or synthetic substances that inhibit growth of, or destroy, bacteria that are responsible for infectious diseases.

anticonvulsant Agent that prevents or stops convulsions.

antigen Protein recognized by the immune system which causes an allergic reaction.

antipyretic An agent that reduces fever.

antivenin A serum that counteracts the effect of venom from an animal or insect.

anxiolysis Reduction of anxiety, agitation, or tension.

apnea A temporary cessation of breathing.

apneic Characterized by absence of breathing.

asphyxia A condition caused by insufficient oxygen.

assessment Evaluation.

assisted ventilation To provide ventilation mechanically.

asthma A disease caused by increased responsiveness of the tracheobronchial tree to various stimuli. The result is paroxysmal constriction of the bronchial airways. Clinically, there is severe dyspnea accompanied by wheezing.

asymmetric Without symmetry.

asystole Cardiac standstill; absence of contractions of the heart.

ataxia An abnormal gait.

atrioventricular heart block Blockage of the electrical impulse from the atrium of the heart to the ventricle.

atrium One of two (right and left) upper chambers of the heart. The right atrium receives blood from the vena cava and delivers it to the right ventricle, which, in turn, pumps blood into the blood vessels of the lungs. The left atrium receives blood from pulmonary veins and delivers it to the left ventricle, which, in turn, pumps blood into the body.

auscultated To listen, as with a stethoscope.

auscultation The process of listening for sounds within the body with a stethoscope.

AVPU The components of the AVPU scale are used to assess the level of consciousness: Alert, Voice, Painful, Unresponsive.

avulsion A tearing away of a part or structure.

axial loading Vertical pressure on the spine.

axillary temperature The temperature taken in the armpit.

axonal shearing A tearing of axons or nerve sheaths, caused by sudden movement, to produce severe brain injury.

B

baseline A known or initial value with which subsequent observations can be compared.

basilar skull fracture A fracture into the base of the skull, sometimes associated with brain hemorrhage or brain injury.

Battle sign Bruising behind the ear; an indication of basilar skull fracture.

benzodiazepine A family of sedative-hypnotic drugs useful for treatment of seizures and agitation.

bezoar A hard mass of entangled material sometimes found in the stomach and intestines.

bilateral Pertaining to, affecting, or relating to two sides.

biologic agents Organisms that cause disease, including viruses, bacteria, and toxins.

biologic pathogen A microorganism that can cause disease in a host.

blood pressure The perfusing pressure of blood.

brachial Pertaining to a main artery and vein of the arm.

bradycardia A slow heartbeat.

brain death Cessation of brain function.

brain perfusion Blood circulation in the brain.

brainstem The stemlike part of the brain that connects the cerebral hemispheres with the spinal cord.

brainstem functions Bodily functions controlled by the brain stem that are necessary for life, such as breathing.

brainstem herniation Bulging and compression of brain tissue; causes breathing to stop and death of the patient.

bronchiolitis Inflammation of the bronchioles by a virus.

bronchodilator A drug that helps open the airways to improve air movement and reduce wheezing.

bronchopulmonary dysplasia (BPD) Iatrogenic chronic lung disease that develops in premature infants following a period of oxygen therapy.

bronchovesicular Pertaining to the tree of pulmonary passages.

buccal Between the teeth and mucosa of the mouth.

buckle fracture A minor fracture only partially through the bone, in which the top layer of bone on one side is compressed, forming a slight angle or "buckle" in the surface.

bulging fontanelle An elevation of the immature opening of bone in the front of the skull; this sign may suggest increased intracranial pressure.

C

calcium channel blockers A family of drugs that helps reduce the speed of conduction through the heart and the overall work of the heart.

cannulating To introduce a catheter through a vein or passageway.

capillary refill time (CRT) A test that evaluates distal circulatory system function performed by pushing on an area such as a nail bed and watching the speed of its return of pinkness after releasing the pressure.

capnometry The use of a capnometer, a device that measures the amount of expired carbon dioxide.

cardiac arrest The cessation of cardiac mechanical activity, determined by the inability to palpate a central pulse, unresponsiveness, and apnea.

cardiac dysrhythmia An abnormal cardiac rhythm.

cardiac medication Various medications used to treat for heart disease and cardiovascular conditions.

cardiogenic shock A reduced cardiac output secondary to abnormal cardiac function.

cardiomyopathy Disease of the myocardium, especially due to primary disease of the heart muscle.

cartilage A specialized type of dense connective tissue, softer than bone, that is common in the skeletons of children.

cartilaginous growth plates The horizontal part of the bone which grows as the human body matures.

cathartic A purgative agent for the bowel.

caustic Corrosive and burning; destructive to living tissue.

central cyanosis Slightly bluish, grayish, or dark purple discoloration of the skin (on the trunk and face) due to presence of hypoxia.

central nervous system (CNS) The organ system that consists of the brain and spinal cord; it controls vital body functions.

central venous catheter Catheter inserted into the vena cava to permit intermittent or continuous monitoring of central venous pressure and to facilitate obtaining blood samples for analysis.

cerebral cortex The higher brain; the source of the senses, thinking, feeling, and voluntary movement.

cerebral edema Swelling of the brain.

cerebral palsy A disorder of movement and tone that results from brain injury during fetal development or at birth.

cerebrospinal fluid (CSF) shunt Tube that allows fluid manufactured in the ventricles of the brain from the subarachnoid space to drain in another part of the anatomy outside of the brain, such as the peritoneum. This can lower pressure in the brain.

chest wall The musculoskeletal framework of the chest.

child maltreatment A general term applying to all forms of child abuse and neglect.

child neglect Failure by those responsible for caring for a child to provide for the child's nutritional, emotional, and physical needs.

child protection services (CPS) This agency is the community legal organization responsible for protection, rehabilitation, and prevention of child maltreatment and neglect. CPS has the legal authority temporarily to remove from home children at risk for injury or neglect and to secure foster placement.

child restraint systems (CRS) A child safety device that is designed to secure an infant or child in both motor vehicles and aircraft.

children with special health care needs (CSHCN) Those who have or are at increased risk for a chronic, physical, developmental, behavioral, or emotional condition and who also require health and related services of a type or amount beyond that required by children generally.

choanal atresia A narrowing or blockage of the nasal airway by membranous or bony tissue; a congenital condition (present at birth).

cholinergic crisis A crisis involving cholinergic drugs, pesticides or "nerve gases" designed for chemical warfare. Cholinergic agents overstimulate normal body functions that are controlled by the parasympathetic nerves.

cholinergic impulses Description of a neuron that secretes the neurotransmitter acetylcholine.

circadian rhythm The regular recurrence, in cycles of about 24 hours, of biological processes or activities, such as sensitivity to drugs and stimuli, hormone secretion, sleeping, feeding, etc. This rhythm seems to be set by a biological clock that seems to be set by recurring daylight and darkness.

clavicles The collarbone; a bone, curved like the letter f, that articulates with the sternum and scapula.

coin rubbing Cultural ritual/traditional healing practices intended to treat an illness by rubbing hot coins, often on the back, which produces rounded and oblong red, patch, flat skin lesions.

colostomy The surgical establishment of an opening between the colon and the surface of the body for the purpose of providing drainage of the bowel.

commotio cordis Sudden cardiac arrest from a blunt, nonpenetrating blow to the chest. The basis of the cardiac arrest is ventricular fibrillation (a chaotically abnormal heart rhythm) triggered by chest wall impact immediately over the anatomic position of the heart.

compensated shock A clinical state in which there are clinical signs of inadequate tissue perfusion, but the patient's blood pressure is in the normal range.

compensatory mechanisms Physiologic responses, initiated to help return the body's vital functions to normal after a severe insult to breathing, perfusion, or metabolic function.

complex febrile seizures A self-limited seizure in a previously healthy child between the ages of 6 months and 6 years that is associated with an elevated fever, which lasts longer than 15 minutes, and may have focal motor activity.

complex partial seizures Characterized by alteration of consciousness with or without complex focal motor activity.

compression A squeezing together; state of being pressed together.

concussion A brain injury causing any type of altered state of consciousness.

congenital Present at birth.

congenital anomalies An anatomic structure that is unusual or different at birth.

congenital diaphragmatic hernia A developmental defect of the diaphragm in which the abdominal organs herniate into the chest.

congenital heart disease Heart disease that is present from birth.

congestive heart failure A disorder in which the heart loses part of its ability to effectively pump blood, usually as a result of damage to the heart muscle and usually resulting in a backup of fluid into the lungs.

consent for care Permission to render care.

constipation Infrequent defecation with passage of unduly hard and dry fecal material.

contact burns A thermal burn from direct contact with a hot object, fluid, or gas.

contraindications A condition indicating that a treatment is inappropriate.

core perfusion Blood circulation in the core of the human body.

corrosive Producing corrosion or destruction of tissue.

cortical Pertaining to or of the outer layer of the brain.

crackles Rales; lung sounds that suggest fluid in alveoli.

cranium (physeal plates) The area of the head above the ears and eyes; the skull. The cranium contains the brain.

crepitus The noise or feel of gas in soft tissues.

critical incident stress management (CISM) A process that confronts the responses to critical incidents and defuses them, directing the emergency service personnel toward physical and emotional equilibrium.

crowning Stage in delivery when the fetal head presents at the vaginal opening.

cupping The practice of placing warm cups on the skin to pull out illness from the body. This results in red, flat, rounded skin lesions which are often more intensely red at the borders.

Cushing triad The combination of hypertension, bradycardia and irregular respirations that occurs with increased intracranial pressure.

cyanide A colorless gas that has an odor similar to almonds, and which is a chemical asphyxiant used in many industrial processes; exposure can occur from by-products of combustion at structure fires.

cyanosis Slightly bluish, grayish, slatelike, or dark purple discoloration of the skin due to presence of hypoxia.

cyanotic heart disease A type of congenital heart disease with a right to left shunt resulting in partially oxygenated blood in the systemic circulation.

cyclic antidepressant A type of antidepressant drug that may cause coma, seizures, and conduction disturbances if taken in an overdose.

cystic fibrosis A congenital disorder that results in lung and digestive disorders due to improper functioning of mucus producing or exocrine glands. Patients experience frequent lung infections, pneumothoraces, impaired digestion and absorption of nutrients and poor growth.

D

decerebrate A posture characterized by rigid extension of the arms and legs; indicates pressure on the brain stem at the level of the pons and may appear in patients with severe brain swelling.

decompensated shock A shock state characterized by low blood pressure, which will rapidly progress to cardiac arrest if not rapidly corrected.

decontamination The process of removing a poison.

decorticate A posture characterized by flexion of the arms and extension of the legs; indicates pressure on the cerebral cortex and subcortical white matter with preservation of brainstem function and may appear in patients with severe brain trauma.

defibrillator An electrical device that shocks the heart; it may be used externally or in the form of an automatic implanted defibrillator.

demarcated A defined area in a boundary.

dendrite A projection from a neuron that makes connections with an adjacent cell.

dextrose A form of glucose (or sugar) found naturally in animal and plant tissue and derived synthetically from starch.

diabetes mellitus A metabolic disorder in which the ability to metabolize sugar is impaired, usually because of a lack of insulin.

diabetic ketoacidosis A form of acidosis in diabetes in which certain acids accumulate when insulin is not available.

diaphoretic A state of excessive perspiration because of high physiologic stress.

diaphragm The muscle separating the chest from the abdominal cavity, which allows breathing.

diaphysis The shaft of a long bone.

diastolic pressure The pressure that remains in the arteries during the relaxing phase of the heart's cycle (diastole) when the left ventricle is at rest.

diffuse axonal injury An injury to the brain, resulting in diffuse brain swelling.

dilated Widened.

direct medical control Physician instructions that are given directly by phone or radio.

dirty bomb Name given to a bomb that is used as a radiological dispersal device (RDD).

disaster A widespread event that disrupts community resources and functions, in turn threatening public safety, citizens' lives, and property.

distal Farthest from the center.

distal extremities Structures that are farther from the trunk or nearer to the free end of the extremity.

distention Inflation, enlargement.

distributive A clinical state characterized by maldistribution of blood volume and vascular tone.

diving reflex Submersion of the face and nose in water to produce a vagal reaction; used to terminate an important dysrhythmia of childhood called supraventricular tachycardia.

Do Not Resuscitate (DNR) Written documentation giving permission to medical personnel not to attempt resuscitation in the event of cardiac arrest.

Down syndrome A congenital disorder in which a person is born with three copies of chromosome 21 (trisomy 21). Clinical features include slanting eyes, a broad short skull, broad hands and short fingers. Other congenital abnormalities include heart defects and esophageal atresia.

dressings Protective covering for diseased or injured parts.

drug-assisted intubation (DAI) A method of airway management that uses pharmacologic agents to facilitate endotracheal intubation.

dysphagia Inability to swallow or difficulty in swallowing.

dysrhythmia Abnormal, disordered rhythm.

E

edema A local or generalized collection of tissue fluid.

effortless tachypnea Without the signs of increased work of breathing; this represents the child's attempt to blow off extra carbon dioxide to correct the acidosis generated by poor perfusion.

electrocardiogram (ECG) A 12-lead electrocardiographic recording used to evaluate the heart and its rhythm.

emancipated minor Person legally under age but recognized by the state as having the legal capacity to consent for self (usually over 14 years of age).

emergency information form (EIF) A form that provides patient information to healthcare providers.

emergency protective custody A child taken into a protective custody by a law enforcement officer if the legal guardian continues to refuse consent for lifesaving care.

emesis Vomiting.

emotional abuse The intentional infliction of emotional harm to a child.

emotional neglect The intentional omission of emotional support to a child.

empathy The awareness of and insight into the feelings, emotions, and behavior of another person.

EMS-EMSC Continuum The linked community services set up to prevent and treat childhood emergencies. The continuum includes prevention, the primary physician, out-of-hospital care, ED care, hospital care, and rehabilitation.

encephalitis Inflammation of the brain.

endotracheal intubation A method of intubation in which an endotracheal tube (ETT) is placed through a patient's mouth, directly through the larynx between the vocal cords, and into the trachea, to open and maintain an airway.

enteroviruses Species of virus that causes gastrointestinal or respiratory disease in children.

envenomation The act of injecting venom, such as by a snake or insect.

environment The surroundings, conditions, or influences that affect an organism or an injury.

environmental assessment Evaluation of the scene to draw clues about what is wrong and the best route to take for treatment. Gathering information by observing things like damage to a vehicle or medication bottles in the patient's home.

epiglottis A leaf or omega-shaped structure located immediately posterior to the root of the tongue that prevents food and secretions from entering the trachea.

epiglottitis Inflammation of the epiglottis.

epilepsy A condition of recurrent seizures.

epinephrine A substance produced by the body (commonly called adrenaline) and that has a vital role in the function of the sympathetic nervous system; also a drug produced by pharmaceutical companies that increases blood pressure and causes bronchodilation; the drug of choice for an anaphylactic reaction.

epiphysis The ends of the bone that are the secondary ossification centers.

esophagus A muscular canal that carries food from the pharynx to the stomach.

etiology Cause and origin of disease.

evaporation Change from liquid to vapor.

exhalation The process of breathing out.

extensor posturing See decerebrate.

extraocular Movement of the eyes in various directions.

F

feeding tube A tube placed into the stomach through the mouth, nose, or skin.

fetus A human or mammal in an early form of intrauterine development.

flaccidity Weak, lax, and soft.

flail chest An unstable condition of the chest wall due to two or more fractures of the ribs resulting in ineffective breathing.

flexion The act of bending.

flexural creases The creases behind the knees or inside the elbows.

focal Limited to a part of the body.

fontanelle A soft spot of undeveloped bone lying between the cranial bones of the skull of a fetus or infant.

fulminant pneumonia Sudden and intense inflammation of the lungs with infection.

G

gag reflex The protective reflex that keeps food, fluid, or secretions from getting into the trachea.

gastric decompression The removal of air and other contents from the stomach.

gastric feeding tube A tube that provides a channel directly into a patient's stomach, allowing removal of gas, blood, and toxins, or insertion medications and nutrition.

gastroenteritis Inflammation of the stomach and intestinal tract.

gastrointestinal (GI) decontamination The removal of poison from the stomach.

gastrostomy tube (G-tube or "button") A feeding tube placed directly through the wall of the abdomen.

generalized seizure Characterized by movements (often tonic-clonic) that indicate involvement of both cerebral hemispheres.

gestation The length of time from conception to birth.

glial cells Specialized cells that surround neurons, providing mechanical and physical support and electrical insulation between neurons.

glottis The sound-producing apparatus of the larynx, consisting of two vocal folds.

glucagon a hormone that has the property of increasing the concentration of sugar in the blood.

greenstick fracture a fracture involving only part of the outer layer or cortex of a bone.

grunting a short, low-pitched sound at the end of exhalation, present in children with moderate to severe hypoxia; it reflects poor gas exchange because of fluid in the lower airways and air sacs.

H

hazardous materials (HazMat) Any substance that is toxic, poisonous, radioactive, flammable, or explosive and causes injury or death with exposure.

head bobbing The head lifts and tilts back during inspiration, then moves forward during expiration; a sign of increased work of breathing.

health information exchanges (HIEs) The sharing of healthcare information electronically across organizations within a region, community, or hospital system.

hematoma A swelling or mass of blood confined to a organ, tissue, or space and caused by a break in a blood vessel.

hemodialysis A form of dialysis in which the blood is removed from the patient through a catheter or fistula, and then returns to the body through another needle, removing various toxins, electrolytes, and fluid in the process.

hemodynamically stable Not changing or fluctuating in relation to the mechanics of blood circulation.

hemopericardium Accumulation of blood around the heart muscle in the pericardial sac.

hemophilia A congenital condition in which the patient lacks one or more of the blood's normal clotting factors.

hemostat Instrument clamp; in its closed position it squeezes tissues or vessels and arrests the flow of blood.

hepatomegaly Enlargement of the liver.

hives Wheals; an itchy rash caused by contact with or ingestion of an allergic substance or food.

homeostasis The maintenance of a relatively stable internal physiologic environment.

host The organism acted upon in an injury or illness process.

hydrocarbon A basic organic compound made up only of hydrogen and carbon.

hydrocephalus The increased accumulation of cerebrospinal fluid within the ventricles of the brain.

hydrochloric acid A powerful and corrosive aqueous solution of hydrogen chloride (HCl).

hyperalimentation The administration of nutrients by intravenous feeding.

hyperoxia Increased oxygen in the blood.

hyperthermia Unusually elevated body temperature.

hypertrophic cardiomyopathy (HCM) A condition in which the heart muscle is unusually thick, which means that the heart has to pump harder to get blood to leave.

hypnotic drug Pertaining to sleep or sedation.

hypocarbia Decreased carbon dioxide in the blood, usually from an excess rate of ventilation.

hypoglycemia Low blood glucose.

hypoperfusion Inadequate circulation.

hypotension Decrease of systolic and diastolic blood pressure below normal for age, representing decompensated shock.

hypotensive shock A shock state characterized by low blood pressure, which will rapidly progress to cardiac arrest if not rapidly corrected.

hypothermia Having a body temperature below normal range.

hypotonia Reduced muscular tension.

hypovolemia Diminished blood volume.

hypovolemic shock A clinical state of reduced intravascular volume.

hypoxemia A decreased oxygen saturation in blood detected by pulse oximetry or direct measurement of oxygen saturation in an arterial blood gas sample.

hypoxia A pathological condition in which the body as a whole (generalized hypoxia) or region of the body (tissue hypoxia) is deprived of an adequate oxygen supply.

hypoxic stress A subnormal concentration of oxygen.

I

ileostomy The surgical establishment of an opening between the small bowel and the surface of the body for the purpose of providing drainage of the bowel.

impending brainstem herniation When brain tissue, cerebrospinal fluid, and blood vessels are moved or pressed away from their usual position inside the skull.

impending herniation syndrome Clinical state in which there is severely abnormal brain pressure, just before the moment of tissue herniation and compression of brain tissue.

implementation phase Second of the three phases in disaster response. Activities during this phase include: search and rescue, victim triage, initial stabilization and transport, and definitive management of scene hazards and victims.

implied consent A type of consent in which a patient who is unable to give consent is given treatment under the legal assumption that he or she would want treatment if thinking in a normal way.

in utero Within the uterus.

indirect medical control Existing or standing orders, written policies, procedures, and protocols.

indwelling central venous catheter Small, flexible plastic tube inserted into a large vein above the heart, usually the subclavian vein, through which access to the blood stream can be made. This catheter is left in place and allows drugs and blood products to be given and blood samples withdrawn painlessly.

infusion A liquid substance introduced into the body for therapeutic or diagnostic purposes.

inspiratory The process of moving air into the lungs.

insulin A hormone produced by the islet of Langerhans (an exocrine gland in the pancreas) that enables sugar in the blood to enter the cells of the body; used in synthetic form to treat and control diabetes mellitus.

intercostal Between the ribs.

intercurrent Intervening.

intra-abdominal Within the abdomen.

intracranial Within the cranium or skull.

intracranial hypertension/increased intracranial pressure Increased pressure of the cerebrospinal fluid that impairs brain function.

intramuscular medications Injections into a muscle; a medication delivery route.

intranasally Within the nasal cavity; a medication delivery route.

intraosseous Within the marrow cavity of a bone; intramedullary; a medication delivery route.

intravascular volume The water portion of the circulatory system surrounding the blood cells.

ipecac An oral medicine to induce vomiting; this medicine is no longer recommended for use by prehospital professionals.

ischemia Deficiency of blood supply.

J

jaundice A condition characterized by yellowness of skin, whites of eyes, mucous membranes, and body fluids due to deposition of excess bilirubin in the blood (hyperbilirubinemia).

jugular venous distension A prominence of the jugular veins as they fill with blood; if patient is not supine, indication that the blood may be having difficulty flowing back into the right side of the heart. This can be caused by pericardial tamponade, tension pneumothorax, or right-sided heart failure.

K

ketogenic diet A diet that eliminates foods with glucose; may be utilized in children with severe, uncontrolled epilepsy to keep the child in a state of ketosis to help control seizures.

L

lactic acidosis The metabolic acidotic state resulting from the accumulation of lactic acid secondary to anaerobic cellular metabolism.

laryngoscope An instrument for examining the larynx.

laryngoscopy An examination of the interior of the larynx.

larynx The enlarged upper end of the trachea, below the root of the tongue, that contains the vocal cords.

lateral Pertaining to the side.

lateral decubitus position The position with the patient on his or her side.

legal authority The ability to make medical decisions under the law.

lethargy Listlessness; weakness.

leukemia A cancerous condition in which certain cell lines begin to grow abnormally fast.

leukocyte (white blood cell) count Measured to determine whether an infectious process is present.

localizing When a patient is able to respond to the site of a specific noxious or painful stimulus (e.g., when a patient reaches for and pushes away the hand that is pinching them during a neurologic exam).

long QT syndrome A condition characterized by a QT interval exceeding approximately 450 ms.

lordosis Forward curve of the lumbar spine.

lye Corrosive, alkaline cleaning liquid.

M

malaise Discomfort, uneasiness, or generalized ill feeling, often indicative of infection.

malposition When something is in an incorrect or abnormal position.

mandible The horseshoe-shaped bone forming the lower jaw.

mass-casualty incident (MCI) An emergency situation involving more than one patient, and which can place such great demand on equipment or personnel that the system is stretched to its limit or beyond.

mature minor A person without the formal legal status of an emancipated minor, but having similar characteristics: married, pregnant, on active-duty status in the armed service, or 15 years or older and living separate and apart from his or her guardians. This person has the legal right to give consent for treatment as well as the legal right to refuse.

meconium The bowel contents of a fetus. The presence of meconium in amniotic fluid means the fetus may have suffered some type of stress, such as hypoxia, and may be depressed and need to be resuscitated.

mediastinum The space between the lungs, in the center of the chest, that contains the heart, trachea, mainstem bronchi, part of the esophagus, and large blood vessels.

medical control Physician instructions that are given directly by radio (online or direct) or indirectly by protocols or guidelines (off-line or indirect), as authorized by the medical director of the service program.

medical home An approach to providing health care services in a high quality and cost-effective manner. Children and their families who have a medical home receive the care that they need from a pediatrician or family physician that they know and trust. The pediatric health care professional and parents act as partners in a medical home to identify and access all the medical and nonmedical services needed to help children and their families achieve their maximum potential.

medical responsibility The moral and legal duty to provide medical care in an emergency.

meninges A set of three tough membranes, the dura mater, arachnoid, and pia mater, that encloses the entire brain and spinal cord.

meningitis Inflammation of the membranes of the spinal cord or brain.

meningococcal sepsis Bloodborne infection with the bacteria *Neisseria meningitidis* leading to sepsis (fever or hypothermia, shock, and hypotension).

meningococcemia Infection of the blood stream by the bacteria *Neisseria meningitidis*. This is usually a severe infection characterized by fever, shock and a characteristic purpuric rash (bruising of the skin) with or without meningitis.

metabolic acidosis A metabolic state of acidosis resulting from retention of hydrogen or other positively charged ions not related to respiratory compromise.

midaxillary lines Imaginary vertical line drawn through the middle of the axilla (armpit), parallel to the midline.

minor A person not of legal age and thus requiring consent from a legal guardian for medical or surgical care.

minute ventilation The volume of air exchanged per minute [minute ventilation = tidal volume × respiratory rate].

miosis Abnormal contraction of pupils.

Mongolian spots Blue-gray areas of discoloration of the skin caused by abnormal pigment, not by trauma or bruising.

mortality Death.

motor activity Muscle use.

mottling A condition of abnormal skin circulation, caused by vasoconstriction or inadequate circulation.

multisystem trauma Injury involving more than one organ system, such as combined injury to the chest, abdomen, and brain.

Munchausen syndrome by proxy A psychological disorder marked by attention-seeking behavior by a caregiver through those who are in their care.

muscular dystrophy A genetic muscle disorder that results in muscle weakness and wasting; patients are at risk for aspiration and pneumonia.

myocardial depression When the heart muscle is not working adequately.

myocardial function A measure of how well the heart is working.

myocardial infarction The death of part of the heart muscle caused by partial or complete occlusion of one or more of the coronary arteries.

myocarditis Inflammation of the myocardium.

N

narcotic An opiate drug that produces analgesia and sedation, as well as euphoria when used for recreational purposes.

nasal cannula An oxygen-delivery device in which oxygen flows through two small, tubelike prongs that fit into the patient's nostrils.

nasal flaring Out of the nostrils, indicating increased work of breathing and hypoxia.

nasopharyngeal airway (NPA) Airway adjunct inserted into the nostril of a conscious patient who is not able to maintain a natural airway.

needle decompression The removal of air from a closed space, such as from the pleura.

neonatal seizures Seizures that occur in neonates.

nerve agents A class of chemicals including organophosphates; they function by blocking an essential enzyme in the nervous system, which causes the body's organs to become overstimulated.

neurogenic shock Shock caused by paralysis of the nerves that control the size of the blood vessels, leading to widespread dilation and pooling of blood in the peripheral vessels to the extent that adequate perfusion cannot be maintained; seen in patients with spinal cord injuries.

neurovascular Concerning both the nervous and vascular systems.

nonpulsatile fontanelle When the fontanelle or "soft spot" on an infant's head is full, usually tense and does not seem to beat or pulse with each beat of the heart.

nuclear bomb A bomb which is extremely powerful due to its use of atomic energy as a source of its explosive nature. In addition to the actual explosive force of the bomb, injury is caused in a wider area by the radiation released by the explosion.

O

obstetric Having to do with pregnancy, delivery of a baby.

obstructive shock Shock or inadequate tissue perfusion that is caused by a restriction to blood flow out from the heart (e.g., shock due to a critical coarctation or severe narrowing of the aorta, tension pneumothorax, or cardiac tamponade).

obturator An inner stabilizing structure that gives stiffness to a hollow tube, to allow insertion or clearing of an obstruction.

occlusion The closure of a passage.

occlusive dressing A dressing that covers completely.

occult illness An illness that is not immediately obvious or is "hidden." An illness that does not have obvious symptoms.

operations Administrative processes.

opiates See narcotics.

oral glucose A simple sugar that is readily absorbed by the bloodstream; it is carried on the EMS unit.

organophosphate insecticide A type of poison with cholinergic properties, used as an insecticide.

oropharyngeal airway An airway adjunct inserted into the mouth to keep the tongue from blocking the upper airway and to make suctioning the airway easier.

oropharynx The part of the pharynx lying between the soft palate and upper portion of the epiglottis.

ossification The formation of bone. An ossification center is an area where cartilage is transformed through calcification into a new area of bone.

osteogenesis imperfecta A genetic disorder in which the bones are brittle, and results in fractures.

ostomies A surgical opening made in the skin as a way for waste products to leave the body.

otorrhea Any flow or discharge from the ear.

P

pallor Lack of color; paleness.

palpation Physical touching for the purpose of obtaining information.

paradoxical irritability A marker for possible serious pediatric illness, consisting of a particular type of irritability where attempts to console further distress the child.

pathology The study and diagnosis of disease.

pathophysiology The study of how disease or injury affects the body.

pedal Related to the foot (e.g., pedal pulses are pulses found in the foot).

pediatric assessment triangle (PAT) Assessment tool that allows rapid formation of a general impression of the type and level of illness or injury in an infant or child without touching him or her; consists of assessing appearance, work of breathing, and circulation to the skin.

pediatric critical care center A type of specialized center for children with advanced resources (such as a pediatric intensive care unit) for care of the critically ill.

pediatric trauma center A type of specialized center for children with advanced resources for care of critically injured children.

pelvic fractures Breaks through one or more bones of the pelvis (the hip bones and the sacrum and coccyx or lower parts of the spine).

percutaneous endoscopic gastrostomy (PEG) A procedure that places a tube through the abdominal wall and into the stomach.

perfusion Blood circulation.

pericardial tamponade Compression of the heart due to a buildup of blood or other fluid in the pericardial sac.

periosteum The membrane, made up of a double layer of connective tissue, that covers all bones, except the articular surfaces.

peripheral cyanosis Slightly bluish or dark purple discoloration of the skin (on the hands and feet only).

peripheral vasoconstriction When the blood vessels in the outer extremities (hands and feet especially) constrict (get smaller in size through the contraction of the smooth muscle in the blood vessel walls) and therefore lead to a decrease in blood flow to those areas. This may produce peripheral cyanosis (bluish discoloration of the hands and feet) and prolonged capillary refill time.

peripherally inserted central catheter (PICC) An indwelling line that is partially implanted under the skin and partially exposed above the skin.

peritoneal dialysis A type of dialysis in which a special solution is instilled through a catheter into the patient's abdomen, and that draws toxins, electrolytes, and other fluids from the body through the peritoneal membrane.

peritoneum The membrane lining the abdominal cavity (parietal peritoneum) and covering the abdominal organs (visceral peritoneum).

peritonsillar abscess A collection of pus adjacent to the tonsil.

petechiae Small, purplish, nonblanching spots on the skin that appear in certain severe fevers and may be indicative of possible sepsis.

petechial rash Rash which contains petechiae, small areas of hemorrhage into the skin that do not blanch when they are pressed on.

pharynx Passageway for air from nasal cavity to larynx and food from mouth to esophagus.

phencyclidine (PCP) A hallucinogen, referred to as PCP or angel dust. Moderate doses cause elevated blood pressure, rapid pulse, increased skeletal muscle tone, and, sometimes, myoclonic jerks.

physeal plate Pertaining to growth or to the segment of bone that is concerned with growth.

physical abuse See child maltreatment.

physical neglect See child neglect.

Physician Orders for Life-Sustaining Treatment (POLST) A document outlining the treatment that is permitted when the patient still has a pulse and is breathing.

physiologic Concerning body function.

Pierre Robin syndrome A condition present at birth marked by a small lower jaw (micrognathia). The tongue tends to fall back and downward (glossoptosis), and there is a cleft soft palate.

placenta The tissue attached to the uterine wall that nourishes the fetus through the umbilical cord.

plague An illness caused by infection with the bacteria *Yersinia pestis*. The disease is characterized by fever and chills followed by a severe illness with pneumonia, headache, and delirium. It is transmitted to humans by the bites of fleas from infected rodents and has a high fatality rate. It is an agent that could possibly be used as a weapon of bioterrorism.

pleura The serous membrane that enfolds both lungs and is reflected upon the walls of the thorax and diaphragm.

pleural space The space between the parietal and visceral layers of the pleura.

pneumomediastinum Air or gas in the mediastinal tissues.

pneumonia An inflammation of the lungs caused primarily by bacteria, viruses, and chemical irritants.

pneumothorax A collection of air in the pleural cavity, which if under pressure may cause severe physiologic changes with poor venous return and inadequate cardiac output.

policies Medicolegal operational standards to guide prehospital professionals intended to help with decision-making in difficult or legally sensitive field situations.

polydipsia A condition in which a person has extreme thirst.

polyphagia Medical term for excessive or extreme hunger.

polyuria Excessive or an abnormally large production or passage of urine.

positive-pressure ventilation (PPV) Assisted ventilation.

posteriorly From the back, from behind, or from underneath.

postictal state The confused state of a patient after having a seizure.

postpartum After childbirth.

posturing Abnormal body positioning after a brain injury; it may be in response to painful stimuli.

preeclampsia A condition during pregnancy characterized by gestational hypertension, typically accompanied by edema and proteinuria.

preterm labor Labor beginning prior to the 37th week of gestation.

primary brain injury Injury resulting from the direct biomechanical effects of the impact forces on the brain which result in direct impact or sudden movement causing shear stress of the brain.

procedure A physical intervention.

prone Lying horizontal with face downward.

propylene glycol A solvent in medicines.

protocol A step-by-step process for treatment.

proximal Nearest the point of attachment, center of the body, or point of reference; opposite of distal.

pulmonary contusion A bruise of the lung.

pulmonary edema A build-up of fluid in the lungs.

pulmonary intoxicants Toxins or poisons which may be absorbed through (e.g., by inhalation) or cause harm to the respiratory system.

pulseless electrical activity (PEA) An organized cardiac rhythm on the cardiac monitor in absence of a palpable pulse.

purpura A rash that looks like bruising of the skin that is usually seen in overwhelming infections (sepsis) or when a patient has an inflammation of the blood vessels (vasculitis).

purpuric Pertaining to bruising of the skin.

pus The liquid product of inflammation, generally yellow in color.

Q

QRS complex The electrical shape of a major portion of the heart rhythm on the cardiac monitor, representing ventricular electrical activity.

quadriplegia A condition that causes paralysis of all four extremities (both arms and both legs) usually due to an injury in the upper cervical portion of the spinal cord.

quality improvement (QI) A system of internal and external reviews and audits of all aspects of the system.

R

racemic Including all isomers of a drug, such as epinephrine.

radial Pertaining to the radius, the larger and more lateral of the two bones in the forearm.

reactivity The tendency of a substance to undergo chemical reaction, either by itself or with other materials, and to release energy.

recovery phase Final of three phases in disaster response. Activities include: scene withdrawal, return to normal operations, and debriefing.

renal dialysis A technique for filtering the blood of its toxic wastes, removing excess fluids, and restoring the normal balance of electrolytes.

respiratory arrest The absence of respirations (i.e., apnea) with detectable cardiac activity.

respiratory depression A condition in which there is a slowing of the respiratory rate and decreased respiratory effort usually due to some effect on the respiratory center in the medulla of the brain. This may be caused by trauma, illness, or the effects of drugs (e.g., morphine or diazepam) or toxins (e.g., ethanol).

respiratory distress A clinical state characterized by increased respiratory rate, effort, and work of breathing.

respiratory failure A clinical state of inadequate oxygenation, ventilation, or both.

respiratory syncytial virus (RSV) A virus that commonly causes bronchiolitis.

retractions Physical drawing in of the chest wall between the ribs that occurs with increased work of breathing.

retropharyngeal abscess Swelling of the retropharyngeal nodes located between the cervical vertebrae and esophagus; can mimic the presentation of epiglottitis.

rhinorrhea Thin watery discharge from the nose.

ricin Neurotoxin derived from mash that is left from the castor bean. When introduced into the body, ricin causes pulmonary edema and respiratory and circulatory failure, leading to death.

Robin sequence See Pierre Robin syndrome.

S

salivation The act of secreting saliva.

saphenous veins Two superficial veins, the great and small, passing up the leg.

scald A burn to skin or flesh caused by moist heat and hot vapors, as steam.

scaphoid The wrist bone that is found just beyond the most distal portion of the radius.

scoliosis A lateral curvature of the spine.

scopolamine An anticholinergic agent with action similar to atropine.

secondary assessment A step in the patient assessment process in which a systematic physical examination of the patient is performed. The examination may be a systematic full-body evaluation or an assessment that focuses on a certain area or region of the body, often determined through the chief complaint.

secondary brain injury Injury to the brain resulting from factors occurring after the initial biomechanical effects of the primary brain injury (such as hypoxia and hypotension).

secretion The process of producing liquid materials into the blood or body cavities.

sedative An agent that relaxes.

semi-Fowler's position The position of a patient who is lying in a bed in a supine position with the head of the bed at approximately 30 degrees.

sepsis A pathological state, usually in a febrile patient, resulting from the presence of invading microorganisms or their poisonous products in the bloodstream.

septic shock Shock from infection, involving hypotension and signs of inadequate organ perfusion.

serial examinations The act of repeatedly examining a patient to carefully watch and document the progression

of signs or symptoms in an attempt to develop a diagnosis (e.g., serial examinations of the abdomen to decide if someone with abdominal trauma may have a perforation of the intestine) or to watch for a change in their condition (e.g., serial examinations of a child with a head injury to monitor their neurologic status and watch for signs of increasing intracranial pressure).

serum glucose The level of blood sugar.

sexual abuse Rape, sexual assault, or sexual molestation.

shock A clinical syndrome in which the blood flow and oxygen delivery are inadequate for normal organ function.

sickle cell disease A hereditary disease characterized by abnormal clumping together of deformed red blood cells. The patients have painful crises, anemia, infection-risks, strokes, and other serious complications.

simple febrile seizure A brief (less than 15 minutes), self-limited, generalized convulsion in a previously healthy child between the ages of 6 months and 6 years that is associated with an elevated fever. Children with simple febrile seizures have relatively short postictal periods after which they return to their baseline with a nonfocal neurologic examination.

simple partial seizures A focal (localized) seizure which involves a motor or sensory abnormality (e.g., twitching of one hand or a visual disturbance) in a patient who remains conscious. In children, partial seizures are usually motor seizures and frequently will progress to generalized seizures.

Simple Triage and Rapid Treatment (START) A triage system.

Sims position A semi-prone position with the patient on her side, with her opposite knee and thigh drawn well up to facilitate delivery of a baby.

sinus arrhythmia A variation in the resting heart rate often seen in children and adolescents. As the child breathes in the heart rate increases slightly and as they exhale the heart rate decreases. This is a normal variation in children and not truly an arrhythmia. On ECG each QRS complex is preceded by a P wave and there are no missed or skipped beats.

sinus tachycardia Rapid heart rate in a child with normal conduction.

slurry A thin, watery mixture.

smallpox A rare, highly contagious viral disease; it is most contagious when blisters begin to form.

sniffing position An upright position in which the patient's head and chin are thrust slightly forward to keep the airway open; the child appears to be sniffing.

soft-tissue injuries Injuries to the skin, fat, muscles, ligaments, and tendons.

Sort, Assess, Lifesaving interventions, and Treatment and/or Transport (SALT) Sort, assess, livesaving interventions, and treatment/transport: a triage system.

spasticity Increased tone or contractions of muscles causing stiff and awkward movements.

spina bifida A congenital anomaly where the posterior elements of the vertebrae have failed to fuse together. The spinal cord and its associated coverings (meninges) may protrude through this defect in the vertebrae leading to a range of neurologic impairment in the lower extremities depending on the degree and level of the protrusion. When the defect is isolated to the bony structures without spinal cord or meningeal abnormality this is termed spina bifida occulta.

spine The vertebral column.

spleen The major abdominal organ involved in the production and destruction of red blood cells and immune cells. It is filled with blood and can hemorrhage after injury.

splinting Fixation with a splint.

status epilepticus A state of continuous seizures or multiple seizures without an intervening return to consciousness.

sterile gauze Basic tool used to stop bleeding and keep wounds clean.

stress Forces that disrupt equilibrium or produce strain.

stridor A harsh sound during inspiration, high-pitched due to partial upper airway obstruction.

subcostal Beneath the ribs.

subdural hemorrhage Bleeding beneath the dura mater.

subglottic Beneath the glottis.

substernal Situated beneath the sternum.

sucking chest wound An open or penetrating chest-wall wound through which air passes during inspiration and expiration.

sudden unexpected infant death (SUID) The sudden death of an infant younger than 1 year that cannot be explained because a thorough investigation was not conducted and cause of death could not be determined.

superior vena cava One of the two largest veins in the body that carries blood from the upper extremities, head, neck, and chest into the heart.

supine Lying on the back with the face upward.

supraclavicular Located above the clavicle.

supraglottic The area above the glottis or true vocal cords.

suprasternal Above the sternum.

suprasternal retractions When the muscles and skin above the sternum sink in above the manubrium as the patient attempts to breathe.

supraventricular tachycardia (SVT) An abnormal heart rhythm with a rapid rate and narrow QRS complex.

symmetry Correspondence in shape, size, and relative position of parts on opposite sides of a body.

sympathomimetic agents Adrenergic drugs; producing effects resembling those resulting from stimulation of the sympathetic nervous system, such as effects following the injection of epinephrine.

symphysis pubis The junction of the pubic bones in the midline on the lower part of the abdomen.

symptomatic ventricular dysrhythmias Abnormal ventricular electrical impulses (e.g., ventricular tachycardia) that are associated with symptoms on the part of the patient.

synaptic connections Connections between two or more nerves (i.e., synapses).

systemic inflammatory response syndrome (SIRS) An inflammatory state affecting the entire body.

T

tachycardia Rapid heart rate.

tachypnea Rapid respiration.

tamponade Compression of tissues.

tension pneumothorax An accumulation of air or gas in the pleural cavity that progressively increases and causes serious hemodynamic changes.

terrorism A violent act dangerous to human life, in violation of the criminal laws of the United States or of any state, to intimidate or coerce a government, the civilian population, or any segment thereof, in furtherance of political or social objectives.

thermoregulation Heat regulation.

thoracic Pertaining to the chest or thorax.

thoracic excursions The movements of the chest wall (rib cage and muscles) associated with respirations.

thoracostomy Opening of the chest wall to allow drainage of the chest cavity.

tidal volume The amount of air that is exchanged with each breath.

titratable The ability to adjust the desired effect of an agent by giving more or less of that agent as needed over time (e.g., using an intravenous catheter to slowly give more analgesic or sedative agents until a patient is just quiet enough to effectively complete a procedure).

tonic-clonic A seizure that features rhythmic back-and-forth motion of an extremity and body stiffness.

totally implanted device A catheter totally implanted and not visible to the eye (mediport).

trachea A cylindrical cartilaginous tube from the larynx to the bronchial tubes. It extends from the 6th cervical to the 5th thoracic vertebra, where it divides at a point called the carina into two bronchi, one leading to each lung.

tracheitis An inflammation of the trachea.

tracheostomy Operation of incising the skin over the trachea and making a surgical wound in the trachea in order to permit an airway during tracheal obstruction.

tracheostomy tube A tube inserted into the trachea in children who cannot breathe or maintain a clear airway on their own.

transdermal Through the skin.

transient Not lasting; of brief duration.

transmucosal To pass across a mucous membrane (e.g., the absorption of a toxin or pharmaceutical agent across the mucous membranes of the mouth).

traumatic brain injury (TBI) The preferred term for head trauma.

tripoding An abnormal position to keep the airway open; it involves leaning forward onto two arms stretched forward.

trismus Tonic contraction of the muscles of mastication.

tympanic temperature Body temperature measurement made by the use of a device which measures the reflectance of infrared light from the tympanic membrane (ear drum).

U

umbilical cord The attachment connecting the fetus with the placenta.

umbilical vein catheterization Placing a cannula into the umbilical artery or vein.

universal precautions Protective measures that have traditionally been developed by the Centers for Disease Control and Prevention (CDC) for use in dealing with objects, blood, body fluids, or other potential exposure risks of communicable disease.

universal standards for pediatric emergency care Standards of care agreed upon and promoted by experts in pediatric emergency care and the organizations they represent for the management of children throughout the emergency medical system.

urostomy Surgical creation of a stoma to allow the elimination of urine.

V

vagal Pertaining to the vagus nerve.

vagal nerve stimulator (VNS) A small device implanted under the skin near the collarbone as a treatment for epilepsy.

vaginal introitus The vaginal opening.

vagus nerve The cranial nerve (X) that provides motor functions to the soft palate, pharynx, and larynx and carries taste bud fibers from the posterior tongue, sensory fibers from the inferior pharynx, larynx, thoracic, and abdominal organs, and parasympathetic fibers to thoracic and abdominal organs.

varicella (chicken pox) An acute viral disease with mild constitutional symptoms (headache, fever, malaise) followed by an eruption appearing in crops and characterized by macules, papules, and vesicles.

vascular tone The amount of constriction in a blood vessel or more generally, the overall amount of constriction in the blood vessels of the body. This is a reflection of the acute cardiovascular health of the patient. Patients in shock often have marked vasoconstriction in an attempt to increase their vascular tone and blood pressure to maximize perfusion to vital organs. When there is a loss of vascular tone (e.g., in sepsis or spinal shock) there is often generalized vasodilatation and severe hypotension.

vasculitis Inflammation of the blood vessels which usually is associated with pain, swelling, and often leakage of fluid and blood from the vessels into other organs. When this occurs in the skin a purpuric rash often develops.

vasoconstriction Decrease in the caliber of blood vessels.

vasodilatation Dilatation of blood vessels.

vasomotor Pertaining to the nerves having muscular control of the blood vessel walls.

vasopressor agent A drug that increases vascular tone and increases blood pressure.

ventilation-perfusion mismatch A pathologic state where the oxygen going into the lungs is not mixing appropriately with the blood circulating through the lungs.

ventilator A mechanical device for artificial ventilation of the lungs.

ventricle One of two (right and left) lower chambers of the heart. The left ventricle receives blood from the left atrium (upper chamber) and delivers blood to the aorta. The right ventricle receives blood from the right atrium and pumps it into the pulmonary artery.

ventricular fibrillation (VF) Disorganized, ineffective twitching of the ventricles, resulting in no blood flow and a state of cardiac arrest.

ventricular tachycardia (VT) A rapid heart rhythm in which the electrical impulse begins in the ventricle (instead of the atrium), which may result in inadequate blood flow and eventually deteriorate into cardiac arrest.

vertebral bodies The 33 bones that make up the spinal column.

vesicants Blister agents; the primary route of entry for vesicants is through the skin.

viral myocarditis A viral infection of the heart which frequently leads to dysrhythmias, especially ventricular dysrhythmias and poor muscle function which produces congestive heart failure.

visual analogue scores (VAS) Scales generated by asking a patient or subject to quantify the amount of a sensation they are feeling (usually pain) by pointing to where on a line their sensation is. By measuring how far along the line the patient points one can use this as a measure of that sensation. A frequently used technique for the measurement of pain in research studies.

vital signs The key signs that are used to evaluate the patient's overall condition, including respirations, pulse, blood pressure, level of consciousness, and skin characteristics.

vocal cords Two small folds of tissue in the larynx which vibrate as air moves across them to produce sound.

volume resuscitation Replenishing the blood volume.

W

wheezing Production of whistling sounds during expiration such as occurs in asthma and bronchiolitis.

work of breathing An indicator of oxygenation and ventilation. Work of breathing reflects the child's attempt to compensate for hypoxia.

Index

Note: Page numbers followed by '*f*' and '*t*' denote figures and tables.

A

AAP. *See* American Academy of Pediatrics
ABCDEs (airway, breathing, circulation, disability, exposure), 11–18, 77–79, 95–96, 145–151. *See also* assessment; initial assessment
  adaptations in, 196–198
  auscultation, 53
  pulse oximetry, 53–54
  respiratory rate, 52
abdomen, 140, 141, 141*f*
  anatomic changes, 36
  physical examination of, 23
abdominal excursions, 33
abdominal injuries, 145*t*
abnormal airway sounds, 7–8, 56
  auscultation for, 53
  interpretation of, 14*t*
abnormal appearance, 120–121
  child with, 6
abnormal circulation to skin, 10
abnormal lower airway sounds, 7
abrasions, 139
absorption, 171
abuse. *See also* child maltreatment
  emotional, 213
  vs. neglect, 213
abusive head trauma, 150, 218
acceleration-deceleration event, 139
accessory muscles, use of, 50
accidents
  defined, 322
  vs. injuries, 322
ACEP. *See* American College of Emergency Physicians
acetaminophen, 126, 168, 185–186, 445
  overdose, 6
acid ingestions, 169
acidosis, 10, 23, 253
ACM. *See* Arnold-Chiari malformation
acrocyanosis, 10, 248
ACTH. *See* adrenocorticotropic hormone
activated charcoal, 171–172, 445
  bindable toxins, 172*f*
  guidelines for use, 172*t*
  toxins poorly adsorbed by, 171, 171*t*
activation phase (disaster response), 273
active labor, patients in, 239
acute burn, 221
acute dystonic reactions, 187
acute illness, caregiver responses to, 32*t*

acute injuries, 137. *See also* trauma
additional assessment (SAMPLE), 2
  cardiovascular emergencies, 79, 79*t*, 94, 96, 97*t*
  child maltreatment, 219–220
  endocrine disorders, 125–126
  history taking, 20–21
  physical examination, 21–26
  respiratory emergencies, 71
  toxic emergencies, 169–170
  trauma, 153–154
additional monitoring devices, 26
adenoidal bleeding, 153
adenosine, 100, 446
adequate protocols, lack of, 277
ADHD. *See* attention-deficit/hyperactivity disorder
adolescents
  approaching, 43*f*
  assessment of, 43
  common conditions in, 43
  EMS provider, tips for, 45
  growth and development characteristics, 42–43
adrenaline release, 37
adrenergic agents, 83
adrenocorticotropic hormone (ACTH), 125
adult airways
  child airways *vs.*, 36*f*
  pediatric airway and, 373
adult cardiac disease, β-blockers for, 173
advanced airway techniques (procedure 13), 69, 153, 389–397
  gum elastic bougie, 396–397
  King Airway, 394–396
  LMA, 390
    insertion, 391–392
advanced life support (ALS), 12, 19, 31, 261
  activated charcoal, 171
  air embolism, 204
  airway management of pediatric burn patient, 157
  AMS, 122
  anxiety, pharmacologic management of, 158*t*
  asystole/PEA, 106
  basilar skull fracture, 149
  BLS *vs.*, 51
  bradycardia, 197
  bronchodilator administration, 197
  cardiac arrest, 102–103
  cardiopulmonary arrest, transport after failed ALS treatment in, 262

clamping a leaking central venous catheter, 203
cold-related emergencies, 132
contraindications for NG insertion, 149
CSHCN, 197
diazepam, 157
drug therapy for bradycardia, 98
elevated intracranial pressure, management of, 151
endotracheal drugs administration, 98
endotracheal intubation, 152*t*
  and epinephrine administration, 249
gastric decompression, 149
gastroenteritis, 128
hyperventilation for suspected increased intracranial pressure, 206
hypoglycemia, 204
inverted pyramid for depressed newborns, 249
IVs and shock, 85–89
midazolam, 157
morphine, 141
naloxone, 158
nonvigorous newborn, treatment of meconium aspiration in, 251
optimal cardiopulmonary resuscitation, 256
pain management, 157, 158*t*
pediatric trauma patient, volume resuscitation of, 149
pleural space, 148
postpartum hemorrhage, 245
removing a feeding tube, 205
for respiratory emergencies, 58, 61, 67
seizures, 116
sepsis and meningitis, 129
shock in newly born, 253
SVT treatment, 99–100
tension pneumothorax, management of, 148
tracheostomy care, 196
transport decision, 308
transport of newly born: hypoglycemia, 254
vascular access, 254
VF/pulseless VT, 106
volume resuscitation, 149
advocacy
  emancipated minors, 296
  for Emergency Medical Services for Children, 331–332
AED. *See* automated external defibrillator
AEIOU TIPPS (causes of AMS), 120, 121*t*
afebrile seizures, 114

age
   minimum blood pressure by, 16t
   normal heart rate for, 14t
   normal respiratory rate for, 12t
agent, 323
agonist, 58
AHA guidelines. *See* American Heart
      Association guidelines
AICD. *See* automated internal cardiac
      defibrillator
air embolism, 204
air movement, auscultation for, 53
air transport, 315
airway, 11–12. *See also* asthma; lower
      airway obstruction; respiratory
      emergencies; upper airway
      obstruction
   anatomic changes, 35–36
   clearing in newborns, 246–247
   CSHCN, 196
   management
      of pediatric burn patient, 156–158
      of pediatric trauma patient, 153
      in seizing children, 116, 116f
   obstruction, 56–65, 145, 146f
      above thoracic inlet, 57
      children, 347
   occlusion, 246
   pediatric and adult, 373
   poor air movement, causes of, 53t
   toxic emergencies, 161
airway adjuncts, 67, 146
airway adjuncts (procedure 5), 67. *See
      also* advanced airway techniques
      (procedure 13)
   NP airway insertion, 353, 354–355
   OP airway insertion, 353, 354–355
airway injuries, 145–146, 145t, 146f
   special considerations in pediatric
      trauma, 152–153
airway sounds, abnormal, 7–8
albuterol (salbutamol), 63, 63t, 65, 84t,
      134, 157, 210, 360, 361, 446
alcohol abuse, 163
alert, verbal, painful, unresponsive
      (AVPU) scale, 5, 17, 17t, 121, 150,
      151, 198
alkali ingestions, 171
allergies, 153t
ALS. *See* advanced life support
altered mental status (AMS), 17,
      111, 173
   AEIOU TIPPS (causes of), 120, 121t
   assessment of, 120, 121f
   common causes of, 167
   description, 120, 126
   management of, 122, 122f
alternative breathing, 69
alveoli, 7, 9, 33
ambulance, 308. *See also* transport
      decisions
   child restraint systems in, 310–315
   taking caregivers in, 309–310

American Academy of Pediatrics (AAP),
      2, 247, 325, 332
   EIF, 195
American Association of Poison
      Control Centers Toxic
      Exposure Surveillance System,
      161, 162t
American College of Emergency
      Physicians (ACEP), 195, 332
American Heart Association (AHA)
      guidelines, 101, 104f
amiodarone, 100, 446
amniotic fluid, 237, 240
AMS. *See* altered mental status
analgesia, 24
analgesic dose, 150t
anaphylactic reaction, 133
anaphylactic shock, 83
anaphylaxis, 76, 77, 82, 133. *See also*
      shock
   treatment of, 88
anatomic changes
   abdomen, 36
   chest and lungs, 35
   heart, 35–36
   musculoskeletal system, 36
   neck and airway, 35
   nervous system, 36
   through childhood, 37
anatomic features, 323
   of infants, 37t
ancillary services, 302
antecubital fossa, 14, 254
anterior fontanelle of infant, 22f
anthrax, 284
antibiotics, 127
anticonvulsant administration, 19
antidotes, 173, 173t
antigen, 83
antipyretics, 126
antivenin, 133
anxiety, 183
   pharmacologic management, 158t
   during transport, 309, 309f
anxiolysis, 24
   methods of, 25t
APAP, 445
APGAR score, 246, 247t
apnea, 38, 118
apneic baby, 247
appearance, 338t
   characteristics of, 5, 76–77, 77f, 94
   CSHCN, 196
   respiratory emergencies, 51
   techniques to assessment, 5–7
   "tickles" (TICLS) mnemonic, 5t
   trauma, 144, 144t
Arnold-Chiari malformation, 197
arteriovenous (AV) fistula, 208
ASD. *See* autism spectrum disorder
asphyxia, 106, 253
aspiration, 7–8
aspirin, 127, 166, 167, 447

assessment, 2, 322. *See also* additional
      assessment; general assessment;
      initial assessment
   ABCDEs (airway, breathing,
      circulation, disability, exposure),
      11–18, 77–79, 95–96,
      145–151
   additional. *See* additional assessment
      (SAMPLE)
   of adolescents, 43
   AMS, 120–121, 121f
   bites and stings, 133–134
   bradycardia, 97–98
   burns, 155–156
   cardiac arrest, 102–103
   cardiovascular, 79, 96
   circulation. *See* circulation assessment
   cold-related emergencies, 132–133
   CSF shunts, 205–206
   CSHCN, 44–45, 195–198
   diabetes mellitus, 123
   of distributive shock, 82–83
   environmental, 3f, 330
   factors associated with maltreatment,
      216t
   fever, 126–127, 127f
   gastroenteritis, 128
   general assessment (PAT), 3–11,
      76–77, 80, 89
   history taking, 20–21
   hyperglycemia, 123
   hypoglycemia, 123–124
   hypothermia, 132–133
   of infants, 38–39
   of injured child (trauma), 143
   meningitis, 129–130
   newborns, 246–248
   pain of, 24–26
   pediatric. *See* pediatric assessment
   perineum, 237
   postictal child, 119–120, 120t
   prearrival preparation, 3
   of preschoolers, 41
   primary. *See* primary assessments
   SAMPLE mnemonic, 20, 20t
   scene size-up, 3
   of school-aged children, 42
   seizures, 116–119, 116f, 116t–117t,
      119t
   sepsis, 129–130
   shock, 80–89
   summary of assessment flowchart, 2
   tachycardia, 98–99
   of toddlers, 40
   toxic emergencies, 165–170
   tracheostomy tube, 201
assisted ventilation, 13, 52, 97, 117,
      148, 247
asthma, 8, 64, 194
   in children, 49
   treatment, 61, 62t
asymmetric pupils, 151
asystole, 101, 103

asystolic arrest, 102
ataxia, 121
atrioventricular heart block, 98
atropine, 63, 98, 174, 282, 423, 447
attention-deficit/hyperactivity disorder
(ADHD), 182, 182f, 194
auscultation, 7, 13, 34, 53
autism, 194
autism spectrum disorder (ASD),
180–182, 181t
automated external defibrillator (AED),
101–102, 101f
automated internal cardiac defibrillator
(AICD), 207
automatic external defibrillator (AED)
and defibrillation (procedure 19),
420–424
conventional use, 421–422
electrical charge for countershock,
421t
one rescuer with, 423
paddle size, 421t
two rescuers with, 424
AV fistula. See arteriovenous fistula
AVPU scale. See alert, verbal, painful,
unresponsive scale
avulsion, 242
axial loading, 141
axillary temperature, 35

B

Bacillus anthracis, 284
back, physical examination of, 23
bacterial pneumonia, 65
bacterial toxins, 76, 82
bacterial upper airway infections, 58
bag-mask device, 200
attached to tracheostomy tube adapter,
200, 201f
on newborn, 249f
vs. endotracheal tube (ET), 152
bag-mask ventilation, 60f, 65, 67,
152t, 248
in place, 148f
prolonged, 252
bag-mask ventilation (procedure 8), 67,
363–366
using one-rescuer technique, 365
using two-rescuer technique, 366
BAL. See British anti-lewisite
baseline general appearance, 195
basic life support (BLS), 299
algorithm, pediatric, 104f
foreign body obstruction maneuvers,
356, 357
transport decision, 19
vs. ALS, 51
basilar skull fracture, 22, 149
Battle sign, 23
β-blockers, 173
bedside blood glucose test, 122, 122f

behavioral emergencies, 179–190
description of, 179–180
pediatric psychiatric and behavioral
conditions, 180–185
anxiety, 183
attention-deficit/hyperactivity
disorder, 182, 182f
autism spectrum disorder,
180–182, 181t
bipolar disorder, 184
conduct disorder, 183
depression, 183–184
oppositional defiant disorder, 183
schizophrenia, 185
psychiatric medications, adverse
reactions of, 186–187
acute dystonic reactions, 187
neuroleptic malignant syndrome, 187
suicide attempt/intentional ingestions
or exposures, 185–186
acetaminophen, 185–186
history taking, 185
selective serotonin reuptake
inhibitors, 186
serotonin syndrome, signs and
symptoms, 186t
tricyclic antidepressants, 186
transport and, 187–189
chemical restraint, 188
emotional well-being, 189
physical restraint, 188–189
verbal restraint, 188
benzodiazepines, 25t, 157, 173
for seizures
administration routes of, 117, 117t
diazepam, 118
lorazepam, 118
midazolam, 118
bilateral air movement, 197
bindable toxins, 172f
biologic agents, assessment and treatment
of, 283–284
biologic disease, treatment of, 285–287
biologic pathogens, 283
biologic weapons, 283
bioterrorism, 164
medical management of, 286t
bipolar disorder, 184
bites, 133–134
bladder, 141
bleeding, 145
bleeding disorders, 222
blind nasotracheal intubation, 153
blizzards, 272t
blood loss, 142
blood pressure, 15–16, 78–79, 96
minimum by age, 16t
systolic, 78
values for age, 34, 35t
blow-by oxygen, 86, 200, 342, 344t, 345
BLS. See basic life support
blunt injuries, 81, 137, 141
to chest, 85

body homeostasis, 5
body temperature, 35
booster seat, 312
botulism, 285
bowels, 143f
BPD. See bronchopulmonary dysplasia
brachial pulse, 78, 95
anatomic position of, 14, 15f
bradycardia, 14, 78, 95, 97–98, 173,
198, 247
assessment, 98
treatment, 98
brain death, 149
brain injuries, 6, 9. See also head injuries
brain ischemia, 150
brain perfusion, 5, 6, 9
brainstem, 16
functions for AMS, 120–121
brainstem herniation, 121, 129, 147,
149, 151
breastfeeding, 245–246
breathing, 12, 146–148
breath sounds, 14t
listening for, 56
CSHCN, 197
disordered control of, 65, 66
ensure adequate, 116–117
in newborns, 247
patterns, 264
toxic emergencies, 162
trauma and, 146–148
breech birth, 237f
breech deliveries, 237–238
breech presentation, 236
brief resolved unexplained event (BRUE)
clinical interventions, 264–265
common clinical presentation of, 264
defined, 264
SUIDS and, 264
summary of, 265
British anti-lewisite (BAL), 283
bronchiolitis, 8, 61, 64, 64t
bronchoconstriction, 61
bronchodilators, 197
treatment, 52, 63
bronchodilator therapy (procedure 7),
63, 360–362
inhalation therapy, 361
intramuscular therapy, 362
bronchopulmonary dysplasia (BPD),
194, 196
bronchovesicular, 35
bruises, 139
maltreatment and, 220–222
buccal route, seizures, 118
buckle fractures, 141
bulb syringes, 347
oropharyngeal/nasopharyngeal
suctioning with, 348–349
bulging fontanelle, 126
burns, 137
assessment, 155–156
child maltreatment, 221–222

burns, 137 (*Continued*)
  management, 156–158, 158*t*
  summary of, 158
buttons. *See* feeding tubes

C

CAH. *See* congenital adrenal hyperplasia
calcium channel blockers, 84, 173
calcium chloride, 173, 447
calcium gluconate, 173, 448
cancer, 194
cannulating peripheral veins, 86
capillary refill time (CRT), 15, 75, 78, 78*f*,
  95–96
capnography, 122, 379, 380
capnometry, 54
car bed for children, 312*f*
carbon dioxide detector device, 70*f*, 384,
  386, 387*t*
carbon monoxide poisoning, 162, 367
cardiac arrest, 102–103
  assessment, 103
  causes, 103
  chest compressions, 103, 104*f*
  length-based drug dosage, 103, 106*f*
  transport decision, 106–107, 107*f*
  treatment, 103, 107
cardiac contusion, 149
cardiac dysrhythmia, 103
cardiac medication, 84
cardiogenic shock, 76, 77, 79*t*, 83–85,
  88–89
  assessment of, 84–85
  symptoms and signs of, 84*t*
  treatment of, 88–89
cardiomyopathy, 98
cardiopulmonary arrest (CPA), 262–263,
  415
cardiopulmonary resuscitation (CPR), 261
  AED with, 101*f*
cardiopulmonary resuscitation (CPR)
  (procedure 18)
  chest compression, 416*t*
  on child, 417–418
  ETCO₂ for quality of compressions,
    417–419
  high-quality, 416
  on infant, 417
  pediatric assessment, 415–416
  ventilation ratios, 416*t*
cardiovascular assessment, summary of,
  79, 96–97
cardiovascular emergencies. *See also* shock
  additional assessment (SAMPLE), 79,
    79*t*, 94
  AED, 101–102, 101*f*
  bradycardia, 97–98
  cardiac arrest, 102–103
  drowning, 108, 108*f*
  dysrhythmias, 97–102
  evaluation, presenting complaint, 76,
    94, 97*t*

general assessment (PAT), 76–77,
    94–95
  prearrival preparation, 76, 94
  primary assessment (ABCDEs), 77–79,
    95–96
  scene size-up, 76, 94
  tachycardia, 98–101
  transport decisions, 89, 106–107, 107*f*
caregivers
  in ambulance, 309–310
  behavior of, 217
  child maltreatment, 217
  communication with, 33
  emotional responses of, 281
  refusal of care or transport, 292–293
  responses to acute illness/injury, 32*t*
  response to infant death, 265–266, 266*f*
  who disagree about care and transport,
    294–295
carotid pulse, 78
car seats in ambulances, 311
  securing to stretcher, 313–314,
    313*f*, 314*f*
  using after collision, 313, 313*t*
cartilage, 139
cartilaginous growth plates, 36, 141
catastrophic events, 271
cathartic charcoal, 172*t*
catheter
  central venous, 202–204
  site infection, 203
  sizes per tracheal tube, 425*t*
  suction, 22
caustic agent, 166
central cyanosis, 248
central nervous system (CNS)
    function, 5
central venous catheters, 202–204
  complications of, 203–204
  types of, 203
cephalopelvic disproportion, 244–245
cerebral cortex, 16
cerebral edema, 123, 149
cerebral palsy, 194, 196, 210
cerebral spinal fluid (CSF) shunts,
    205–206
cerebrospinal fluid, 22
cervical collar, 139, 154
cervical spine injuries, 147
Chain of Survival, Pediatric, 102
CHD. *See* congenital heart disease
chemical weapons, 281
chest, 139–140, 139*f*, 140*f*
  anatomic changes, 35
  injuries, 145*t*
  physical examination of, 23
chest compressions, 103, 104*f*
  to ventilation ratios, 416*t*
chest wall, 139, 139*f*
CHF. *See* congestive heart failure
Child Abuse Prevention and Treatment
    Act (CAPTA), 224
child airways *vs.* adult airways, 36*f*
child care facilities, 278

child maltreatment, 302
  abuse *vs.* neglect, 213
  additional assessment, 219–220
  assessing caregiver's behavior, 217
  assessment factors, 216, 216*t*
  background, 213–214
  child neglect, 213
  communication with child and
    caregivers, 217
  complications of, 214*t*
  CPS, 213, 223–224
  defined, 213
  documentation of, 217–218
  duties, communication and assessment
    in, 223
  emotional abuse, 213
  emotional neglect, 213
  fact *vs.* fiction, 220, 220*t*
  human trafficking, 225–227, 226*t*–227*t*
  mandatory obligation to report,
    216–217
  physical abuse, 213
  physical examination, 220–222
    bruises, 220–221
    burns, 221–222
    deceptive skin signs masquerading
      as abuse, 222
    fractures, 222
  prehospital professional in,
    216–218, 217*t*
  questions and considerations in
    evaluating, 219, 219*t*
  risk factors for, 216
  scene assessment, 217–218
  sexual abuse, 213
  SUIDS and, 260
  transport decision, 218
  victims by race/ethnic group, 216*t*
child neglect, 213
child protective services (CPS), 213,
    223–224
  initial actions, 224*t*
  for protection against child
    maltreatment, 223–224
child refusal of transport, medicolegal
    issues, 292–293
children
  additional assessment, 169–170
  airway obstruction, 347
  babies born to narcotic-addicted
    mothers, 122
  characteristics of, 389
  in disasters, 271
  effective emergency care of, 2
  emotional responses of, 281
  endotracheal intubation, 347
  general assessment, 165
  illness/injury, family's response to,
    32, 32*f*
  initial management of toxic
    exposures, 168
  iron poisoning in, 168
  mental health needs of, 281
  modified anatomic diagram of, 155, 156*f*

poisoning in, 162, 163
primary assessment, 165–167
toxicologic emergencies in, 174
with tracheostomy tubes, 347
transport decision, 169
unique anatomic features of
    abdomen, 140–141, 141f
    chest, 139–140, 139f, 140f
    extremities, 141–142, 141f
    head injury, 138–139, 140f
    skin, 142
    spinal column, 139
children assisted by technology. *See*
    technology, children assisted by
children with special health care needs
    (CSHCN), 32, 43–44, 280. *See also*
    disabled children
additional EMS considerations for,
    209–210
approaching, 44f
assessment of, 44–45, 198–199
    initial assessment (ABCDEs), 196–198
    modifications, 195–196
    PAT, 196
care coordination for, 209
children assisted by technology
    central venous catheters, 202–204
    CSF shunts, 205–206
    dialysis shunts, 208
    feeding tubes, 204–205
    ICD, 207
    internal pacemakers, 207
    ostomies, 206–207
    tracheostomy tubes, 199–202
    VNS, 207–208
chronic conditions, 194
cognitive disabilities, 193–194
defined, 193
evaluation of, 195
growth and development
    characteristics, 43–44
medical home for, 209
physical disabilities, 194–195
transport, 199, 208
child restraint systems (CRS) in
    ambulance
    car seats, 313–314
    choosing, 311–313, 312f
    dangers of, 310–311, 314
    integrated, 311, 311f
    stretcher, securing to, 313–314,
        313f, 314f
    summary of, 315
choanal atresia, 252
cholinergic crisis, 168
cholinergic impulses, 34
chronic respiratory illness, 54
circadian rhythm, 34
circulation, 13–16, 264
    CSHCN, 197
    functional components of, 80
    hypothermia and, 132
    toxic emergencies, 166–167
    trauma and, 149

circulation assessment
    blood pressure, 78–79, 96
    heart rate, 95
    HR, 77–78
    pulse quality, 78, 95
    skin temperature and CRT, 78, 78f,
        95–96
    using PAT, 76–77, 94–95
circulation to skin, 77, 94, 95
    characteristics of, 9–10, 10t
    CSHCN, 196
    PAT characteristics, 77, 94–95
    respiratory emergencies, 52
    signs of, 15
    techniques to assessment, 10
    trauma, 144–145, 145f
CISM. *See* critical incident stress
    management
clamping down, 76, 77
clavicles, 23
clean delivery surface, selecting, 242
clean dry sheets, 156
clinical problem, 20
closed head injuries, 144, 154
Clostridium botulinum, 285
coin rubbing, 222, 223f
cold circulating air temperature, 10
cold-related emergencies
    assessment, 132
    management, 132, 132f
color assessment, 248
colorimetric exhaled carbon dioxide
    detector, 387t
colostomy, 206
coma, 167
comfort level, transport decision, 19
commotio cordis, 101, 103
communication
    with child and caregivers, 33, 217
    from medical home, 326
    skills, 32
community, prevention role and, 330–331
Community Emergency Response Team
    (CERT), 330
community resources, for critical
    incident stress, 268
compensated shock, 81
    IV fluid treatment of, 87
compensatory mechanisms, 6, 79, 81
complex febrile seizure, 114
complex partial seizures, 115
compression, 139
concussion, 11, 151
conduct disorder, 183
confidentiality, 295
confirmation of endotracheal tube and
    end-tidal capnography (procedure
    12), 70, 383–388
    carbon dioxide detector device,
        384, 386, 387t
    clinical assessment, 384–385
    esophageal detector bulb or
        syringe, 383
    quantitative end-tidal CO$_2$, 388

confusion, symptoms of, 151
congenital adrenal hyperplasia (CAH),
    124
congenital anomalies, 103
congenital cardiovascular defects, 253
congenital diaphragmatic hernia,
    252–253, 253f
congenital disorders, 252–253
congenital heart block, 98
congenital heart disease (CHD), 38, 76,
    107–108, 194
    causing CHF, 108t
congenital problems, 193
congestive heart failure (CHF), 77
    congenital heart disease causing, 108t
consent for care, 174
constipation, 172t
contact burns, 156
continuous positive airway pressure
    (CPAP), 63
contraindications for NG insertion, 149
convertible child safety seat, 312f
copious secretions, 197
core body temperature, 132
core perfusion, 6
coroners, SUIDS and, 264t
corrosive substance ingestion, 172t
cortical functions for AMS, 120
cortisol deficiency, 124
counseling, for critical incident stress,
    268–269
CPA. *See* cardiopulmonary arrest
CPAP. *See* continuous positive airway
    pressure
CPR. *See* cardiopulmonary resuscitation
CPS. *See* child protective services
crackles, 13
cranium, 36
crash testing of ambulances, 314
crepitus, 147
cricothyrotomy, 69t
criminal activity, 279
critical incident stress management
    (CISM), 267t, 271, 287
    community resources, 268
    risk reduction activities and risk
        counseling, 268–269
croup, 7, 9, 65
    invasive airway management for, 58
    pharmacologic treatment of, 58
crowning, 237
CRS in ambulance. *See* child restraint
    systems in ambulance
CRT. *See* capillary refill time
crystalloid fluid, 46, 157, 197
CSF shunts. *See* cerebral spinal fluid
    shunts
CSHCN. *See* children with special health
    care needs
cultural differences, respect for, 295–296
cupping, 222, 222f
curvature of spine, 36
cyanide, 282
cyanosis, 9, 52, 248

D

cyanotic heart disease, 193
cyclic antidepressant, 167
  overdose, 6
cystic fibrosis, 53, 194–195

dark-skinned children, 11*f*
data management, 328–329
death
  causes of, 137
  injury-related, 138*t*
  responses to an infant, 265–267
deceptive skin signs, 222
decerebrate posturing, 121
decompensated shock, 6, 81
  IV fluid treatment of, 87
decontamination, 275, 286–287
  toxicologic management, 174
    eyes, 170–171
    gastrointestinal, 171–172
    skin, 170
decorticate posturing, 121
decubitus position, lateral, 116
defibrillator, 100. *See also* automated
    external defibrillator
dehydration, 280
delivery
  breech deliveries, 237–238
  of infant, 233
  obstetric pack, 241*t*
  performing, 242–245
  perineum assessment, 237
  positioning of mother, 241–242
  preparation for, 240–242
  resuscitation-oriented history,
    240–241
  risks and benefits of, 238*t*
  safe maternal position for, 241, 241*f*
  selecting a clean delivery surface, 242
  triage of patient in labor, 236–239
  vaginal
    complications during, 244–245
    steps for, 242–244
  warming environment, 241
demarcated creases, 221
dendrites, 36
depressed newly born resuscitation, 247
depression, 183–184
developmental characteristics
  of adolescents, 42–43
  CSHCN, 43–44
  infants, 37–38
  preschoolers, 40–41
  school-aged children, 41
  toddlers, 39
dexamethasone, 448
dextrose, 124, 125, 198, 249, 452
diabetes mellitus. *See also* hypoglycemia
  assessment of, 123
  management of, 123
  types 1 and 2, 123–124
diabetes (type 1), 123

diabetes (type 2), 123, 124
diabetic ketoacidosis (DKA), 23, 123
diagnostic testing, 27
dialysis shunts, 208
diaphoresis, 168
diaphoretic shock, 85
diaphragm, 35, 67, 140, 140*f*
diaphysis, 36
diarrhea, 128–129
diastolic pressure, 34
diazepam, 25, 157, 328, 427, 448
  for seizures, 118
diffuse axonal injury, 149
dilated pupil, 151
dinitrogen oxide, 456
diphenhydramine, 88, 449
diphenhydramine hydrochloride, 134
direct medical control, 302, 302*f*, 303*t*
dirty bomb, 285
disability
  assessment of, 16–17
  CSHCN, 198
  hypothermia, 132
  management of, 117, 117*t*
  toxic emergencies and, 167
  trauma and, 149–151
disabled children, 44, 215. *See also*
    children with special health care
    needs
disasters
  anthrax, 284
  biologic agents, 283
  biologic disease, treatment of,
    285–287
  chemicals, 281
  children in, 271
  CISM, 287
  cyanide, 282
  defined, 271
  explosives, 287
  family reunification, 277
  man-made, 272, 272*t*, 279
  natural, 272, 272*t*
    disease epidemics, 279
    earthquakes, 277–278
    floods, 278
    hurricanes, tornados, and severe
      storms, 278–279
  nerve agents, 281–282
  nuclear, 285–287
  plague, 284
  planning, 273
  pulmonary intoxicants, 283
  response to
    overall strategy, 273–274
    phases, 273
    staging, 274
    triage, 274–275
  ricin, 284
  roles of prehospital professional in,
    273–274
  smallpox, 283–284, 284*f*
  staging, 274
  transport and tracking, 277

  treatment, 275–277
    bioterrorism infections, 286*t*
    vesicants, 283
  triage in, 274–275
  types of, 272
  vulnerable pediatric physiologic and
    psychologic characteristics in,
    280–281
disease epidemics, 279
distal extremities, 36
distal femur site, 413
distal tibia site, 413
distention of abdomen, 23
distraction techniques, 25*f*
distributive shock, 76, 81*t*, 88
  assessment of, 82–83
  treatment of, 88
  types of, 82–83
diving reflex, 100, 100*f*
DKA. *See* diabetic ketoacidosis
Do Not Resuscitate (DNR) order, 297, 297*f*
donut burn, 221, 222*f*
dopamine, 88, 449
DOPE (dislodgment, obstruction,
    pneumothorax, equipment), 68*t*
Down syndrome, 195, 196, 197
dressings, 156
drowning, 108*f*, 137, 138*t*
  prevention of, 108
  treatment of, 108
drug dosage, length-based, 103, 106*f*
drug intoxication, shock from, 83, 83*t*
drugs
  endotracheal administration of, 98
  ET delivery of, 426
drug use, life-threatening complications
    of, 174
dual lumen airways, 57, 69*t*
DUMBELS mnemonic, 168, 174
dysphagia, 166
dysrhythmias, 76, 84. *See also*
    cardiovascular emergencies
  AED, 101–102, 101*f*
  bradycardia, 97–98
  cardiac, 103
  summary of, 102
  symptomatic ventricular, 102
  tachycardia, 98–101, 99*t*

E

EAP. *See* employee assistance programs
early (compensated) hypovolemic
    shock, 81
  IV fluid treatment of, 87
ears, physical examination of, 22–23
earthquakes, 277–278
E-C clamp technique, 147, 148*f*
ECG. *See* electrocardiogram
edema, 23, 145
effective emergency care of children, 2
effectiveness, 329
efficiency, 326

effortless tachypnea, 10, 77, 94
EHRs. *See* electronic health records
EIF. *See* emergency information form
electrical charge for countershock, 421*t*
electrocardiogram (ECG), 35
    of sinus arrhythmia, 34*f*
    of sinus tachycardia, 100*f*
electrocution, 103
electronic health records (EHRs), 209
elevated intracranial pressure,
        management of, 151
emancipated minors, 292, 294
    advocacy, 296
    characteristics of, 294*t*
emergencies. *See* medical emergencies
emergency information form (EIF), 195,
        280, 326, 327*f*
emergency medical services (EMS),
        31–32, 137, 216, 233, 261–263, 336
    on consent, 295
    pediatric calls and response from, 32–33
    policy, 295, 300
    professionalism, ethical considerations
        and, 234
    protocols, 57, 163, 164
    system, 271, 272, 278–279, 301
        status epilepticus, 114
        transport decision, 19
    tips for, 45
    transport, 155
Emergency Medical Services for Children
        (EMSC), 273, 320
    advocacy for, 331–332
    data and information management,
        328–329
    data collection, importance of, 329
    EMS-EMSC continuum, 320, 321*f*
    medical home, 325–326
    prehospital professional's roles for
        prevention, 329–331
        common injuries and prevention
            strategies, 331*t*
        in community, 330–331
        safe transport, 330
        on scene, 330
    prevention, 322–325
    quality and safety in, 326, 328
Emergency Nurses Association, 332
emergency protective custody, 293
emesis, 145
emotional abuse, 213
emotional crises, in disasters, 278
emotional distress of children, 309
emotional neglect, 213
empathy, 263*t*
employee assistance programs (EAP), 138
EMS. *See* emergency medical services
EMSC. *See* Emergency Medical Services
        for Children
EMS-EMSC continuum, 320, 321*f*, 325
encephalitis, 21
endocrine disorders
    additional assessment, 125–126
    CAH, 124

cortisol deficiency, 125
    diabetes mellitus, 123–124
    hospital transport, 125
    hyperglycemia, 123
    panhypopituitarism, 125–126
endotracheal drugs administration, 98
endotracheal intubation (ETI)
        (procedure 11), 68–69, 88, 152*t*,
        249, 373, 389. *See also* confirmation
        of endotracheal tube and end-tidal
        capnography (procedure 12)
    children with, 347
    extubation, 382
    indications for tube removal, 380
    insertion, 382
    management with, 67
    reconfirming placement, 381
    securing, 381
    selecting sizes, 377*t*
    suggestion of, 376*t*
endotracheal tube drug instillation
        (procedure 20), 98, 425–426
    catheter sizes, 425*t*
    endotracheal drug delivery, 426
endotracheal tube (ETT), 396
    placement, confirmation of, 69–70
    troubleshooting, 68*t*
end-tidal carbon dioxide ($ETCO_2$), 418–419
    for AMS, 122
    detectors, 70, 70*f*
    for quality of compressions, 418–419
enteroviruses, 129
envenomation, 133
environment, of injuries, 323
environmental assessment, 3*f*, 330
environmental emergencies, 111
    bites and stings, 133–134
    cold-related, 132–133, 132*f*
    heat-related, 130–131, 131*t*
environmental factors, SUIDS cases, 260
epiglottis
    changes, 35
    inflammation of, 58
epiglottitis, 58
epilepsy, 113
epinephrine, 58, 65, 88, 98, 106, 133, 157,
        249, 361, 422, 426, 450. *See also*
        anaphylaxis
epiphysis, 36
equipment for premature infant
        resuscitation, 240*f*
equity, 326
esophageal detector bulb or syringe, 383
esophageal intubation, 394
esophagus, 59
$ETCO_2$. *See* end-tidal carbon dioxide
ethical considerations. *See also*
        medicolegal considerations
    and EMS professionalism, 234
    ETI. *See* endotracheal intubation
etiology, 75
ETT. *See* endotracheal tube
evaporation, 246
event factors, injury phases, 324, 324*f*

exhalation, 7
expiratory wheezing, 13
explosives, 287
exposure, 17–18
    CSHCN, 198
    trauma, 151
extension, 139
extensor posturing, 17
external radiation exposure, 285
extraocular muscle movements, 21
extreme flexion, 139
extreme hyperventilation, 151
extremities, physical examination, 23–24
extremities injuries, 141–142, 141*f*
eye contact, 6, 6*f*
eyes, physical examination of, 21
eyes, toxic treatment, 170–171, 171*f*
EZ-IO insertion, 411–412

F

facial bruises, 220
falls, 139, 142*t*
family
    communication with, 33
    pediatric calls and response from,
        32–33
    reunification, 277
fatal injuries, 138. *See also* injuries; trauma
FBAO. *See* foreign body airway
        obstruction
febrile respiratory infections, 126
febrile seizures, 113–114
feeding tubes, 199
    complications of, 205
    removal of, 205
    types of, 204
fenestrated tubes, 200
fentanyl, 25, 141, 157, 158*t*, 450
fetal-placental transfusion, 253
fetus, 240
fever, 126–127
    age and, 127
    assessment, 126–127, 127*f*
    description, 126
    management, 127
field reporting (procedure 1), 27, 336–339
    template, 339*t*
    terminology, 338*t*
fires, 138, 138*t*
flaccidity, 16, 121
flail chest, 139
flexor posturing, 17
flexural creases, 221
floods, 278
fluid resuscitation, 253
flumazenil, 173, 173*t*, 450
focal, 113
fontanelle, 21
foreign body airway obstruction (FBAO)
    in children, 356
    maneuvers, 60, 60*f*, 60*t*
foreign body aspiration, 59, 64, 65*f*, 66

foreign body obstruction (procedure 6), 60
  BLS maneuvers, 356, 357
  laryngoscopy and Magill forceps, 358
foreign body removal, 60
fosphenytoin, 119, 119*t*, 451
fractures, 141
  maltreatment and, 222
fulminant pneumonia, 50
furosemide, 451

G

gag reflex, 122
gastric decompression, 149
gastric distention, 147, 148–149
gastric feeding tube, 44
gastric tube insertion, 369
gastroenteritis, 81
  assessment, 128
  description, 128
  management, 128–129
gastrointestinal decontamination, 171–172
gastrostomy tube, 204
general assessment (Pediatric Assessment
      Triangle), 2, 5–11
  cardiovascular emergencies, 80, 94–95
  respiratory emergencies, 51–52
  toxic emergencies, 165
  trauma, 144–145
generalized seizures, 113, 115
general observations, 21
genital growth, 35
gentle bulb suction, 22, 22*f*
gestation, 234–235, 240
GH. *See* growth hormone
Glasgow Coma Scale, 198
glial cells, 36
glottis, 7
glove distribution, 156, 157*f*
glucagon, 122, 124, 204, 451
glucose, 452
greenstick fractures, 141
growth hormone (GH), 125
growth plates, cartilaginous, 141
grunting, 7, 65
G-tube. *See* gastrostomy tube
guardian refusal of transport,
      medicolegal issues, 292–293
gum elastic bougie, 69*t*, 396
  device, 397
gunshot wounds, 85
gurgling, 7

H

Haemophilus influenzae type B vaccine, 129
hazardous materials exposures, 164,
      279, 279*t*, 281. *See also* Toxic
      emergencies
  common materials, 279*t*
hazardous materials (HazMat), 281

HCM. *See* hypertrophic cardiomyopathy
head, physical examination, 21, 22*f*
head bobbing, 8, 196
head injuries, 138–139, 142, 147. *See also*
      brain injuries
head-tilt/chin-lift maneuver, 56, 57*f*
health information exchanges (HIEs), 209
healthy infant, 254
hearing impairment, 194
heart
  anatomic changes, 35–36
  congenital heart disease, 76, 107–108
  congestive heart failure, 77
  heart rate (HR), 13–14
    by age, 14*t*, 34, 34*t*
    assessing in newborns, 247–248
    circulation assessment, 76–77, 95
heat cramps, 130, 131
heat exhaustion, 130, 131
heat-related emergencies assessment, 131
  clinical presentation of, 131*t*
  description, 131
  management, 131
heat stroke, 130, 131
hematomas, 21
hemodialysis, 208
hemodynamically stable child, 155
hemopericardium, 85
hemophilia, 195, 222
hemorrhage, 144–145
hemostat, 203
hepatomegaly, 84
HIEs. *See* health information exchanges
highest level MCI, 272
hives, 83, 83*f*
hoarse speech. *See* muffled speech
homeostasis, 5
hospital destination, 300–301
hospital transport. *See also* transport
      decisions
  cardiac arrest, 107
  endocrine disorders, 125
  hyperglycemia, 125
  seizures, 119
host, 323
HR. *See* heart rate
human health, common chemicals
      detrimental to, 281*t*
human trafficking, pediatric, 225–227,
      226*t*–227*t*
hurricanes, 278–279
hydrocarbon, 23
  inhalation, 166
hydrocephalus, 205
hydrochloric acid, 168
hydrocortisone, 124, 452
hydroxocobalamin, 282
hymenoptera, 135
hyperalimentation, 204
hypercapnia, 53
hyperglycemia. *See also* diabetes
  assessment of, 123
  defined, 123

hospital transport, 125
  management of, 123
  signs and symptoms of, 123
  treatment of, 123
hyperoxia, 255
hypertension, b-blockers, 173
hyperthermia, 130
hypertrophic cardiomyopathy (HCM),
      101
hypnotic drug, 166
hypocarbia, 10
hypoglycemia, 6, 38
  newborn, 254
  treatment, 204
hypoperfusion, 76, 144–145
  SAMPLE components in child with,
      79, 79*t*
hypotension, 26, 82
hypothermia, 46, 132, 142, 241
  assessment, 132
  in newborns, 255
  treatment, 132, 132*f*
hypotonia, 121
hypovolemia, 75, 81, 82, 254
  treatment of, 86
hypovolemic shock, 46, 81, 81*t*, 82
  compensated stage of, 81
  decompensated stage of, 81–82
  treatment of, 87
hypoxemia, 26
hypoxia, 77, 150, 151, 197, 247, 342
  conditions causes, 7
  evaluation for hypovolemia and, 102
  moderate to severe, 9*f*
  placement of oximetry probe,
      53–54, 54*f*
  suctioning (procedure 4), 348
hypoxic stress, 9, 50

I

ibuprofen, 126, 452
ICD. *See* internal cardiac defibrillator
ICS. *See* Incident Command System
IDDM. *See* insulin-dependent diabetes
      mellitus
ileostomy, 206
illness
  PAT to evaluation, 10–11
  preventing, 322–325
  responses to, 32*t*
IM. *See* intramuscular injections
impaled objects, 147–148
impending brainstem herniation, 16, 151
impending herniation syndrome, 151, 152
implanted devices, 203
implementation phase (disaster
      response), 273
implied consent, 292
Incident Commander, 273
Incident Command System (ICS), 273
indirect medical control, 302–303, 303*t*

indwelling central venous catheters, 199
infant death. *See also* sudden infant death syndrome
　caregiver's response to, 265–266, 266*f*
　prehospital professional's response to, 266–267, 267*t*
infants, 37–38
　anatomic and physiologic features of, 37*t*
　approaching, 38*f*
　assessment of, 38–39
　common conditions in, 38
　delivery of, 233
　developmental characteristics, 37–38
　EMS provider, tips for, 45
　growth rates of, 35
　monitoring, 255
infections, 6
inflicted burns, 221
inflicted injury, 220*f*
information management, 328–329
informed consent, 291
infusion, 204
inhalation therapy, 361
initial assessment (ABCDEs), 2, 11–18
　CSHCN, 196–198
　toxic emergencies, 165–167
injections, 398–401. *See also* intramuscular injections (procedure 14)
injured child, assessment of, 143
injuries. *See also* trauma
　caregiver responses to, 32*t*
　causes of increased work, 144, 145*t*
　child, assessment of, 143
　common injuries and prevention strategies, 331*t*
　components of an injury event, 322–323, 323*f*
　elements of injury control, 322*t*
　head and cervical spine, 146–147
　mechanism of, 142, 142*t*, 143*f*
　patterns. *See* children, unique anatomic features of
　phases of, 323–324, 325*t*
　to physeal plate, 142
　preventing, 322–325
　related death, 138*t*
　vs. accidents, 322
　1-4 years of age, 139
inspiratory crackles, 13
Institute of Medicine (IOM), 209
insulin, 123
insulin-dependent diabetes mellitus (IDDM), 123
intellectual disability, 194
intentional injuries, 222. *See also* child maltreatment
intercostal area, 8
intercurrent illness, 205
internal cardiac defibrillator (ICD), 207
internal pacemakers, complications of, 207
internal radiation exposure, 285
　management of, 287

intestinal bezoar, 172*t*
intoxication, 9, 11
intra-abdominal injury, 23
intracranial bleeding, 21
intracranial hypertension, 149
intracranial pressure, 98, 206
intramuscular injections (IM), 63
intramuscular injections (procedure 14), 63, 398–401
　needle length for, 398
　sites for, 399*t*
intramuscular medications, 25
intramuscular therapy, 362
intranasal dose, midazolam, 118
intranasal medication administration (procedure 15), 118, 402–404
　limitations, 402–403
　preparations, 403
　rationale, 402
　utilization of drip method, 404
　utilization of MAD, 403–404
intraosseous infusions, 320
intraosseous (IO), 373
intraosseous (IO) needle insertion, 86
intraosseous (IO) needle insertion (procedure 17), 86, 409–414
　distal femur site, 413
　distal tibia site, 413
　EZ-IO insertion, 411–412
　proximal humerus site, 414
　proximal tibia site, 415
　traditional IO insertion, 410
intravascular volume, 78
intravenous (IV) access (procedure 16), 86, 405–408
intravenous (IV) delivery, 26
intravenous (IV) fluids, 239
intravenous (IV) route, 375
intubation
　preparation for, 58
　techniques, 69
in utero, 248
inverted pyramid, for depressed newly borns, 249
IOM. *See* Institute of Medicine
IO needle insertion. *See* intraosseous needle insertion
ipecac, 171
ipratropium, 63, 63*t*, 361, 453
iron poisoning in young children, 168
ischemia, 98, 103
isotonic saline, 149
IV access. *See* intravenous access
IV fluids. *See* intravenous fluids
IV fluid treatment
　of hypovolemic shock, 87

J

jaundice, 127
jaw-thrust maneuver, 56, 57*f*
jugular vein distention (JVD), 23

jugular venous distention, 84
JumpSTART triage system, 274, 275*f*

K

ketamine, 453
kidneys, 141, 141*f*
kinetic energy, 323
King Airway, 394–395
　insertion, 395–396
knee-chest position, 244, 244*f*
Kussmaul respirations, 124

L

labor, triage of patient in, 236–239
lactic acidosis, 10
language, toddlers, 39
large-bore rigid suction catheter, oropharyngeal suctioning with, 352
laryngeal mask airway (LMA), 390
　insertion, 391–392
laryngeal tube, 69*t*
laryngoscopy, 60, 98, 240, 358
larynx, 35, 153
last food or liquid, 79*t*
late (decompensated) hypovolemic shock, 81–82
　IV fluid treatment of, 87
lateral decubitus position, 116
lateral movement, 154
LEAN. *See* lidocaine, epinephrine, atropine, and naloxone
legal authority, 301
legal mandate, 216
length-based resuscitation tape, 340, 341
　computerized calculations, 341
L-epinephrine, 58
lethal toddler ingestions, 169*t*
lethargy, 126
leukemia, 222
levalbuterol, 63
Level C respiratory protection, 274
lewisite liquid, 283
lidocaine, 98, 426, 454
lidocaine, epinephrine, atropine, and naloxone (LEAN), 375
lifelong paralysis, 146
lifesaving interventions, 275
lighted stylet, 69*t*
liver, 141, 141*f*
lividity, 261
LMA. *See* laryngeal mask airway
localizing, 17
longitudinal bone growth, 36
long QT syndrome, 103
lorazepam, 427, 454
　for seizures, 118
lordosis of spine, 36

lower airway obstruction. *See also*
    asthma; bronchiolitis
  asthma, 61, 62*t*, 65
  breathing, disordered control of, 65, 66
  bronchiolitis, 61, 64, 64*t*
  bronchodilator treatment, 63
  causes of, 65
  foreign body aspiration, 59, 64, 65*f*, 66
  lung disease, 65
  treatment of, 61–64
lower airway problems, 66
low level MCI, 272
lungs
  anatomic changes, 35
  diseases, 65
lye, 166

M

Magill forceps, 358
malaise, 126
malposition, 98
maltreatment. *See* child maltreatment
mandible, 56
man-made disasters, 272, 272*t*. *See also*
    disasters
  criminal activity and terrorism, 279
  hazardous materials exposures, 279
  structural failures, 279
mannitol, 151, 152, 454
mass-casualty incident (MCI), 272
  pediatric considerations in, 272
maternal assessment, 235
maternal medical history, 236
maternal physical assessment, 236–237
mature minors, 294
  characteristics of, 294*t*
MCI. *See* mass-casualty incident
McRoberts maneuver, 244, 245*f*
MDI. *See* metered dose inhaler
mechanism of injury (MOI), 51
meconium, 235, 240, 244
  aspiration, 251
  aspirator, 251, 252*f*
meconium-stained amniotic fluid, 251
mediastinum, 85
medical control, 302–303
medical emergencies, 111
  AMS, 120–122, 126
  bites and stings, 133–134
  cold-related emergencies, 132–133,
    132*f*
  communicable diseases, 127–128
  endocrine disorders
    additional assessment, 125–126
    CAH, 124
    cortisol deficiency, 125
    diabetes mellitus, 123–124
    hospital transport, 125
    hyperglycemia, 123
    panhypopituitarism, 125–126
  environmental emergencies, 130
  fever, 126–127, 127*f*

gastroenteritis, 128–129
heat-related emergencies, 130–131, 131*t*
seizures
  afebrile, 114
  assessment and treatment, 116–119,
    116*f*, 116*t*–117*t*, 119*t*
  causes of, 113
  classification of, 115, 115*t*
  complications of, 115
  description, 120
  febrile, 113–114
  generalized, 113
  postictal child assessment,
    119–120, 120*t*
  status epilepticus, 114
sepsis and meningitis, 129–130
medical examiners, SUIDS and, 264*t*
medical home, 325–326
medical responsibility, 301
medicolegal considerations
  caregivers who disagree about care and
    transport, 294–295
  child maltreatment and sexual abuse, 302
  child refusal of transport, 293–294
  confidentiality, 295
  consent, 291–295
  cultural/religious differences, 295–296
  Do Not Resuscitate (DNR) order,
    297, 297*f*
    guardian refusal of transport,
      292–293
  hospital destination, 300–301
  off-line (indirect) medical control,
    302–303
  on-line (direct) medical control, 302
  organ donation, 299
  pediatric policies and procedures,
    301–302
  physician on scene, 300
  resuscitation, 299
  treatment protocols examples, 301*t*
  truth-telling in difficult situations,
    299–300
medicolegal expectations, 301
meninges, 82
meningitis, 21
  assessment, 129
  management, 130
meningococcal sepsis, 129
meningococcemia, 3, 222
meningococcus, 129
metabolic acidosis, 77, 94, 144
metered dose inhaler (MDI), 360, 362
methylprednisolone, 88, 455
midaxillary lines, 13, 13*f*
midazolam, 157, 455
  for seizures, 118
minors, 291
  emancipated. *See* emancipated minors
  mature. *See* mature minors
  transport, 292*f*
minor trauma, 137. *See also* trauma
minute ventilation, 53
miosis, 168

moderate level MCI, 272
modifiable factors in injury phases, 327*t*
MOI. *See* mechanism of injury
Mongolian spots, 222, 222*f*
monitoring devices, 2
  secondary assessment, 26
morphine, 25*t*, 455
morphine sulfate, 141, 158*t*
mortality, SUID, 330
mother, positioning for delivery,
    241–242
motor activity, 121
mottling, 9–10
mouth, physical examination of, 23
muffled speech, 7
multiparas mothers, 236
multiple gestations, 235
multisystem pediatric trauma, 149
multisystem trauma, 137, 142. *See also*
    trauma
Munchausen syndrome by proxy,
    163, 217
muscle growth, 36
muscular dystrophy, 195, 210
musculoskeletal system, anatomic
    changes, 36
mustard gas, 283
mutual aid agreements, 272
myocardial depression, 76
myocardial function, 76
myocardial infarction, 103
myocarditis, 76, 84, 101, 103

N

naloxone, 98, 122, 158, 173, 173*t*, 247,
    426, 456
narcotics, 122, 158
  reversal of, 247
narrow complex tachycardia, 99
nasal cannula, 55, 55*f*, 342, 343, 344*t*
nasal flaring, 8, 9*f*, 196
nasogastric insertion, 67
nasogastric (NG) tube
  insertion, 369–372
  placement, 148–149
nasopharyngeal airway (NPA), 52
National Highway Traffic Safety
    Administration (NHTSA), 2, 313
National Incident Management System
    (NIMS), 273
natural disasters, 272, 272*t*, 277–279.
    See also disasters
nature of illness (NOI), 51
nausea, 128–129
nebulized bronchodilator, 62*f*, 65
nebulized drug therapy, 63
nebulized epinephrine, 58, 65
nebulized medications, 72
neck
  anatomic changes, 35
  physical examination of, 23
needle decompression, 140, 148

needle thoracostomy (procedure 23), 69, 89, 140, 148, 435–436
neglect. *See also* Child maltreatment
abuse *vs.*, 213
Neisseria meningitidis, 129
Neonatal Resuscitation Program (NRP) flow diagram, 250*f*
neonatal seizures, 115
nerve agents, 281–282
treatment for, 282
nerve gas exposure, symptoms of, 282
nervous system, growth of, 36
neurogenic shock, 82
neuroleptic malignant syndrome (NMS), 187
neurologic evaluation systems, 5
neurologic function distal, 151
neurovascular problems, 142
newly born. *See also* delivery
body temperatures, 35
complications, 251–254
hypoglycemia, 254
immediate care of, 246–248
APGAR score, 246, 247*t*
assess breathing, 247
assess color, 248
assess heart rate, 247–248
clear the airway, 246–247
depressed newly born resuscitation, 247
dry and warm, baby, 246
endotracheal intubation and epinephrine administration, 249
inverted pyramid for, 249
meconium aspiration, 251
shock, 253
for transport, 254–255
vascular access, 254
resuscitation, general principles of, 248–251
NG tube placement. *See* nasogastric (NG) tube, placement
NIDDM. *See* non-insulin-dependent diabetes mellitus
NIMS. *See* National Incident Management System
9-1-1 call, infant, 150
nitrous oxide, 25, 456
NMS. *see* neuroleptic malignant syndrome
NOI. *See* nature of illness
non-insulin-dependent diabetes mellitus (NIDDM), 123
noninvasive treatment, 54–56
high-flow oxygen, 54–55
positioning, 54
of shock, 85–86
nonpulsatile fontanelle, 21
nonrebreathing mask, 342, 344*t*
nonvigorous newborn, treatment of meconium aspiration in, 251
norepinephrine, 456
nose, physical examination of, 22
NPA. *See* nasopharyngeal airway

NP airway insertion, 353, 354–355
NRP flow diagram. *See* Neonatal Resuscitation Program flow diagram
nuchal umbilical cord, 244
nuclear, 285–287
nuclear bomb, 285

O

obstetric delivery in prehospital setting, 234
obstetric pack, 241*t*
portable, 241, 241*t*
obstructed tracheostomy tube, 201
obstruction
central venous catheter, 204
symptoms, CSF shunts, 205
tracheostomy tubes, 200–202
obstructive shock, 76, 81*t*, 89
assessment of, 85
treatment of, 89
obturator, 200
occlusion, airway, 246
occlusive dressing, 147, 148*f*
occult illness, 265
ODD. *see* oppositional defiant disorder
off-line (indirect) medical control, 302–303, 303*t*
OG tube placement. *See* orogastric tube placement
older children, securing to stretcher, 314
older preterm infants, 235
one-rescuer technique, bag-mask ventilation using, 365
online (direct) medical control, 292, 302, 302*f*, 303*t*
OPA. *See* oropharyngeal airway
OP airway insertion, 353, 354–355
operations, goal of, 301
opiates, 25
oppositional defiant disorder (ODD), 183
OPQRST mnemonics, 96. *See also* additional assessment
optimal airway management, 152, 152*t*
optimal cardiopulmonary resuscitation, 256
oral glucose, 122
organ donation, 299
statistics, 299*t*
organ growth, 35
organophosphate insecticides, 168
organophosphate poisoning toxidrome, 174
organophosphates, 174
orogastric and nasogastric tube insertion (procedure 10), 67, 148–149, 369–372
check placement of NG/OG tube, 371
methods for determining tube size, 370*t*
NG insertion, 371
OG insertion, 371
technique for distance measuring, 370*f*

orogastric insertion, 67
orogastric (OG) tube placement, 148–149
oropharyngeal airway (OPA), 52, 106
oropharyngeal/nasopharyngeal suctioning with bulb syringe, 348–349
oropharyngeal/nasopharyngeal suctioning with suction catheter, 349–350
oropharyngeal suctioning, 242
with large-bore rigid suction catheter, 352
oropharynx, 7
ossification, 36
osteogenesis imperfecta, 222
ostomies, 206
otorrhea, 22
oval bruises, 219*f*
overdoses, 6
oxygen delivery (procedure 3), 55–56, 342–346
methods to gain child's cooperation for, 346*t*
technique and patient assessment, 344*t*
oxygen-powered nebulizer, 62*f*
oxygen saturation, 12–13
oxygen therapy, 55, 254
oxygen toxicity, 55
oxygen treatment, noninvasive treatment, 54–56, 86

P

pacemakers, internal, 207
pain, 141, 144*t*, 158*t*
additional assessment (OPQRST) of, 96, 97*t*
appearance, 144, 144*t*
assessment of, 24–26
management and sedation, 157–158
pharmacologic management, 157, 158*t*
pallor, 9–10
palpation, 34
panhypopituitarism, 125–126
paradoxical irritability, 82, 126, 127*f*
paranoia, 164, 167
Parkland formula, 157
past medical problems, 79*t*
PAT. *See* Pediatric Assessment Triangle
pathology, 14
pathophysiology, 76
patient-centered care, 326
patients
in active labor, 239
assessment, child maltreatment, 220–222
global sorting of, 275
rights, 296
in supine position, 239
pattern burn, 156
PCP. *See* phencyclidine
PEA. *See* pulseless electrical activity
pedal pulse, 78, 95

pediatric airway and adult airway, 373
pediatric assessment, 2. *See also*
   reassessment
   environmental, 3*f*
   history taking, 20–21
   primary. *See* primary assessments
   secondary. *See* secondary assessment
   summary of flowchart, 2
Pediatric Assessment Triangle (PAT),
      2, 49, 56, 79, 89, 165. *See also*
      assessment; general assessment
   abnormal appearance, 77, 77*f*
   for AMS, 120–121
   appearance, 5–7, 5*t*, 6*f*, 51, 94
   assessment of circulation using, 94–95
   assessment of respiratory status using,
      51–52
   breathing, work of, 52
   circulation to skin, 9–11, 10*t*, 11*f*, 77,
      94–95
   CSHCN, 196
   developing general impression, 4, 4*f*
   evaluation of severity and illness/
      injury, 10–11
   general assessment, 144–145
   pediatric-specific terminology for, 338*t*
   physical characteristics of, 5
   presenting complaint, evaluating, 51
   respiratory status, assessment of, 51–52
   skin, circulation to, 52
   work of breathing, 7–9, 7*t*, 77, 94
pediatric BLS algorithm, 104*f*
pediatric burn patients
   assessment, 155–156
   management, 156–158
pediatric calls, 32–33
Pediatric Chain of Survival, 102
pediatric critical care centers, 320
Pediatric Education for Prehospital
      Professionals (PEPP) course, 2
pediatric emergency care, universal
      standards for, 320
pediatric endotracheal intubation, RSI
      for, 153
pediatric equipment, 3
Pediatric Glasgow Coma Scale (PGCS),
      5, 18*t*, 150, 150*t*
pediatric injury, 142, 142*t*
pediatric patient
   airway, characteristics of, 280
   communication with, 33
   pediatric reporting template, 339*t*
pediatric psychiatric and behavioral
      conditions, 180–185
   anxiety, 183
   attention-deficit/hyperactivity
      disorder, 182, 182*f*
   autism spectrum disorder,
      180–182, 181*t*
   bipolar disorder, 184
   conduct disorder, 183
   depression, 183–184
   oppositional defiant disorder, 183
   schizophrenia, 185

pediatrics, toxidromes in, 165, 166*t*
pediatric scene size-up, 3
pediatric-specific terminology for PAT,
      338*t*
pediatric transport, 307–308. *See also*
      transport decisions
pediatric trauma
   SAMPLE history in, 153–154, 153*t*
   special airway considerations in,
      152–153
pediatric trauma, SAMPLE history in,
      153–154, 153*t*
pediatric trauma centers, 320
PEEP. *See* positive end-expiratory
      pressure
PEG. *See* percutaneous endoscopic
      gastrostomy
pelvic fractures, 141
penetrating chest trauma, 140, 147–148
penetrating injuries, 137, 140
percutaneous endoscopic gastrostomy
      (PEG), 204
perfusion, 5
   evaluation of, 80
   problems in children, 75
pericardial fluid accumulation, 85
pericardial tamponade, 76, 85
perineum, assessing, 237
periosteum, 141
peripheral cyanosis, 248
peripherally inserted central catheter
      (PICC), 202
peripheral vasoconstriction, 76, 78
peripheral veins, cannulating, 87
peritoneal dialysis, 208
peritoneum, 205
persistent hemorrhage, 245
personal protective equipment (PPE),
      51, 273
personal protective measures, 143
petechiae, 219, 221
petechial lesions, 21
petechial line, 221
petechial rash, 82, 129
PGCS. *See* Pediatric Glasgow Coma
      Scale
pharmacologic management
   anxiety, 158*t*
   pain, 157, 158*t*
   of pediatric burn patient, 157, 158*t*
pharmacologic methods for reducing
      pain, 25
pharmacologic treatment
   burns, 157
   of croup, 58
   pain, 157
   seizures, 117–119, 117*t*, 119*t*
   of wheezing, 63
pharynx, 56
phencyclidine (PCP), 166
phenobarbital, 118, 119*t*, 456
phenytoin, 119, 119*t*, 457
physeal plates, 36, 141*f*, 142
physical abuse, 213, 221*f*

physical examination, 21–26
   child maltreatment, 220–222
physician on scene, 300
physiologic features, 323
   of infants, 37*t*
physiologic instability, 3
PICC. *See* peripherally inserted central
      catheter
Pierre Robin syndrome, 252, 253*f*
placenta previa, 235, 235*f*
plague, 284
pleura, 9, 205
pleural space, 148
pneumococcal vaccine, 129
pneumomediastinum, 64
pneumonia, 7, 56, 61, 65, 66. *See also*
      lungs, diseases
   fulminant, 50
pneumonic plague, 284
pneumothorax, 89, 98
   tension, 85
poison centers, 164
poisoning, 6, 98, 103, 163
   in children, 162, 163
poisons, 76, 162
policies, 301–302
polydipsia, 123
polyphagia, 123
polyuria, 123
poor air movement, 53, 53*t*
positioning, 54, 86
   for delivery, 241–242
positive end-expiratory pressure (PEEP),
      7, 144, 385
positive-pressure ventilation, 67
posterior position during delivery,
      243, 243*f*
postevent critical incident stress
      management (CISM), 271
postevent factors, injury phases, 324
postictal child, assessment of,
      119–120, 120*t*
postictal state, 11
postpartum hemorrhage, 245
postterm pregnancy, 235
posturing, 121
PPE. *See* personal protective equipment
pralidoxime (2-PAM), 174
   dosing, 282
prearrival preparation, 3
   for cardiovascular emergencies, 76, 94
   for respiratory emergencies, 51
   toxic emergencies, 164
predisaster, planning, 273
pre-event factors, injury phases, 324, 324*f*
pregnancy, complications during,
      234–236
prehospital analgesia, methods of, 25*t*
prehospital antidotes, 173, 173*t*
prehospital professionals
   duties and communication, 216–218
   evaluation, 2
   medical home and, 325–326
   prevention roles, 329–331

QI case study, 328
   response to infant death, 266–267, 267t
prehospital provider, 260–261
preschoolers, 40–41
   approaching, 41f
   assessment of, 41
   common ailments in, 41
   developmental characteristics, 40–41
   EMS provider, tips for, 45
presenting complaint
   cardiovascular emergencies, 76, 94
   evaluating, 51, 51t
presumptive diagnosis, 252
preterm infants, 252
preterm labor, treatment of patient in,
     234–235
prevention, 2
   before the call, 330
   common injuries and prevention
     strategies, 331t
   drowning, 108
   injuries vs. accidents, 322
   injury control elements, 322t
   injury event components, 322–323, 323f
   phases of, 323–324, 325t
primary assessments (ABCDEs), 2,
     11–18, 153
   cardiovascular emergencies, 77–78,
     95–96
   children, special considerations in,
     165–168
   hands-on, 145, 146t
     airway, 145–146, 146t
     breathing, 146–148
     circulation, 149
     disability, 149–151
     exposure, 151
   PAT. See Pediatric Assessment Triangle
   respiratory emergencies, 52–54, 71
   summary of, 19–20, 152
   transport decision, 19, 153
primary brain injuries, 144, 144t, 149–150
primiparas, first-time mothers, 236
   needle thoracostomy (procedure 23),
     140, 148
   procedures of pediatric, 301–302
profound hemorrhage, 235
prompt transportation, risks and benefits
     of initiating, 238t
prophylactic treatment, 287
propylene glycol, 119
protective custody, emergency, 293
protocols, 301–302
   examples of pediatric treatment, 301t
proximal airway obstruction, 56–57
proximal humerus site, 414
proximal tibia site, 412
psychiatric medications, adverse
     reactions of, 186–187
   acute dystonic reactions, 187
   neuroleptic malignant syndrome, 187
public health interface, 322
pulmonary contusion, 7, 139
pulmonary edema, 7, 77

pulmonary intoxicants, 283
pulseless electrical activity (PEA), 93, 101
pulseless ventricular tachycardia (VT), 101
pulse oximetry, 2, 7, 12–13, 53–54, 96
   placement of, 54f
pulse oximetry (procedure 9), 53–54,
     367–368
pulse quality, 14–15, 78, 95
pulses, 264
pupils
   brainstem function and, 151
   miosis, 168
purpura, 82, 83f, 129
purpuric lesions, 21
purpuric rash, 126
pus, presence of, 23

Q

QA. See quality assurance
QI. See quality improvement
QRS complex, 99
quadriplegia, 146
quality improvement (QI), 326
   prehospital case study, 328
quantitative end-tidal CO_2, 388

R

racemic epinephrine, 58
radial pulse, 78, 95
radiation disasters, 285–287
radiologic dispersal device (RDD), 285.
     See also dirty bomb
radio reporting, 26–27
rapid assessment, 3
rapid sequence intubation (RSI), 58,
     69t, 153
RDD. See radiologic dispersal device
reactivity, 150
reassessment, 2, 26
recovery phase (disaster response), 273
recreational abuse, toxic emergencies
     and, 162–163
rectal administration of benzodiazepines
     (procedure 21), 118, 427–429
rectal diazepam, 25, 328, 427
rectal temperature, 35
rectum, 427
"red flag" caregiver behaviors, 217, 217t
refusal of care, 292–293
religious differences, respect for, 295–296
removing and replacing tracheostomy
     tube (procedure 24), 202, 437–440
renal dialysis, 208
rescue breathing techniques, advantages
     and disadvantages of, 69t
reserve hyperventilation, 151
respiratory arrest, 50
respiratory assessment, general and
     initial, 56
respiratory depression, 118

respiratory disease, 49
respiratory distress, 49, 55f
   high-flow oxygen, 54–56
   positioning, 54
   SAMPLE components in child with, 71t
   treatment for, 56, 65–66
     lower airway obstruction. See lower
      airway obstruction
     upper airway obstruction. See upper
      airway obstruction
respiratory emergencies, 49–72
   additional assessment (SAMPLE), 71
   DOPE (dislodgment, obstruction,
     pneumothorax, equipment), 68t
   general assessment (PAT), 51–52
   noninvasive treatment, 54–56
   prearrival preparation, 51
   primary assessment (ABCDEs),
     52–54, 70
   respiratory arrest, 50
   respiratory distress, 49
   respiratory failure, 50
     management of. See respiratory
      failure, management of
   scene size-up, 51
   treatment, 56
     lower airway obstruction. See lower
      airway obstruction
     upper airway obstruction. See upper
      airway obstruction
respiratory failure, 50
   in bronchiolitis, 64, 64t
   from lung disease, 65
   management of, 66–70
     alternative breathing and intubation
      techniques, 69
     bag-mask ventilation, 67
     endotracheal intubation, 68–69
     endotracheal tube placement,
      confirmation of, 69–70
     nasogastric/orogastric insertion, 67
     rescue breathing techniques,
      advantages and disadvantages, 69t
respiratory infections, febrile, 126
respiratory insufficiency, 65
respiratory rate, 12, 12t, 52
   for age, 33–34, 34t
respiratory status, assessment of, 51–52
respiratory syncytial virus (RSV),
     64, 196
restraint, 188
   in ambulance, 155, 199
   chemical, 188
   physical, 188–189
   verbal, 188
resuscitation, 299
   cardiopulmonary, 415–419
resuscitation-oriented history,
     240–241, 240t
resuscitation tape, 106f
resuscitation tapes, length-based
     (procedure 2), 340–341
retractions, 8, 9f, 11
retropharyngeal abscess, 58

rhinorrhea, 22
ricin, 284
Ricinus communis, 284
right atrium, 202
risk assessment, 168, 168*t*, 169
rocuronium bromide, 457
rotary wing transport for pediatric
    patients, 315
RSI. *See* rapid sequence intubation
RSV. *See* respiratory syncytial virus
rule of palms, 155

S

safe maternal position for delivery,
    241, 241*f*
safety
  in EMSC, 326, 328
  in transport, 330
salbutamol, 63, 63*t*, 65
salivation, 168
SALT triage system. *See* Sort, Assess,
    Lifesaving interventions, and
    Treatment and/or transport triage
    system
SAMPLE mnemonic, 20, 20*t*. *See also*
    additional assessment; assessment
saphenous vein, 254
scald burns, 156
scaphoid abdomen, 36
scene size-up, 3
  cardiovascular emergencies, 76, 94
  child maltreatment, 223
  infant death and, 264
  prevention role and, 330
  respiratory emergencies, 51
  toxic emergencies, 164
schizophrenia, 185
school-aged children, 41–42
  approaching, 42*f*
  assessment of, 42
  common conditions in, 41
  developmental characteristics, 41
  EMS provider, tips for, 45
school shootings, 279
scoliosis, 53
scopolamine, 166
secondary assessment, 2
  monitoring devices, 26
  physical examination, 21–26
secondary brain injuries, 144, 144*t*, 150
secretions, 197
sedation, pain management and, 156–158
sedative/hypnotic drugs, 166
seismic events, 278
seizures, 16, 19, 113–115, 150, 167,
    173, 219
  afebrile, 114
  assessment and treatment, 116–119,
    116*f*, 116*t*–117*t*, 119*t*
  causes of, 113
  classification of, 115, 115*t*
  complications of, 115

description, 120
  febrile, 113–114
  generalized, 113
  hospital transport, 119
  postictal child assessment,
    119–120, 120*t*
  status epilepticus, 114
selective serotonin reuptake inhibitors
    (SSRIs), 186
"self-report" scales, 24, 24*f*
semi-Fowler's position, 308, 330
separation anxiety, 39
sepsis, 11, 38, 76, 82–83
  assessment, 129
  management, 130
septic shock, 203
serial examinations, 141
serotonin syndrome, signs and
    symptoms, 186*t*
serum glucose, 122
severe storms, 278–279
sexual abuse, 213, 302
shaken baby syndrome, 218, 224
shelter management, pediatric aspects
    of, 281
shock, 10, 76, 253. *See also* cardiovascular
    emergencies
  abdomen injuries and, 140–141
  anaphylactic, 83
  anaphylaxis, 88
  assessment to identify, 80–81
  cardiogenic. *See* cardiogenic shock
  CSHCN, 197
  distributive. *See* distributive shock
  from drug intoxication, 83, 83*t*
  electrical charge for countershock, 421*t*
  hypovolemic. *See* hypovolemic shock
  neurogenic, 83
  in newly born, 253
  noninvasive treatment of, 85–86
  obstructive. *See* obstructive shock
  summary of, 89
  types of, 81*t*
shoulder dystocia, 244, 245*f*
sickle cell disease, 126
silent tachypnea, 77
simple febrile seizure, 113
simple mask, oxygen delivery device,
    342, 344*t*
simple partial seizures, 115
Simple Triage and Rapid Treatment
    (START) triage system, 274
Sims position, 242, 242*f*
single-wrapped nuchal cord, 244
sinus arrhythmia, 34
  ECG of, 34*f*
sinus tachycardia, 98
  ECG of, 100*f*
  features of, 99*t*
skin, physical examination of, 21
skin, toxic treatment, 170
skin injuries, 142
  circulation to, 144–145, 145*f*
skin temperature, 15, 78, 95–96

slept prone, 330
slurry, 172*t*
smallpox, 283–284, 284*f*
smoke inhalation, 157
sniffing position, 8, 8*f*, 55*f*
snoring, 7
socioeconomic status in SIDS and SUID
    cases, 261
sodium bicarbonate, 173, 426, 458
soft-tissue injuries, 144
somatic growth, 35
sorbitol, 172, 173, 174
Sort, Assess, Lifesaving interventions,
    and Treatment and/or transport
    (SALT) triage system, 275, 275*f*
spasticity, 195
spina bifida, 193, 195, 209
spinal column injuries, 139
spinal compression, 139
spinal injuries, 145, 146, 155
spinal motion restriction, 146, 147*f*,
    154–155
spinal motion restriction (procedure 22),
    146, 430–434
  releasing and monitoring, 433–434
  securing patient to stabilization device,
    432–433
  spinal motion restriction, 431
  spine board, 154
  spleen, 141, 141*f*
  during transport, 154–155
spine, 139
spine board, 154
spleen, 141, 141*f*
splinting, 155, 155*f*
spore-forming bacterium, 285
"squeeze-release-release" timing
    technique, 147
SSRIs. *See* selective serotonin reuptake
    inhibitors
staging, 274
standards for pediatric emergency
    care, 320
START triage system. *See* Simple Triage
    and Rapid Treatment triage
    system
state-of-the-art care for children, 273
status epilepticus, 427
  definition of, 114
sterile gauze, 200
stings, 133–134
stocking distribution, 156, 157*f*
stomach, 141
stomas, 199, 200, 206–207
stranger anxiety, 39
Streptococcus pneumoniae, 129
stress, 267, 267*f*
stretcher
  securing car seat to, 313–314, 313*f*, 314*f*
  securing older children, 314
stridor, 7, 53, 58, 65
structural failures, 279
subcostal, baseline retractions, 196
subdural hemorrhage, 11

subglottic level, 58
sublingual administration, 118
substernal area, 8
succinylcholine, 69t, 458
sucking chest wounds, 140, 147, 148f
suction catheter
    oropharyngeal/nasopharyngeal
        suctioning with, 349–350
    sizes, suggestion of, 376t
    tracheal tube suctioning with, 350–351
suctioning, 66
    tracheostomy tube, 201–202
suctioning (procedure 4), 66, 347–352
    based on age and type of obstructing
        material, 347, 348t
    complications, 348
    oropharyngeal/nasopharyngeal
        suctioning with bulb syringe,
        348–349
    oropharyngeal/nasopharyngeal
        suctioning with suction catheter,
        349–350
    oropharyngeal with large-bore rigid
        suction catheter, 352
    preparation, 348
    tracheal tube with suction catheter,
        350–351
sudden unexpected infant death (SUID),
    103, 259–260, 299, 330. See also
    infant death
    actions in suspected, 261–263
    ALTE, 264
    Caregiver's response to, 265–266,
        266f
    clinical presentation, 261–262
    common clinical presentation of,
        261–262
    communication about, 263, 263t
    decreasing mortality, 330
    defined, 259–260
    definition of, 259–260
    documentation, 263
    epidemiology and risk factors, 260
    epidemiology and risk factors of, 260
    external appearance of SUIDS
        victims, 261t
    flowchart of what to do in suspected
        cases, 263t
    history collection, 261t
    infants, pros and cons of transporting
        suspected, 262, 262t
    medical examiner/coroner and
        local health department
        responsibilities, 264t
    prehospital professional's response to,
        266–267, 267t
    risk of, 268–269
    scene size-up, 264
    summary of, 263
suicide, toxins and, 162–163
suicide attempt/intentional ingestions or
    exposures, 185–186
    acetaminophen, 185–186
    history taking, 185

selective serotonin reuptake
        inhibitors, 186
    serotonin syndrome, signs and
        symptoms, 186t
    tricyclic antidepressants, 186
SUID. See sudden unexpected infant
    death
superior vena cava, 202
supine position, 330
supraclavicular area, 8
supraglottic airway devices, 57, 69t,
    390–392
supraglottic structures, 7
supralaryngeal airway, 69t
suprasternal, baseline retractions, 196
suprasternal retractions, 39
supraventricular tachycardia (SVT),
    84, 420
    features of, 99t
    treatment of, 99–100
suxamethonium, 458
SVT. See supraventricular tachycardia
sweating, 80
symmetry, 23
sympathomimetic agents, 166
sympathomimetic drugs, 166
symphysis pubis, 243
symptomatic ventricular
        dysrhythmias, 102
synaptic connections, 36
systolic blood pressure, 16t, 35t, 78

T

tachycardia, 13–14, 77, 95, 149, 196
    assessment, 98–99
    narrow complex, 99
    sinus. See sinus tachycardia
    SVT. See supraventricular tachycardia
        (SVT)
    treatment of, 99–101
    wide complex, 101
tachypnea, 10
tamponade, 149
    pericardial, 76
TART chart, 165, 166t
TBI. See traumatic brain injury
teamwork, 2, 326
technology, children assisted by
    central venous catheters, 202–204
    CSF shunts, 205–206
    dialysis shunts, 208
    feeding tubes, 204–205
    ICD, 207
    internal pacemakers, 207
    ostomies, 206
    tracheostomy tubes, 199–202
    VNS, 207–208
temperature, 35
TEN-4 bruising rule, 220
tenderness, 139
tension pneumothorax, 76, 85, 140
    management of, 148

terminology, 338t
terrorism, 279
thermoregulation, 39
thoracic excursions, 33
thoracic inlet, airway obstruction
        above, 57
thoracic spine, 139
thoracostomy, 89
thyroid-stimulating hormone
        (TSH), 125
"tickles" (TICLS) mnemonic. See TICLS
    mnemonic
TICLS mnemonic, 5t, 121, 338t
    respiratory emergencies, 51
tidal volume, 53
timeliness, 326
titratable method, 26
toddlers, 39–40
    approaching, 40f
    assessment of, 40
    common ailments in, 39
    developmental characteristics, 39
    EMS provider, tips for, 45
tonic-clonic activity, 113
tornados, 278–279
totally implanted devices, 203
tourniquet application (procedure 25),
        441–444
    complications, 443
    preparation, 442
    rationale, 441
toxic cases (2017), 162t
toxic emergencies
    additional assessment (SAMPLE),
        169–170
    age-related differences, 161–163
    cases (2017), 162
    common toxidromes in, 166, 166t
    general assessment (PAT), 165
    initial management of, 168
    lethal toddler ingestions, 169t
    medicolegal issues, 174
    organophosphates, 174
    poison centers, 164
    prearrival preparation and scene
        size-up, 164
    primary assessment, 165–168
    recreational abuse and, 162–163
    risk assessment, 168–169, 168t
    statistics, 162t
    suicide and, 162
    toll-free number for
        (1-800-222-1222), 165
    toxic exposure defined, 162
    toxicologic management. See
        toxicologic management
    transport decision, 169
    treatment
        antidotes, 173
        decontamination, 171–172
        enhancement of elimination, 173
toxic exposures, pediatric SAMPLE for,
    169–170, 170t
toxicologic emergencies, 6

toxicologic management
  antidotes, 173
  decontamination
    eyes, 170–171
    gastrointestinal, 171–172
    skin, 170
  enhancement of elimination, 173
toxidromes, signs and symptoms of,
    165, 166*t*
toxins, appearance and, 144, 144*t*
trachea, 35
  examination of, 23, 23*f*
tracheal tube suctioning with suction
    catheter, 350–351
tracheitis, 58
tracheostomy, 44, 197, 199, 200*f*
  complications, 200–202
  indications for, 199, 199*t*
tracheostomy tubes, 199. *See also*
    removing and replacing
    tracheostomy tube (procedure 24)
  children with, 347
  obstruction, 200–202
  oxygen delivery and assisted
    ventilation, 200
  replacement, 202
  types of, 199–200
trach tube. *See* tracheostomy tubes
transdermal route, 25
transmucosal route, 25
transplants, 194
transport
  considerations
    for infants, 254–255
    for patient in labor, 239
  disasters, 277
  restraint during, 154–155
  safety in, 330
  stabilization and splinting for, 154–155
transport decisions, 19
  beginning transport, 308–309
  behavioral emergencies, 187–189
    chemical restraint, 188
    emotional well-being, 189
    physical restraint, 188–189
    verbal restraint, 188
  cardiac arrest, 107, 107*f*
  cardiovascular emergencies, 89
  child maltreatment, 218
  child restraint systems in ambulances,
    310–315
  CSHCN, 199
  dangers of, 310–311, 314
  destination, 315
  hospital destination, 300–301
  hyperglycemia, 125
  multiple pediatric patients, 315
  for newly born, 254–255
  pediatric, 307–308
  pouch replacement, 206–207
  refusal of care or transport, 292–293
  respiratory emergencies, 70–71

seizures, 119
summary of, 315
taking caregivers in ambulance,
    309–310
toxic emergencies, 169
transport mode, 315
transport time, 19
trauma, 19, 20. *See also* injuries
  abdomen, 140–141, 141*f*
  additional assessment (SAMPLE),
    153–154
  airway considerations, 152–153
  burn
    patients, 155–158
    summary of, 158
  chest, 139–140, 139*f*, 140*f*
  child, assessment of, 143
  children, unique anatomic features of.
    See children, unique anatomic
    features of
  extremities, 141–142, 142*f*
  fatal injury mechanisms, 138
  general assessment (PAT), 144–145
  head, 138–139
  mechanisms and associated patterns of
    pediatric injury, 142, 142*t*
  pediatric burn patients, 155–158
  physical examination, 21–24
  primary assessment, 153
  skin, 142
  special airway considerations in
    pediatric, 152–153
  spinal column, 139
  stabilization and splinting for
    transport, 154–155, 155*f*
traumatic brain injury (TBI), 138, 145,
    149, 150
traumatic emergencies, 6
traumatic hemorrhage, 75
treatment
  AMS, 122, 122*f*
  anaphylaxis, 88
  for bioterrorism infections, 286*t*
  bites, 133–134
  bradycardia, 98
  cardiac arrest, 103, 107
  cardiogenic shock, 88–89
  cold-related emergencies, 132, 132*f*
  CSF shunts, 205–206
  decompensated shock, 87
  diabetes mellitus, 123
  disasters, 275–277
  distributive shock, 88
  drowning, 108
  expected benefits of, 19
  feeding tubes, 205
  fever, 127
  gastroenteritis, 128–129
  hyperglycemia, 123
  hypoglycemia, 204
  hypothermia, 132, 132*f*
  hypovolemia, 86

of infant born, 247
of meconium aspiration in
    nonvigorous newborn, 251
meningitis, 130
for nerve agents, 282
obstructive shock, 85
of pediatric patients, 275–277
of postpartum hemorrhage, 245
for respiratory distress, 56–65
seizures, 116–119, 116*f*, 116*t*–117*t*,
    119*t*
sepsis, 130
of shock in newly born, 253
stings, 133–134
suctioning a tracheostomy tube,
    201–202
SVT, 99–100
tachycardia, 99–101
toxic emergencies, 170–173
triage, 274–275
  algorithms, 275
  JumpSTART, 274, 275*f*
  of patient in labor, 236–239
  START, 274
tricyclic antidepressants, 186
tripod position, 8, 8*f*, 55*f*, 196
truth, in difficult situations,
    299–300
TSH. *See* thyroid-stimulating hormone
two-person bag-mask ventilation
    technique, 58, 60*f*
2-pyridine aldoxime methochloride
    (2-PAM), 457
two-rescuer technique, bag-mask
    ventilation using, 366
"two thumb encircling hand"
    technique, 249
tympanic temperature, 35

U

umbilical catheterization, 254
umbilical cord, 242, 242*f*, 244
universal precautions, 143
universal standards for pediatric
    emergency care, 320
upper airway obstruction, 7
  airway obstruction above thoracic
    inlet, 57
  bacterial upper airway infections, 58
  cause of, 65
  foreign body aspiration, 59, 64,
    64*f*, 66
  and foreign body removal, 60
  proximal airway obstruction, 56–57
  treatment of, 60
urination, 168
urostomy, 206
uterine contractions, 237
uterine massage, 245, 245*f*
uterus (womb), 243

V

vagal nerve stimulator (VNS), 207–208
vagal stimulation, 98, 100
vaginal delivery. *See also* delivery
    contents of portable obstetric pack for, 241, 241*t*
    maternal and newborn complications during, 244–245
vaginal introitus, 237
vagus nerve, 34
varicella, 3
VAS. *See* visual analogue scores
vascular access, 254
vascular tone, 76
vasculitis, 222
vasoconstriction, 10, 77, 80, 94
    peripheral, 76, 78
vasodilation, 10
vasomotor, 10
vasopressor agent, 88
vehicular trauma, 138*t*
ventilation, 63–65
ventilation-perfusion mismatch, 61
ventilation ratios, chest compressions to, 416*t*

ventilator, 44
ventricle, anatomic changes in, 35
ventricular fibrillation (VF), 94, 106, 420
    AED and, 101–102
ventricular tachycardia (VT), 94
    features of, 99*t*
    pulseless, 106
vertebral bodies, 36
vesicants, 283
VF. *See* ventricular fibrillation
vigor, 246
viral myocarditis, 76
visual analogue scores (VAS), 24
visual impairment, 194
visual signs, increased work of breathing, 8–9
vital signs, 2, 80, 96–97, 239
    changes through childhood, 37
    physical examination, 24
    through ages, 33–35
VNS. *See* vagal nerve stimulator (VNS)
vocal cords, 11
volume resuscitation, 149
vomiting, 128–129
VT. *See* ventricular tachycardia
vulnerable pediatric characteristics, 280*t*

W

weapons of mass destruction (WMD), 174
wheezing, 7–8, 61, 64, 144, 157
    from bronchospasm, 360
    management of, 63*t*
    pharmacologic treatment of, 63
wide complex tachycardia, 101
withdrawing, GCS motor categories, 17
WMD. *See* weapons of mass destruction
womb (uterus), 243
Wong-Baker FACES Scale, 24, 24*f*
work of breathing, 338*t*
    abnormal airway sounds, 7–8
    characteristics of, 7, 7*t*
    CSHCN, 196
    PAT characteristics, 76–77, 94
    respiratory emergencies, 52, 56
    techniques to assessment, 9
    trauma, 144, 145*t*
    visual signs of increased, 8–9

Y

Yersinia pestis, 284

V

vagal nerve stimulator (VNS), 205–208
vagal stimulation, 98, 100
vaginal delivery. See also delivery
  contents of portable obstetric pack for, 281, 281t
  maternal and newborn complications during, 244–245
vaginal infections, 237
vagus nerve, 34
varicella, 3
VAS. See visual analogue scores
vascular access, 254
vascular tone, 76
vasculitis, 232
vasoconstriction, 10, 77, 80, 94
  peripheral, 76, 78
vasodilation, 10
vasomotor, 10
vasopressor agent, 68
velander trauma, 181
ventilation, 63–65
ventilation-perfusion mismatch, 81
ventilation ratios, chest compressions to, 316t

ventilation, 64
ventricles, anatomic changes in, 35
ventricular fibrillation (VF), 94, 106, 420
  AFD and, 101–102
  supraventricular tachycardia (VT), 94
  features of, 99t
  pulseless, 106
vertebral bodies, 36
vesicants, 234
VF. See ventricular fibrillation
vigor, 246
viral myocarditis, 76
visual analogue scores (VAS), 24
visual impairment, 194
visual signs, increased work of breathing, 8–9
vital signs, 2, 80, 96–97, 239
  changes through childhood, 37
  physical examination, 24
  through ages 33–35
VNS. See vagal nerve stimulator (VNS)
vocal cords, 11
volume resuscitation, 149
vomiting, 128–129
VT. See ventricular tachycardia
vulnerable pediatric characteristics, 280t

W

weapons of mass destruction (WMD), 174
wheezing, 7–8, 61, 63, 141, 157
  from bronchospasm, 380
  management of, 62t
  pharmacologic treatment of, 62
wide complex tachycardia, 101
withdrawing, GCS motor categories, 17t
WMD. See weapons of mass destruction
womb (uterus), 243
Wong-baker FACES scale, 24, 24f
work of breathing, 63t
  abnormal airway sounds, 7–8
  characteristics of, 7
  GSHCN, 196
  PAT characteristics, 76–77, 99
  respiratory emergencies, 72, 96
  techniques to assessment, 9
  trauma, 144, 157
  visual signs of increased, 8–9

Y

Yersinia pestis, 284